MedStudy

2022–2023

Internal Medicine
REVIEW SYLLABUS

© 2022 MedStudy
ALL RIGHTS UNDER THE COPYRIGHT ARE RESERVED BY:
MedStudy Corporation
1455 Quail Lake Loop, Colorado Springs, CO 80906
medstudy.com

Deepen Your Understanding
of the Concepts in These Sessions

Reviewing and practicing recall of a topic using different formats deepens your understanding and memory of that topic. Expand your understanding of the topics in these lectures with **Study Strong Digital Essentials**:

- **Digital Core**—A more comprehensive review of topics covered in the lectures
- **Q&As**—Board-style questions with complete explanations of the most testable concepts
- **Core Scripts**—Common illness presentations in a flashcard format
- **Personal Trainer**—Optimizes your time with adaptable plans built around your goals and study pace

We've interlinked content in each of these digital learning tools. For example, read about pericardial disease in the Core and immediately jump to related questions in the Q&As or Flashcards—it works in reverse, too!

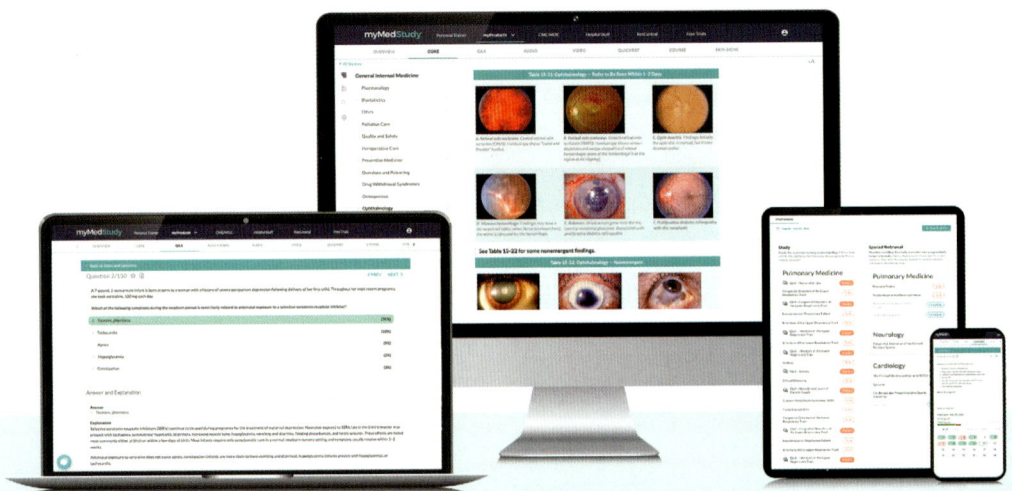

Board-Style Q&As

1,700+ board-style Q&As improve your recall as you self-test in Study Mode or Test Mode.

Up to 100 CME credits/MOC points available

Digital Core

The source of truth for all MedStudy Internal Medicine material. Comprehensively covers everything you need to know in a concise yet casual style.

Up to 150 CME credits/MOC points available

Core Scripts® Flashcards

A powerful way to exercise your recall of diseases, syndromes, and fundamental facts.

Up to 50 CME credits/MOC points available

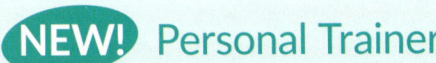 **NEW!** Personal Trainer

Your super-smart, personalized learning guide processes Core and Q&A content using the best evidenced-based learning techniques.

- Creates weekly study plans
- Adapts to your goals and pace
- Tracks your progress
- Organizes it all on your Study Board (Complete all your work from here!)

To learn more go to **medstudy.com/products/IM** or call **1-800-841-0547**

MedStudy products come with free shipping (standard ground shipping to 48 contiguous states) and free CME.

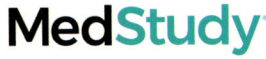

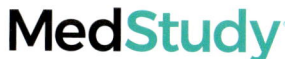

INTERNAL MEDICINE REVIEW

Table of Contents

Disclaimers

Notice

Medicine and accepted standards of care are constantly changing. We at MedStudy do our best to review and include in this publication accurate discussions of the standards of care and methods of diagnosis. However, the authors, reviewers, section editors, medical editors, editor in chief, publisher, and all other parties involved with the preparation and publication of this work do not guarantee that the information contained herein is in every respect accurate or complete. We recommend that you confirm the material with current sources of medical knowledge whenever considering presentations or treating patients.

Speakers

This program includes a diversity of presenters sharing their knowledge and expertise with viewers, listeners, and readers. The views and opinions expressed by these presenters are their own and not necessarily those of MedStudy.

ABIM and AOBIM

For over 30 years, MedStudy has excelled in determining and teaching what a clinically competent internist should know. The American Board of Internal Medicine (ABIM) and the American Osteopathic Board of Internal Medicine (AOBIM) test this same pool of knowledge. MedStudy's expertise, demonstrated by the superb pass rate of those who use MedStudy products, is in the teaching of this knowledge in a clear, learner-friendly manner that results in a stronger knowledge base, improved clinical skills, and better board exam results. Although what we teach is in sync with what the boards test, MedStudy has no affiliation with the ABIM or AOBIM, and our authors, reviewers, and editors have no access to ABIM or AOBIM exam content. Our material is developed as original work by MedStudy physician authors, with additional input from expert contributors, based on their extensive backgrounds in professional medical education. This content is designed to include subject matter typically tested in certification and recertification exams as outlined in the ABIM and AOBIM publicly available exam blueprints but makes no use of, and divulges no details of, the ABIM or AOBIM proprietary exam content.

MedStudy

INTERNAL MEDICINE REVIEW

Allergy & Immunology

Presented by

Peter Huynh, MD

TABLE OF CONTENTS

Why We Moved Some Slide Information to the Audience Response Answers Page

At MedStudy, we do all we can to optimize your self-testing and learning.

In this presentation, the speaker will give some extra information after their AR questions to help explain the correct and incorrect answers. To keep from interfering with your self-testing, we've moved that explanatory text to the Audience Response Answers page(s) at the end of the section.

Be assured, all the content on the slides is in your syllabus—so you can focus on the teaching instead of taking detailed notes.

ABIM Content Specification
- Allergy and immunologic disorders approximate percent in examination = 2%
  - Derm = 3%
  - Endocrine = 9%
  - Heme = 6%
  - Neuro = 4%
  - Renal = 6%

A&I Outline
- Hypersensitivity
  - Type 1
  - Type 2
  - Type 3
  - Type 4
- Anaphylaxis / Anaphylactoid
- Urticaria
- Angioedema
- Eczema
- Contact Dermatitis
- Rhinosinusitis
- Drug Allergy
- Radiocontrast Reactions
- Insect Allergy
- Food Allergy
- Immunodeficiencies

HYPERSENSITIVITY REACTIONS

Audience Response 1
A 45-year-old man with a history of peanut allergy develops shortness of breath and abdominal pain after accidentally eating a cookie containing peanuts. His blood pressure is 130/80 mmHg and heart rate is 110 bpm. On exam, there are audible wheezes. Skin exam is normal.

What is the most appropriate next step?

A. Give albuterol.
B. Give diphenhydramine.
C. Give solumedrol.
D. Give epinephrine.
E. Observation only

Answer:_____

Hypersensitivity Reactions
- Type 1: immediate hypersensitivity
  - IgE-mediated
  - Onset: **minutes to 2 hours**
- Type 2: cytotoxic
  - IgM- or IgG-mediated
  - Onset: **days**
- Type 3: immune complex
  - Antibody-antigen complex
  - Onset: **weeks**
- Type 4: delayed
  - T-cell-mediated
  - Onset: **48–96 hours**

TYPE 1 — IMMEDIATE HYPERSENSITIVITY
- Immediate
  - Onset: **minutes to 2 hours**
  - **IgE-mediated**
- Example: classic "allergies"
  - Hives, allergic rhinitis, asthma, food allergies, latex allergies
- Acute phase
- Late phase

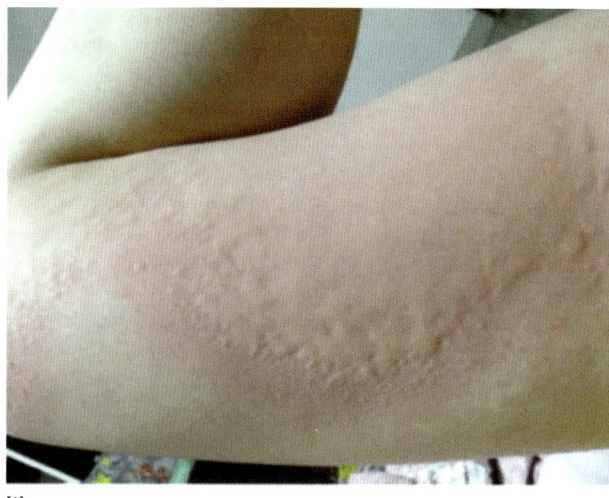

[1]

Type 1 — Acute Phase
- Occurs **within minutes to 2 hours** of exposure
  - Antigen binds to IgE antibodies, then
  - IgE binds to receptors on mast cells
  - Mast cell degranulation
  - Histamine, leukotrienes, prostaglandins, and cytokines
    - H_1 = wheal and flare, bronchoconstriction, pruritus
    - H_2 = increased gastric acid secretion

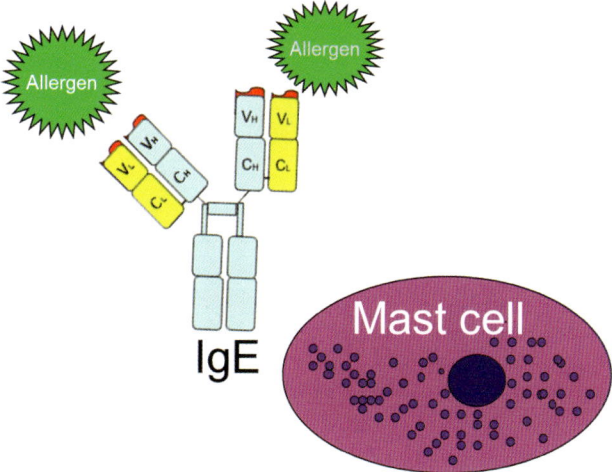

[2]

Type 1 — Late Phase
- Occurs 3–12 hours after acute phase
  - Can last hours to days
  - Release of cytokines during acute phase causes recruitment of **eosinophils** and **basophils**
  - Probability of late-phase response increases with severity of acute-phase reaction

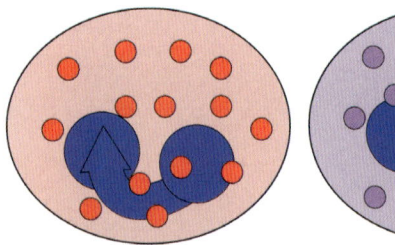 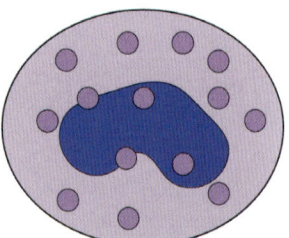

Eosinophils   Basophils

Anaphylaxis
- **Life-threatening IgE-mediated reaction**
- Common causes
  - Antibiotics
    - PCN, cephalosporins
  - Foods
    - Peanuts, tree nuts, shellfish
  - Latex
    - Health care workers, spina bifida, urogenital malformation
  - Anesthetic agents
    - Induction agents, neuromuscular blocking agents
  - Insect stings

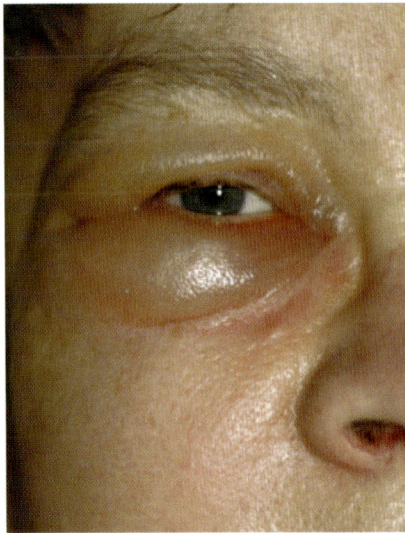

[3]

Anaphylaxis Diagnosis
1) Sudden onset with involvement of the skin or mucosal tissue and either:
   - Sudden respiratory symptoms or
   - Hypotension
2) **≥ 2 of the following occur suddenly after exposure to a likely allergen:**
   - Skin or mucosal tissue involvement
   - Respiratory involvement
   - Hypotension
   - GI symptoms
3) Hypotension after exposure to a known allergen

Anaphylactoid Reactions
- Clinically indistinguishable from anaphylaxis
- Now called "**non**-IgE-mediated anaphylaxis"
- Results from direct mast cell degranulation
  - IgE receptor-independent
  - C3a, C4a, C5a (anaphylatoxins)
- Examples
  - ASA/NSAIDs, opioids, radiocontrast, sulfites

Anaphylaxis / Anaphylactoid
- Usually **minutes** (up to 2 hours) after antigen exposure
- Multisystemic symptoms
  - Cutaneous symptoms most common (90%)
    - Angioedema and urticaria
      - **Lack of cutaneous symptoms does <u>not</u> rule out anaphylaxis!**
  - Respiratory symptoms (50%)
    - Wheezing, shortness of breath, throat tightness
  - Cardiac (30%)
    - Hypotension, dizziness, syncope
      - **Lack of hypotension does <u>not</u> rule out anaphylaxis!**
  - GI (25%)
    - Abdominal pain, nausea, and vomiting

Anaphylaxis — Treatment
- **Epinephrine! Epinephrine! Epinephrine!**
  - Fatalities from anaphylaxis
    - Failure to recognize anaphylaxis
    - Failure to give epinephrine early
  - **Epinephrine 0.2–0.5 mL of 1:1,000 dilution IM** anterolateral thigh
    - Adrenaline autoinjector = 0.3 mL IM
  - α- and β-Adrenergic effects
    - Bronchial relaxation, vasoconstriction, decreased vascular permeability

What about Patients on β-Blockers?
- β-Blockers are relatively contraindicated in patients at risk for anaphylaxis
  - Example: patient with food allergy and HTN
- **Epinephrine <u>still</u> 1st line**
- **Glucagon** for patients on β-blockers nonresponsive to epinephrine

Anaphylaxis — Treatment
- **A**irway
  - Inhaled albuterol for wheezing
- **B**reathing
  - Intubate if needed
- **C**irculation
  - Volume resuscitation for hypotension
- **D**rugs
  - **Epinephrine** is always **1st line**
  - H_1 and H_2 antagonists
  - Steroids may prevent late-phase reaction

TYPE 2 — CYTOTOXIC HYPERSENSITIVITY
- Onset: **days**
- IgM or IgG antibodies bind to **fixed tissue antigen** or **cell receptors**
- Binding of antibody causes target cell destruction
  - Complement activation
  - Opsonization from production of C3b
  - Phagocytes can attack antibody-coated cells

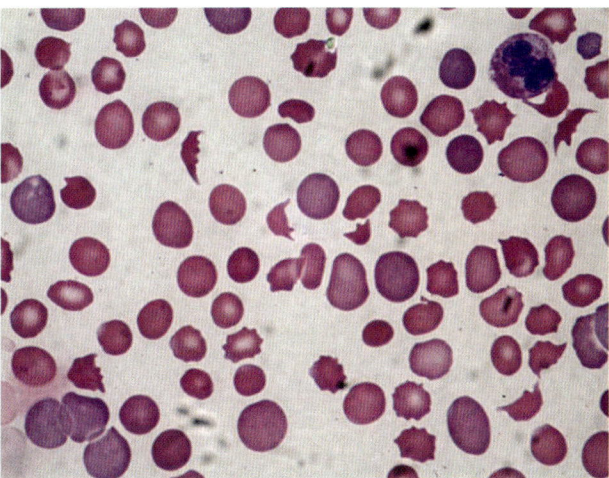

- Example: **fixed tissue antigen**

Fixed Tissue Antigen	Disease
Basement membrane	Goodpasture's
ACh receptor on muscle	Myasthenia gravis

- Example: **target cell receptors**

Target Cell Receptors	Disease
Platelets	Thrombocytopenia
RBCs	Hemolytic anemia
WBCs	Leukopenia

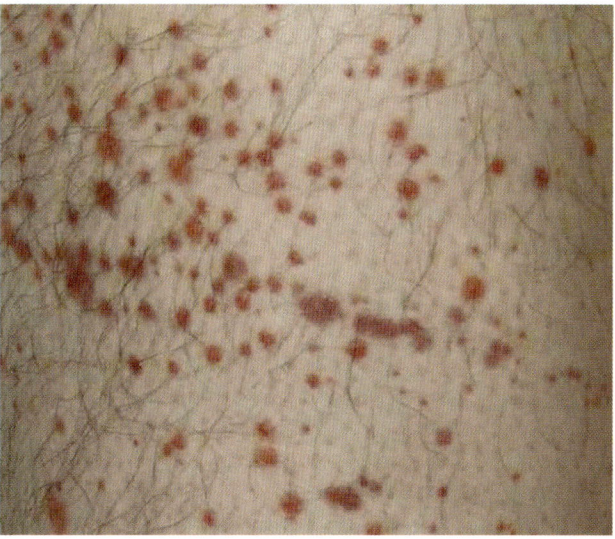

[4]

TYPE 3 — IMMUNE COMPLEX HYPERSENSITIVITY
- Onset: **weeks (usually 1–3 weeks)**
- Think vasculitis!
  - Immune complexes form when antibodies combine with antigen
    - Immune complexes precipitate in small vessels
      - Activates complement, inflammatory cascade
      - Results in necrosis of small blood vessels
        = **leukocytoclastic vasculitis**
        » Hemorrhagic indurated lesions

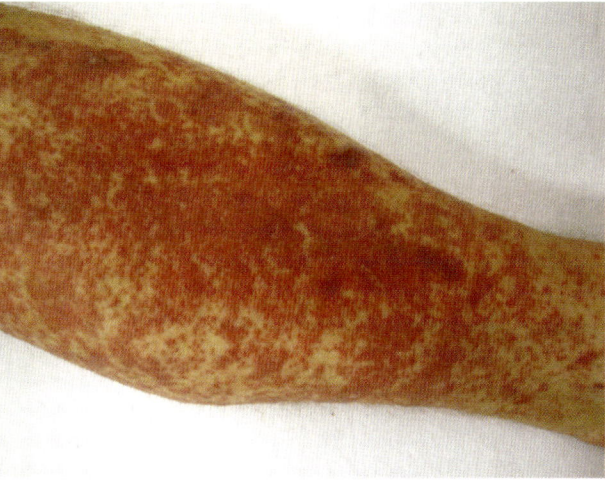

[5]

- Serum sickness (systemic reaction)
  - Large amount of antigen is injected into nonimmunized person
- Arthus reaction (local reaction)
  - Person is hyperimmunized, then given injection of antigen
    - Many circulating IgG antibodies
    - Immune complexes form

TYPE 4 – DELAYED CELL-MEDIATED HYPERSENSITIVITY

- **Onset: 24–96 hours**
- Previously **sensitized T cells** interact with antigen
- Examples
  - Contact dermatitis
  - Tuberculin sensitivity

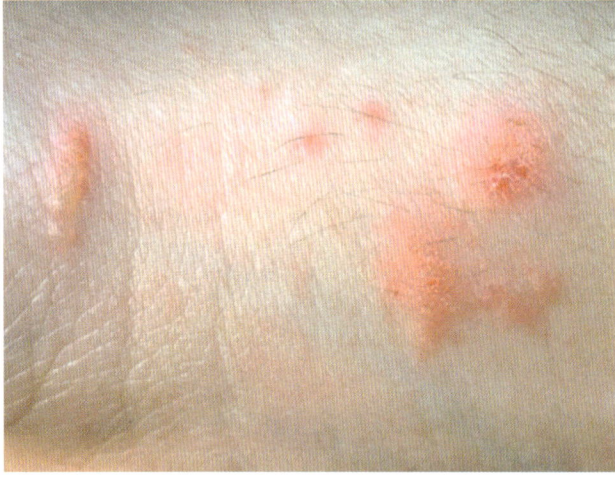

[6]

URTICARIA

AR 2

A 68-year-old woman has had daily hives for the past 8 weeks. Lesions last < 24 hours, but reappear in a different location. She denies any fevers, arthritis, or weight loss.

Which of the following is the most appropriate next step?

A. Prescribe topical corticosteroids.
B. Prescribe nonsedating antihistamines.
C. Prescribe sedating antihistamines.
D. Measure C1 inhibitor levels.
E. Refer to a dermatologist for skin biopsy.

Answer:_____

Urticaria

- <u>Acute</u>: hives lasting < 6 weeks
  - Foods, drugs, pollen, insect sting
- <u>Chronic</u>: hives lasting > 6 weeks
  - > 90% idiopathic
    - Of causes identified
      - Thyroid disease
      - Autoimmune disease
      - Malignancy
      - Chronic infection
- Treatment
  - **Nonsedating antihistamine** is 1st line therapy

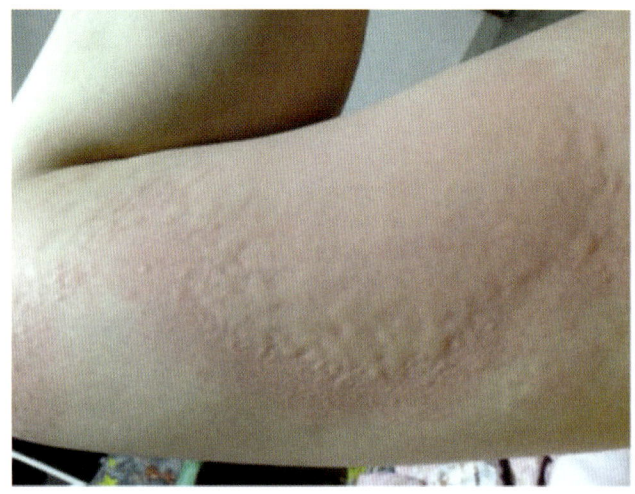

Dermatographism

- "Writing on the skin"
- Exaggerated hives occur after the skin is stroked or gentle pressure is applied

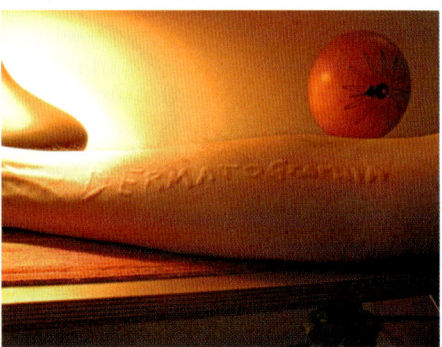

[7]

Physical Urticaria

- Acquired cold urticaria
  - Precipitated by **cold** exposure
    - Shock may occur if the patient is immersed in cold water!
    - Test with a 5-minute skin ice cube challenge
- Cholinergic urticaria
  - Precipitated by **heat** (e.g., hot shower, hot day, exercise)
  - Punctate hives that are very pruritic

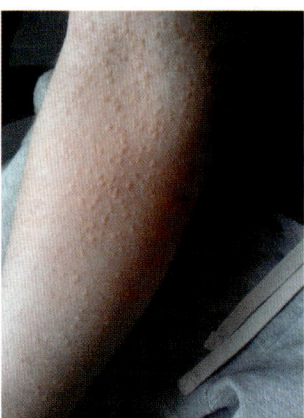

[8]

Urticarial Vasculitis

- Autoimmune disease
  - **Red flags**
    - Lesions last > 24 hours in a fixed location
    - Residual ecchymosis, hyperpigmentation, or purpura
    - Hives are nonpruritic, tender, and burn
    - Arthritis, fever, fatigue, weight loss
- Dx: skin biopsy
- Labs: decreased C3/C4 level and antibodies to C1q
- Rx: immunosuppressive agents such as cyclosporine

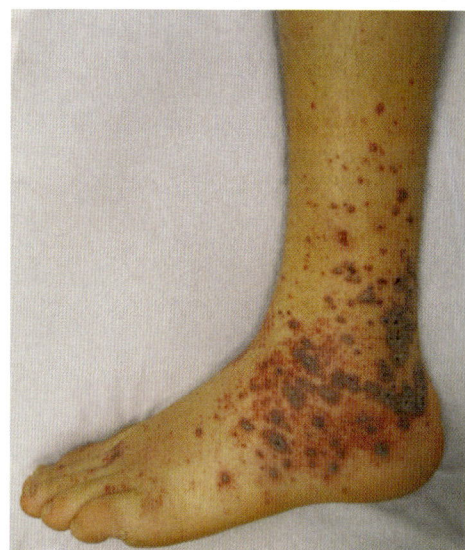

[9]

ANGIOEDEMA

- Sudden, temporary edema of localized area of skin or mucosa
  - Lips, face, hands, feet, larynx
- **Type 1 IgE-mediated angioedema**
  - Food allergy, insect sting allergy, drug allergy, latex allergy
- **ACEI-induced angioedema**
  - Can occur weeks to months after starting ACE inhibitor
  - Occurs in 0.1–0.7%
  - More common in African Americans
- **Non-IgE-mediated angioedema**
  - Idiopathic, virally induced, hereditary angioedema

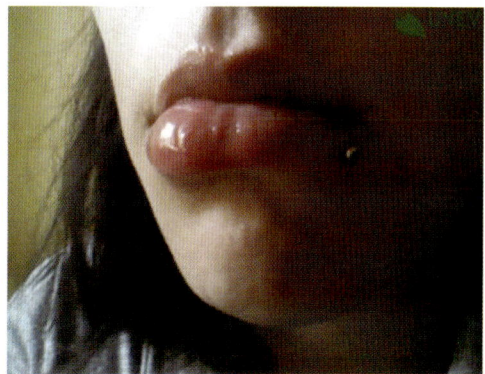

[10]

HEREDITARY ANGIOEDEMA

- Due to defect in **C1 inhibitor function**
  - Autosomal dominant
  - Type 1: low levels of C1 inhibitor protein
  - Type 2: normal levels of C1 inhibitor protein, but nonfunctioning
- Recurrent episodes of **angioedema**, abdominal pain, extremity swelling, laryngeal edema
  - **No urticaria!**
- **Erythema marginatum**

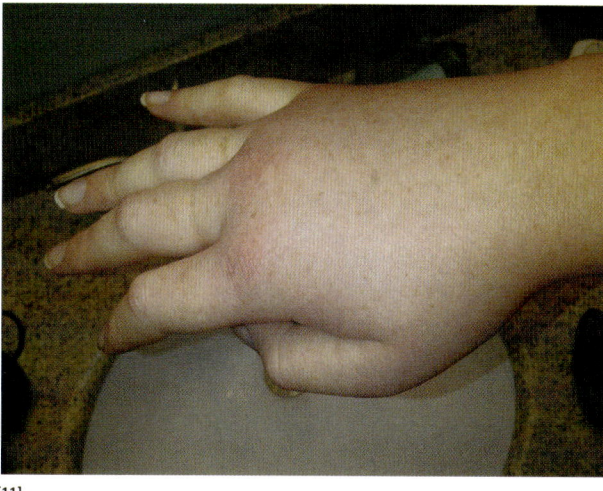

[11]

- Diagnosis
  - Screen: **low C4 level**
  - Type 1
    - Low C1 inhibitor level
    - Low C1 inhibitor functional level
  - Type 2
    - Normal C1 inhibitor level
    - Low C1 inhibitor functional level

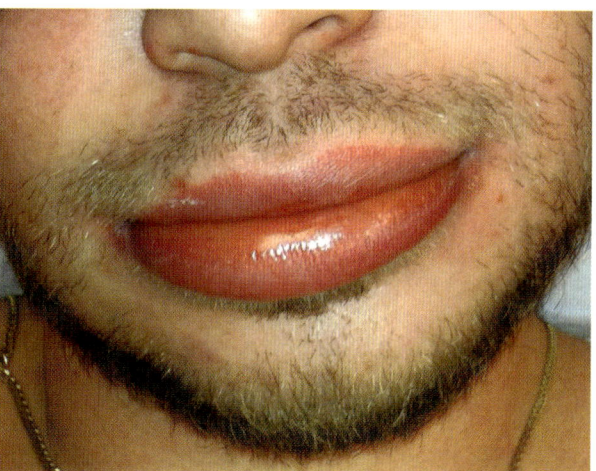

[12]

ALLERGY & IMMUNOLOGY

- Treatment
  - Attenuated androgens (danazol)
  - ε-Aminocaproic acid
  - **Plasma-derived C1-esterase inhibitor** protein
  - Bradykinin receptor antagonist (icatibant)
  - Kallikrein inhibitor (ecallantide, lanadelumab)

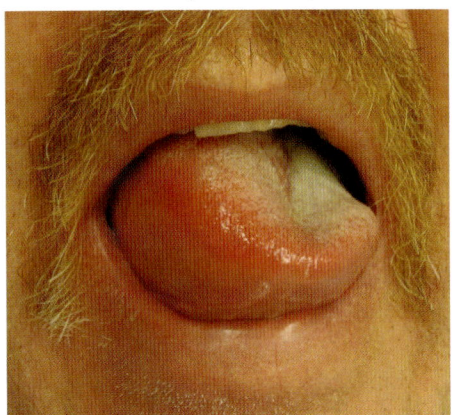

[13]

ATOPIC DERMATITIS (AD)

AR 3

A 28-year-old woman has had eczema since she was a child. She complains of a dry, scaly, and very pruritic rash on her antecubital fossa despite using emollients.

What is the most appropriate next step?

A. Start oral corticosteroid.
B. Start topical corticosteroid.
C. Start pimecrolimus.
D. Start tacrolimus.
E. Start oral antihistamine.

Answer:_____

Atopic Dermatitis (AD; a.k.a. Eczema, Atopic Eczema)
- Occurs in ~ 1–3% of adults
- Presents as a dry, red, scaly, and very pruritic rash
- Refer to a dermatologist for new-onset adult AD that is refractory to conventional therapy
  - Skin biopsy to rule out T-cell lymphoma

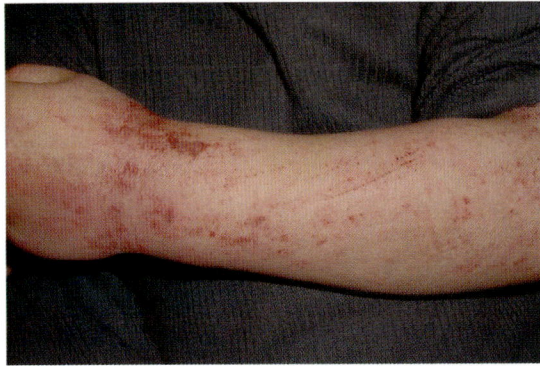

[14]

AD — Treatment

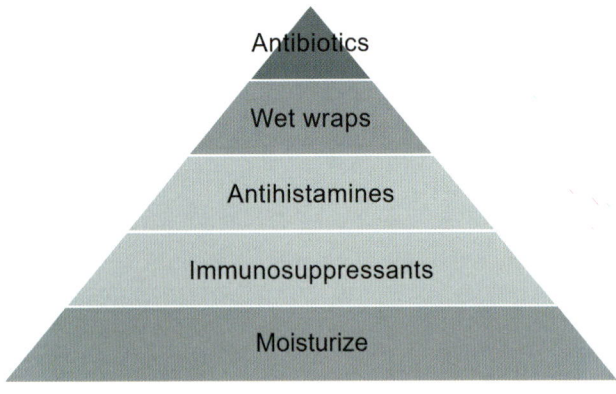

Layered approach to treatment

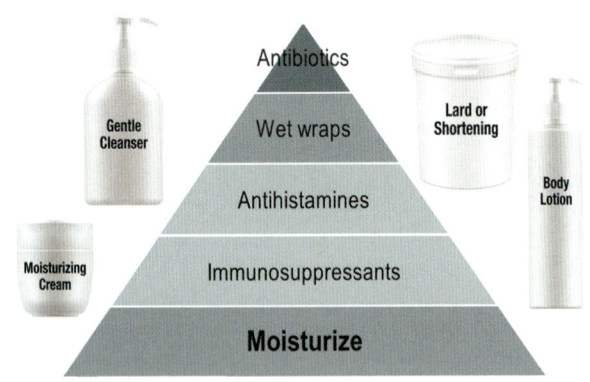

Tx — Moisturize
- Aggressive application of **emollients is key!**
- Atopic skin has enhanced transepidermal water loss
  - Impaired function of the water permeability barrier
  - Transepidermal water loss is increased from both involved and normal-appearing atopic skin
  - Water content in skin is decreased

AD — Treatment

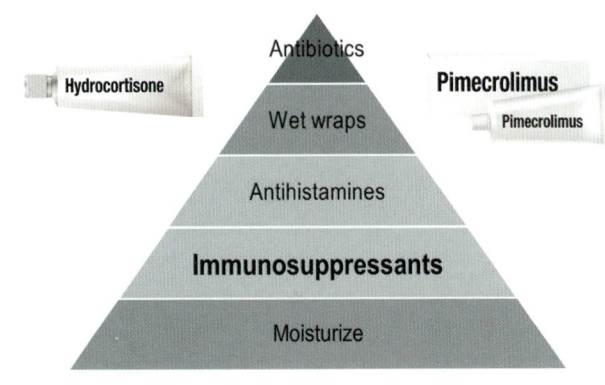

Rx — Immunosuppressants
- **Topical corticosteroids**
- **1st line** treatment
  - Ointments > creams in bioavailability
  - Ointments are most occlusive, but during excessive heat or humidity increased occlusion may cause itching or folliculitis
  - Creams may be better tolerated during heat
- Chronic use of high-potency topical steroids can cause **skin atrophy**
- **Topical calcineurin inhibitors**
  - Tacrolimus and pimecrolimus bind to FK506-binding protein
  - **2nd line** treatment
    - Inhibits signal transduction and gene transcription of various proinflammatory cytokines
      - Tacrolimus (Protopic)
      - Pimecrolimus (Elidel)
  - Does <u>not</u> cause skin atrophy

AD — Treatment

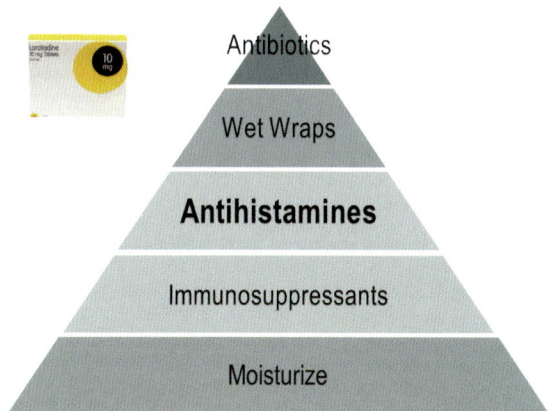

Rx — Antihistamines
- Break scratch-itch-scratch cycle
  - H_1 and H_2 blockers
    - 1st generation H_1 blockers more effective than newer ones, but have sedative and anticholinergic effects
      - **Avoid in older patients**
    - H_2 receptors on skin, so H_2 blockers are of value
  - Topical antihistamines should be avoided because of potential sensitization

AD — Treatment

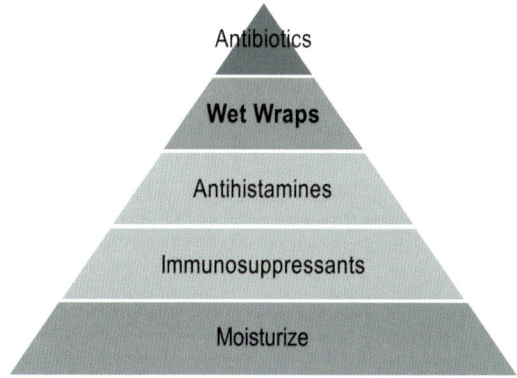

Tx — Wet Wraps[15]
- Wet dressings
  - Reduce pruritus and inflammation by cooling skin
  - Acts as barrier to trauma associated with scratching
  - Improves penetration of topical steroids and topical calcineurin inhibitors

AD — Treatment

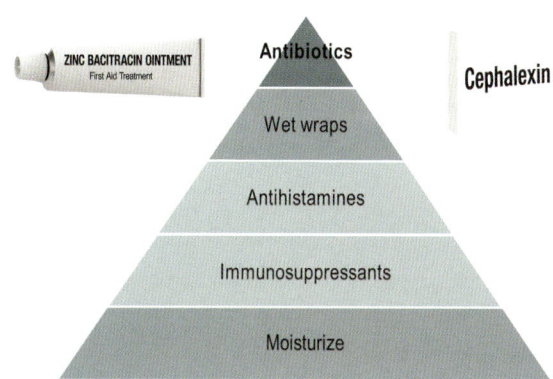

Role of Infections[16]
- Patients with AD are frequently colonized by *S. aureus* that secrete enterotoxins and toxic shock syndrome toxin (TSST-1)
  - *S. aureus* detected in > 90% of AD skin lesions (in contrast, only 5% of normal patients harbor this organism)
  - 50% of the *S. aureus* cultured produced enterotoxins and TSST-1

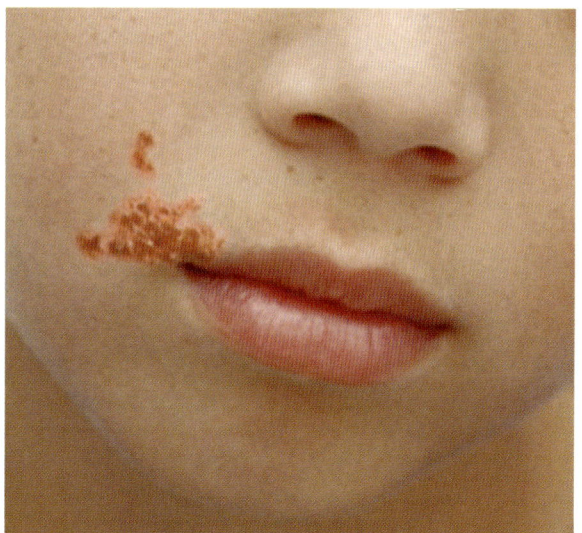

[17]

Treatment — Antibiotics
- Systemic antibiotic therapy against *S. aureus* secondary infection
  - Semisynthetic penicillin or 1st generation cephalosporin
  - Topical antibiotic mupirocin for local involvement
  - Maintenance antibiotic therapy should be avoided 2/2 MRSA colonization

CONTACT DERMATITIS

AR 4
A 45-year-old woman develops linear vesicles and blisters 3 days after going hiking on a forest trail.

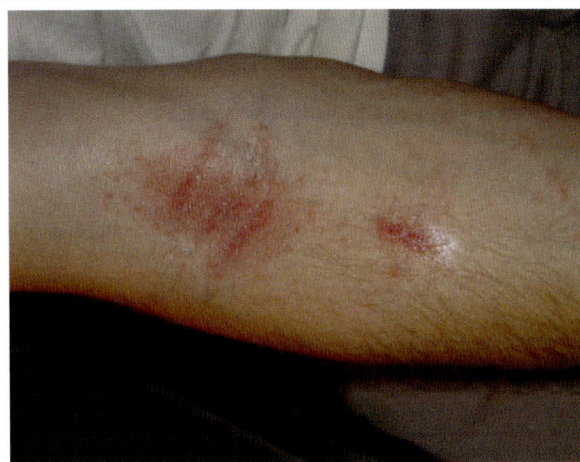

Her reaction is most likely categorized by which type of hypersensitivity reaction?

A. Type 1
B. Type 2
C. Type 3
D. Type 4

Answer:_____

Contact Dermatitis
- Type 4: delayed hypersensitivity reaction
  - T-cell-mediated
  - Onset: **48–96 hours**
  - Common causes
    - **Poison oak and poison ivy**
    - Nickel, rubber, hair products, and makeup
  - Patch testing if suspect chemical or metal allergy

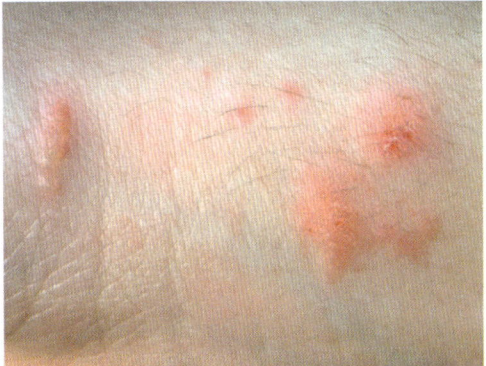

RHINITIS

AR 5
A 42-year-old man reports runny nose, sneezing, and itchy nose occurring every April. He has carpets in his home and has 2 dogs. Symptoms last for about 8 weeks. He denies symptoms during other times of the year.

Which of the following allergens is most likely the cause of his symptoms?

A. Dog dander
B. Tree pollen
C. Grass pollen
D. Weed pollen
E. Dust mites

Answer:_____

Rhinitis
- Allergic rhinitis
  - Seasonal
  - Perennial
  - Perennial with seasonal exacerbation
- Nonallergic rhinitis with eosinophilia syndrome (NARES)
- Vasomotor rhinitis
- Rhinitis medicamentosa
- Atrophic rhinitis

Allergic Rhinitis
- Cardinal symptoms of <u>nasal congestion</u>, <u>rhinorrhea</u>, <u>sneezing</u>, <u>nasal pruritus</u>
- **IgE-mediated**
- Nasal smear shows **eosinophilia**
- **2 main types**
  - Seasonal
    - Grass, tree, weed pollens
  - Perennial
    - Dust mites, molds, animal dander
  - Perennial with seasonal exacerbation

Allergic Rhinitis — AAAI Tx
- **A**voidance
  - Do skin prick test or radioallergosorbent assay (RAST) to determine sensitization
- **A**ntihistamines
  - 2nd generation antihistamines
- **A**llergen-specific immunotherapy (allergy shots)
- **I**ntranasal corticosteroids
  - 1st line therapy

Avoidance
- Do skin prick test or RAST to determine sensitization
  - Pollen avoidance
    - **Tree** pollens highest in **spring**
    - **Grass** pollens in **summer**
    - **Weeds** in **fall**
      - Close windows
      - Home air filtration systems
  - Dust mites
    - Impermeable mattress/pillow covers
    - Decrease humidity to < 50%
    - Wash sheets in 140.0°F (60.0°C) water
  - Removal of pet
    - But cat allergen can be detectable even 4 months after removal!

Antihistamines

- Early-generation antihistamines cause sedation
  - **Avoid in older patients**
  - Diphenhydramine, chlorpheniramine, and hydroxyzine
  - Cross blood-brain barrier
    - Interact with dopamine, serotonin, acetylcholine receptors in the brain
    - Anticholinergic effects
      - Blurry vision, dry mouth, urinary retention
- 2nd generation less likely to cross blood-brain barrier
  - Cetirizine, fexofenadine, loratadine, desloratadine
  - Cause little-to-no sedation

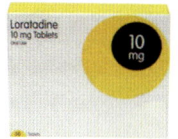

Allergen Immunotherapy

- Only works for **IgE**-mediated conditions
  - Give increasing doses of allergens via subcutaneous (SQ) route to induce immune tolerance to allergens
    - T regulatory cells
    - Increase in regulatory/suppressive cytokines such as IL-10 and TGF-β
    - Production of blocking antibodies IgG isotype to IgE

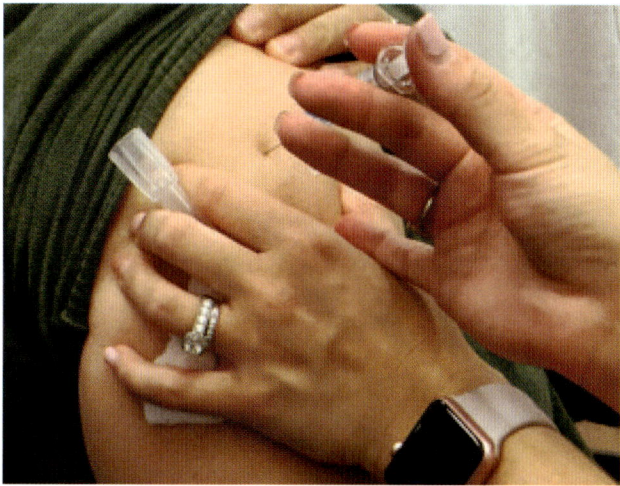

[18]

Nonallergic Rhinitis with Eosinophilia Syndrome (NARES)

- Chronic nasal congestion
- Nasal smear shows **eosinophilia**
- Do **not** demonstrate sensitization to any allergens
  - **Negative** RAST and skin prick test

Vasomotor Rhinitis

- Reaction to neurogenic/vagal stimuli
- Sneezing attacks followed by nasal congestion on exposure to cold, sunlight, spicy foods
  - Examples:
    - Skier's nose (cold)
    - Gustatory rhinitis (food)

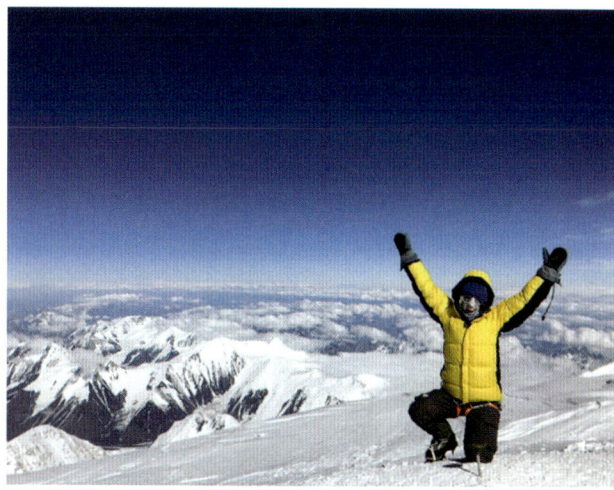

Rhinitis Medicamentosa

- Rebound congestion caused by overuse of vasoconstricting nasal drops
  - Phenylephrine, oxymetazoline, naphazoline
- Exam shows beefy red nasal mucosa
- Treatment: Discontinue nasal decongestant and start intranasal corticosteroid instead

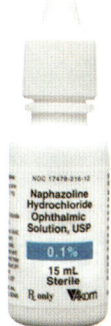

AR 6

A 28-year-old pregnant woman in her last trimester complains of nasal congestion that keeps her up at night and affects her quality of life.

Which of the following is the most appropriate next step?

A. Prescribe intranasal budesonide.
B. Prescribe oral budesonide.
C. Prescribe intranasal decongestant.
D. Prescribe oral decongestant.
E. Refer to an allergist for skin testing.

Answer:_____

Rhinitis and Pregnancy

- Pregnancy rhinitis
  - Nasal congestion in the last 6 weeks of pregnancy
- Choose pregnancy Category B medications
  - Budesonide intranasal spray
  - Cetirizine, loratadine
  - Cromolyn
  - Montelukast
- Avoid oral decongestants
  - Increased risk of congenital malformations
    - Gastroschisis
    - Intestinal atresia

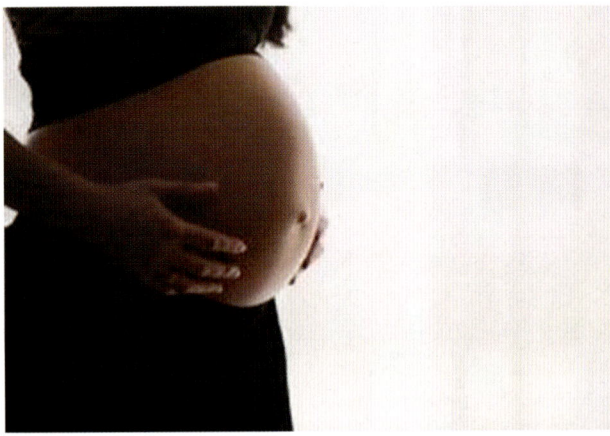

RHINOSINUSITIS

AR 7

A 35-year-old man complains of purulent rhinorrhea, sinus headache, and cough for the past 2 days. His children are also sick at home. He is afebrile.

What is the most appropriate next step?

A. Order allergy testing.
B. Prescribe amoxicillin.
C. Prescribe oral corticosteroid.
D. Prescribe topical decongestant.
E. Reassurance only

Answer:_____

Rhinosinusitis

- Sinus mucosa considered extension of nasal mucosa = "rhinosinusitis"
- Acute rhinosinusitis
  - Symptoms lasting < 4 weeks
- Chronic rhinosinusitis
  - Symptoms lasting > 12 weeks

Acute Rhinosinusitis

- Rhinorrhea, nasal congestion, facial pain, and sinus tenderness
- Vast majority are **viral in etiology**
  - < 2% are bacterial
- Do **not** routinely order sinus CT or x-ray!
  - <u>Cannot</u> distinguish between bacterial vs. viral etiology
- Bacterial sinusitis is a <u>clinical</u> diagnosis!

Acute Bacterial Rhinosinusitis

- When to give antibiotics
  - **Severe** initial symptoms with high fever (> 102.0°F [38.9°C]), purulent nasal discharge, and facial pain
  - **Worsening** symptoms after initial improvement (a.k.a. "double sickening")
  - **Persistent symptoms** with no improvement after 10 days
- 1ˢᵗ line treatment is amoxicillin + clavulanic acid
  - Use doxycycline for patients with PCN allergy

Chronic Rhinosinusitis

- Symptoms > 12 weeks
  - Mucopurulent discharge, obstruction, nasal congestion, sinus pressure and pain, and loss of smell
- CT sinus = sinusitis
- Rhinoscopy = mucopurulent discharge from ostiomeatal complex
- Treatment: intranasal steroids and saline lavage to restore ostiomeatal patency

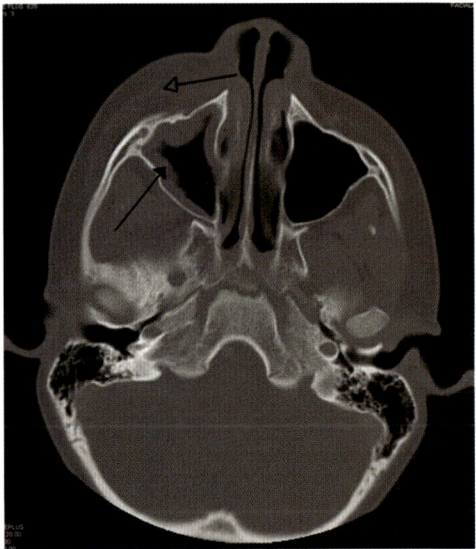

ADVERSE DRUG REACTIONS

OVERVIEW

AR 8

Drug desensitization allows for a temporary state of tolerance.

Which of the following would be an indication for drug desensitization?

A. Cephalosporin-induced Steven-Johnson syndrome
B. History of toxic epidermal necrolysis
C. Epilepsy and a history of DRESS syndrome
D. Pregnant woman with history of contact dermatitis due to neomycin
E. Neurosyphilis and a history of PCN anaphylaxis

Answer:_____

AR 9

A 25-year-old woman develops rash, fever, arthralgia, and lymphadenopathy 3 weeks after starting cefaclor for a urinary tract infection.

Her reaction is most likely categorized by which type of hypersensitivity reaction?

A. Type 1
B. Type 2
C. Type 3
D. Type 4

Answer:_____

Adverse Drug Reactions

- World Health Organization (WHO) definition
  - "Any noxious, unintended, and undesired effect of a drug that occurs at doses used for prevention, diagnosis, or treatment"
  - Cutaneous reactions are most common
    - 15% of patients sustained ADRs during their hospitalizations
    - 7% of patients experienced serious reactions

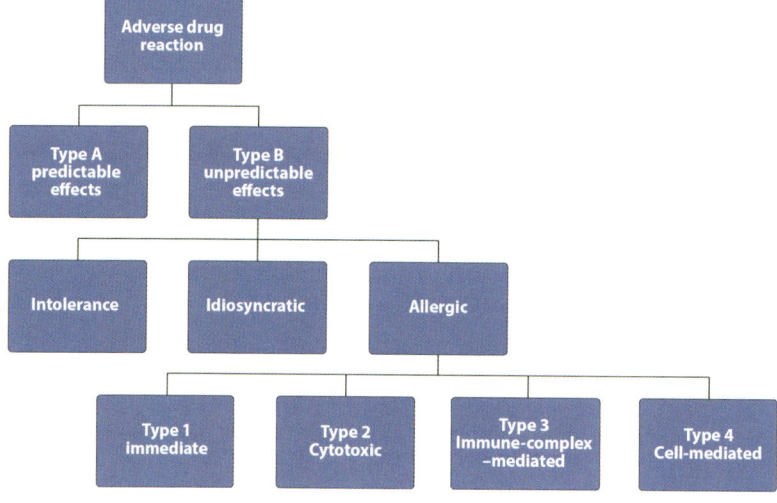

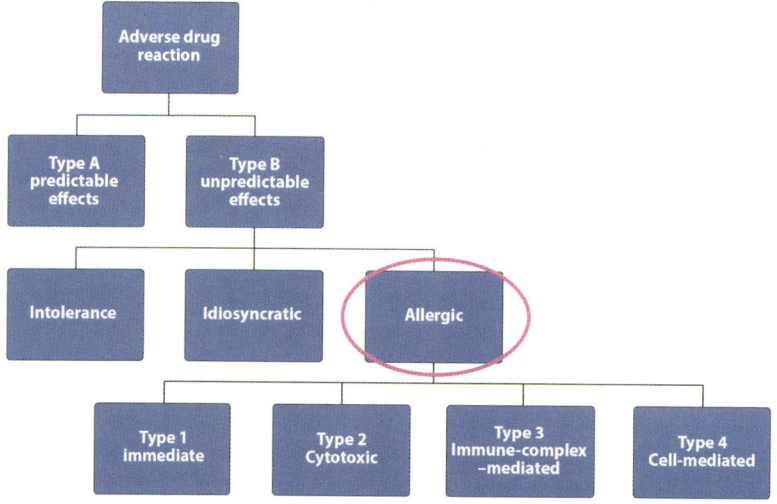

TYPE 1 — DRUG REACTION

- Timing: **immediate**
  - Within **minutes to hours**
- Type: specific **IgE** hypersensitivity
  - Cross-linking of IgE causes the release of mediators from mast cells
- Reaction
  - Urticaria, anaphylaxis
- Example: PCN
  - PCN acts as hapten

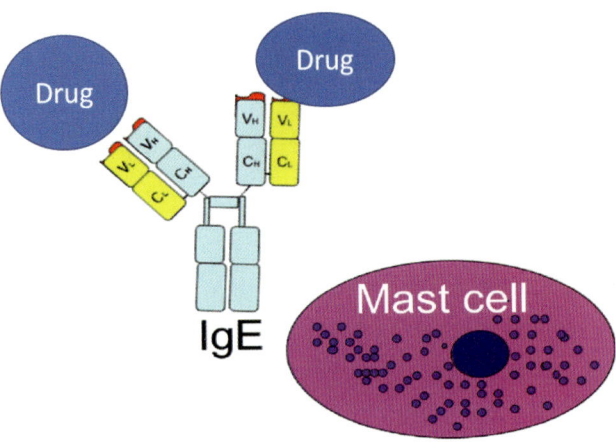

β-Lactam Drug Allergy

- <u>Most common</u> drug allergy
- PCN cross-reacts with cephalosporins at a rate of only 1–3%
  - Safe to give 2nd and 3rd generation cephalosporins to patients with PCN allergy
- Desensitization can be performed if needed
  - Neurosyphilis
  - Pregnancy and syphilis
  - Multidrug-resistant organism

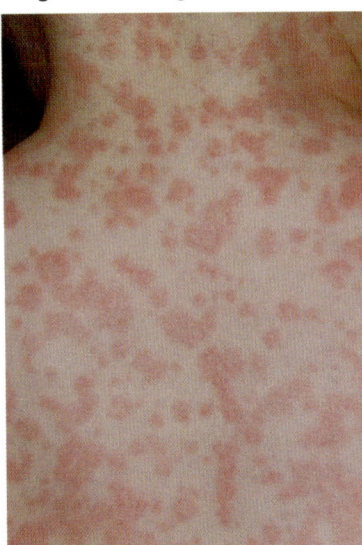

[19]

Drug Desensitization

- Allows for <u>temporary</u> state of tolerance
- Necessary if the drug is the only available effective therapy
  - Pregnant woman with syphilis with PCN allergy
  - Neurosyphilis
- Involves slow introduction of increasing amounts
  - 1st dose usually 1/10,000 of the full dose
  - Dose increased every 15 minutes
  - Usually takes 4–8 hours
- Contraindicated for serious non-IgE-mediated reactions
  - SJS, TEN, DRESS

TYPE 2 — DRUG REACTION

- Timing: days
- Type: **cytotoxic** reaction
  - IgG or IgM antibodies recognize drug antigen on cell membranes
  - Antibody-coated cell cleared by the monocyte-macrophage system
- Drug: drug-induced hemolytic anemia and thrombocytopenia
- Examples: methyldopa, PCN, cephalosporins

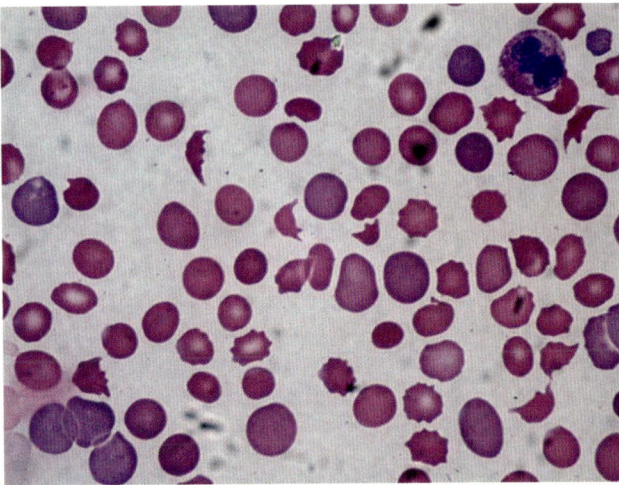

TYPE 3 — DRUG REACTION

- Timing: **1–3 weeks**
- Type: **immune complex**-mediated
  - Immune complexes are deposited in blood vessel walls and cause injury by activating the complement cascade
- Reaction: **fever, rash, urticaria,** lymphadenopathy, and arthralgias
- Example: serum sickness
  - Antithymocyte globulin (ATG), thiouracils, and phenytoin

TYPE 4 — DRUG REACTION

- Timing: **48–72 hours**
- Type: delayed type
  - Mediated by drug-specific T lymphocytes
- Reaction: contact dermatitis
- Example
  - Neomycin, local anesthetics, and topical antihistamines

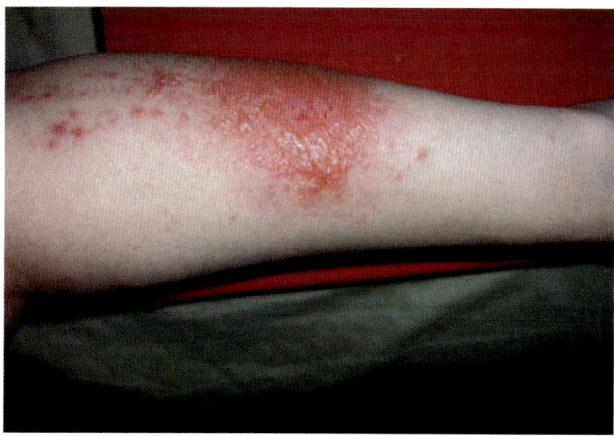

VANCOMYCIN HYPERSENSITIVITY

- Constellation of symptoms
  - Pruritus, flushing, erythroderma
- Secondary to **nonspecific histamine release** that is rate dependent
- Severity correlates with amount of histamine
- Released into plasma
  - Nothing to do with vancomycin levels
- Treat by:
  - Reducing rate
  - Premedicating with H_1 antagonists

DRESS SYNDROME

- **D**rug **r**eaction/**r**ash **e**osinophilia with **s**ystemic **s**ymptoms
- Causative drugs
  - Antiseizure medications, sulfonamides, allopurinol
- Associated with HHV-6 infection/reactivation
- Treatment
  - Stop offending drug
  - Glucocorticoids ± IVIG

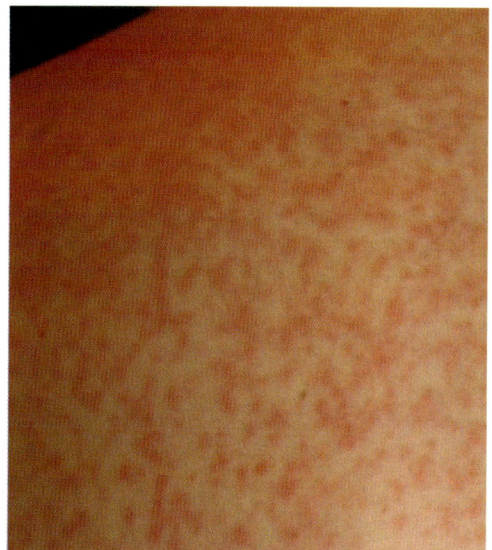

[20]

SERUM SICKNESS

- Appears 1–3 weeks after administration of drug
- Clinically: **fever, rashes, joint pain, lymphadenopathy,** muscle aches, and proteinuria
- Skin findings are universal
  - Classic serpiginous rash of the hands and feet
  - Itching, redness, urticaria, angioedema
- Arthralgia
  - Involves multiple joints: knee, ankles, fingers, and toes
- GI
  - Nausea and vomiting
- Causes
  - Equine antitetanus
  - Antibiotics
    - Cefaclor
    - Penicillin
  - Antithymocyte globulin (ATG)
  - Muromonab-CD3 (Orthoclone OKT3) monoclonal antibodies
  - Venom stings (bees, wasps)

RADIOCONTRAST MEDIA (RCM) REACTIONS

AR 10

A 42-year-old woman develops generalized urticaria and pruritus after undergoing a CT scan of the abdomen with contrast.

Which of the following increases the risk of radiocontrast media (RCM) reactions?

A. Seafood allergy
B. Iodine allergy
C. Coronary artery disease
D. Diabetes

Answer: _____

RCM Reactions

- Direct mast cell degranulation
  - Non-IgE-mediated; some IgE-mediated
- <u>Not</u> associated with seafood or iodine allergy (**myth**!)
- Risk factors
  - Female
  - Asthma
  - Prior reaction to radiocontrast
  - Cardiovascular disease

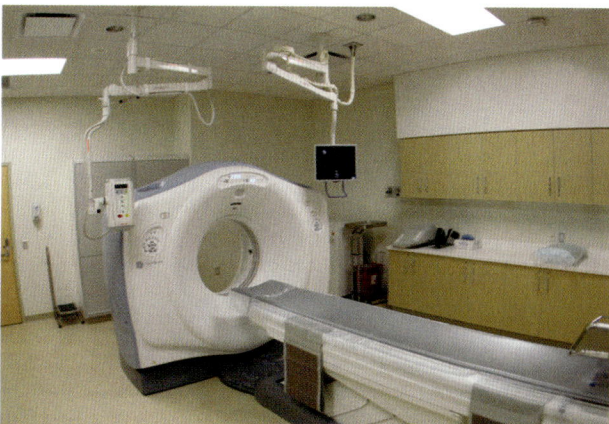

[21]

RCM Reactions — Treatment
- Nonionic or hypoosmolar radiocontrast
- Treatment
  - Prednisone 50 mg
    - 13, 7, and 1 hour prior
  - Diphenhydramine 50 mg 1 hour prior
  - Albuterol PRN

STINGING-INSECT HYPERSENSITIVITY

Insect Allergy
- Most common from *Hymenoptera* order
  (bees, yellow jackets, hornets, wasps, fire ants)
- Large local reactions do not require any additional
  workup
- Venom anaphylaxis requires further testing
  to allergy tests
- Venom immunotherapy is 98% effective in preventing
  future systemic reactions to stings

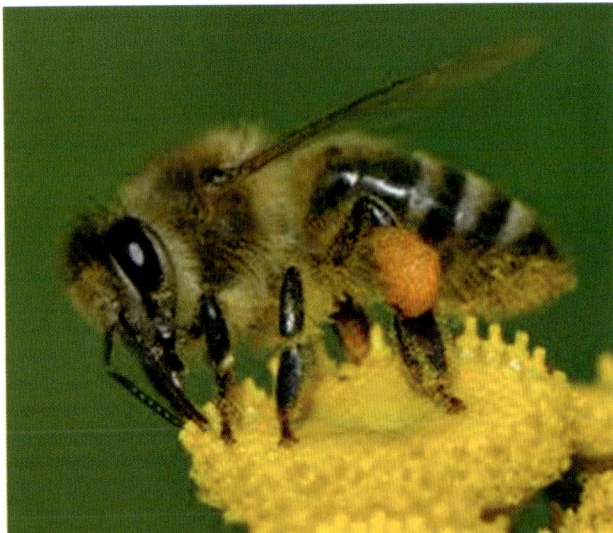

[22]

Natural History of Insect Stings[23]

Severity	Age	Risk of Future Systemic Reaction (in 10 years)*
No reaction	All	17%
Large local reaction	All	10%
Cutaneous systemic	Child	10%
	Adult	20%
Anaphylaxis	Child	40%
	Adult	60%

*Risk of systemic reaction in untreated patients
with a history of sting reaction and positive skin test

FOOD ALLERGY
- Affects ~ 1–5% adults
- Leading cause of anaphylaxis outside of hospitals
- Nuts and seafood most common

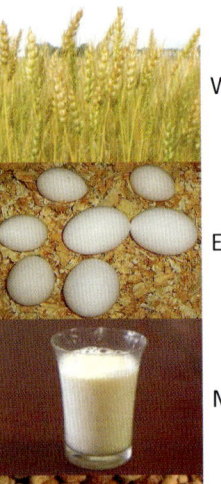
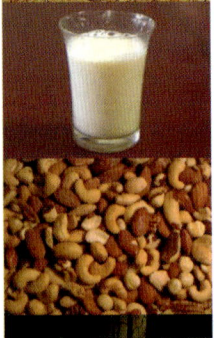

Wheat

Eggs

Milk and soy

Peanuts and tree nuts

Seafood (fish and shellfish)

Food Allergy Testing
- Diagnosis
  - History and physical
  - Skin prick test (SPT)
    - Negative predictive value > 95%
    - Low specificity = 50%, very sensitive > 90%
      - Indicates sensitization, not clinical reactivity
- RAST
  - Less sensitive than SPT
  - But, with certain cutoffs, has high positive
    predictive value

Food Allergy[24]

Food	RAST Level	PPV
Egg	7 kU/L	96–98%
Milk	15 kU/L	95%
Peanut	14 kU/L	100%
Codfish	20 kU/L	100%

- Diagnosis
  - Compatible history with confirmatory allergy test
- Treatment
  - Avoidance
  - Epinephrine autoinjectors for high risk

Oral Allergy Syndrome
- <u>Localized</u> food allergy syndrome
  - Raw fruits and vegetables
- Symptoms confined to lips, mouth, and throat
- Pruritus, tingling of lips, tongue, roof of mouth, and throat
- Tolerate cooked fruits and vegetables

IMMUNODEFICIENCIES

AR 11
A 22-year-old woman is admitted to the hospital for her 3rd episode of *Neisseria* meningitis.

What is the most appropriate next step to establish the diagnosis?

A. Order HIV testing.
B. Order CH50.
C. Order quantitative immunoglobulins.
D. Order B cell subsets.

Answer:_____

Immunodeficiencies
- Think about immunodeficiency in patients with **recurrent or opportunistic infections**
- Primary immunodeficiency (PI) is most commonly found in children, but increasingly recognized in adults
- **Inherited**
  - Agammaglobulinemia
  - Common variable immunodeficiency
  - IgA deficiency
- **Acquired**
  - HIV
  - Cancer
  - Asplenia

When Should You Suspect Primary Immunodeficiency?

Any 2 or More of the Following:
2 or more new ear infections within 1 year
2 or more new sinus infections within 1 year, in the absence of allergy
1 pneumonia per year for more than 1 year
Chronic diarrhea with weight loss
Recurrent viral infections (colds, herpes, warts, condyloma)
Recurrent need for intravenous antibiotics to clear infections
Recurrent, deep abscesses of the skin or internal organs
Persistent thrush or fungal infection on skin or elsewhere
Infection with normally harmless tuberculosis-like bacteria
A family history of primary immunodeficiency

Congenital Agammaglobulinemia
- a.k.a. Bruton's or X-linked
- Mutation in Bruton tyrosine kinase → arrested B-cell development
- Recurrent **sinopulmonary** and ear infections
- **Encapsulated organisms**
  - *Staphylococcus, Streptococcus, Meningococcus, Haemophilus*
- **Enteroviral** infection; *Giardia* infection
- Diagnosis: no antibodies; no B cells
- Treatment: IVIG or SQIG ± prophylactic antibiotics

Common Variable Immunodeficiency
- Failure of B-cell maturation into plasma cells
- Recurrent **sinopulmonary** and ear infections
- **Encapsulated organisms**
  - *Staphylococcus, Streptococcus, Meningococcus, Haemophilus*
- Bronchiectasis
- **Enteroviral** infection; *Giardia* infection
- Increased risk of autoimmune disease and malignancy
- Diagnosis: low IgG with low IgA or low IgM; low B cells
- Treatment: IVIG or SQIG ± prophylactic antibiotics

IgA Deficiency
- Most common 1° "immunodeficiency"
  - 1:300 persons
  - Most asymptomatic
- Prolonged or recurrent **upper respiratory infections**
- Giardiasis
- Increased **autoimmune disease**
  - Celiac disease and thyroid disease
- Diagnosis: undetectable IgA
- Treatment: usually does not require Tx

Complement Disorders
- **Early complement deficiency**
  - Pyogenic infections
  - Increased risk of autoimmune disease
- **Terminal complement deficiency**
  - Recurrent bacterial infections
  - *Neisseria* **meningitis**
- Dx
  - **Screen CH50**
  - If CH50 undetectable, check individual complement factors
- Rx
  - Prophylactic antibiotics
  - Immunization

HIGH-YIELD PEARLS

- Anaphylaxis can occur without cutaneous manifestations
- Anaphylaxis can occur without hypotension
- Do not confuse SQ and IV doses of epinephrine
  - **Epinephrine (0.2–0.5 mg)** intramuscularly is the **1st line** treatment for anaphylaxis
- Do **not** routinely order sinus CT or x-ray for acute rhinosinusitis
- Do **not** routinely prescribe antibiotics for uncomplicated acute rhinosinusitis
- A positive allergy test only indicates sensitization but not necessarily clinical reaction
- Consider T-cell lymphoma (mycosis fungoides) for new-onset adult AD that is refractory to conventional therapy
- Radiocontrast media reactions are <u>not</u> associated with seafood or iodine allergy (**myth**!)
- Consider immunodeficiency in patients with **recurrent or opportunistic infections**

AUDIENCE RESPONSE ANSWERS AND EXPLANATORY INFORMATION

Audience Response 1
D. Give epinephrine.

Explanation: The correct answer is D.
The patient has 2-organ involvement after consuming a known allergen; therefore, he has anaphylaxis. The 1st line treatment of choice for anaphylaxis is epinephrine.
A. Albuterol will help with bronchoconstriction; however, epinephrine is still 1st line.
B. Diphenhydramine will help with itch.
C. Solumedrol may help with the late-phase reaction.
D. **Epinephrine is 1st line therapy for anaphylaxis.**
E. Observation only is inappropriate because the patient is experiencing an anaphylactic event.

AR 2
B. Prescribe nonsedating antihistamines.

Explanation: The correct answer is B.
The diagnosis is chronic urticaria. Nonsedating antihistamines are 1st line therapy. Topical steroids are not beneficial. Sedating antihistamines should be avoided in older patients. Measuring C1 inhibitor levels is not useful because this patient has urticaria. Hereditary angioedema is associated with isolated angioedema, not urticaria. Referral to a dermatologist is not indicated in the absence of red flags such as fever, arthritis, and weight loss.

AR 3
B. Start topical corticosteroid.

Explanation: The correct answer is B.
Topical agents are the mainstay of therapy for eczema. Moisturizers are the cornerstone of treatment and topical steroids are the mainstay of antiinflammatory therapy.
A. Oral corticosteroids are reserved only for severe eczema due to the risk of adverse side effects.
B. **Topical corticosteroids are the 1st line agents for eczema.**
C. Pimecrolimus: calcineurin inhibitors are 2nd line agents.
D. Tacrolimus: calcineurin inhibitors are 2nd line agents.
E. Oral antihistamines are adjunctive therapy to help with pruritus.

AR 4
D. Type 4

Explanation: The correct answer is D.
The patient most likely developed contact dermatitis from poison oak/ivy, consistent with a Type 4 delayed hypersensitivity reaction.
A. Type 1: Describes IgE-mediated reactions like anaphylaxis.
B. Type 2: Describes immunoglobulin- or antibody-mediated reactions like ITP purpura.
C. Type 3: Describes immune complex (antibody:antigen)-mediated disorders like serum sickness.
D. **Type 4: Describes delayed cell-mediated immune reactions like contact dermatitis.**

AR 5
B. Tree pollen

Explanation: The correct answer is B.
Patients with allergic rhinitis present with runny nose, sneezing, and itchy nose upon exposure to allergens. Tree pollen allergens occur during the spring.
A. Dog dander allergens occur year-round.
B. **Tree pollen allergens occur during the spring.**
C. Grass pollen allergens occur during the summer.
D. Weed pollen allergens occur during the fall.
E. Dust mites are year-round allergens.

AR 6
A. Prescribe intranasal budesonide.

Explanation: The correct answer is A.
The patient has pregnancy rhinitis which typically occurs in the last 6 weeks of pregnancy. Intranasal budesonide is the only treatment choice that is Category B in pregnancy. Oral budesonide and intranasal decongestants are Category C in pregnancy. Oral decongestants are associated with gastroschisis and should be avoided in pregnancy. Referral to an allergist without a trial of empiric therapy would not be appropriate.

AR 7
E. Reassurance only

Explanation: The correct answer is E.
Reassurance. The patient has acute rhinosinusitis. The vast majority of cases are caused by viral infection and antibiotics are not recommended. While giving oral corticosteroids may reduce symptoms, it significantly increases the risk of adverse events. Topical decongestants may cause rhinitis medicamentosa. Allergy testing is unnecessary because the cause is likely viral in etiology.

AR 8
E. Neurosyphilis and a history of PCN anaphylaxis

Explanation: The correct answer is E.
Drug desensitization is performed for IgE-mediated reactions and is only performed if the drug is the only clinically effective therapy. Neurosyphilis in a patient with a history of PCN anaphylaxis would be an indication for PCN drug desensitization. Desensitization is contraindicated in serious non-IgE-mediated reactions such as SJS, TEN, and DRESS.

AR 9
C. Type 3

Explanation: The correct answer is C.
This vignette describes a classic case of serum sickness.
A. Type 1: Describes IgE-mediated reactions like anaphylaxis.
B. Type 2: Describes immunoglobulin- or antibody-mediated reactions like ITP purpura.
C. **Type 3: Describes immune complex (antibody:antigen)-mediated disorders like serum sickness.**
D. Type 4: Describes cell-mediated immune reactions like celiac disease.

AR 10
C. Coronary artery disease

Explanation: The correct answer is C.
Risk factors for RCM reactions include female sex, asthma, cardiovascular disease, and a prior history of RCM reactions.
A. There is no association between seafood allergy and RCM reactions.
B. There is no association between iodine allergy and RCM reactions.
C. **Coronary artery disease is a risk factor for RCM reactions.**
D. Diabetes is not a risk factor for RCM reactions.

AR 11
B. Order CH50.

Explanation: The correct answer is B.
Patients with terminal complement deficiency are 10,000 times more likely to develop *Neisseria* meningitis. Therefore, one should suspect terminal complement deficiency in a patient with recurrent episodes of *Neisseria* meningitis.
A. HIV patients are not at higher risk for developing *Neisseria* meningitis, so HIV testing would not be helpful.
B. **CH50 is the correct test to screen for terminal complement deficiency.**
C. Quantitative immunoglobulins are used to evaluate for antibody deficiency.
D. B cell subsets are used to evaluate for congenital agammaglobulinemia.

ENDNOTES

[1]   john [CC BY-SA 3.0 (https://creativecommons.org/licenses/by-sa/3.0)], from Wikimedia Commons

[2]   Breck Nichols, MD

[3]   Klaus D. Peter [CC BY-SA 3.0 (https://creativecommons.org/licenses/by-sa/3.0)], from Wikimedia Commons

[4]   Hektor [CC-BY-SA-3.0 (http://creativecommons.org/licenses/by-sa/3.0/)], via Wikimedia Commons

[5]   James Heilman, MD [CC BY-SA 3.0 (https://creativecommons.org/licenses/by-sa/3.0)], from Wikimedia Commons

[6]   Britannic124 [CC BY-SA 3.0 (https://creativecommons.org/licenses/by-sa/3.0)], from Wikimedia Commons

[7]   R1carver [CC BY-SA 3.0 (https://creativecommons.org/licenses/by-sa/3.0)], from Wikimedia Commons

[8]   PKeMcG [CC BY 3.0 (https://creativecommons.org/licenses/by/3.0)], via Wikimedia Commons

[9]   James Heilman, MD [CC BY-SA 3.0 (https://creativecommons.org/licenses/by-sa/3.0)], from Wikimedia Commons

[10]   Allergyresearch [CC BY-SA 4.0 (https://creativecommons.org/licenses/by-sa/4.0)], from Wikimedia Commons

[11]   LucyHAE [CC BY-SA 3.0 (https://creativecommons.org/licenses/by-sa/3.0)], from Wikimedia Commons

[12]   James Heilman, MD [CC BY-SA 3.0 (https://creativecommons.org/licenses/by-sa/3.0)], from Wikimedia Commons

[13]   James Heilman, MD [CC BY-SA 3.0 (https://creativecommons.org/licenses/by-sa/3.0)], from Wikimedia Commons

[14]   Eisfelder [CC-BY-SA-3.0 (http://creativecommons.org/licenses/by-sa/3.0/)], via Wikimedia Commons

[15]   Kagi, et al. *Dermatology*. 2001;203:280–283.

[16]   Leung, et al. *J Clin Invest*. 1993;92:1374–1380.

[17]   CNX OpenStax [CC BY 4.0 (https://creativecommons.org/licenses/by/4.0)], via Wikimedia Commons

[18]   NIAID CC BY 2.0 (https://creativecommons.org/licenses/by/2.0)

[19]   Skoch3 [CC BY-SA 4.0 (https://creativecommons.org/licenses/by-sa/4.0)], from Wikimedia Commons

[20]   Matibot [CC BY-SA 3.0 (https://creativecommons.org/licenses/by-sa/3.0)], from Wikimedia Commons

[21]   daveynin [CC BY 2.0 (https://creativecommons.org/licenses/by/2.0)], via Wikimedia Commons

[22]   Andreas Trepte [CC BY-SA 2.5 (https://creativecommons.org/licenses/by-sa/2.5)], via Wikimedia Commons

[23]   Golden DB, et al. Natural history of *Hymenoptera* venom sensitivity in adults. *J Allergy Clin Immunol*.100:760, 1997.

[24]   Sampson, HA. *J Allergy Clin Immunol*. 107:891–896, 2001.

MedStudy®

INTERNAL MEDICINE REVIEW

Cardiology

Presented by

John P. Higgins, MD

TABLE OF CONTENTS

About Myself

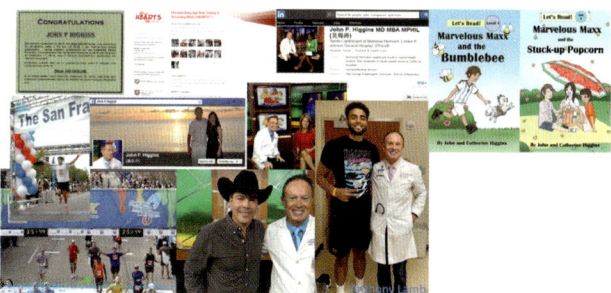

Cardiology Outline
- 5 Segments = 5 hours
- Each PPT 55 mins, and contains
  - Multiple choice questions intermixed, then
  - 5-minute break (please get up, stretch, and relax)

Q: My board prep?
A: MedStudy

Results for Dr. John P. Higgins

Examination Results			
Examination	Consecutive Attempts	Results	Score Reports
September 29, 2016 Maintenance of Certification examination in Cardiovascular Disease	Not Applicable	Pass	View Score Report
May 9, 2014 Maintenance of Certification examination in Internal Medicine	Not Applicable	Pass	

"Neo, sooner or later you're going to realize, just as I did: There's a difference between knowing the path and walking the path."

WHO AM I?
I AM DR. STARLORD, & U ARE

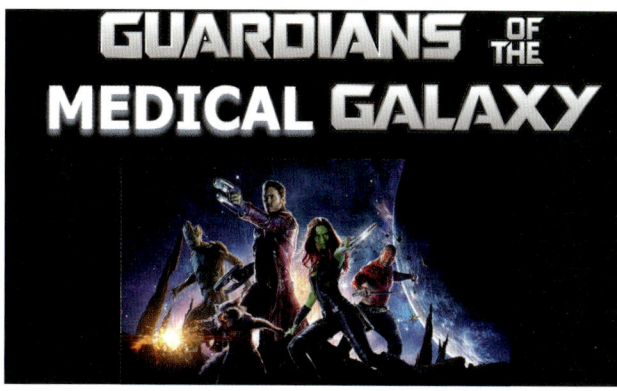

&
I HAVE A PLAN . . .
I HAVE PART OF A PLAN!
Our **NEMESIS**:
The Board Exam!!!

My presentation will directly mirror the ABIM exam content for Cardiology

While I can't answer questions during this presentation (due to traveling at **TURBO SPEED**), you can send questions to speakers by clicking on "Ask the Speaker" in the participation panel

"I Will Never Let You Down" — Rita Ora

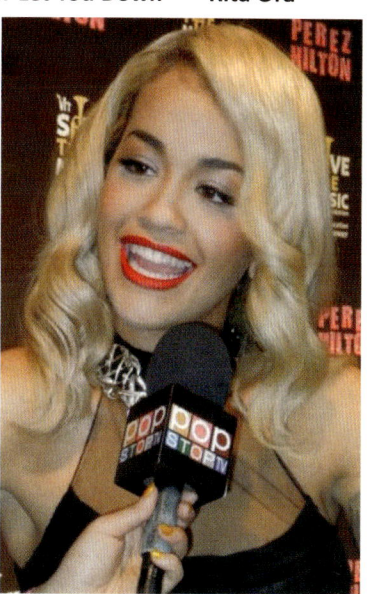

[1]

If you <u>enjoy</u> my presentation, I would be <u>honored</u> to receive a **great feedback score** on your evaluation of me!

Lecture 1

L1 Outline
- Chest X-Rays (CXRs)
- TransThoracic Echocardiography (TTE)
- TransEsophageal Echocardiography (TEE)
- Cardiac Stress Tests
- Cardiac Catheterization, Coronary Computed Tomography Angiography (CCTA), Coronary Artery Calcium Scoring (CACS), Cardiac Magnetic Resonance (CMR)
- Pericardial Effusion
- Physical Exam

CHEST X-RAYS (CXRs)

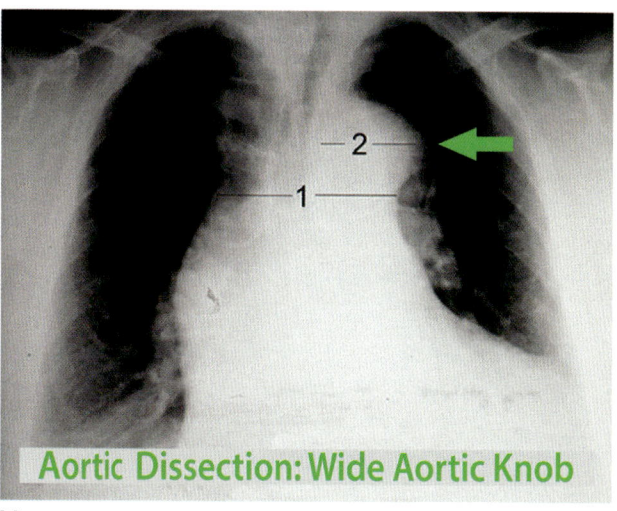

Aortic Dissection: Wide Aortic Knob

[2]

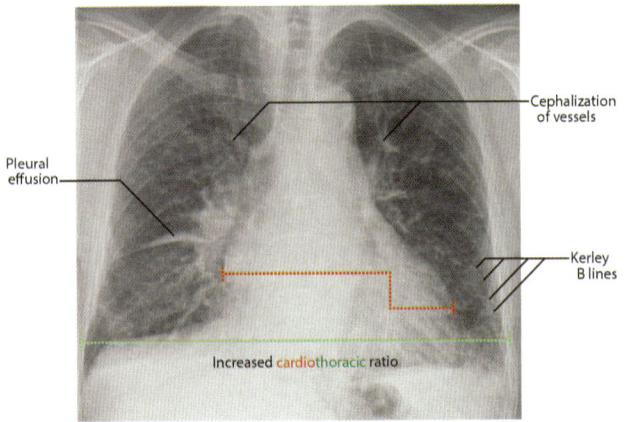

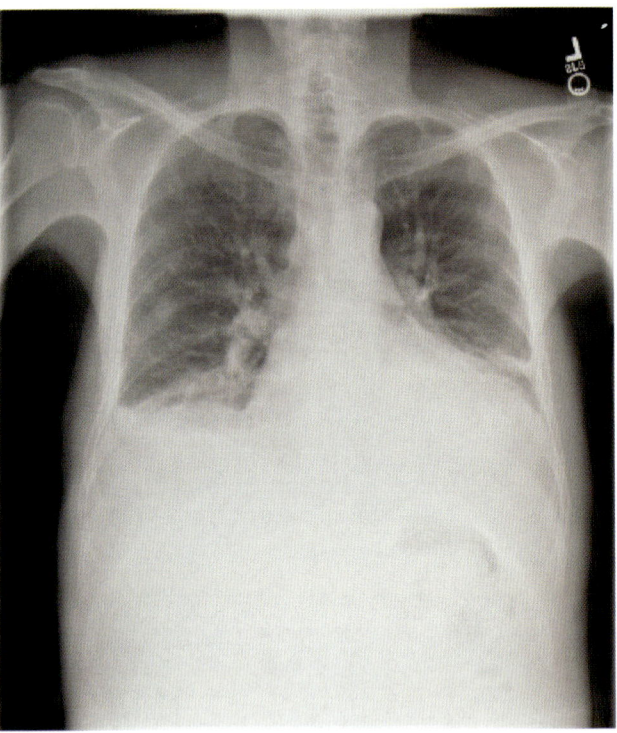

Normal CXR — PA and Lateral

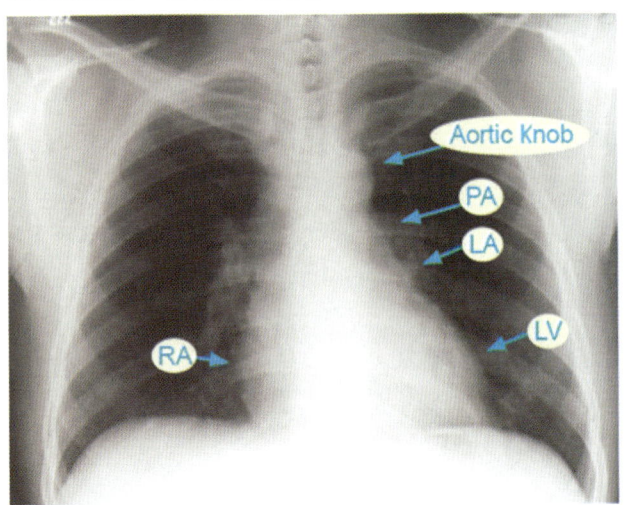

75-year-old male with dyspnea and pedal edema; worse last 2 weeks

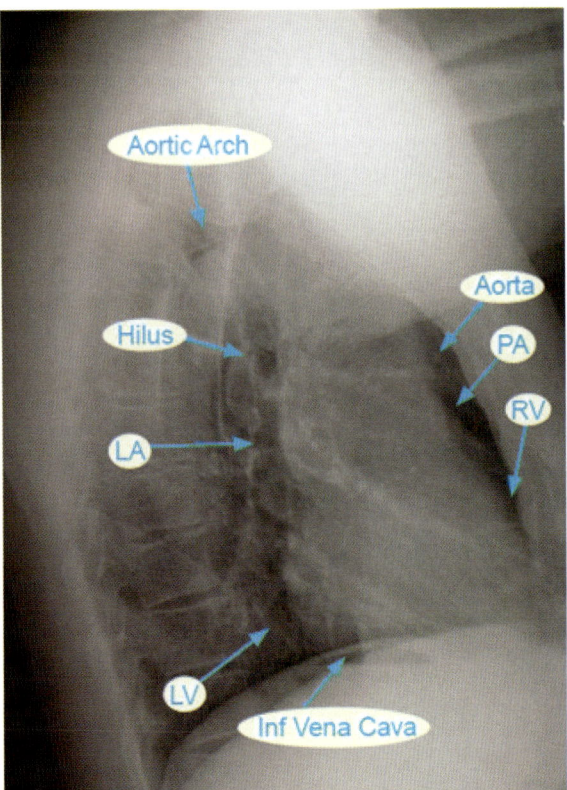

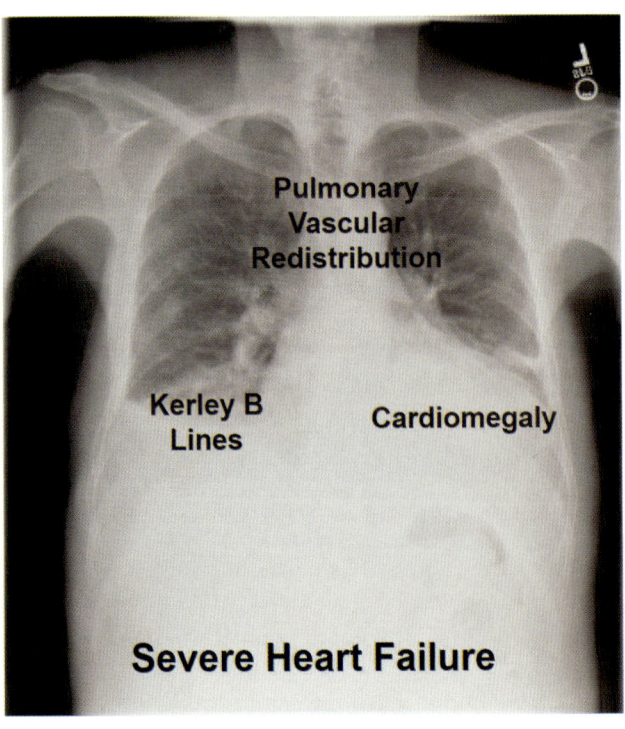

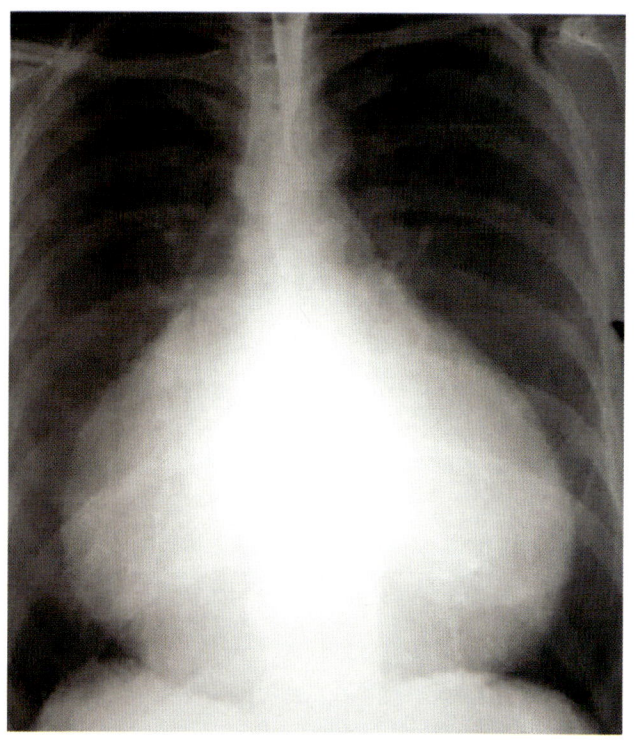

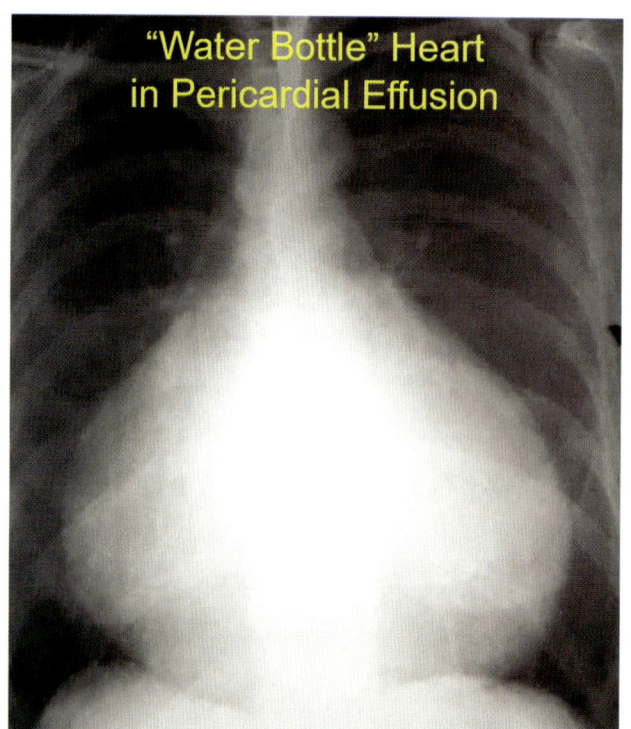

"Water Bottle" Heart
in Pericardial Effusion

25-year-old ESRD male with dyspnea over past 2 months; he missed multiple dialysis sessions

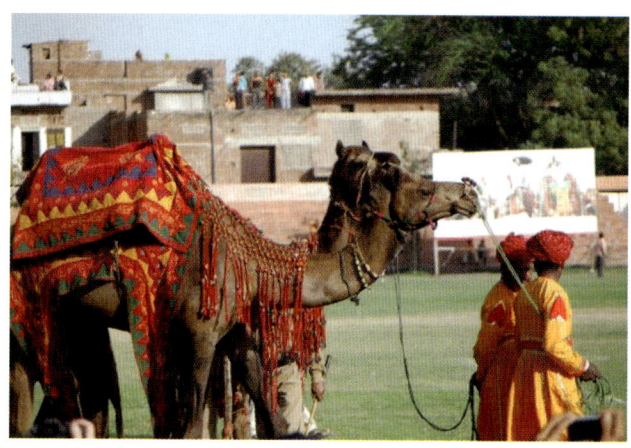

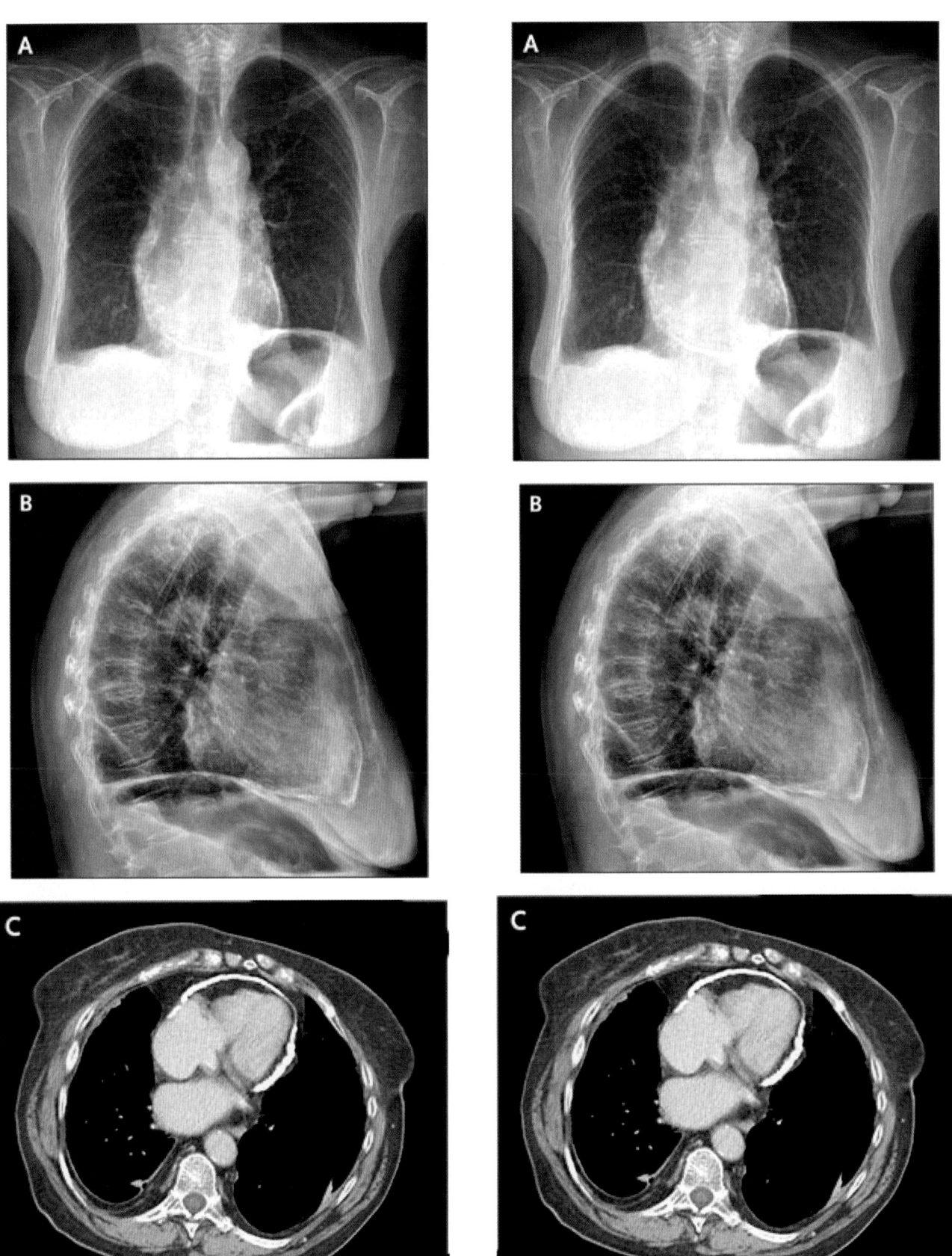

45-year-old female with lymphoma S/P mediastinal radiation with peripheral edema, ascites, and hepatomegaly

*Pericardial calcification on x-ray and CT; **constrictive pericarditis** (a.k.a. skull heart!)*

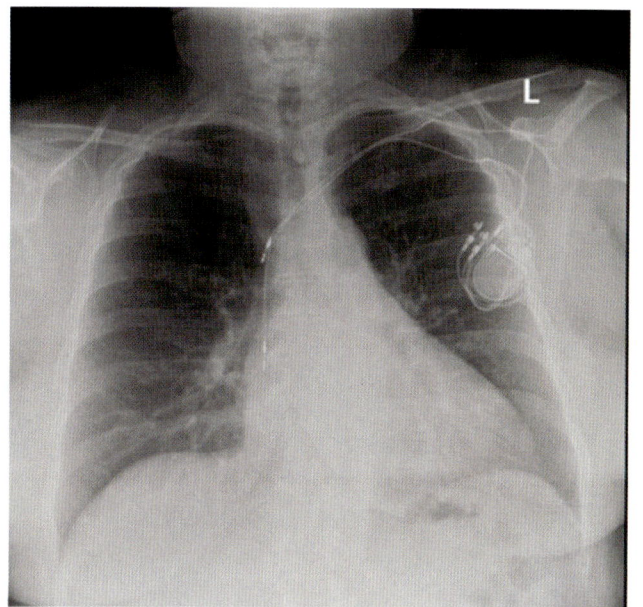

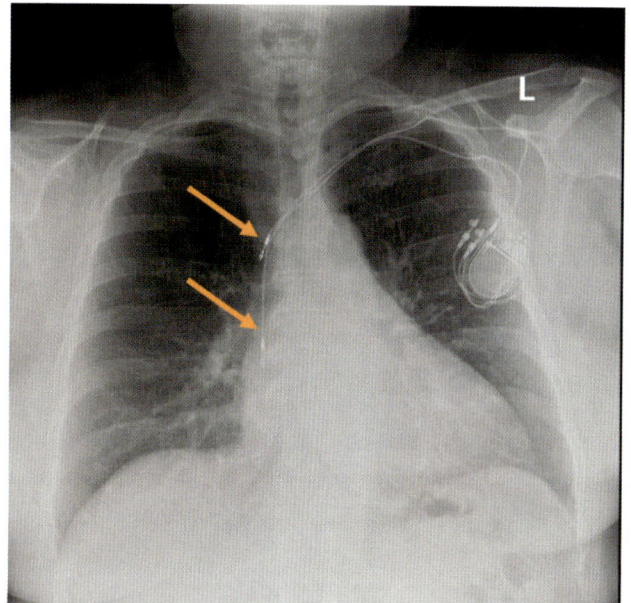

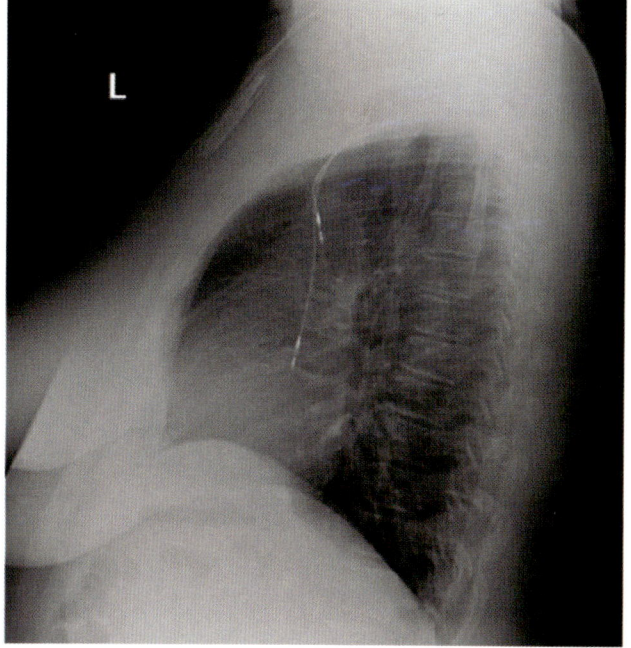

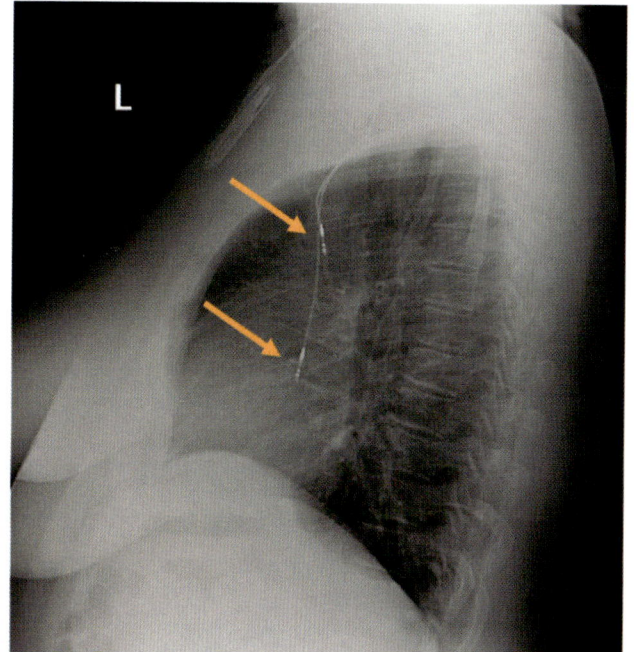

51-year-old female with a dual-chamber pacemaker fell down an embankment and presents with hiccups, a stuttering voice, and chest wall twitching.

Pacemaker lead displacement. *May present with lightheadedness, syncope, or symptoms from extra cardiac pacing.*

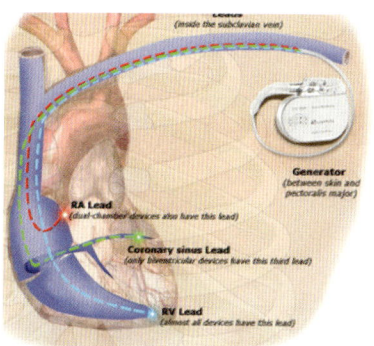

[3]

Normal position

Audience Response 1

A 19-year-old man presents for high blood pressure. PMH: bicuspid aortic valve, HTN. Meds: metoprolol. PE: BP is 200/90 mmHg in both arms; an ejection click and systolic murmur are heard at the left sternal border; a different systolic murmur is heard under the left clavicle. The radial-to-femoral artery pulse is delayed. No abdominal bruits are noted. Lab is normal. CXR is shown:

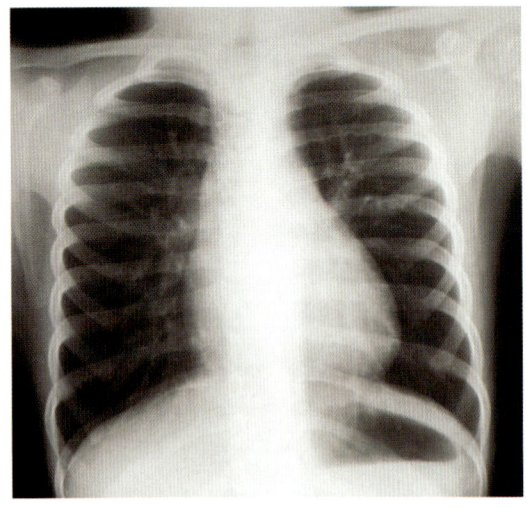

Which is the likely cause of his hypertension?

A. Essential hypertension
B. Coarctation of the aorta
C. Renovascular hypertension
D. Tetralogy of Fallot

Answer:_____

Coarctation of the Aorta[4]

- **70% bicuspid aortic valve:** Early systolic click and murmur!
- **Upper-extremity HTN** and radiofemoral delay; claudication; systolic/continuous murmur left infraclavicular area; Dx: CTA/MRI
- CXR: **rib notching**; **figure 3 sign**
- MRI brain: Look for <u>intracranial</u>/**berry aneurysms**!
- Avoid contact sports and isometric exercise
- **Turner Broadcasting Co. — Turner** Syndrome (XO)-associated: **b**icuspid AV and **co**arct
- <u>**Sx or stent if**</u>
  - **Peak-to-peak gradient ≥ 20 mmHg,**
  - **Hypertension, or**
  - **Heart failure**

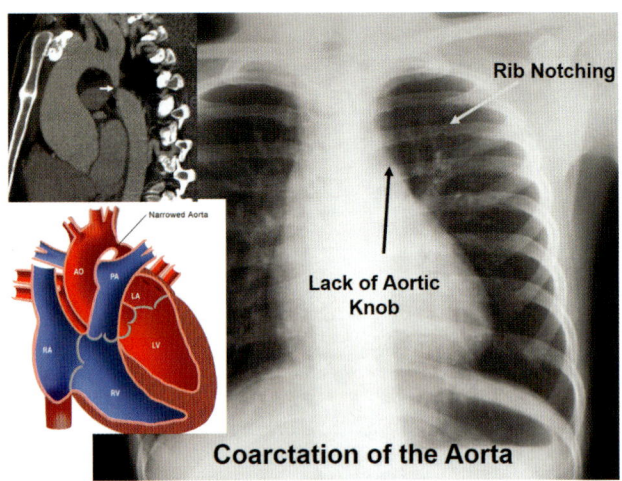

Coarctation of the Aorta

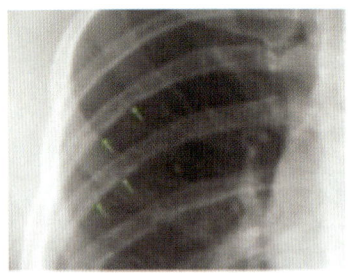

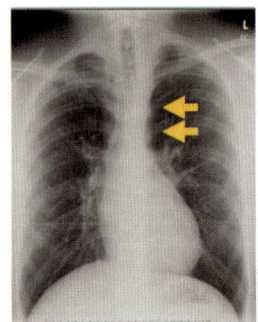

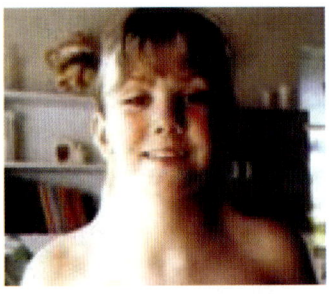

[5]

ECHOCARDIOGRAPHY

TransThoracic Echocardiography (TTE)

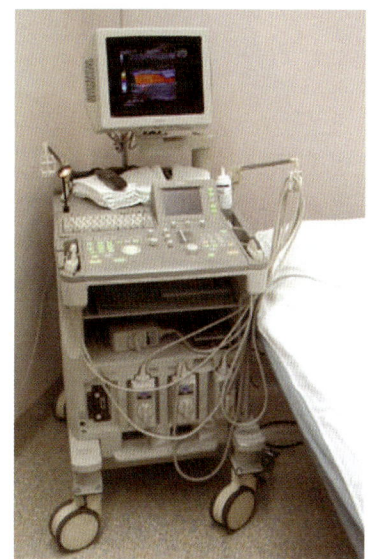

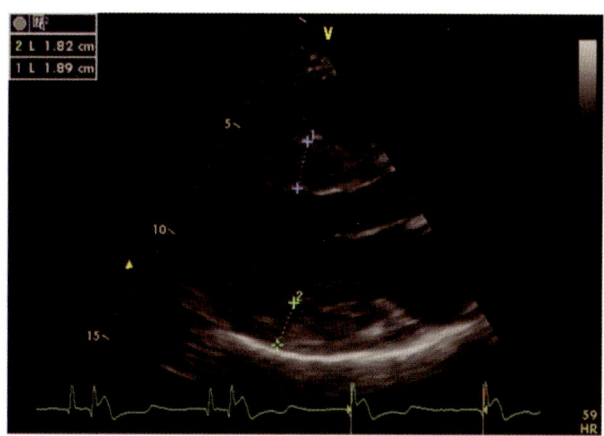

Fabry disease: diffuse LVH

Anatomy

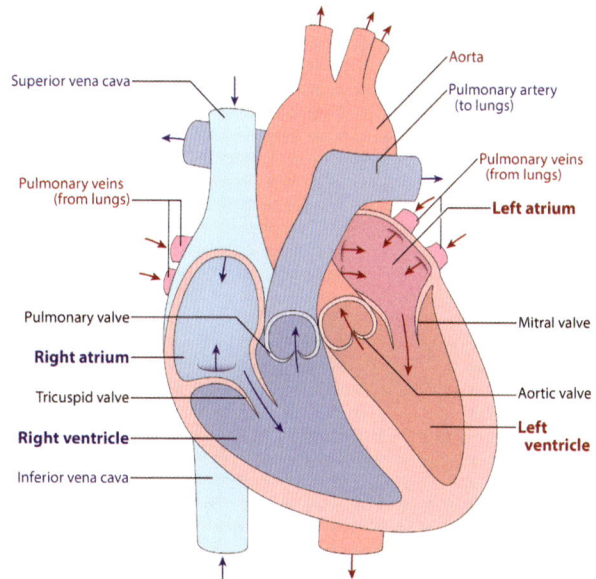

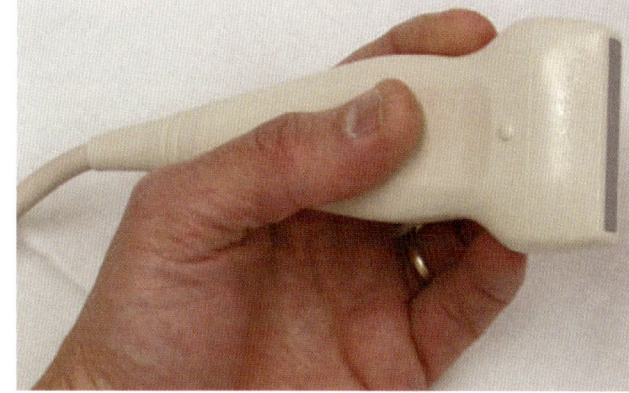

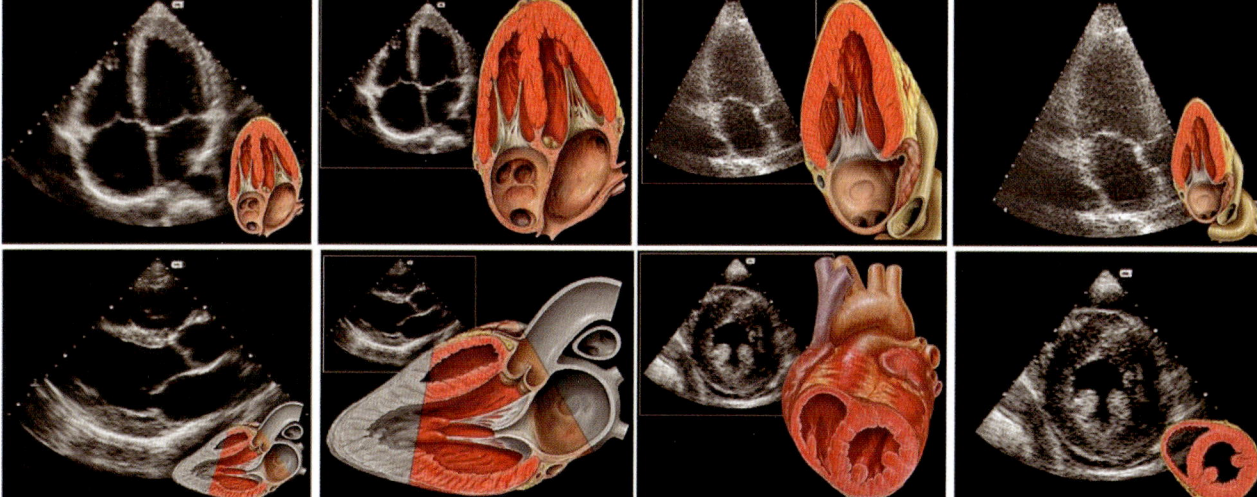

CARDIOLOGY

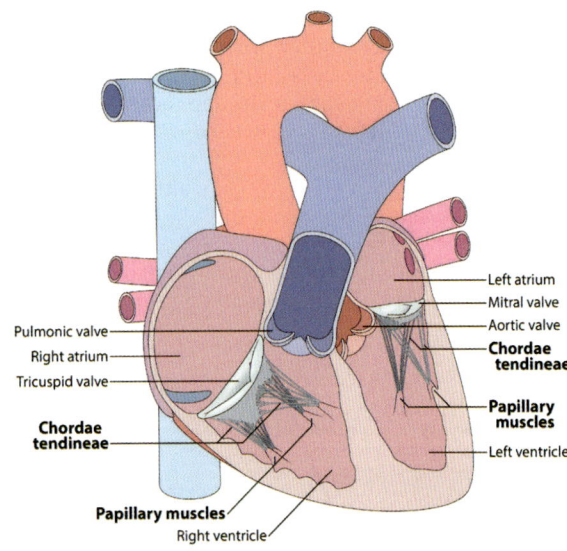

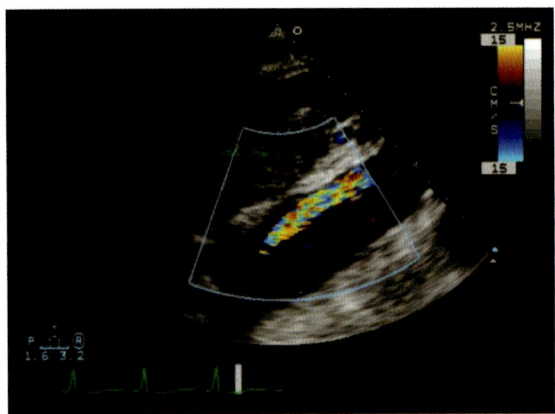

Aortic dissection (Type A): Longitudinal view

TTE Indications[8][9][10]

1) **Cardiac Structure and Function** — chest pain; e.g., RV mid-wall dyskinesis with sparing of apex = **pulmonary embolism**
2) **Arrhythmias** — AFib, new LBBB, 2nd/3rd degree AV block
3) **Pulmonary Hypertension** — loud P_2 and TR murmur
4) **Acute Setting** — hemodynamic instability
5) **Valvular Function** — murmur (> grade 2/6, late holosystolic, diastolic, or continuous)
6) **Intra-/Extracardiac Structures and Chambers** — embolus
7) **Aortic Disease** — Marfan syndrome
8) **Hypertension, HF, or Cardiomyopathy** — hypertrophic
9) **Adult Congenital Heart Disease** — fixed split S_2 = **ASD**

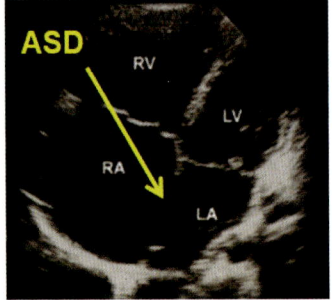

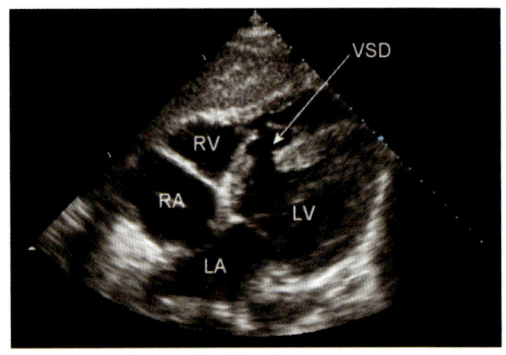

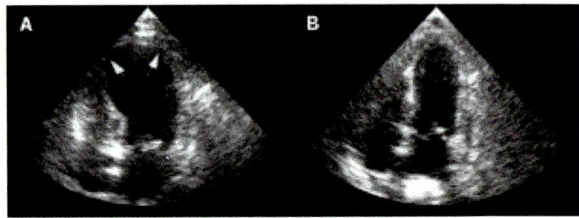

(A) *Apical ballooning akinesis with basal hyperkinesis in Takotsubo cardiomyopathy*

(B) *Resolution of LV function 6 days later.*

TTE — Just DON'T DO IT![11]

- **Asymptomatic patients** with mild **innocent-sounding** murmurs; e.g.,
  - **1/6–2/6 short, well-localized, systolic mid-peaking murmur at left sternal border (benign — from RVOT/PA/pulmonary valve; leaflets or aortic valve sclerosis!)**
  - **Continuous murmur over breast = venous hum or mammary soufflé (in lactating women)**
- **Repeatedly on chronic HF** patients, **unless** clinical change
- Yearly echoes on **mild valvular** stenosis/regurgitation or prosthetic valves with no change in clinical status **(rather q 3 years)**

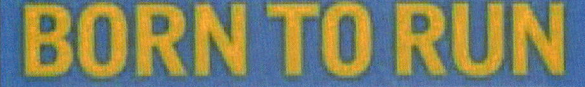

[12]

TransEsophageal Echocardiography (TEE)

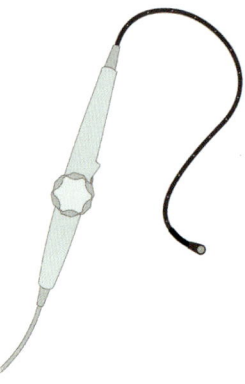

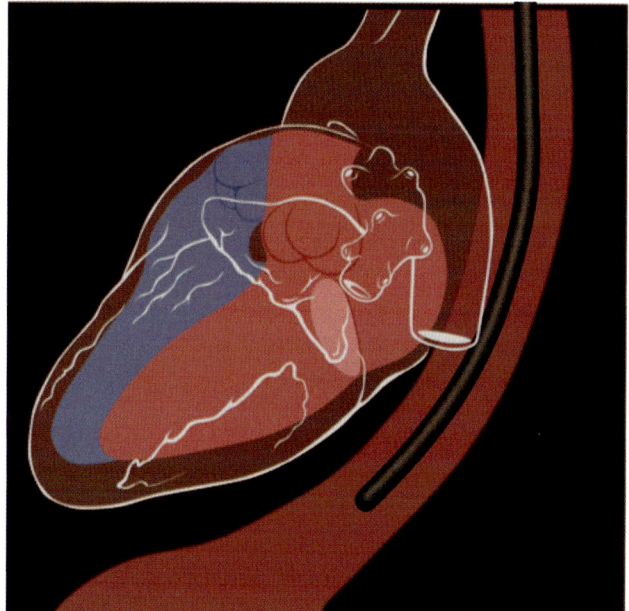

[13]

TEE Indications[14]
1) **Cardiac and aortic structure and function**
   - Aorta and left atrial appendage
   - Prosthetic heart valves
   - **Paravalvular abscesses**
   - On ventilator
   - Chest wall injuries
   - Body habitus → inadequate TTE
   - Unable to move into left lateral decubitus position
2) **Intraoperative TEE**
   - **All open heart** (i.e., valvular) and thoracic aortic surgical procedures
   - Some CABGs
   - Noncardiac surgery if cardiovascular pathology may impact outcomes

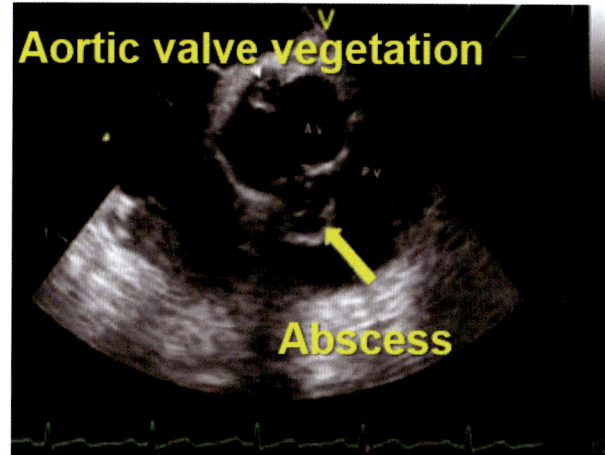

[15]

TEE Indications[16][17]
3) **Guidance of transcatheter procedures**
   - **Guiding catheter-based intracardiac procedures** (septal defect closure, atrial appendage obliteration, and **transcatheter valve procedures**)
4) **Critically ill patients**
   - **If TTE inadequate** and data can alter management

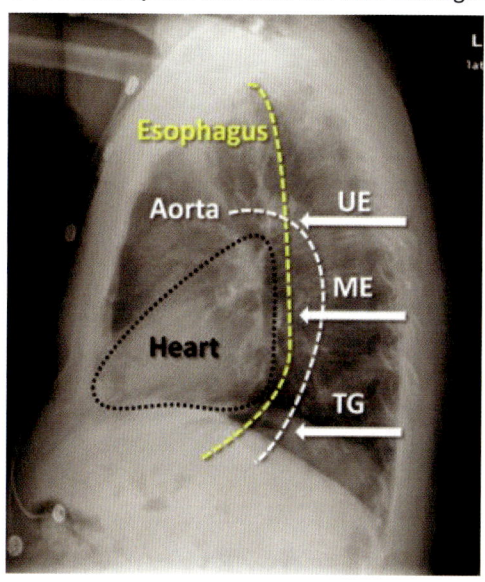

Lateral CXR. Arrows indicate the upper esophageal (UE), midesophageal (ME), and transgastric (TG) positions of the TEE probe

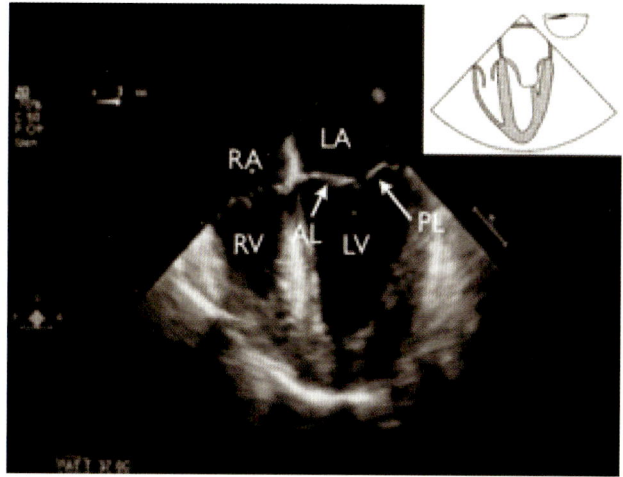

ME 4-chamber view:

AL, anterior leaflet of the MV
LA, left atrium
LV, left ventricle
PL, posterior leaflet of the MV
RA, right atrium
RV, right ventricle

CARDIOLOGY

CARDIAC STRESS TESTS

Cardiac Stress Tests — Introduction[18]
- Best if **intermediate** (10–90%) pretest probability of disease
  - **Younger typical CP**
  - **Older atypical CP**
- A number of moderately raised risk factors = **a higher risk** than a single very elevated risk factor
- Women lower sensitivity and specificity
- Normal stress test warranty = 1 year

Exercise Treadmill Test (No Imaging) — a.k.a. Exercise Electrocardiography[19][20]
- Ischemia, functional capacity, arrhythmia, prognosis (post-MI)
- Sensitivity ~ 65%, specificity ~ 75%
- **Good if normal ECG and achieve 85% MPHR**
- **Contraindications:**[21]
  - **Active** MI (≤ 2 days)/unstable angina/endocarditis/myocarditis/pericarditis/aortic dissection/PE/DVT; decompensated HF, inability to exercise, symptomatic severe AS, hemodynamically unstable arrhythmia

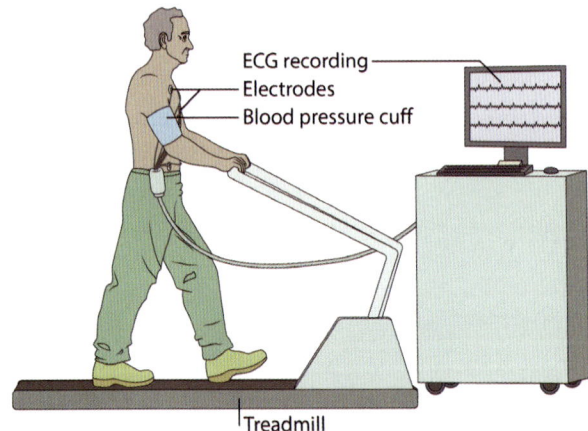

ECG recording
Electrodes
Blood pressure cuff
Treadmill

- **High-risk findings**:
  - Poor **capacity** (< 5 METS)
  - **Low-peak SBP** (< 130 mmHg) or an exercise fall in SBP ≥ 10 mmHg below standing rest values
  - Exercise-induced **angina**
  - ≥ 2 mm of ischemic **ST-segment depression** at low workload (≤ Bruce Stage 2 or HR ≤ 120/bpm)
  - **Early onset** (Bruce Stage 1) or prolonged (> 5 minutes) or multiple leads (≥ 5) with ST-segment depression
  - Exercise-induced **ST-segment elevation** (excluding aVR or leads with Q waves)
  - Ventricular **couplets**, triplets, sustained (> 30 seconds) or symptomatic ventricular tachycardia
  - Abnormal **heart rate recovery:** drop of < 12/minute in first minute after exercise stops

ECG Baseline

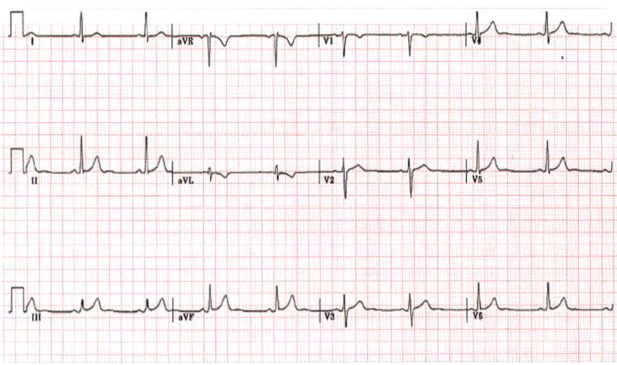

Normal baseline ECG

ECG During Exercise

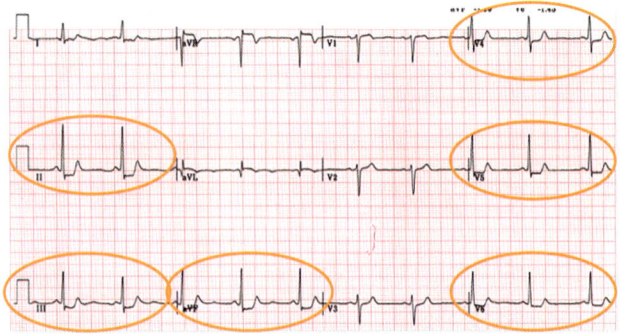

Positive test *is at least 1 mm of horizontal or downsloping ST depression in 2 contiguous leads*

AR 2
A 56-year-old male patient with HTN presents with chest pain on moderate exertion. He is a delivery driver and walks 2 miles a day. Myocardial infarction is ruled out. His baseline ECG shows LVH with 1- to 2-mm ST-segment depression in the lateral leads:

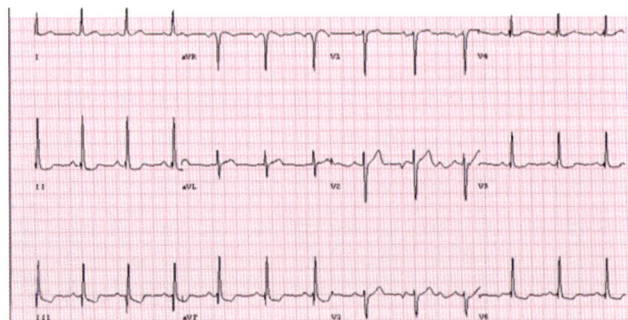

To evaluate for CAD, what test do you order?

A. A regular exercise treadmill stress test
B. An exercise test with imaging (nuclear or echo)
C. An ST-segment–sensitive Holter monitor
D. Cardiac magnetic resonance imaging

Answer:_____

Cardiac Stress Tests + Imaging

- Unable to exercise, <u>or</u>
- Certain baseline abnormalities on ECG

<u>So</u>:

What ECGs are uninterpretable for ischemia on a standard treadmill ECG test?

Left Bundle-Branch Block

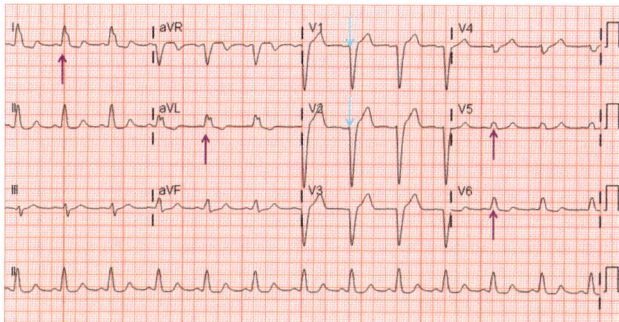

<u>Broad R waves</u> *in I and aVL and left precordial leads (V5, V6)*

<u>Large S or Q wave</u> *in right precordial leads (V1, V2)*

Paced Rhythm

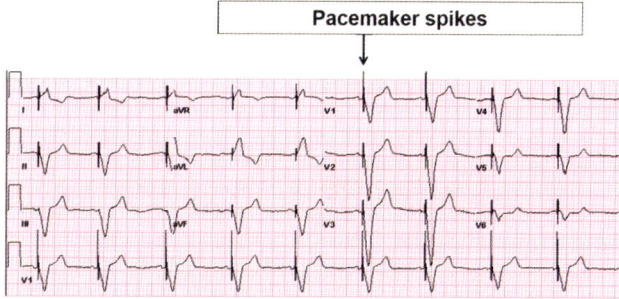

Preexcitation — Wolff-Parkinson-White (WPW) Pattern

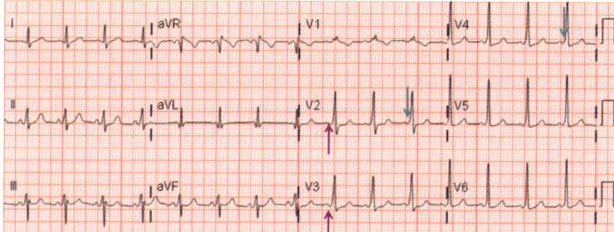

Resting ECG ST Changes ≥ 1 mm

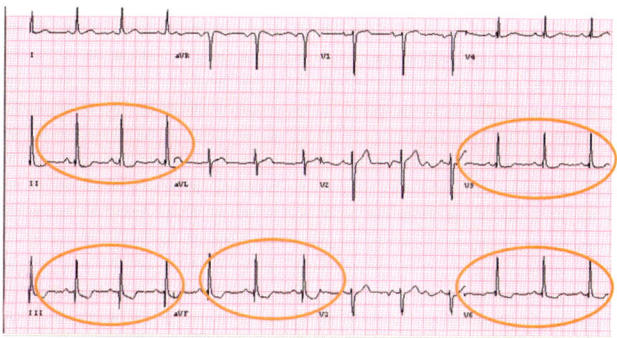

Stress Imaging Tests[22]

- **Stress echo** or **nuclear stress** if:
    - **Left bundle-branch block (LBBB)***
    - **Paced rhythm**
    - **Preexcitation — WPW pattern**
    - **Resting ECG ST changes ≥ 1 mm**
- Relative indications
    - Left ventricular hypertrophy (LVH)
    - Digoxin therapy
    - Location of ischemia
    - Cannot get to 85% MPHR

*LBBB: Use vasodilator stress because exercise/dobutamine leads to false-positive perfusion defect in septum

Myocardial Perfusion Imaging (MPI) — a.k.a. Nuclear Stress[23]

- **Stress** = increased **contractility and O$_2$ demand** (exercise [treadmill], dobutamine + atropine) <u>or</u> **regional hypoperfusion** via coronary vasodilation (adenosine, regadenoson, dipyridamole [Persantine])
- **Technetium-99m** goes where blood flow is good
- Induced abnormalities in myocardial **function or perfusion** suggest significant coronary stenosis
- e.g., **anteroseptal ischemia** consistent with LAD stenosis

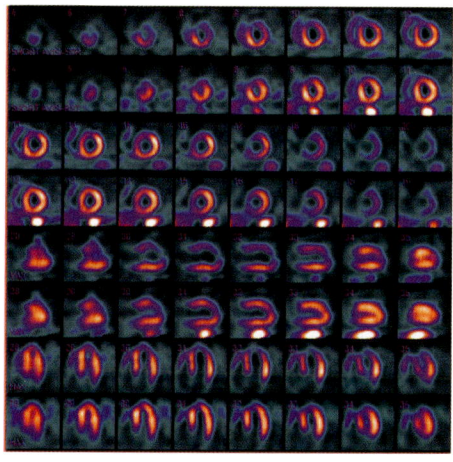

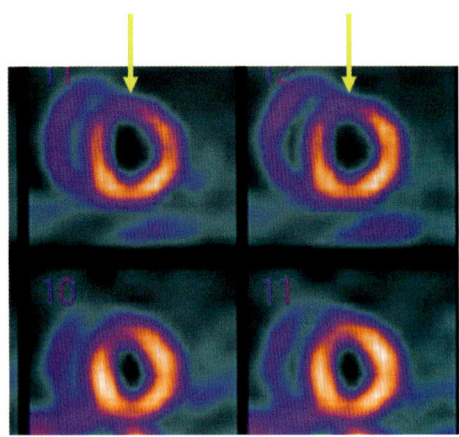

Stress Echocardiography[24]

- Stress = increased **contractility and O₂ demand** (exercise [treadmill, stationary bike], dobutamine + atropine)
- **Wall motion abnormalities** indicate either **ischemia** (**stress** images only) or **infarction** (**stress and rest** images)
- Also get **valve function** and pulmonary pressures
- NB: Image quality poor in obese or COPD patients

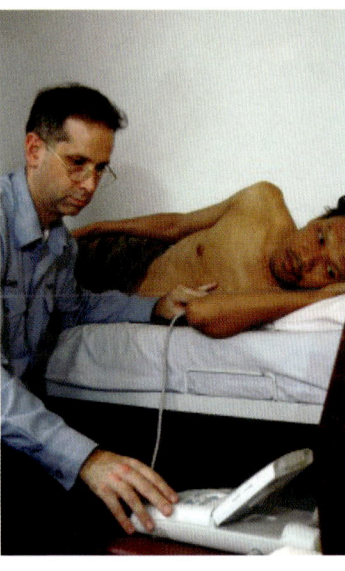

[25]

CARDIAC CATHETERIZATION AND OTHER CARDIAC IMAGING TESTS

Cardiac Catheterization,
Coronary Computed Tomography Angiography (CCTA),
Coronary Artery Calcium Scoring (CACS),
Cardiac Magnetic Resonance (CMR)

Cardiac Catheterization — a.k.a. "Left Heart Cath"

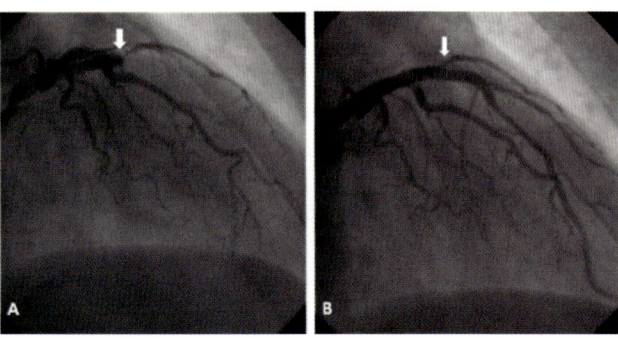

Total occlusion of the mid-left anterior descending artery — successfully stented!

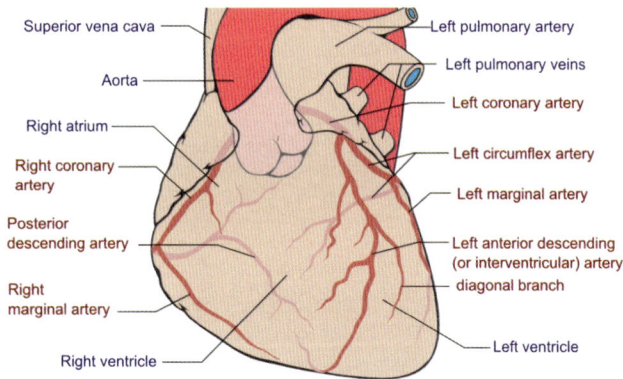

[26]

Cardiac Catheterization[27][28][29][30]

- If angina progressing despite optimal/maximal medical Tx **or** high-risk stress test findings
- Normal study warranty period: 2 years
- All contraindications are relative
- Mortality < 0.1%; morbidity < 6.0%
  - Hematoma, hemorrhage, MI, CVA, emergency CABG, femoral artery pseudoaneurysm, **arteriovenous fistula**, arrhythmias, allergic reactions (dye, medication), arterial dissection, cholesterol emboli syndrome, **retroperitoneal bleeding (Grey-Turner sign)**, renal damage/dysfunction, infection, thrombosis

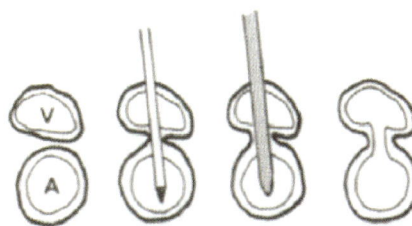

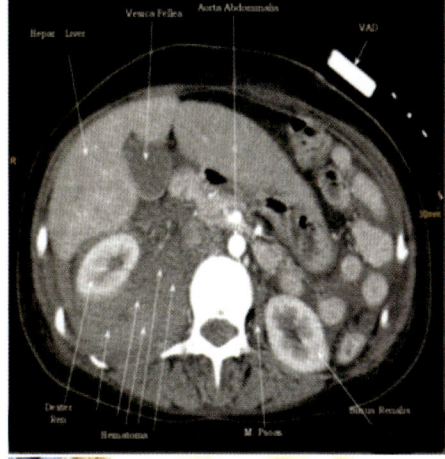

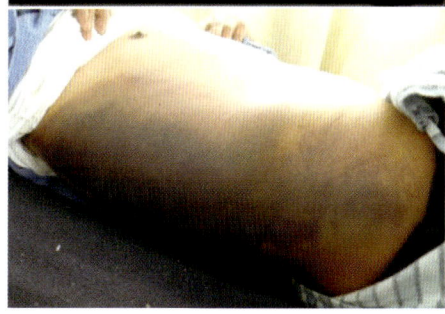

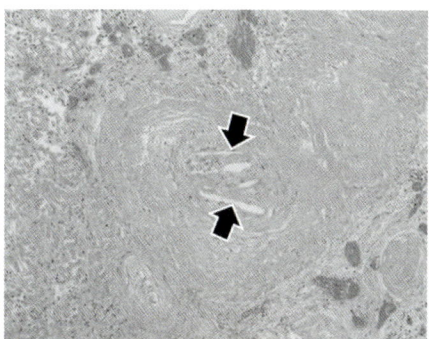

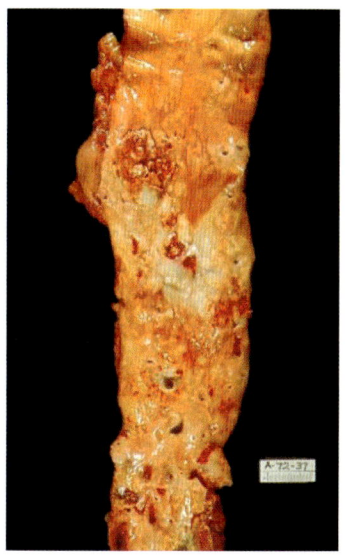

Coronary Computed Tomography Angiography (CCTA)
Let's call a radiologist and order a CCTA

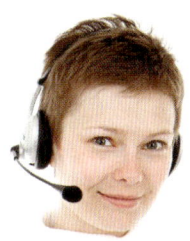

Cholesterol Embolization Syndrome[31]
- Endovascular manipulation → embolization of cholesterol crystals and atheroma
- Fever, fatigue, myalgias
- **Red/Purple/Blue** toes, digital gangrene
- Livedo reticularis, Hollenhorst plaque
- Leukocytosis (**+eosinophilia**), ↑ ESR
- Acute kidney injury, **eosinophiluria** (+Hansel stain)

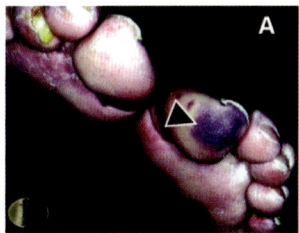
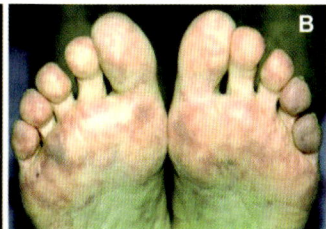

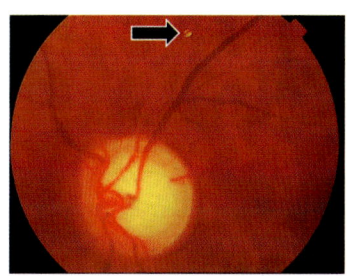

CCTA[32]
- IV contrast
- HR < 60 bpm and regular*
- Hold breath 15 sec
- Dx:
  - Aortic disease
  - Coronary disease (**sensitivity 95–99%**)
  - Cardiac masses
  - Pericardial disease
  - Ventricular structure/fn
- ↑ Ca^{2+} blooming artifact

*50–100 mg oral metoprolol 2 hours prior; 5 mg IV slowly on scan table

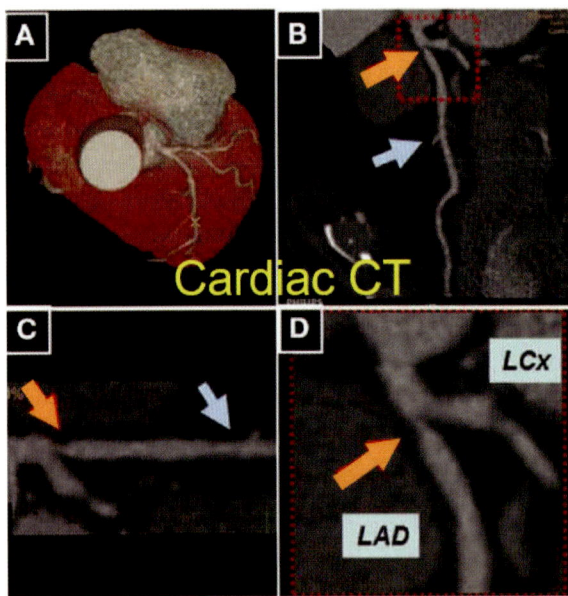

Older male with atypical chest pain: a **high-grade proximal (orange arrows)** and an intermediate lesion (blue arrows) of the mid LAD.

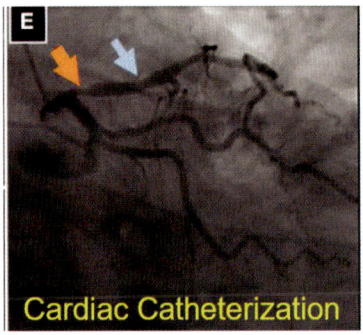

Coronary Artery Calcium Scoring (CACS)[33]
- <u>No</u> contrast (but radiation → **CI: pregnancy**)
- Helpful if **intermediate risk** of CAD
- <u>Don't do it</u> in asymptomatic patients at very low/high risk of coronary event
- **CACS = 0 = no disease = low risk** for CAD
- **> 400 = severe disease = high risk** for CAD (~ 3-fold) and 10-fold increased risk of cardiac events!

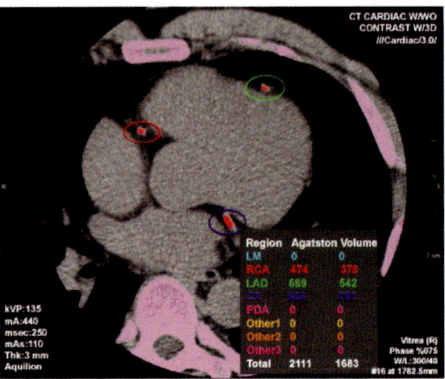

Cardiac Magnetic Resonance (CMR)[34][35][36]
- Good at everything **but CAD**!
- **Congenital** heart and **aortic** disease
- **Perfusion and viability** (DE-MRI)
- **Tissue characterization** — infiltrative; e.g., hemochromatosis, myocarditis (giant cell), HCM, arrhythmogenic RV cardiomyopathy
- **LV/RV mass, function,** and blood flow (including adult congenital heart disease)
- **Nephrogenic systemic fibrosis** = skin/organ fibrosis = gadolinium + severe chronic kidney disease (eGFR < 30 mL/min/1.73 m^2)

A 66-year-old man with dyspnea and palpitations; MRI tissue appearance characteristic of myxoma (proven by histology)

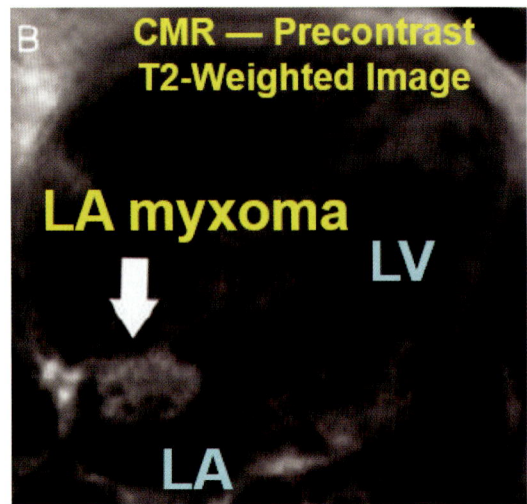

PERICARDIAL EFFUSION

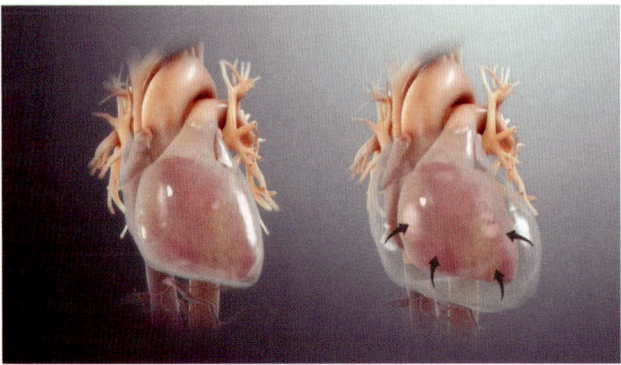

[37]

AR 3

Moments after a temporary transvenous pacemaker was placed into the RV of a 50-year-old male with complete heart block, he developed hypotension, chest pain, and elevated neck veins. Heart sounds became muffled, but lung fields are clear. You note an inspiratory fall of systolic BP of 15 mmHg.

What would an echocardiogram show?

A. Atrial septal defect
B. Acute mitral regurgitation
C. Hypertrophic cardiomyopathy
D. Cardiac tamponade

Answer:_____

Pericardial Effusion

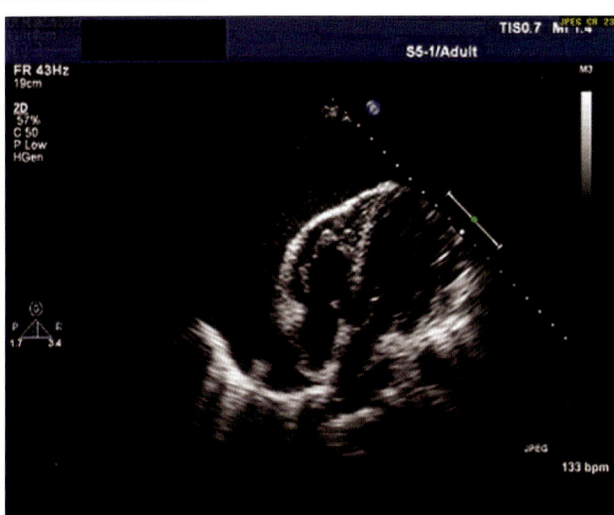

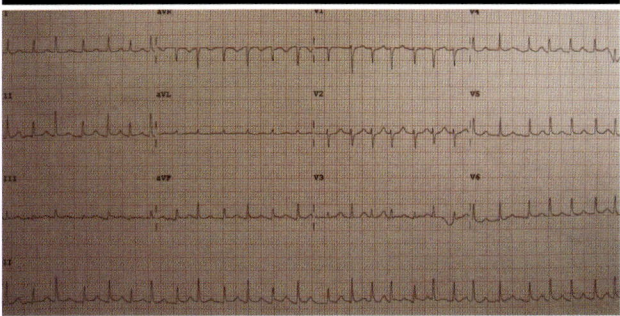

Effusion Size	Depth	Volume
Normal	< 5 mm	< 100 mL
Moderate	15–30 mm	400–1000 mL

- ECG: low voltage, electrical alternans

Pericardial Effusion[38]

- <u>Etiology</u>: postviral, infection (TB, bacteria), uremia, post-cardiothoracic surgery, chest trauma, minoxidil/ hydralazine, neoplasm **LMNOO → P: L**ung, **L**eukemia, **M**elanoma, **N**HL, **OO** Breast, **P**ericardial effusion
- Clinical impact depends on speed of accumulation
- CBC, lytes, BUN, TSH, ANA, TB skin tests
- **If idiopathic pericardial effusion > 3 months → pericardiocentesis**
- ~ 50% idiopathic effusions are cured
- Surgical drainage for malignant effusions and from aortic dissection
- **Effusive constrictive pericarditis = findings of constrictive pericarditis and effusion (tap: intrapericardial pressure normal, intracardiac pressures remain elevated); Rx: NSAIDs + colchicine**

TAMPONADE

Cardiac Tamponade[39]

- **Beck at the HELM**: <u>Beck Triad</u> — **H**ypotension, **EL**evated neck veins, **M**uffled heart sounds; **pulsus paradoxus**
- **TTE mitral inflow > 25% decrease** in passive diastolic flow during inspiration (reflects enhanced ventricular interdependence)
- JVD elevated with no collapse during diastole; **blunted *y* descent** = early diastolic filling impaired from extrinsic restraint from effusion/tamponade
- **Tx: if SBP < 100 mmHg then volume load; pericardiocentesis/surgical pericardial drain**
- **JVD absent if severely hypovolemic!**

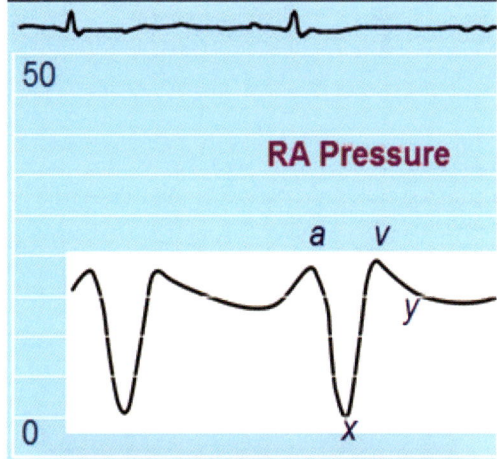

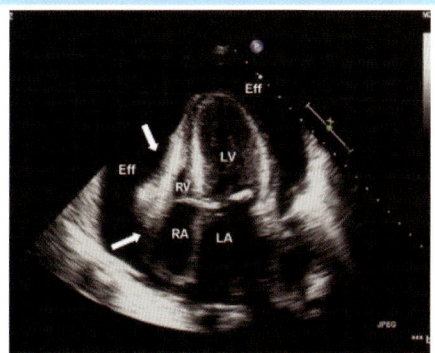

PHYSICAL EXAM

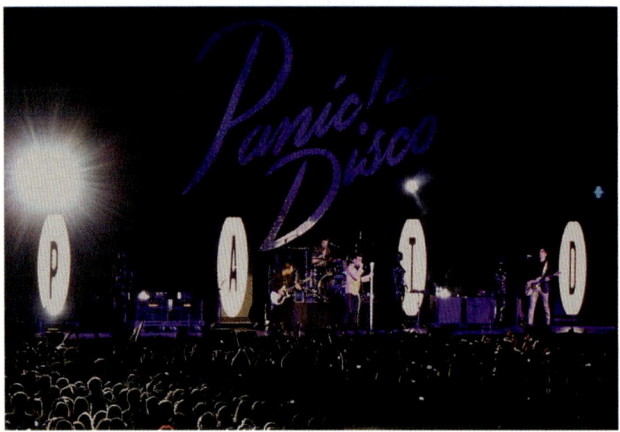

[40]

Physiologically Split S$_2$
- Inspiration →
- Increased venous return →
- Increased RV volume →
- Delayed RV emptying →
- Delayed P$_2$

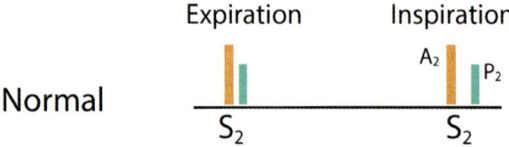

Normal

| Expiration | Inspiration |

AR 4
A 43-year-old woman reports dyspnea for 6 months. Echocardiography shows severe mitral regurgitation and pulmonary HTN.

What would you auscultate regarding her second heart sound?

A. Normally split second heart sound
B. Widely split second heart sound
C. Paradoxically split second heart sound
D. Fixed split second heart sound

Answer:_____

Widely Split S$_2$
- **A$_2$ early**
- **Early closure of the aortic valve**
  - Severe MR
- **P$_2$ late**
- **Delayed RV emptying**
  - Pulmonic stenosis
  - Pulmonary embolism
  - PVCs in LV
  - RBBB

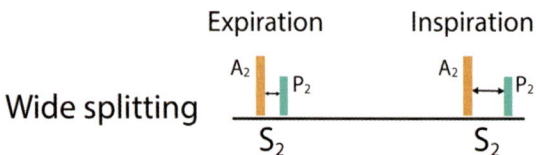

Wide splitting

| Expiration | Inspiration |

AR 5
An 18-year-old female patient from Honduras says she has had a murmur since birth, and she was told she had a hole in her heart. You detect a split second heart sound that does not vary with respiration. There is a 3/6 systolic flow murmur in the pulmonary area. ECG shows right axis deviation and RBBB.

What is the likely diagnosis?

A. Mitral stenosis
B. Aortic coarctation
C. Atrial septal defect
D. Mitral regurgitation
E. Hypertrophic cardiomyopathy

Answer:_____

Fixed Split S$_2$ "Fixed FAST as a FLASH!"[41][42]

F	**F**ixed Split
AS	**AS**D
T	**T**wo (S$_2$)

- Systolic flow murmur (increased pulmonary blood flow) and holosystolic murmur (increased TR)
- Fixed split **S$_2$** (RV overloaded systole and diastole)
- Ostium secundum = most common!
- ECG: **R**AD + I**R**BBB/**R**BBB
  (think **secund**um/**sec**ond = 2 = **2 Rs**)
- **Sx: Reduced functional capacity or RA/RV enlargement with > 1.5:1 Qp:Qs without PAH = close**

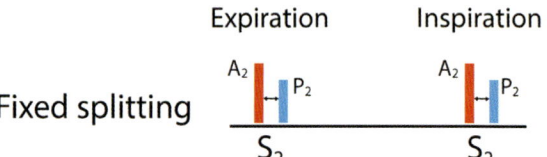

Fixed splitting

| Expiration | Inspiration |

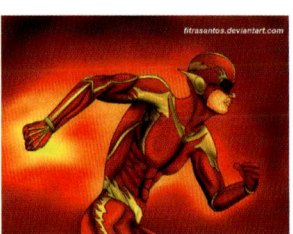

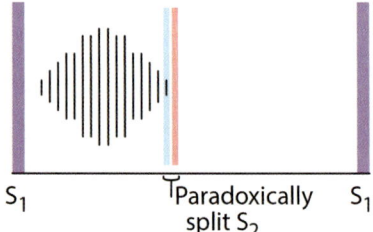

S$_1$ — Paradoxically split S$_2$ — S$_1$

— Aortic valve closure (A$_2$)
— Pulmonic valve closure (P$_2$)

S₃

- Early diastole: S_1 S_2 **S_3** lub dub **DUH!** Dull thud
- **Sudden termination** of early rapid diastolic filling into a **stiff dysfunctional ventricle/tensing of CT**
- **L**-sided S_3: **LV apex** (left lat. decub. position) with **bell** during **ex**piration
- HFrEF, AR, MR, TR, VSD, ASD, PDA
- Physiological < 40 years of age or **HYPER FAT HIP**: **HYPER**dynamic circulation; **F**ever, **A**nemia, **A**V fistula, **T**hiamine deficiency, **H**yperthyroidism, **I**nfection, **P**aget disease, **P**regnancy

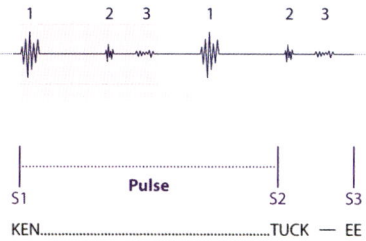

Murmurs — Valsalva (Strain Phase)

Louder
MVP (and moves closer to S_1)
HCM
Valsalva
Amyl nitrate
STanding
Little (decreased preload) → decreased LV volume

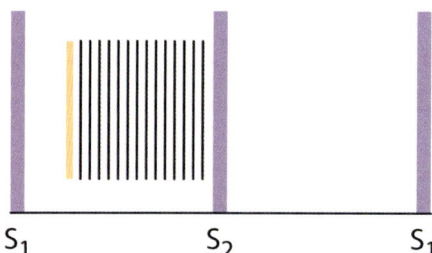

Systolic click

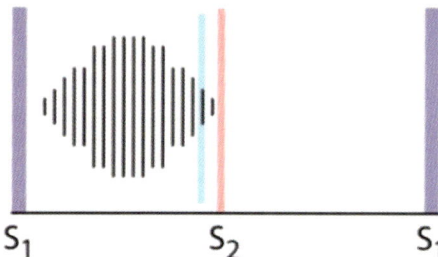

Aortic valve closure (A_2)
Pulmonic valve closure (P_2)

Elevated Jugular Venous Pressure (JVP)[44]

- **Internal jugular vein**
- Occurs at RAP ≥ 7 cm H_2O (5 mmHg)

THE CVP
TR/TS
HF (R-sided)
Embolism (pulmonary)
Constrictive pericarditis
Vena cava obstruction (SVC obstruction)
Pericardial effusion/tamponade

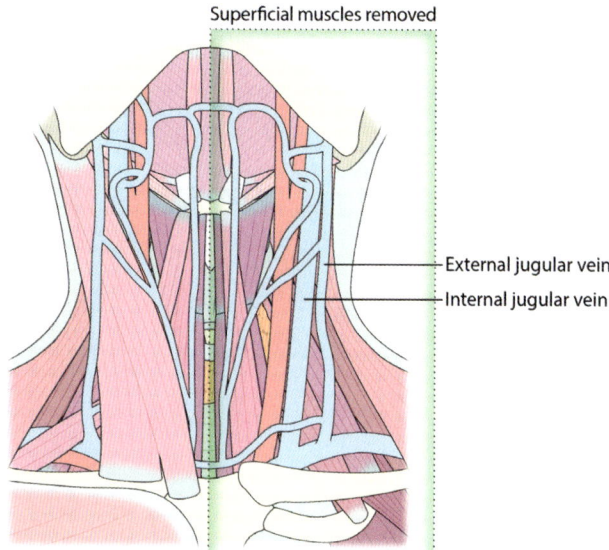

Superficial muscles removed

External jugular vein
Internal jugular vein

Purring Paralytic Pulsus Paradoxus

Car driving
C
A
T
- An "inspiratory fall in systolic blood pressure"
  - **Car**diac tamponade
  - **C**onstrictive pericarditis
  - **A**sthma/emphysema
  - **T**ension pneumothorax

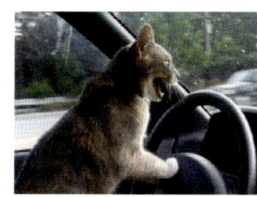
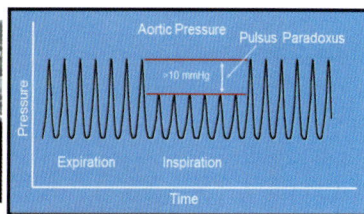

[45]

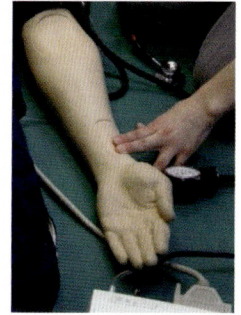

Lecture 2

L2 Outline
- **Acute Coronary Syndrome (ACS)**
- **Markers for Acute Coronary Syndrome (ACS)**
- **ACS Tx — Management of Non–ST-Elevation Acute Coronary Syndrome (NSTE-ACS)**
- **ACS Tx — Management of ST-Segment Elevation Myocardial Infarction (STEMI)**
- **Complications of ACS**
- **Stable Ischemic Heart Disease (SIHD)**
- **Hyperlipidemia**

ACUTE CORONARY SYNDROME (ACS)

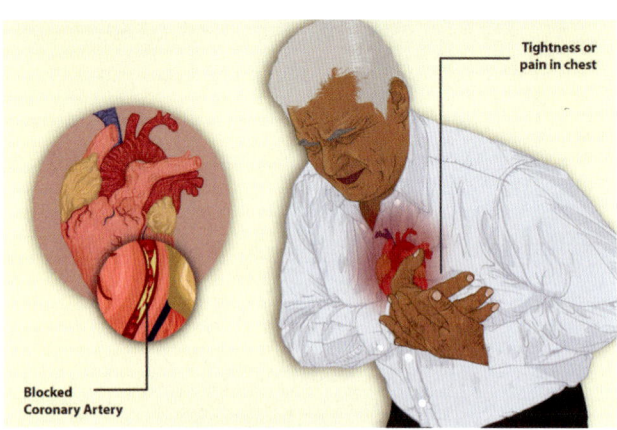

Tightness or pain in chest

Blocked Coronary Artery

[46]

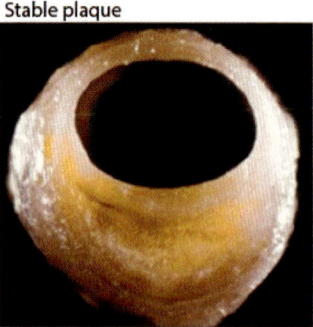

Stable plaque

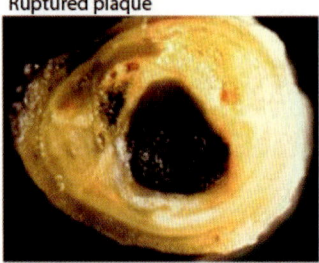

Ruptured plaque

ACS — Symptoms and Signs[47][48][49][50][51][52]
- Nontraumatic central chest ("tightness," "pressure," "squeezing," "gripping," or "heaviness") ± dyspnea, nausea/vomiting, diaphoresis
- **Older adults/Diabetics/Women: SOB, heart failure, confusion, fatigue, nausea**
- Dyslipidemia and smoking = most important risk factors for MI; **positive family history or diabetes doubles risk (ACS)**!
- **Preeclampsia**, pregnancy-induced hypertension, gestational diabetes, premature menopause (< 40 years of age), chronic inflammatory conditions e.g., psoriasis, rheumatoid arthritis (RA), lupus (2× risk CAD), HIV (2× risk CAD), chronic kidney disease are CVD risk factors

ACS — ED ≤ 10 mins
1) **Chew:** aspirin (162–325 mg)
2) **Electrode sticker:** ECG interpreted
3) **Chat you up:** focused Hx and PE
4) **Stick you:** cardiac markers drawn
5) **How hot are you?** Risk evaluation — TIMI

ACS — Spectrum

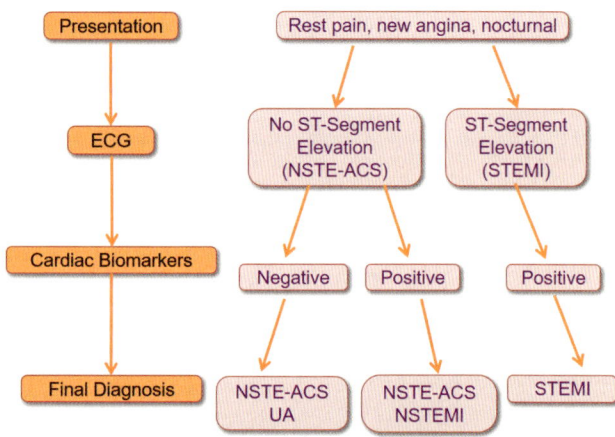

Non-ST-Segment Elevation Acute Coronary Syndrome (NSTE-ACS) — ECG[53]
- T-wave inversion
- ST-segment depression

Unstable Angina/Non–ST-Elevation Myocardial Infarction

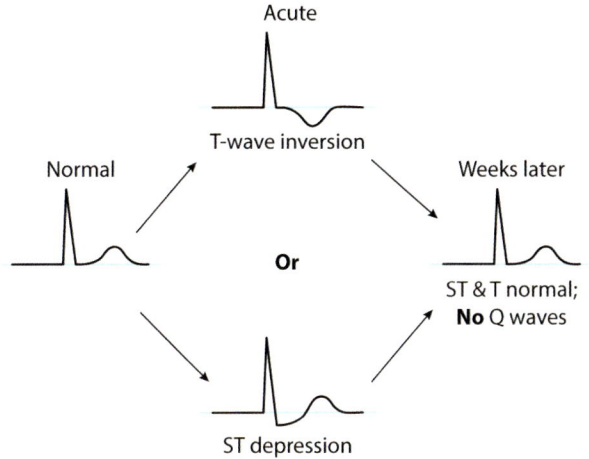

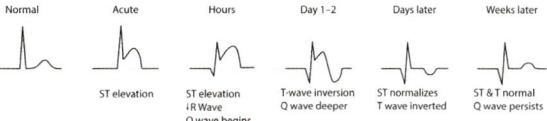

STEMI — Artery Location

Location	ST Elevation	Artery
Anterior	V1–V4 (or new LBBB)	LAD
Lateral	V5, V6, I, aVL	LCX
Inferior	II, III, aVF	RCA (or LCX)
Right	V4R	RCA
Posterior	**V1, V2 (ST dpn) V7–V9***	**PDA**

*Leads: Posterior axillary line to left border of spine.
LAD = left anterior descending; LCX = left circumflex;
RCA = right coronary artery;
PDA = posterior descending artery = branch of the RCA or LCX

NSTE-ACS

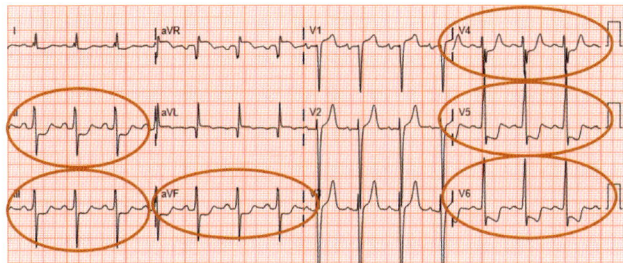

60-year-old African American male with chest pain

Anterolateral STEMI — V1–V6, I, aVL

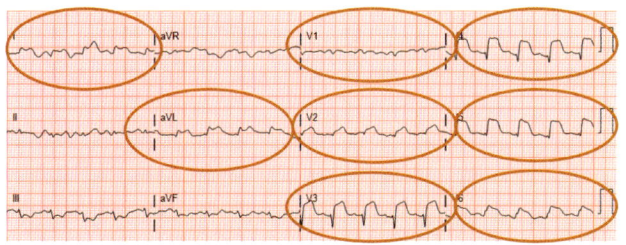

68-year-old Caucasian male with severe chest pain

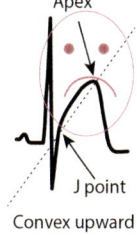

ST-Segment Elevation Myocardial Infarction (STEMI) — ECG[54][55][56]

- Peaked T waves → Elevated ST segments
- Loss of R waves → Q waves
- T-wave inversion
- Weeks later: Resolution of ST-segment elevation
- **If new LBBB and hemodynamic instability/HF = STEMI equivalent**
- **If old LBBB and Sgarbossa criteria = STEMI equivalent**

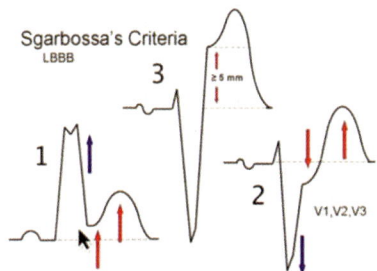

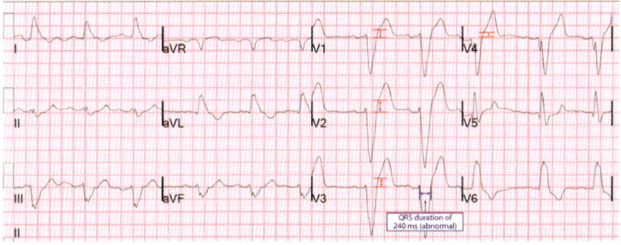

MARKERS FOR ACS

Troponins[57]

- **Gold** standard = sensitive (not specific) for acute myocardial infarction
- Rule of **4**s
  - Elevated @ **4** hours
  - Peaks @ **24–44** hours
  - Normalizes by **14** days

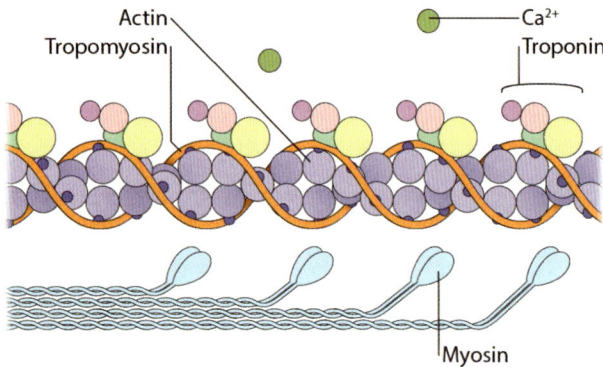

MANAGEMENT OF NSTE-ACS

ACS Tx — Management of Non–ST-Elevation Acute Coronary Syndrome (NSTE-ACS)

AR 6

A 41-year-old African American female presents with chest pain. Last night, she has had 3 episodes at rest, each lasting an hour, described as a severe 9/10 "chest squeezing."

PMH: Hyperlipidemia, diabetes, HTN, tobacco use, and GERD. Father had bypass surgery at 40 years old.

Meds: Aspirin, lisinopril, HCTZ, and rosuvastatin.
Vitals: Signs and physical exam are normal.
Cardiac: troponin I 1.1 ng/mL.
ECG: Sinus rhythm 75 bpm and 1-mm ST depression in V4–V6.

Metoprolol, nitrates, clopidogrel, and heparin were initiated. She reports still having chest pressure at 6/10 severity, and she is diaphoretic and nauseous.

What would you recommend doing now?

A. IV thrombolytic therapy
B. Exercise stress electrocardiography
C. Urgent coronary angiography
D. Regadenoson nuclear stress testing

Answer:_____

NSTE-ACS[58]

- Aspirin (inhibits COX-1 ↓ TxA_2 and prostacyclin)
- $P2Y_{12}$ ADP PLT RI (inhibits platelet cross linkage) — European Society of Cardiology guideline says hold (no benefit and excess bleeding)[59]
- O_2: Sat < 90%, respiratory distress, or other high-risk features of hypoxemia
- β-Blocker
- High-intensity statin (atorvastatin 80 mg daily)
- Nitrate prn: **CI with recent intake of sildenafil/ vardenafil (< 24 hr) or tadalafil (< 48 hr), severe aortic stenosis, HCM, RV infarction, SBP < 90 mmHg or 30 mmHg below baseline**
- IV anticoagulant
- Telemetry
- **Hotness level/Risk stratify**

Hotness Level

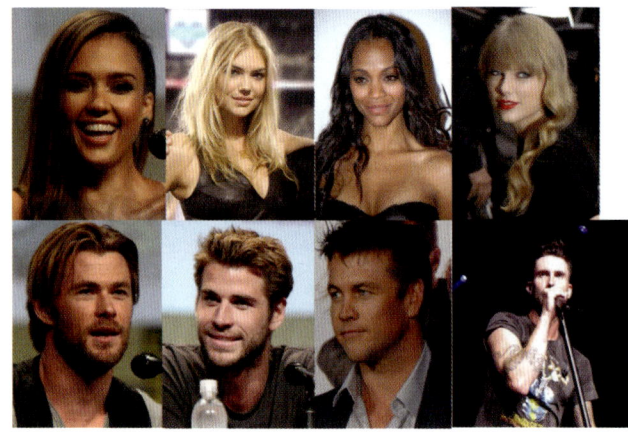

[60]

TIMI AMERICA[61][62]

Age ≥ 65 years
Markers elevated (cTn-I CKMB)
ECG ST deviation (new or transient) ≥ 0.5 mm
Risk factors* ≥ 3
Ischemia: ≥ 2 anginal episodes in past 24 hrs
CAD (known stenosis ≥ 50%)
Aspirin use in prior 7 days

*HTN (> 140/90 mmHg or on Rx); DM; H/lipid (LDL ≥ 190 mg/dL, TC ≥ 240 mg/dL, HDL < 40 mg/dL, TG ≥ 200 mg/dL); active smoker; family Hx premature CAD = fatal/nonfatal MI, coronary revascularization, or sudden death < 55 years of age (father/1st degree male relative) or < 65 years of age (female/1st degree relative)

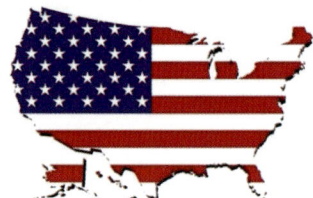

TIMI Prognosis and Tx[63][64]

TIMI Score (Risk)	Risk Death / MI / Urgent Revascularization at 14 Days; i.e., major adverse cardiac events (MACEs)
0–2 (low)	5% ischemia-guided strategy
3–4 (intermediate)	20% early invasive
5–7 (high)	40% early invasive

NSTE-ACS — Early Invasive = Coronary Angiography "Cath"[65][66][67][68][69]
- TIMI risk score ≥ **3**
- GRACE score > 1**4**0
- New onset HF/EF < **4**0%
- Recurrent/Refractory angina (dynamic ST changes, rise/fall troponins)
- Hemodynamic/Electrical instability
- Moderate-severe ischemia on stress test
- PCI within 6 months/Prior CABG

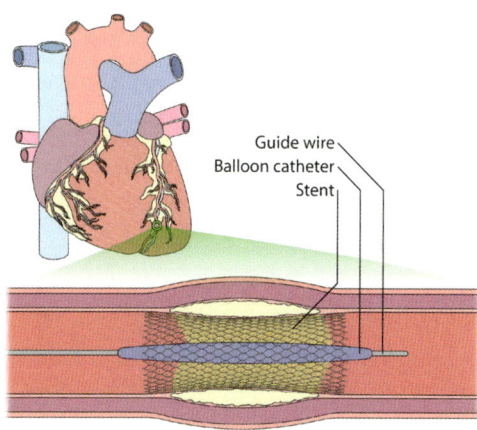

Guide wire
Balloon catheter
Stent

NSTE-ACS Initial Antiplatelet Rx[70][71]
- **Aspirin** 162–325 mg load then 81–162 mg daily indefinitely (if intolerant, then clopidogrel)
- **P2Y$_{12}$ receptor inhibitor** load:
  - Clopidogrel (Plavix) 300–600 mg (reversed with platelets; associated with TTP)
  - **P**rasugrel (Effient) 60 mg (reversed with platelets) if going for **P**CI
  - Ticagrelor (Brilinta) 180 mg (**not** a prodrug so faster & direct effect; reversible); **NB: ticagrelor-related dyspnea ~ 15%, normal BNP (consider switch to clopidogrel)**
- **P2Y$_{12}$ inhibitor for up to 1 year** (if no PCI); for **1 year (BMS or DES):**
  - Clopidogrel 75 mg daily
  - **P**rasugrel 10 mg daily; **5 mg daily if wt < 60 kg [132.3 lb] (contraindicated: Hx stroke/TIA, active bleeding)**
  - Ticagrelor 90 mg twice daily (aspirin 81 mg daily)

NSTE-ACS — Initial Anticoagulant Rx Options[72]
- **Unfractionated heparin (UFH) (antithrombin [AT; formerly antithrombin III] stimulator, 9a & 10a inhibitor)**: IV bolus 60 U/kg (max **4**,000 U) then infusion 12 U/kg/hr (max **1**,000 U/hr) for 48 h or until PCI performed: **4 − 1 = 3 letters** <u>UFH</u>
  - **Side effects:** HIT, OP, elevated LFTs, alopecia, hypoaldosteronism
- **Enoxaparin (2a & 10a inhibitor)**: IV bolus 30 mg then SC injections (1 mg/kg q 12 h; 1 mg/kg daily, if CrCl < 30 mL/min; CI: dialysis patients) for duration of hospitalization or until PCI performed
- **Bivalirudin (direct thrombin inhibitor)** until diagnostic angiography or PCI is performed if early **inva**sive strategy only (DTIs: no antidote)
- **Fondaparinux (10a inhibitor)** SC for the duration of hospitalization or until PCI performed (CI: dialysis patients); no antidote

NSTE-ACS — Stent: BMS or DES (Early Invasive)[73][74]
- Antiplatelet Rx: **HOT!!!**
  - In patients with high-risk features (e.g., elevated troponin) not adequately pretreated with clopidogrel or ticagrelor → give **GP 2b/3a inhibitor^** = double-bolus eptifibatide, or high-dose bolus tirofiban) at time of PCI

^ Block final common pathway of platelet activation; stop GP 2b/3a inhibitor and/or heparin if platelet < 100,000 cells/mm^3 or > 50% drop from baseline

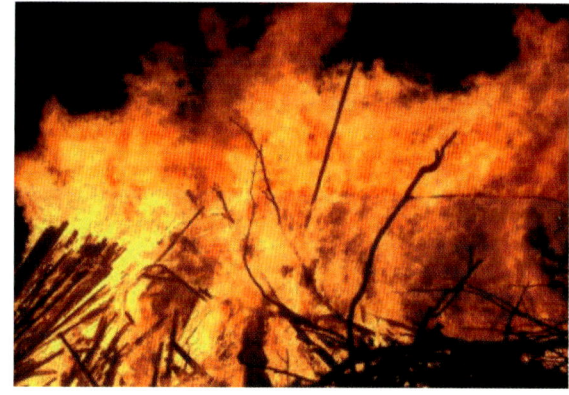

[75]

NSTE-ACS — Stent: BMS or DES (Early Invasive) Anticoagulant Rx Options[76][77]
- Reduce risk of intracoronary and catheter thrombus formation
- **Unfractionated heparin** (UFH): IV*****
- **Enoxaparin**: IV bolus then SC injections
- **Bivalirudin**

*Protamine sulfate 1 mg: Neutralizes 100 U UFH; IV heparin half-life 60 mins

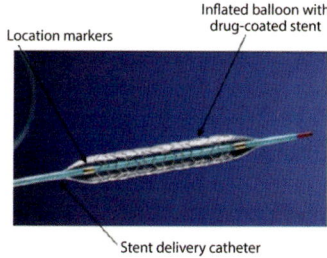

Inflated balloon with drug-coated stent
Location markers
Stent delivery catheter

NSTE-ACS — Cocaine and Methamphetamine Users[78]
- Treat the same
- **Exception**: Patients with signs of **acute intoxication** e.g., euphoria, tachycardia, hypertension **should not be given BBs** due to the risk of coronary spasm & ↑BP (unopposed α-adrenergic effect)
- **Benzodiazepines** and/or **nitroglycerin** for management of hypertension and tachycardia

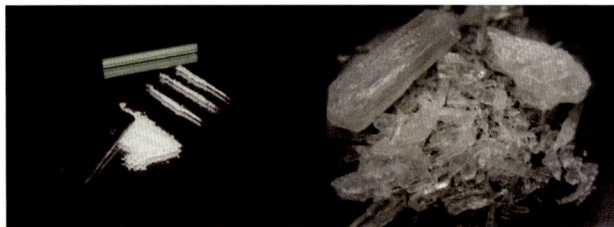

[79]

MANAGEMENT WITH STEMI

ACS Tx — Management of ST-Segment Elevation Myocardial Infarction (STEMI)

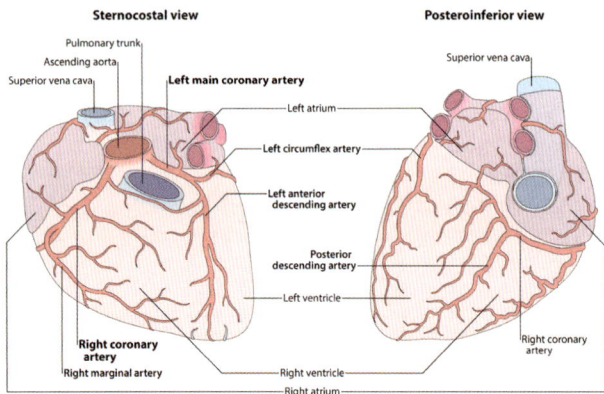

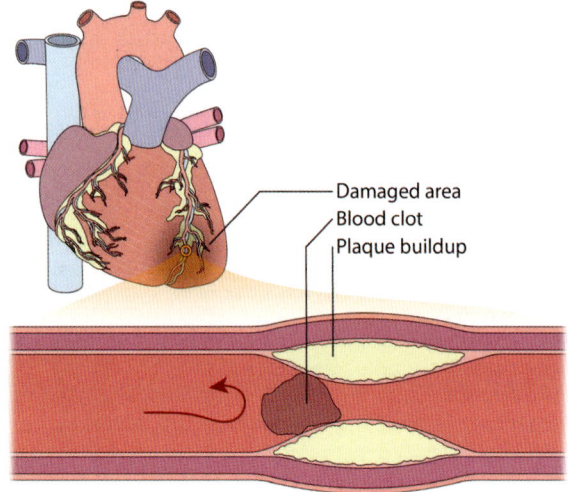

Damaged area
Blood clot
Plaque buildup

AR 7

A 51-year-old woman is seen in the emergency department for chest pressure and nausea that started 90 mins ago.

PMH: hypertension, hyperlipidemia, cigarette smoking.

Meds: pravastatin, HCTZ. PE: BP 110/70 mmHg, heart rate 88 bpm, afebrile, O₂ sat 97% on room air; rest unremarkable.

Labs: initial cTnI 2.5 ng/mL; ECG is shown:

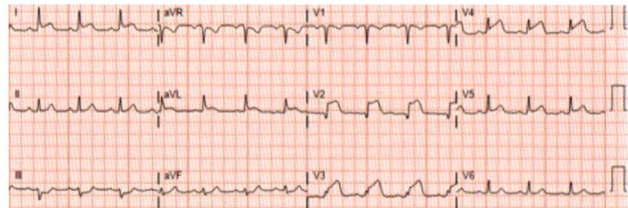

You start aspirin, clopidogrel, and IV heparin. The nearest PCI hospital is 3 hours away.

What is the most appropriate treatment?

A. Admit to ICU and observe.
B. Full-dose reteplase (rPA), then transfer to PCI-capable hospital.
C. Transfer for primary PCI.
D. Half-dose reteplase with eptifibatide, then transfer to PCI-capable hospital.

Answer:_____

STEMI[80][81]
- Aspirin (inhibits cyclooxygenase → platelet aggregation)
- P2Y₁₂ ADP PLT RI (inhibits platelet cross linkage)
- O₂ Sat < 90%, respiratory distress, or other high-risk features of hypoxemia
- β-Blocker (**↓ ventricular arrhythmias, ↑ survival**)
- High-intensity statin (atorvastatin 80 mg daily)
- **ACEI/ARB, aldosterone antagonist (EF ≤ 0.40)**
- Nitrate prn (IV: Recurrent angina, uncontrolled HTN, or heart failure)*
- IV anticoagulant
- Telemetry
- **Emergent reperfusion therapy**

***CI with recent intake of sildenafil/vardenafil (< 24 h) or tadalafil (< 48 h); severe aortic stenosis, or HCM**

STEMI Reperfusion Therapy

Consider emergent reperfusion (primary PCI/fibrinolytic therapy) in all who present with a STEMI or new LBBB

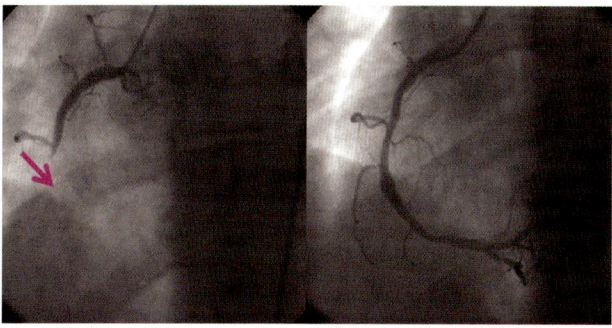

[82]

Inferior STEMI: Occlusion in middle right coronary artery (RCA) 100%.
Underwent PCI.

STEMI — Primary PCI[83][84]

- **Better** than fibrinolytic therapy in reestablishing flow
- Within **90 minutes** of the first medical contact (FMC) with patient if taken to a PCI-capable hospital (**120 minutes** if non-PCI hospital)
- > 75 yo: ↑ complic., ↓ efficacy
- Radial access (INR < 2.2) over femoral (< 1.8) preferred

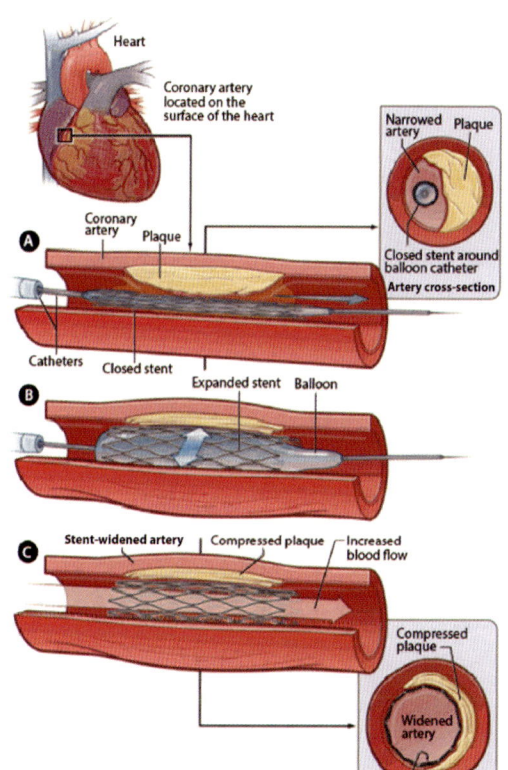

STEMI — Primary PCI Bare Metal Stents (BMS)[85][86]

- High **bleeding** risk
- Inability to **comply** with 1-year dual antiplatelet therapy (DAPT)
- Invasive/surgical **procedure** in next year

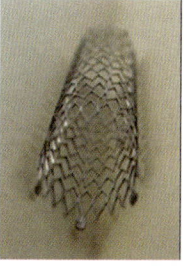
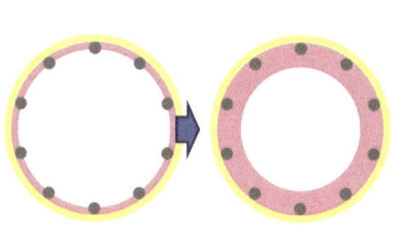

STEMI — Antiplatelet and Anticoagulant Rx[87]

- **Same as NSTE-ACS**
- **Aspirin + P2Y$_{12}$ receptor inhibitor (for load, clopidogrel 600 mg; fibrinolysis: 300 mg ≤ 75 years old, 75 mg > 75 years old)**
- **Unfractionated heparin, enoxaparin, or bivalirudin**

STEMI — Fibrinolytic Rx[88]

- If primary PCI not available and/or FMC-to-device time at a PCI-capable hospital > **12**0 minutes and patient presents within **12** hours of symptom onset; **intracranial hemorrhage ~ 0.8%**

Fibrin specific (80% TIMI 2/3 flow)
- **Tenecteplase (TNK-tPA)**: 30–50 mg single IV weight-based **bolus**
- **Reteplase (rPA)**: 10-U + 10-U IV **bolus** given 30 min apart
- **Alteplase (rtPA)**: Up to 100 mg in 90-min weight-based **infusion**

Non-fibrin specific (60% TIMI 2/3 flow)
- **Streptokinase** 1.5 million units **infusion** over 30–60 minutes
- **After thrombolytics, transfer to PCI facility:** Allows for rescue PCI in case of failure to reperfuse (e.g., lack of at least 50% resolution of ST elevation)

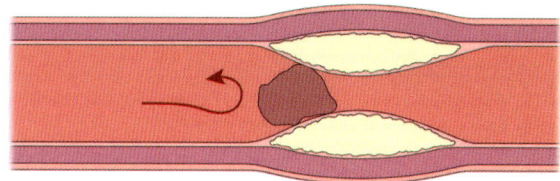

Fibrinolytics — Absolute Contraindications[89][90]

- Any prior **ICH**
- Known structural **cerebral vascular** lesion (e.g., arteriovenous malformation)
- Known malignant **intracranial neoplasm** (primary or metastatic)
- Ischemic stroke within 3 months, <u>except</u> acute ischemic stroke < 4.5 h; Rx IV rtPA (alteplase 0.9 mg/kg, max dose 90 mg over 60 minutes with initial 10% of dose given as bolus over 1 minute)*
- Suspected **aortic dissection**
- Active **bleeding** or bleeding diathesis (excluding menses)
- Significant **closed-head or facial trauma** within 3 months
- **Intracranial or intraspinal** surgery within 2 months
- Severe uncontrolled **hypertension** (unresponsive to emergency therapy) = based on repeated measurements SBP > 185 mmHg or DBP > 110 mmHg
- For streptokinase, prior treatment within the **previous 6 months**

*If ineligible, give aspirin within 24–48 hours of acute ischemic stroke to reduce risk of recurrent ischemic stroke

STEMI — CABG and Antiplatelet Rx[91]

- Aspirin should **not** be withheld before urgent CABG

Stop:

- **Clopidogrel** or **ticagrelor** at least **24 hours** before urgent CABG, if possible
- Short-acting intravenous GP 2b/3a receptor antagonists (**eptifibatide, tirofiban**) at least **2–4 hours** before urgent CABG

NSTE-ACS and STEMI — β-Blockers[92][93]

- Start oral β-blockers (metoprolol tartrate, carvedilol) within 24 hours (↓ **reinfarction/ventricular arr.**) if **no**:
  - **HF**/Low-output state
  - Risk for **cardiogenic shock***
  - Prolonged **1st degree** heart block (PR interval > 0.24 seconds)
  - **2nd or 3rd degree** HB without a pacemaker
  - Active **asthma**/reactive airways disease (use diltiazem)
- IV metoprolol tartrate 5 mg q 5 min × 3 for refractory HTN or ongoing ischemia

*Age > 70 years, systolic BP < 120 mmHg, sinus tachycardia > 110 bpm or heart rate < 60 bpm, and increased time since onset of symptoms of STEMI

STEMI — Renin-Angiotensin-Aldosterone System (RAAS) Inhibitors[95]

- **ACEIs** (lisinopril, captopril, ramipril, trandolapril) within **24 hours** to all with **anterior STEMI, HF, EF ≤ 0.40**
- **ARB** (valsartan*) if ACEI intolerant
- **Aldosterone antagonist** (eplerenone) for those already on ACEI + BB and **EF ≤ 0.40 and HF symptoms or DM — NB:**

CI: K > 5.0 mEq/L, Cr > 2.5 mg/dL men/Cr > 2.0 mg/dL women, concomitant K-sparing diuretic (amiloride, triamterene) or K supplement

*All valsartan medicines containing the active substance from Zhejiang Huahai Pharmaceuticals have been recalled, but several other valsartan medicines not affected by the impurity are available

Right Ventricular (RV) Myocardial Infarction[96][97]

- **RIGHT ON, CHER!!!**:

Suspect **RIGHT** V STEMI if:

  - **C**lear lung fields
  - **H**ypotension
  - **E**levated JVP (Kussmaul sign)
  - **R**V Infarction (50% of INFERIOR STEM)
- Dx: ST-elevation R-sided chest leads (V4R ≥ 1 mm)
- RV dysfunction → preload to left heart reduced → cardiac output is reduced! Rx:
  - **Fluids** (wide open normal saline!)
  - **Dobutamine** if hypotension persists
  - **Avoid** preload reducers (e.g., **nitrates, morphine**)

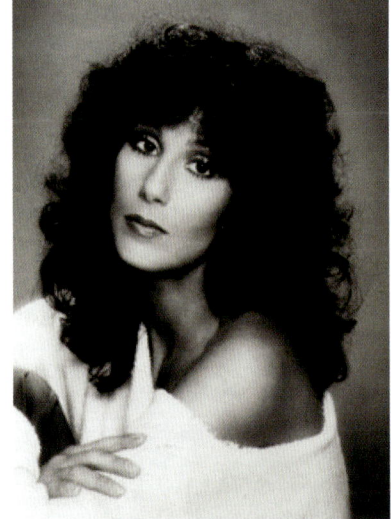

Activation of Mineralocorticoid Receptor[94]

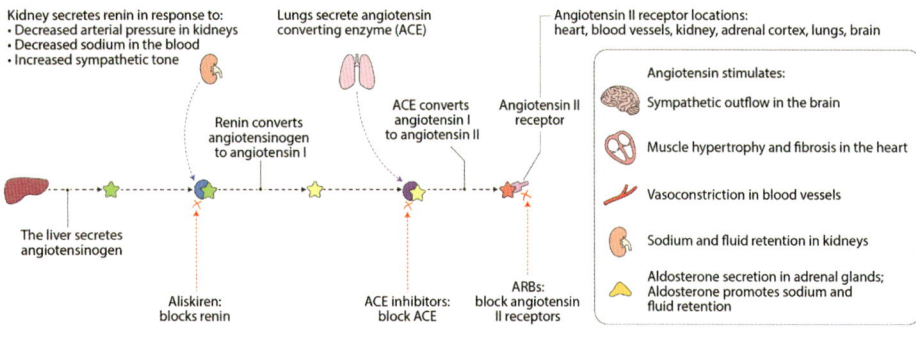

COMPLICATIONS OF ACS

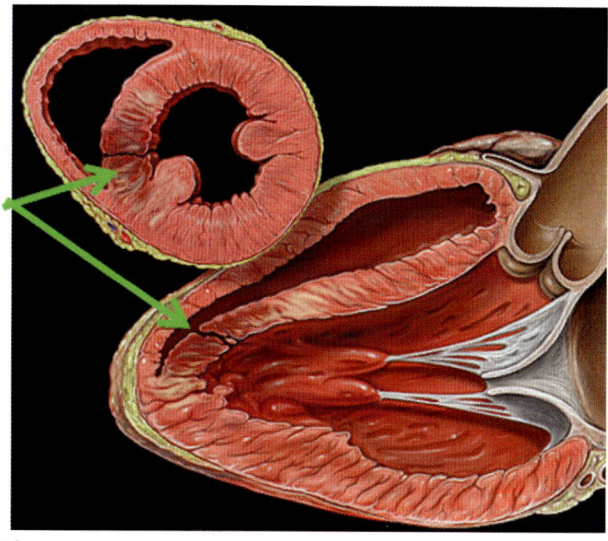

[98]

Rupture of Interventricular Septum

AR 8

A 56-year-old Hispanic male with chest pain to neck has the following ECG i.e., INFERIOR STEMI:

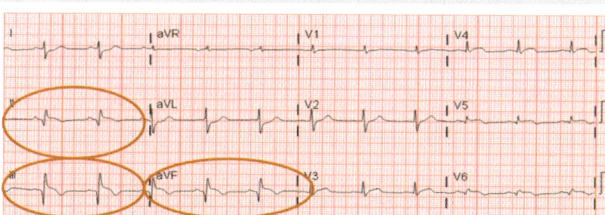

Which complication is he at higher risk for?

A. LV free wall rupture
B. Papillary muscle rupture/severe MR
C. Cardiogenic shock
D. Torsades de pointes
E. None of the above

Answer:_____

Mechanical Complications — Shock 2–7 Days Post Event

	LV Free Wall Rupture	MR— Papillary Muscle Rupture	Rupture of Interventricular Septum	Extensive LV Infarction / Cardiogenic Shock
Setting	**Anterior MI, older, women, on NSAIDs, delay reperfusion > 12 hours**	Inferior MI **1 PM: 1** blood supply = RCA = **P**ostero-**M**edial **P**apillary **M**uscle	Large anterior MI, **lie flat due to hypotension**	Large anterior MI or MI with previous LV dysfunction
Physical Exam	BECK @the **HELM**: **H**ypotension, **EL**evated JVD, **M**uffled heart sounds (tamponade)	Holosystolic murmur at APEX with radiation; pulmonary edema **(sit up)**	Loud holosystolic systolic murmur **LSB**, heard widely	Signs of left heart failure, kidney failure, cool extremities
Echo	Pericardial effusion with tamponade, RWMA, defect in myocardium	Flail mitral valve leaflet with papillary muscle head attached, severe MR	High-velocity L-R systolic jet within V septum	Severe LV systolic dysfn
Management	CT surgery	Nitroprusside + IABP + CT surgery	Nitroprusside + IABP + CT surgery	Supportive measures, primary PCI
Mortality	95%	50%	50%	85% (50% with primary PCI)

Ventricular Tachyarrhythmias[99]

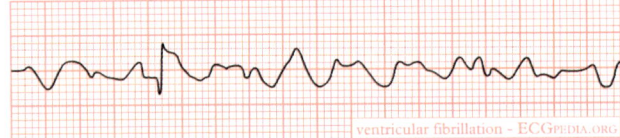

ventricular fibrillation - ECGPEDIA.ORG

- Cardiovert VFib and unstable VT
- Polymorphic VT or VFib with STEMI → emergency catheter with PCI/CABG
- Stable VT Rx amiodarone
  - Bolus 150 mg infused over 10 mins, repeated every 10–15 minutes, <u>or</u>
  - Infusion: 1 mg/min 6 hours, 0.5 mg/min next 18 hours

STEMI — Implantable Cardioverter Defibrillator (ICD) [100][101][102]

- Before discharge if develop sustained VT/VFib > 48 hours after STEMI and not due to transient/reversible ischemia, reinfarction, metabolic abnormalities (or wearable cardioverter-defibrillator; e.g., LifeVest if infection)
- **Prolong survival in post-MI patients with:**
  - **LVEF ≤ 35%** @ 40 days post-MI (nonrevascularization) or 90 days post-MI (revascularization)
  - **Survival ≥ 1 year**

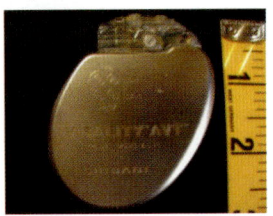

[103]

Implantable Cardioverter Defibrillator (ICD)[104][105]
1° Prevention
- Ischemic CMP 40 <u>days</u> post-MI & 90 days post-revascularization with:
  - EF ≤ 35% NYHA II, III HF (EF ≤ 30% NYHA I HF); NSVT EF ≤ 40% SusVT/VF EPS
- Nonischemic CMP:
  - EF ≤ 35% NYHA II, III HF

2° Prevention (SCA VT/ VFib, unstable VT/syncope from VT)
- Structural heart disease (e.g., HCM)
- Ischemic/Nonischemic CMP, or EF ≤ 35%
- NB: Not due to reversible causes

2 Zones & 2 Therapies
- VT zone 170–200 bpm: antitachycardia pacing
- **VFib** zone > 200 bpm: **Shock 35J**
- BB, amiodarone, or catheter ablation for recurrent arrhythmia

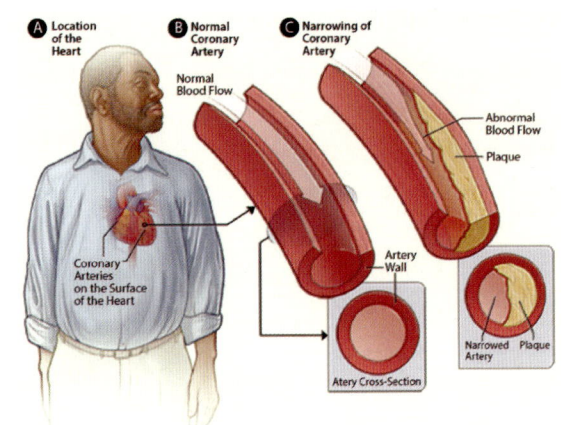

STABLE ISCHEMIC HEART DISEASE (SIHD)

AR 9

Your CAD patient has persistent exertional angina despite being on maximal doses of isosorbide mononitrate, metoprolol succinate, lisinopril, aspirin, and atorvastatin.

Providing there are no contraindications, which medication could you add to the current medication to improve the angina?

A. Amiodarone
B. Candesartan
C. Vitamin E
D. Niacin
E. Ranolazine

Answer:_____

SIHD Tx[106]

- **Nitrates, BBs, and DHP-CCBs* (nife-, amlo-, felodipine)**: Decrease myocardial O_2 demand and afterload
- **Ranolazine (Ranexa)** if **persistent angina** on maximal med Rx, or a **BB substitute** (side effects/CI)
- Ra**N**olazine inhibits myocytes late **Na** current → improves myocardial relaxation and reduces LV diastolic stiffness → enhances contractility and perfusion (caution if kidney/liver damage; prolongs QT); **reduce ranolazine dose used with moderate CYP3A inhibitors (e.g., diltiazem, verapamil)**

STRONG STRONG CYP3A inhibitors

N	**N**efazodone
P	**P**rotease inhibitors (nelfin-, riton-, indin-, saquinavir)
KICKS	**K**etoconazole, **I**traconazole, **C**larithromycin = **contraindicated with**
RANDY	**RAN**olazine

*Block L-type calcium channel of smooth muscle; peripheral edema

SIHD Tx[107][108][109][110][111]

- **Diet**
  - Saturated (< 7%), trans fatty acids (< 1% total calories)
  - Cholesterol (< 200 mg/day) and sodium (< 1500 mg/day)
  - 5–10 portions **fruit** and **vegetables**/day; 1–2 seafood meals/week
  - **Plant-based** and **Mediterranean** diets (fruit, vegetables, fish, legumes, nuts, whole grains)
- **Statin** for all
- BP < 130/80 mmHg (**SIHD, DM, CKD, post-MI, stroke/ TIA, carotid artery disease, PAD, AAA, HFpEF, ≥ 65 yo, 10-yr ASCVD risk ≥ 10%**); ACEI/ARBs ± BBs first (add thiazide diuretics/CCBs for goal BP)
- **Exercise**: 150 minutes moderate- or 75 minutes vigorous-intensity aerobic exercise/week (↑ nitric oxide, collaterals)
- Men's **waist**: < 102 cm (40"); women's: < 88 cm (35")

SIHD Tx[112][113]

- Smoking cessation: **Ask, Advise, Assess, Assist, Arrange,** and **Avoid** secondhand smoke; Tx behavioral plus nicotine replacement therapy, varenicline, or bupropion
- **Antiplatelet**:
  - Aspirin 75–100 mg daily indefinitely (low dose) — NB: Aspirin resistance caused by noncompliance; Increasing aspirin dose does not help!
  - Clopidogrel if aspirin contraindicated
- **BBs**: Start and continue for 3 years in all with normal LV fn after MI/ACS
- Carvedilol, metoprolol **s**uccinate (**s** for **s**ustained release), or bisoprolol in all with **LV systolic dysfunction (EF < 40%) with HF or prior MI**

SIHD Tx[114][115]

- **ACEI** in all with **HTN, DM, LVEF ≤ 40%, HX MI,** or **chronic kidney disease**; **ARBs** if ACEI intolerant
- **Coronary angiography** if unacceptable ischemic symptoms despite guideline-directed medical therapy (GDMT) and who are revascularization candidates (hold apixaban, rivaroxaban, dabigatran for 24 hours)
- Annual **influenza** vaccine and **Pneumovax 23** for adults ≥ 65 years of age, or adults 19–64 years of age who smoke, with chronic cardiovascular/pulmonary/ renal/liver disease, DM, alcoholism, asplenia, or S/P transplant
- **Microvascular angina = cardiac syndrome X = angina, abnormal stress, women, no significant CAD; likely microvascular dysfunction Tx same**

Percutaneous Coronary Intervention (PCI)[116][117][118][119]

- If **symptoms** despite GDMT, or unable to **tolerate** meds, or **high-risk** findings on noninvasive imaging
- PCI improves **symptoms, not survival** or future CV events
- Fractional flow reserve < 0.8 abnormal (nl 1.0) → needs PCI
- Need for **2nd procedure** higher with PCI vs. CABG
- Elective surgery delayed **30 days** after **BMS, 6 months to 1 year** after **DES** if **SIHD, 1 year** both if **ACS**
- **Safer, newer-generation DES minimum DAPT 3–6 months**
- If require more urgent surgery and on DAPT, hold P2Y$_{12}$RI **5 days prior** and continue ASA

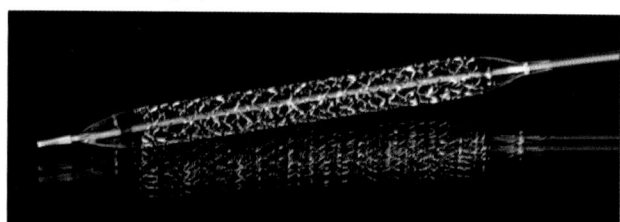

Coronary Artery Bypass Graft (CABG) Surgery[120][121][122]

- Improves **symptoms and survival** for chronic stable angina with:
  - **LMAIN (≥ 50% stenosis)**
  - **3VD/2VD (≥ 70%) with Prox LAD + DM/low EF**
- NB: In other 1 or 2 VD can Rx with either medical therapy, PCI, or CABG

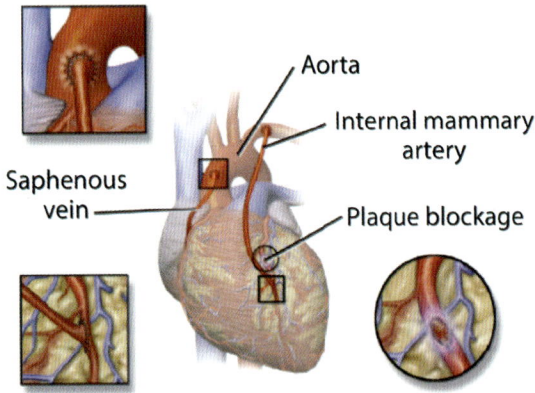

Coronary artery bypass surgery

[123]

HYPERLIPIDEMIA

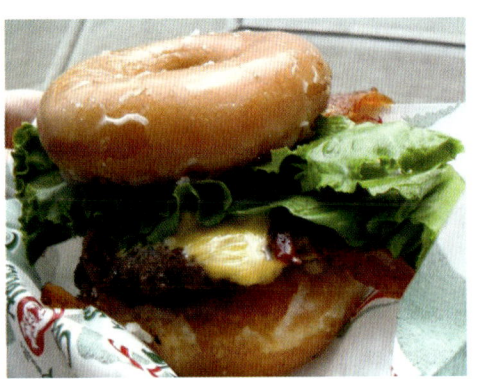

[124]

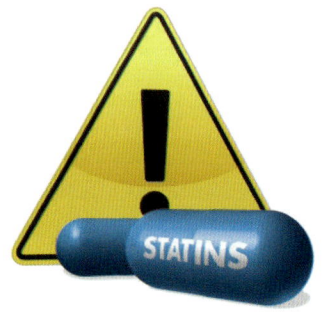

STATINS DON'T WORK:
Hemodialysis, nonischemic HFrEF!

AR 10

A 49-year-old Pakistani female comes in because she heard there are some "new cholesterol guidelines." She has T2DM and is taking metformin. Blood pressure 135/88 mmHg. Total cholesterol 179 mg/dL; HDL 55 mg/dL, 10-year risk ASCVD is 1.9%.

What Rx would you recommend?

A. Fibrate
B. Ezetimibe
C. Niacin
D. Moderate-intensity statin

Answer:_____

In CAL the HIGH DR was MODERN![125][126][127][128]
Cholesterol Rx (Age 40–75)

1) **A**SCVD (Clinical)* #
   - CAD or PAD
   - Hx MI or stable/ unstable angina
   - Acute coronary syndrome
   - Coronary/ other arterial revascularization
   - Stroke/TIA

   HIGH intensity ($\downarrow$ LDL ≥ 50%) **$**
   Atorva 80
   Rosuva 20
   (STATINS + **FACE = BAD**!)
   [**F**ibrates/niacin, **A**zoles, **C**yclosporine, **E**rythro] $\uparrow$ **myositis**

2) **L**DL-C ≥ 190 mg/dL **@**
3) **D**iabetes 40–75 yo
4) **R**isk ≥ **7.5–20**% ASCVD @ 10 y **%**

   HIGH intensity
   MOD intensity
   ($\downarrow$ 30–50%)
   MOD intensity
   Simva 20–40,
   Atorva 10,
   Rosuva 10,
   Prava 40 (cyclosporine)

Intensity of Rx = goal; STOP if LFTS > 3 × ULN or myopathy CK > 10 × ULN; check fasting lipids 1–3 months after starting/ adjusting statin, and every 3–12 months thereafter

* Continue statins in persons > 75 years of age who have clinical ASCVD and are tolerating statin therapy.
$ If HIGH intensity contraindicated/side effects, try moderate-intensity statin therapy
% If 10-yr ASCVD risk ≥ 20 use HIGH-intensity statin (pooled cohort equation at https://clincalc.com/ Cardiology/ASCVD/PooledCohort.aspx).
# Nonstatin Rx: 1st ezetimibe (10 mg) inhib. chol. intestinal absorb.; if LDL not lowered 50%, consider ezetimibe + statin with long half-life 1–3 times/week; e.g., rosuvastatin 20 mg twice/week 2nd PCSK9 inhibitor (evolocumab, alirocumab). If elevated triglyceride levels despite statin therapy and cardiovascular disease or diabetes and multiple other risk factors, add icosapent ethyl (highly purified fish oil).
@ Also consider bile acid sequestrants (colesevelam, cholestyramine, colestipol).

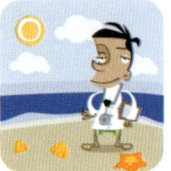

Risk-Enhancing Factors Favoring Rx[129]

- **Family Hx** premature ASCVD (male < 55, female < 65 y)
- Primary hypercholesterolemia (**LDL-C 160–189 mg/dL**)
- **Metabolic** syndrome [**PHATS*** 3/5]
- **CKD:** eGFR 15–59 mL/min/1.73 m^2 **(not dialysis or Txpl)**
- Chronic **inflammation**: psoriasis, RA, HIV
- **Premature menopause** (< 40 years) or Hx preeclampsia
- **South Asian** (Afghanistan, India, Pakistan, Bangladesh, Sri Lanka, Nepal, Bhutan, Maldives) or other high-risk race/ethnicity
- **TRIG** ≥ 175 mg/dl, **hs-CRP** ≥ 2 mg/L, **Lp(a)** ≥ 50 mg/dL, **apoB** ≥ 130 mg/dL, **ABI** < 0.9

*PHATS 3/5: **P**ressure (Blood) > 130/85 mmHg; **H**DL < 40 mg/dL (men), < 50 mg/dL (women); **A**bdominal obesity; **T**RIG > 150 mg/dL; **S**ugar (blood glucose) ≥ 110mg/dL

Lecture 3

L3 Outline
- **Peripheral Arterial Disease (PAD)**
- **Vasospastic Disease**
- **Carotid Artery Disease**
- **Cerebral Embolic Disease**
- **Aortic Disease**
- **Infective Endocarditis (IE)**
- **Aortic Stenosis (AS)**
- **Acute Aortic Regurgitation (AR)**
- **Chronic Aortic Regurgitation (AR)**
- **Mitral Stenosis (MS)**
- **Acute Mitral Regurgitation (MR)**
- **Chronic Mitral Regurgitation (MR)**
- **Prosthetic Heart Valves**

PERIPHERAL ARTERIAL DISEASE (PAD)

Peripheral Arterial Disease (PAD)[130]

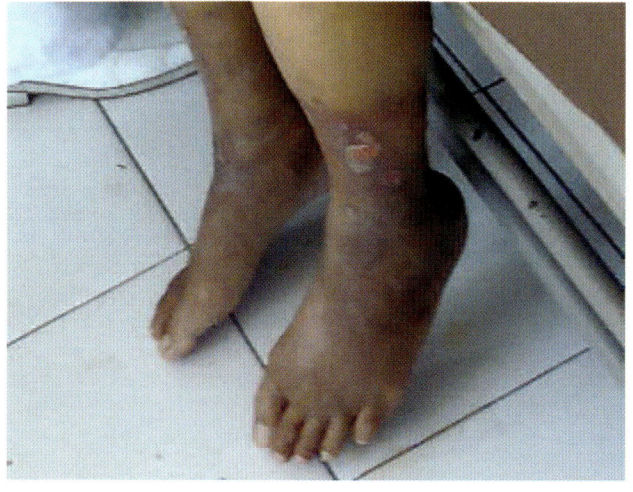

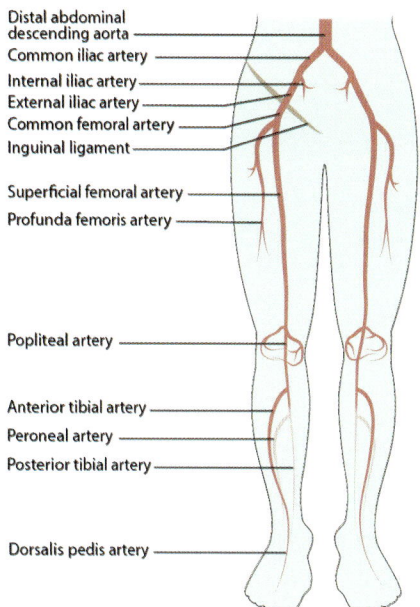

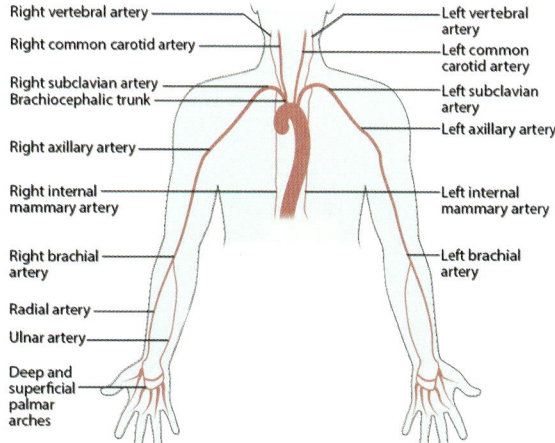

Men: More common and at earlier age; Black race > others
Rarely upper extremity PAD: arm claudication
"PAD die from CAD!"

AR 11

A 73-year-old woman has a 5-month history of calf pain, L > R, that comes on when walking or standing, worse when walking downhill. She does not get the pain when she is pushing a cart buying groceries. She gets relief by sitting down and leaning forward.

Which study will likely reveal the cause of the symptoms?

A. Ultrasound examination of the peripheral arterial circulation
B. Abdominal aortogram
C. Resting ankle brachial index (ABI)
D. MRI of the lumbar spine
E. CT abdomen

Answer:_____

CARDIOLOGY

PAD Screening — Ankle Brachial Index (ABI)[131]

= **A**nkle SBP/**B**rachial artery SBP (highest) obtained lying down

ABI	Interpretation
> 1.40	Noncompressible
1.00–1.40	Normal
0.91–0.99	Borderline
< 0.90	**Abnormal**

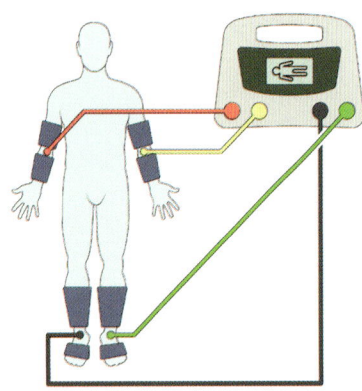

PAD Screening[132]

- **Resting ABI** (**± segmental waveforms**) if:
  - Exertional leg symptoms/rest pain (only 20% have claudication!)
  - Abnormal LE pulses/vascular bruit/nonhealing wounds/gangrene
  - Age < 50 years old with DM + RF; 50–64 years old if RF or FHx PAD; ≥ 65 years old
  - Atherosclerosis elsewhere; e.g., CAD, carotid
- **Exercise ABI** if exertional symptoms and normal/borderline resting ABI: **20% decrease or ≥ 30 mmHg drop ankle pressure = PAD**
- **Toe-brachial index (PAD: < 0.70 or toe SBP < 40 mmHg)** If ABI > 1.4 = noncompressible arteries (e.g., older adults, diabetics, renal disease)
- **Critical limb ischemia**: ABI < 0.40, flat waveform on pulse volume recordings, low/absent pedal flow on ultrasound; Tx: immediate angiography and endovascular revascularization

DDx — Lumbar Spinal Stenosis

- **Nonarterial claudication, a.k.a. pseudoclaudication**
- Bilateral, often paraesthesias
- **Relieved by flexing spine**
  - Sitting down (but not by standing still)
  - Walking while leaning on grocery cart
- Exacerbated by extending spine
  - Standing or walking (especially downhill)
- Absent deep tendon reflexes at ankles
- Dx: magnetic resonance imaging (MRI) of lumbar spine

"Walking is man's best medicine."

— Auguste Rodin

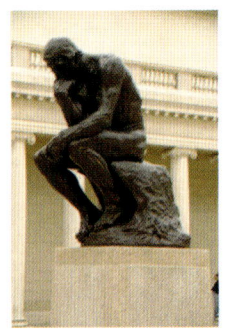

Le Penseur (The Thinker). Auguste Rodin.

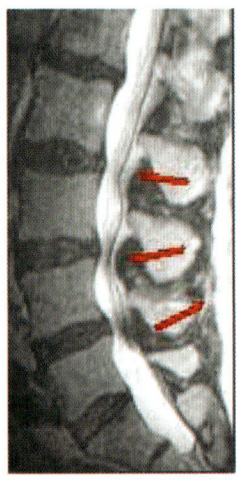

PAD — Highly Symptomatic and Likely Revascularization: Location, Severity[133]

- Duplex ultrasound
- Magnetic resonance angiography (MRA)
- Computed tomographic angiography (CTA); or
- Invasive angiography

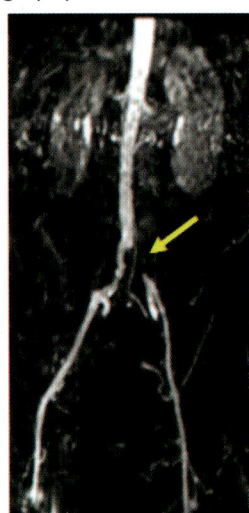

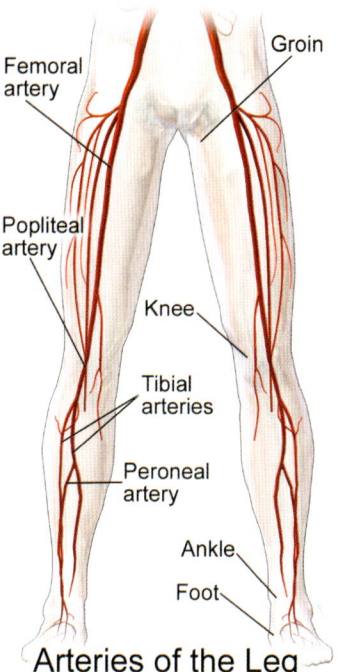

Arteries of the Leg

[134]

PAD — Tx[135][136]

- Aspirin 75–325 mg or clopidogrel 75 mg daily (decrease CV events!!!); statin
- BP: < 130/80 mmHg
- DM — self foot exam; ? infection — Dx/Tx ASAP
- Smoking
  - Advise to quit at every visit
  - Smoking cessation program and med Rx: Varenicline, bupropion, and/or nicotine replacement therapy
  - Avoid secondhand smoke

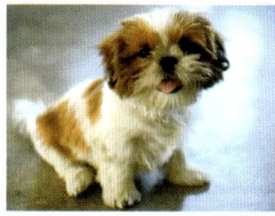

[137]

PAD — Tx[138]

- **1st: Supervised exercise: 30–45 mins ≥ 3 days/week × 12 wks**
- **Cilostazol**, a **phosphodiesterase inhibitor** → Increase cAMP in platelets (↓ aggregation) and blood vessels (↑ vasodilation) → Improves symptoms and walking distance
- Use only if **normal LV function: (CI: HF of any severity!) NYHA III or IV HF patients have increased mortality with any phosphodiesterase inhibitor!**
- **Vorapaxar** (protease-activated receptor-1 inhibitor) reduces hospitalizations for acute limb ischemia in symptomatic PAD
- Annual influenza vaccination

"Cilostazol phosphodiesterase inhibitor normal LV fn!"

PAD — Lifestyle-Limiting Claudication Tx[139]

- **Endovascular Tx (stent):** For **proximal** (aortoiliac and femoropopliteal) stenosis and **short-segment** occlusions (focal aortoiliac occlusive disease), those with comorbidities (CAD, CKD, HF, COPD)
- **Surgery (endarterectomy ± bypass):** For **long lesions** (common femoral artery) and **occlusions** (use autogenous vein or prosthetic graft); e.g., femoral-popliteal bypass
- **Both relieve symptoms + ischemia**

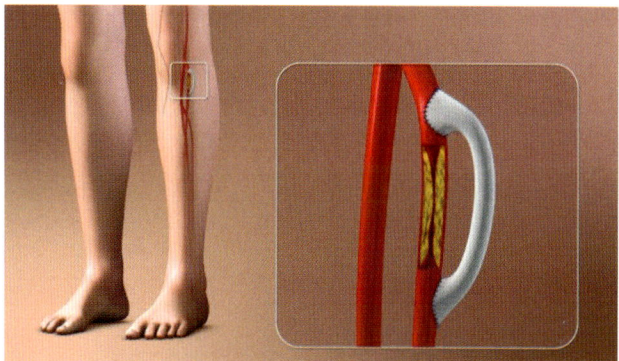

[140]

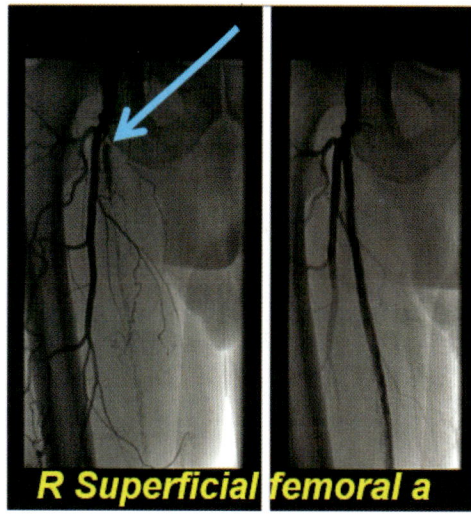

R Superficial femoral a

AR 12

A 59-year-old man presents with acute left leg pain for 3 days, worse with exertion. Today, the pain is now severe, at rest, and his foot is cool and going numb.

PMH: HTN, hyperlipidemia, smoking, Type 2 diabetes.
Meds: aspirin, lisinopril, HCTZ, metformin, atorvastatin.

PE: Vital signs normal. Left foot is pale, cool, with reduced sensation and no palpable pulses; muscle strength is normal. Arterial Doppler ultrasound no pulses. IV Heparin is started.

What is the most appropriate management?

A. Emergent left leg amputation
B. Urgent invasive angiography
C. Intravenous glycoprotein 2b/3a Inhibitors
D. Admit and watchful waiting

Answer:_____

CARDIOLOGY

Acute Limb Ischemia — Cold, Painful[141][142]

- Pain and ↓ pulses → sensory loss → muscle weakness **Pain-Pallor-Pulseless-Paresthesia-Poikilothermia-Paralysis**
- Etiology: thrombosis/embolization
- **IV heparin (stops collaterals thrombosing), immediate invasive angiography!**
- **Salvageable limb (intact sensation, muscle strength): Urgent (< 3 hrs) catheter-directed thrombolysis** then percutaneous transluminal angioplasty (**NB: systemic thrombolysis not beneficial!), or** embol-/thrombectomy and/or **surgical** revascularization
- Monitor and fasciotomy if get compartment syndrome
- **Nonsalvageable limb (gangrene, paralysis) ~ 20%: Tx immediate amputation**

VASOSPASTIC DISEASE

Vasospastic (Prinzmetal) Angina[143][144]

- At rest in younger persons — **The OMG ECG!**
- Tx: CCBs, stop smoking, and risk factor modification
- Coronary angiography recommended if episodic chest pain accompanied by transient ST elevation to rule out CAD

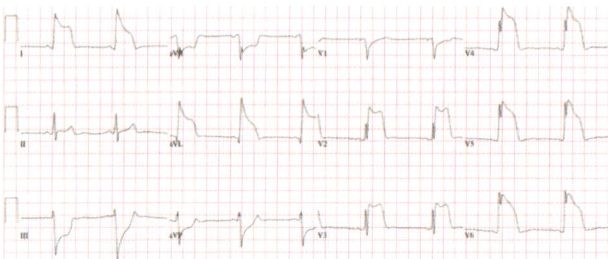

CAROTID ARTERY DISEASE

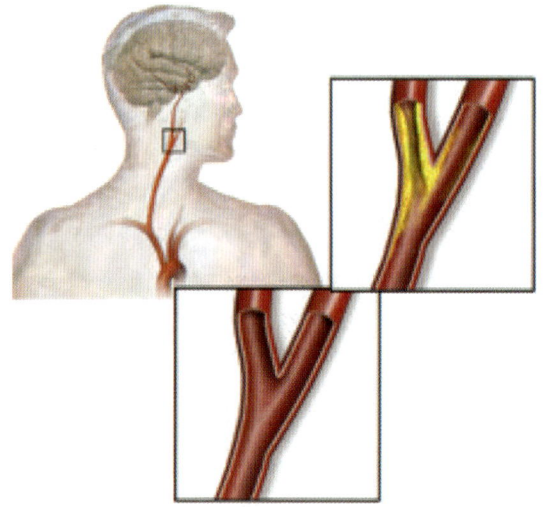

[145]

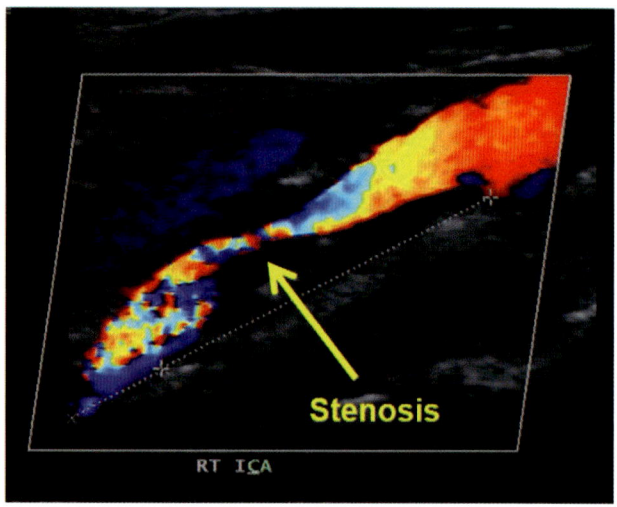

Patients are more likely to have an **MI** than a TIA/Stroke! "Carotid artery disease die from CAD!"

AR 13

A patient who had a TIA 1 month ago and has an ipsilateral internal carotid artery stenosis of 75% on ultrasound should be referred for carotid endarterectomy or stent placement.

A. True
B. False

Answer:_____

Carotid Artery Disease — Dx[146]

- Ultrasound in:
  - Asymptomatic, suspected stenosis: **bruit**
  - Symptomatic: **Focal neurological symptoms** in L or R internal carotid artery territories; sudden weakness and numbness of extremity/face; aphasia, dysarthria, or unilateral blindness (a. fugax); **echo to rule out cardiogenic embolism if don't find severe disease**
- Magnetic resonance angiography or computed tomography angiography when ultrasound:
  - Cannot be obtained, or
  - Yields equivocal/nondiagnostic results

Carotid CT Angio

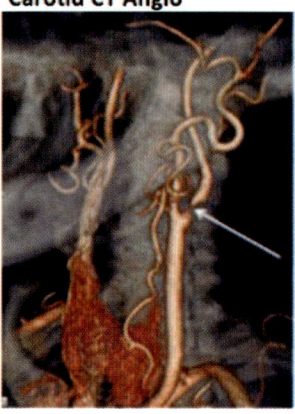

High-grade stenosis (90%) of internal carotid artery

Carotid Artery Disease — Med Rx[147][148]

- Aspirin 75–325 mg daily, or clopidogrel 75 mg daily, or aspirin + extended-release dipyridamole (25 and 200 mg) twice daily
- BP: < 130/80 mmHg
- Statin: high intensity
- Smokers: Quit!

Carotid Artery Disease Tx — Endarterectomy or Stent[149][150]

- Low or average surgical risk patients who experience nondisabling ischemic stroke or TIA symptoms within 6 months should undergo **carotid endarterectomy (more MI)** or **stent (more stroke)** if:
  - Diameter of lumen of ipsilateral internal carotid artery is reduced (**> 70% by noninvasive imaging or > 50% by catheter angiography**), and
  - Perioperative stroke/mortality < 6%
  - **Stent**: Aspirin (81–325 mg) + clopidogrel (75 mg) daily for 1 month; younger patients do better

70% noninvasive,
50% angiography,
+ symptoms = surgery!

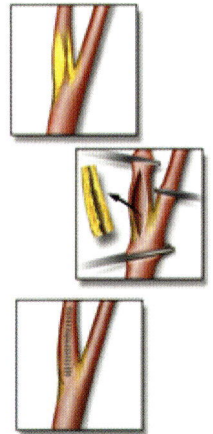

[151]

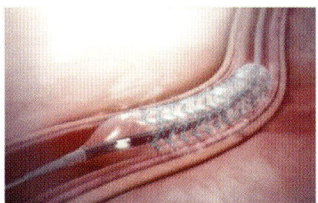

[152]

CEREBRAL EMBOLIC DISEASE

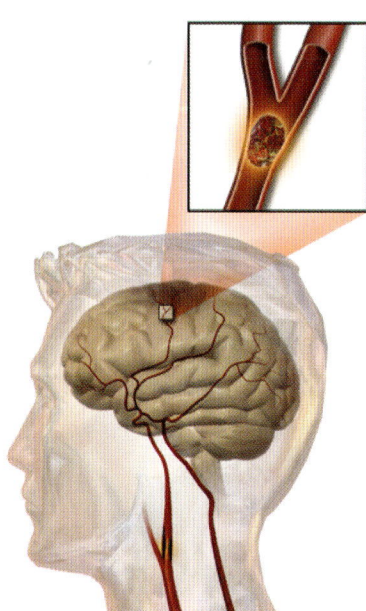

[153]

Cerebral Embolic Disease — Cardiac Causes and Rx[154][155]

- **Atrial fibrillation (AFib) = most common!**
- **NB: In older adult stroke patient in NSR, embolization from occult/low-burden AFib is common, so do long-term monitoring, even if no history of AFib and no AFib is on telemetry at time of stroke; 30-day cardiac event recorder improves detection of AFib 5× over Holter**
- Acute MI, ventricular aneurysm, mechanical valve, valvular heart diseases/endocarditis, patent foramen ovale, dilated cardiomyopathy
- If nothing found → probable cause atherosclerosis, so Rx:
  - Aspirin, or
  - Clopidogrel, or
  - Aspirin + extended-release dipyridamole

AORTIC DISEASE

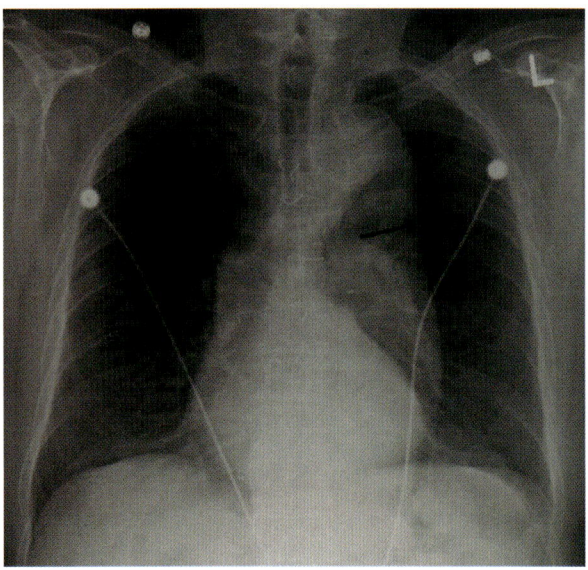

Thoracic aortic aneurysm

Ehlers-Danlos

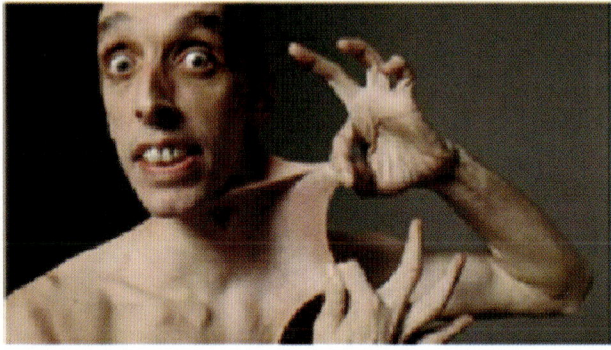

Elongated face, thin nose and lips, large eyes, easy bruising, thin skin with visible veins; rupture of arteries, uterus, intestines

Marfan's

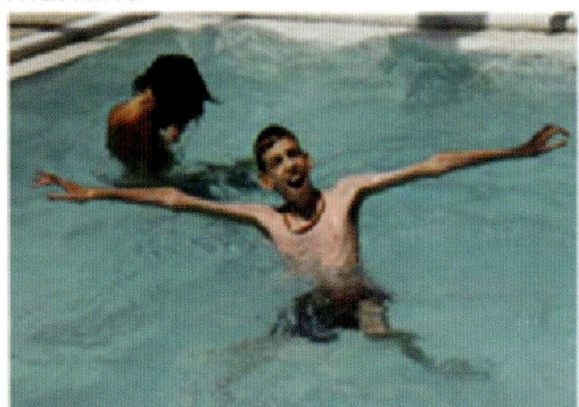

Thoracic Aortic Aneurysm[156][157][158][159][160][161]

- RFs: **Systemic HTN**, Marfan Sd (FBN1), Loeys-Dietz Sd (AD, ~ Marfan's but TGFBR1/2[#]), vascular Ehlers-Danlos Sd (COL3A1), bicuspid aortic valve (Turner 45,X), coarctation of aorta, FTAAD[$], pregnancy 3rd trimester
- Dissection: Ripping chest/interscapular tearing pain 'worst chest pain of my life' in hypertensive patient; **syncope, heart failure, stroke; plasma D-dimer < 500 ng/mL rules out** dissection (& PE)!
- Rx: If not in shock, lower HR (**60** bpm), BP (**120** mmHg): **IV β-blocker 1st** then nitroprusside (minimize reflex tachycardia)
- **Type A dissection: Sx; uncomplicated type B dissection: Rx medically**
- Dx: CT and MRI (TEE if unstable)
- Sx/Thoracic endovascular aortic repair (TEVAR):

– **≥ 5.5 cm***	"≥ 5.5
– **Expands > 0.5 cm in 6 months**	> 0.5 in 6
– **Symptoms (compression nearby structures)**	Symptoms Slash 'em!"

#Transforming growth factor β-receptor 1 or 2
*Aortic root (sinuses) or ascending aorta (nl < 3.7 cm)
(**Marfan's and BAV + other risk factors: Consider fix at ≥ 5.0 cm**; if BAV + severe AS/AR ≥ 4.5 cm); if wanting pregnancy, fix Marfan's > 4.5 cm; BAV aortopathy > 5.0 cm; if requite CABG fix > 4.5 cm. If BAV and > 4.5 cm or grows > 0.5 cm/yr do imaging every 6 months.
$Familial thoracic aortic aneurysm and dissection

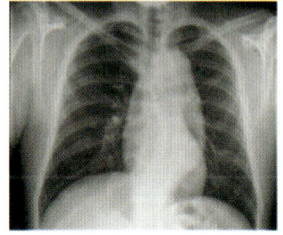

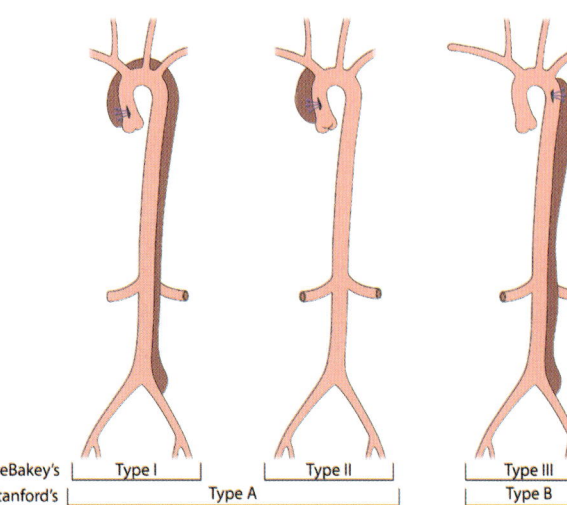

DeBakey's	Type I	Type II	Type III
Stanford's		Type A	Type B

Aneurysm (AAA)[162]

- RFs: **systemic HTN**, male, smoking, emphysema, cholesterol, obesity, genetics
- **65–75 years old**, most asymptomatic
- 80% of 5-cm aneurysms are palpable
- Grows faster (2–5 mm/year) than TAA
- Prefer CT or MRA size and location
- **Rarely chest/abdominal/lower back/scrotal pain or pulsating sensation**
- Sx/Endovascular aneurysm repair:
  - **≥ 5.5 cm (if 4.0–5.4 cm U/S / CT q 6–12 months)**
  - **Expands > 0.5 cm in 6 months**
  - **Symptoms (abdominal/back pain + pulsatile mass + hypotension)**

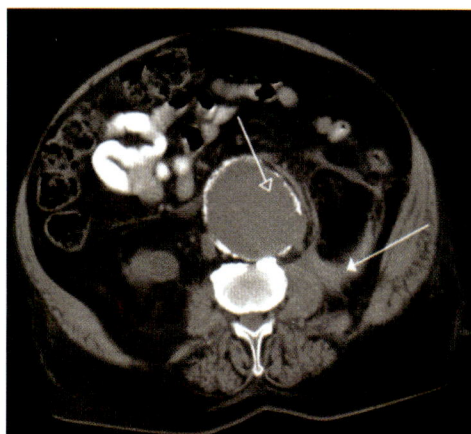

"≥ 5.5
> 0.5 in 6
Symptoms
Slash 'em!"

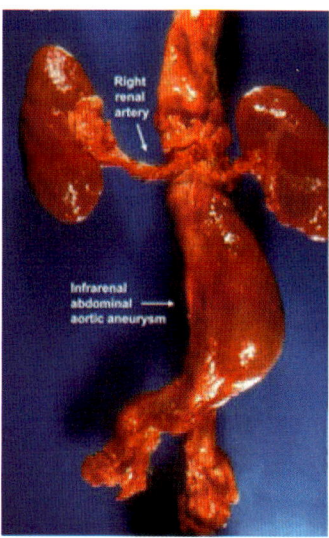

[163]

Endovascular Aneurysm Repair (EVAR)[164][165]

- **Stent** acts as a **sleeve**
- **Infrarenal** and/or **common iliac** aneurysms (supra- and juxtarenal aneurysms: open surgical repair)
- **Significantly improved short-term** (30-day) morbidity and mortality for EVAR (doesn't require operative aortic exposure or aortic clamping), but no significant differences in long-term outcomes **c/w open surgery**
- **Endoleaks** = persistent blood flow in the aneurysm sac after EVAR; incidence 10%: rupture risk 1.0%
- Rx: **Aspirin/Clopidogrel** and annual long-term imaging to monitor endoleak and stability of excluded aneurysm sac

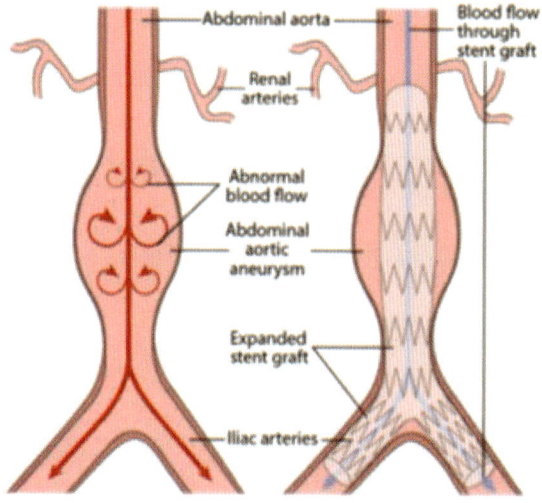

U.S. Preventive Services Task Force

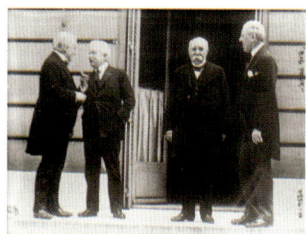

U.S. Preventive Services Task Force Screening AAA — Recommendation[166]

One-time screening for abdominal aortic aneurysm (AAA) by ultrasonography in **men 65–75** years of age who have **ever smoked (at least 100 cigarettes)**

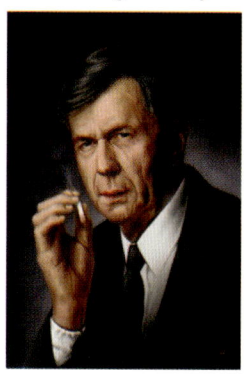

INFECTIVE ENDOCARDITIS (IE)

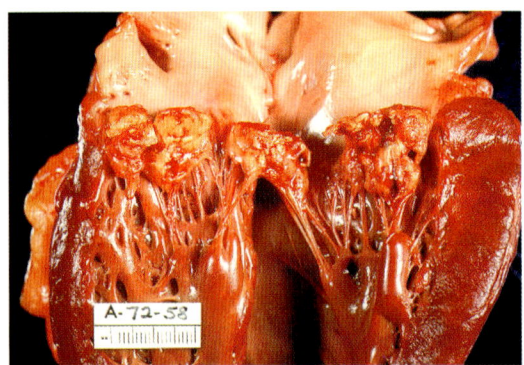

Male:Female Ratio 2:1

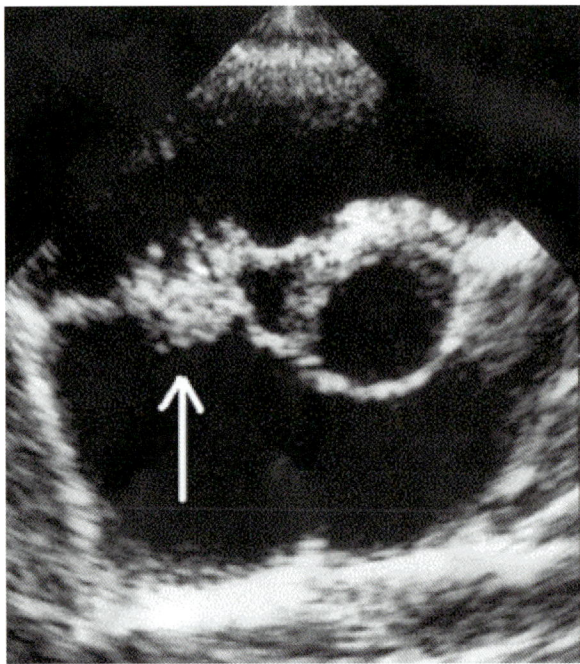

Arrow: tricuspid valve vegetation

IE — Pearls[167][168][169]
- **Staphylococcus** = the "IT" bug
  - No. 1 cause of IE, if:
    - **Native** valve (*S. aureus*)
    - **Prosthetic** valve (**CoNS***)
    - Cardiac **implantable** electronic device (CoNS/*S. aureus*)
- IE clinically suspicious → ≥ **2× blood cultures** then empirically Rx FOG (Fluclox/Ox+Gent) or VG Vanc+Gent (if penicllin allergy/methicillin-resistant staph)
- **Sensitivity: TTE 75% (always 1st line!), TEE 90%**
- IE and change (new murmur, embolism, persistent fever, HF, abscess, AV block) or high risk (extensive/large vegetations, staph/enterococcal/fungal) **reevaluate with TTE/TEE**
- **Modified Duke criteria**

*CoNS = coagulase-Negative *Staphylococcus* (e.g., *S. epidermidis*)

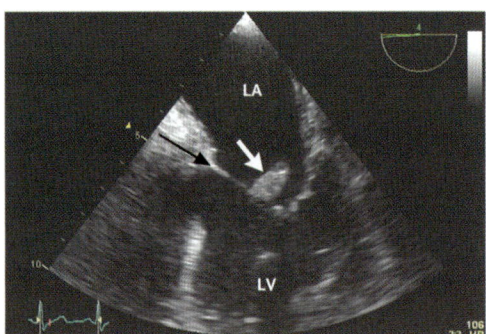

*TEE showing a large vegetation on a native **mitral valve** (most common valve affected)*

	Major Criteria
Bacterial	**Blood culture +ve**: Typical microorganisms (Viridans streptococci, *Streptococcus bovis*, HACEK, *Staphylococcus aureus*, or community-acquired enterococci) in 2 separate cultures or persistently +ve blood cultures drawn 12 hours apart or single +ve blood culture for *Coxiella burnetti*
Endocarditis @	**Endocardial involvement**: +ve echocardiogram (vegetation, abscess or valve dehiscence) or new valvular regurgitation
	Minor Criteria
F	**Fever** > 100.4°F (38.0°C)
I	**Immunologic phenomena**: Glomerulonephritis, Osler nodes, Roth spots, rheumatoid factor
VE	**Vascular emboli**: Major arterial emboli, septic pulmonary infarcts, mycotic aneurysm, intracranial hemorrhage, conjunctival hemorrhage, Janeway lesions, splinter hemorrhages
P	**Predisposition**: Heart condition or IV drug user
M !	**Microbiologic evidence**: + Blood culture — not meeting major criteria
Modified Duke criteria: Definite IE = 2M/5m/1M3m	

Janeway Lesions

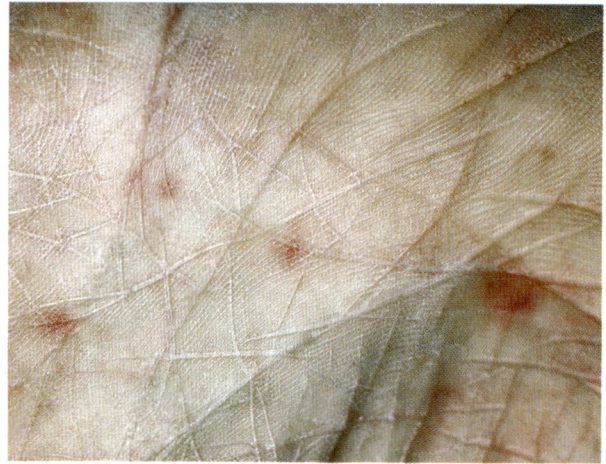

Flat, **painless** lesions on the palms and soles

Splinter Hemorrhage

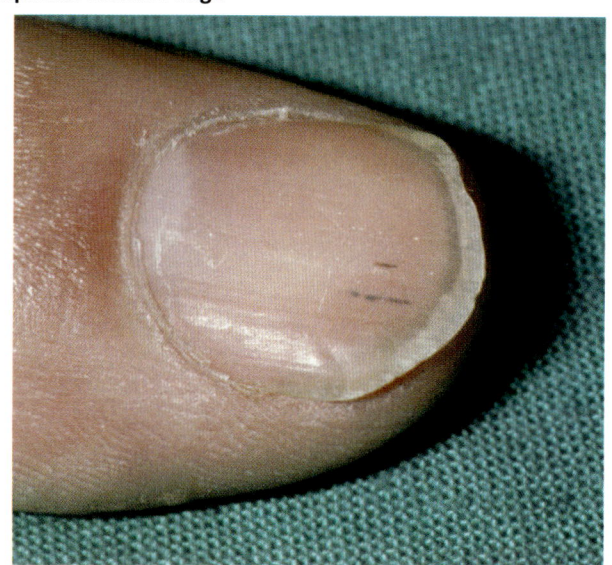

Etiology likely **thrombotic**

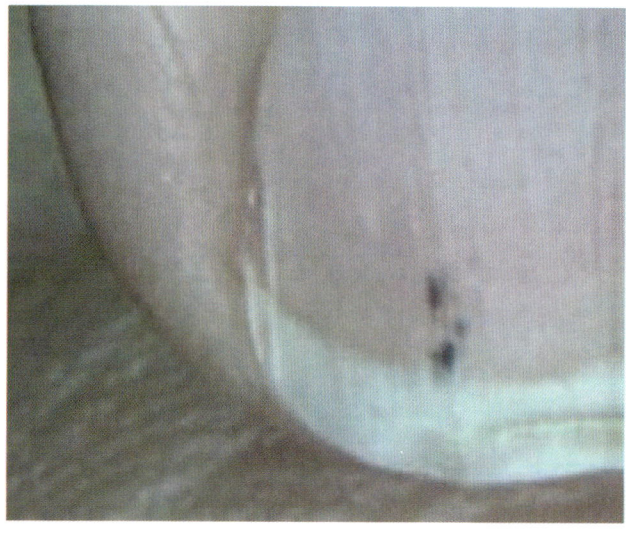

Osler Nodes

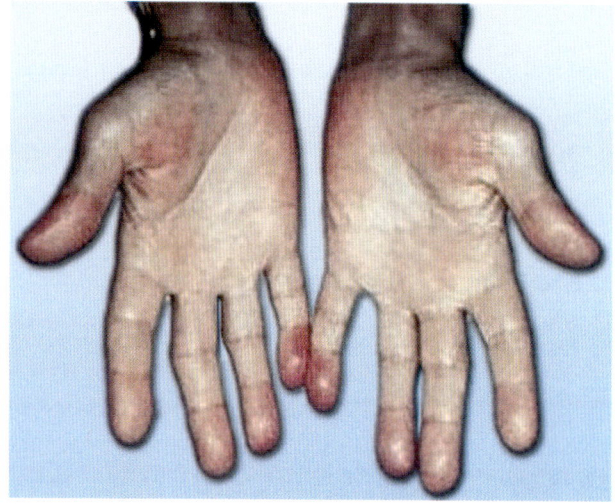

Painful raised lesions on the hands and feet

Osler knew everything — what a **pain**!!!

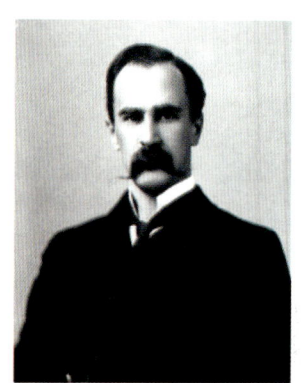

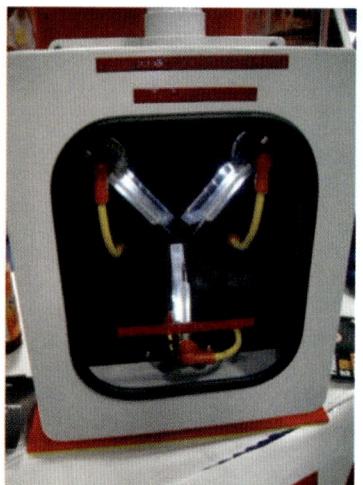

[170]

CARDIOLOGY

Roth Spots

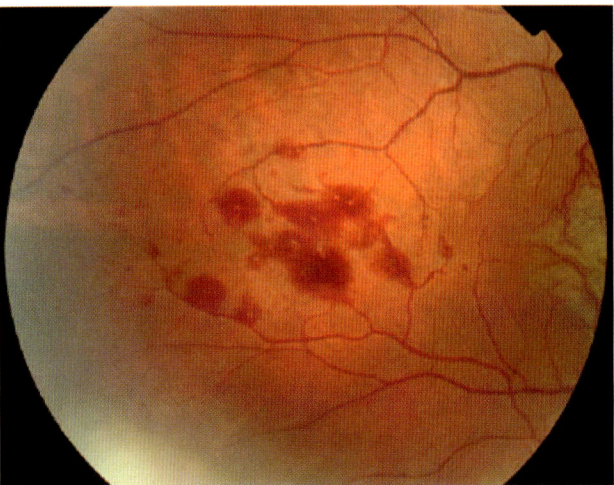

Retinal hemorrhages with white centers

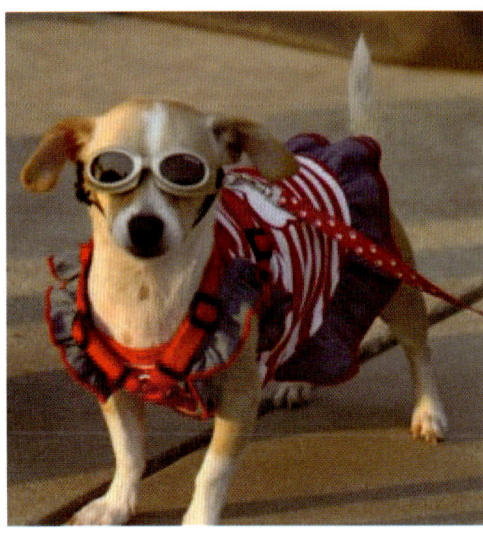

[171]

Endocarditis — Early Surgery[172][173]
- Valve dysfunction → **heart failure**
- L-sided IE from **S. aureus, fungal, highly resistant organism**
- **Heart block**, annular/aortic **abscess, destructive** penetrating lesions
- **Persistent infection > 5 days despite antibiotics**
- **Recurrent emboli/persistent vegetations** despite antibiotics
- **Prosthetic valve** endocarditis and **relapsing infection**

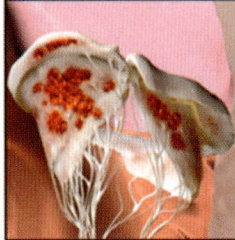

[174]

Mitral valve endocarditis

Cardiovascular Implantable Electronic Device (CIED) Infections[175][176]
Complete device (generator) and lead(s) removal:
1) **Definite CIED infection**: Valvular/lead endocarditis or sepsis
2) **CIED pocket infection**: Abscess formation, device erosion, skin adherence, or chronic draining sinus; <u>do not</u> aspirate device site!
3) **Valvular endocarditis** without involvement of the lead/device
4) **Occult staphylococcal bacteremia**
When infection is not in doubt, take it out!

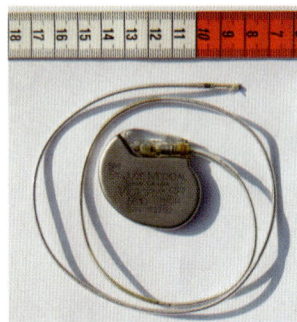

[177]

Antibiotic Prophylaxis — Highest-Risk Dental Patients Only![178][179]
- **Prosthetic valve** including transcatheter valve/prosthetics; e.g., annuloplasty rings or clips
- **Previous** infective endocarditis
- **Congenital heart disease** (CHD)
  - Unrepaired cyanotic CHD
  - Repaired CHD with residual shunts or valvular regurgitation on/near patch/device; **e.g., pulmonary atresia palliated with Blalock-Taussig shunt**
- **Cardiac transplant** with valve regurgitation
- **Only dental (teeth/gingiva/oral mucosa) need it!**
- Amoxicillin 2 g PO/Ampicillin 2 g IM/IV, cefalexin 2 g PO or clindamycin 600 mg PO/IM/IV or azithro-/clarithro-mycin 500 mg **30–60 mins before**

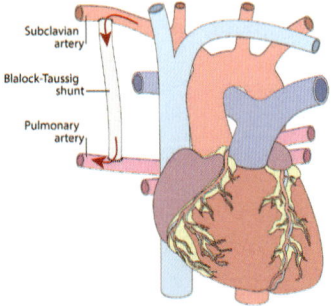

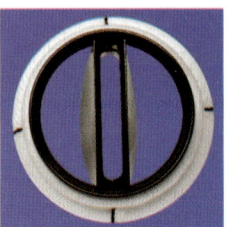

[180]

AORTIC STENOSIS (AS)

Males > Females

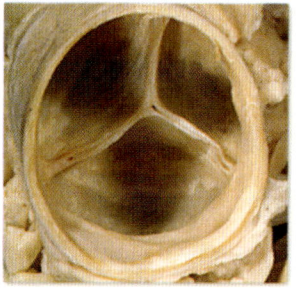 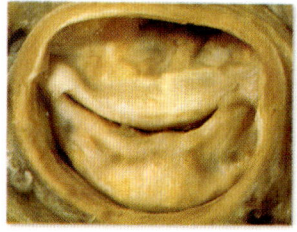

Normal   *Bicuspid valve with severe AS*

Bicuspid aortic valve = most common congenital cardiac anomaly: 1% stenosis 40–70 yo
Many: aortic root dilation
Murmur peaks **after** midsystole

AS Sx: 5 − 4 = 1 Rule![181][182]
- Symptomatic (angina/pre-syncope/HF) with severe **AS** (AVA ≤ **1.0** cm^2) with:
  A) Decreased valve opening and
  B) Aortic velocity ≥ **4.0** m/s (**peak** instantaneous gradient ≥ 64 mmHg) or **mean** P gradient ≥ **40** mmHg
- Asymptomatic with severe **AS** and LVEF < **50**% with velocity ≥ **4.0** m/s or mean P gradient ≥ **40** mmHg (if abnormal stress test, very severe AS, rapid progression, or elevated BNP: prefer **SAVR**)
- Severe **AS** undergoing cardiac surgery for other indications when velocity ≥ **4.0** m/s or mean P gradient ≥ **40** mmHg
- **Severe LV dysfunction with pseudostenosis vs. true AS** — Dobutamine stress if low EF: If velocity ≥ **4.0** m/s or mean P gradient ≥ **40** mmHg at any time → AVR; **discrepancy** clinical vs. echo, do **cardiac catheterization** gradient
- **TAVI (transcatheter aortic valve implantation)** if ≥ 65 years old & prohibitive/high/intermediate risk for surgical AVR and a predicted post-TAVI survival > 1 year risk (riskcalc.sts.org)
- **Heyde syndrome** = **GI bleeding** from **AVM** and AS **Rx** **SAVR** or **TAVI**

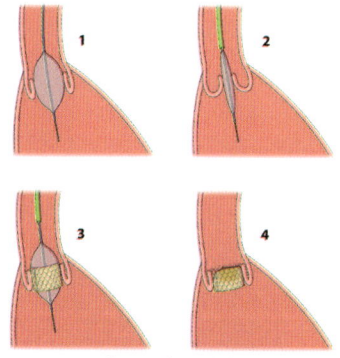

Transcatheter AVR

ACUTE AORTIC REGURGITATION (AR)

- **High index of suspicion** if **endocarditis, trauma, aortic dissection** and presents with tachycardia and hypotension
- PE: decrescendo **short** murmur
- **Sudden huge volume overload** on LV → rapid decompensation, shock, and death
- Dx: echo
- Positive **inotropic** therapy (dobutamine) and peripheral **vasodilation** (nitroprusside)
- Urgent CT **surgical** consult!

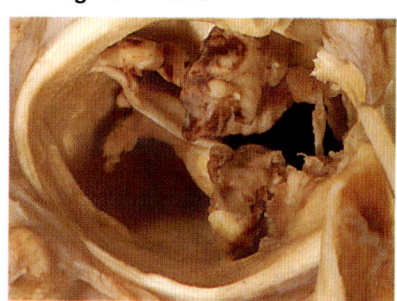

CHRONIC AORTIC REGURGITATION (AR)

Chronic Aortic Regurgitation (AR)[183]
- **Valve**: bicuspid valve (25%), rheumatic fever, endocarditis, degenerative/trauma
- **Aortic root**: Marfan, Loeys-Dietz, Ehlers-Danlos syndrome, pseudoxanthoma elasticum, HTN, osteogenesis imperfecta, ankylosing spondylitis, rheumatoid arthritis, giant cell arteritis, relapsing polychondritis, Behçet disease, syphilis
- Increased **peripheral pulse pressure** e.g., **160/60**
- High-pitched, blowing, **decrescendo murmur**
- **Watson's** water hammer pulse = rapid rise and fall in armor leg pulse; **C**orrigan's pulse ~ **c**arotid artery; **Quincke pulse** = nailbed capillary pulsations; **Duroziez sign** = to & fro murmur over partially compressed femoral artery; **Musset sign** = head bob with each pulse; **Austin Flint murmur**

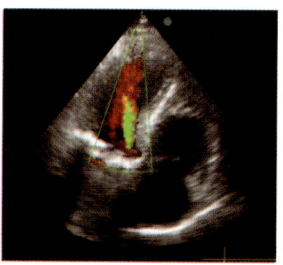

[184]

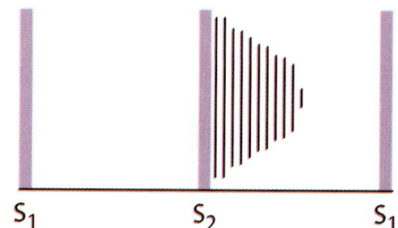

S_1 S_2 S_1

CARDIOLOGY

Chronic AR Sx — RS55 Rule![185][186][187]

- **S**ymptomatic w/ **S**evere A**R** — All!
- Asymptomatic w/ chronic **S**evere A**R** and LVEF < **55**% at rest if no other cause of systolic dysfunction
- Asymptomatic w/ chronic **S**evere A**R** and normal systolic function (LVEF ≥ **55**%) with severe LV dilation (LVESD > **50** mm or LVESD > 25 mm)
- Severe AR having cardiac surgery for other indications
- **Equivocal symptoms — do stress echo:** Exercise-induced increases in pulmonary systolic pressure to > 60 mmHg or 25-mm increase above baseline = hemodynamically significant AR → Sx

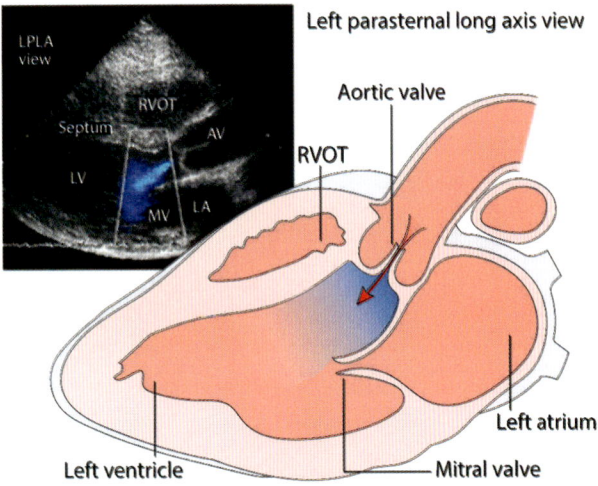

Left parasternal long axis view

MITRAL STENOSIS (MS)

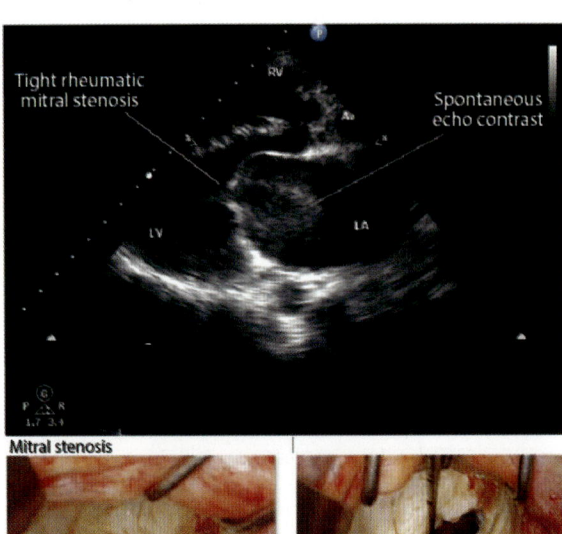

Mitral stenosis

Post commissurotomy

MS — PE

Mitral **S**tenosis

Diastolic **O**pening **S**nap

- **Etiology:** acute rheumatic fever: Group A β-hemolytic streptococci (*Streptococcus pyogenes*) — valvular dysfunction 20 years later
- **S₂-OS:** sudden opening MV → CT tensing → sudden reduction in leaflet motion (then low-pitched middiastolic rumble-bell at apex)
- **More severe MS** → higher LA press → earlier MV forced open in diastole → **smaller S₂-OS** (inverse relationship) & **longer** murmur duration!

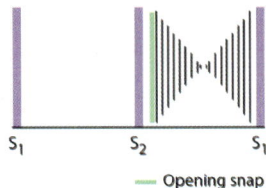

MS — Chest X-Ray

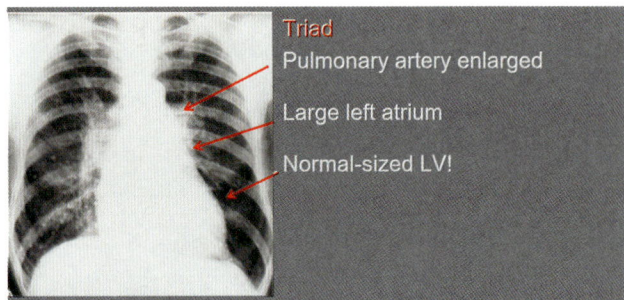

Triad
Pulmonary artery enlarged
Large left atrium
Normal-sized LV!

Fatigue, exertional dyspnea, orthopnea; atrial fibrillation

Chronic Severe MS — Sx[188][189][190]

- **Percutaneous mitral balloon commissurotomy** (PMBC) for symptomatic severe MS patients (**MVA ≤ 1.5 cm²**) and favorable valve morphology — **need TEE** (no LA thrombus, no moderate-to-severe MR; Wilkins score ≤ 8)
- MV surgery (**repair, or valve replacement**) for symptomatic patients (NYHA III–IV) with severe MS who are not high risk for surgery and not PMBC candidates/failed PMBC
- Concomitant MV surgery for severe MS patients undergoing cardiac surgery for other indications
- **Discrepancy** between clinical and echo findings: do **exercise echocardiography** to assess response of mitral gradient and pulmonary pressures

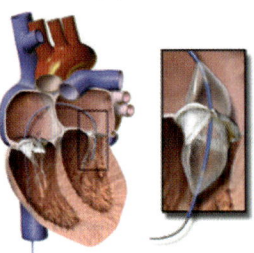

[191]

ACUTE MITRAL REGURGITATION (MR)

Acute MR[192]
- Causes
  - **Rupture of myxomatous chordae = most common cause!**
  - Endocarditis
  - Trauma
  - Ischemia of papillary muscle
- Present with **shock** ~ acute aortic regurgitation
- Positive **inotropic** therapy (dobutamine) and peripheral **vasodilation** (nitroprusside)
- **Intraaortic balloon pump**: Decreases LV afterload, increases forward output, decreases regurgitant volume
- Urgent cardiothoracic **surgical** consult!

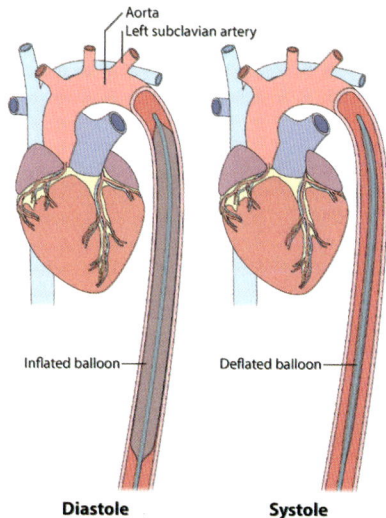

Diastole   Systole

CHRONIC MITRAL REGURGITATION (MR)

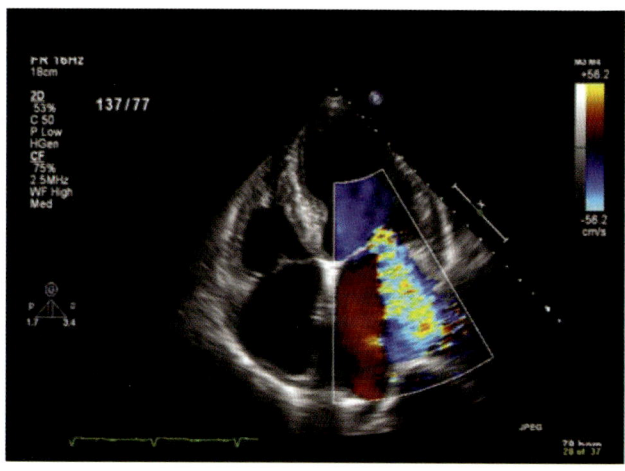

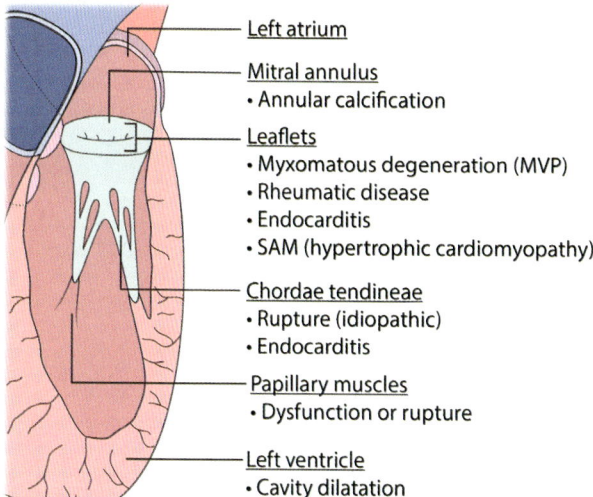

Left atrium

Mitral annulus
• Annular calcification

Leaflets
• Myxomatous degeneration (MVP)
• Rheumatic disease
• Endocarditis
• SAM (hypertrophic cardiomyopathy)

Chordae tendineae
• Rupture (idiopathic)
• Endocarditis

Papillary muscles
• Dysfunction or rupture

Left ventricle
• Cavity dilatation

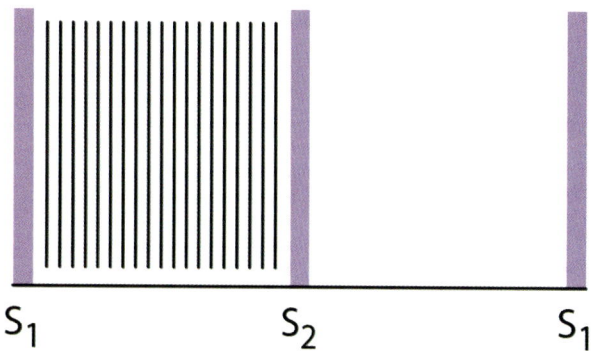

S_1 S_2 S_1

AR 14

A 51-year-old man with MR is inactive and has a desk job. He denies symptoms, watches movies and drinks beer on weekends. PE: BMI 32 kg/m², BP 115/70 mmHg, pulse 80 bpm. CVS: PMI diffuse 5th ICS midclavicular line and forceful, with a grade 4/6 systolic murmur heard loudest at apex, radiating to the axilla. CXR: Prominent LV; ECG: NSR, LAE, borderline LVH.

TTE: Thickened myxomatous mitral valve, severe MR; EF 45%; LV end-systolic diameter (LVESD) = 4.8 cm (normal ≤ 2.6 cm).

What is the most appropriate treatment for this patient?

A. Start lisinopril and repeat TTE in 6 months.
B. Refer for mitral valve repair/replacement.
C. Start long-acting nifedipine and repeat TTE in 6 months.
D. Follow in clinic closely and repeat TTE annually.
E. Refer for percutaneous mitral balloon commissurotomy.

Answer:_____

Chronic MR Sx — 6040 Rule![193][194][195]

- **Sym**ptomatic (HF, DOE, decr. ex toler) with chronic severe primary **MR**
- Asymptomatic with chronic severe primary **MR** and LV EF ≤ **60**% and/or LV end-systolic diameter (LVESD) ≥ **40** mm (consider if serial incr. in LVESD/decr. in EF; **clinical and echo follow-up every 6–12 months**)
- **MV repair preferred** to replacement
- Chronic severe secondary MR (valve/valve apparatus normal) with severe symptoms despite GDMT consider transcatheter interventions — need TEE
- Transcatheter MV repair (**MitraClip**) — high risk/ refused Sx
- Concomitant mitral valve repair/replacement if chronic severe primary MR undergoing cardiac surgery already

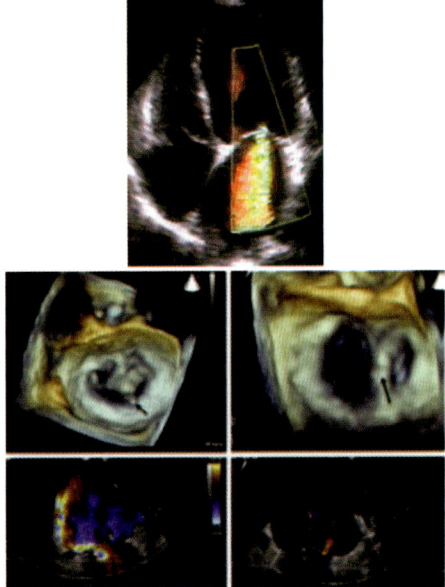

[196]

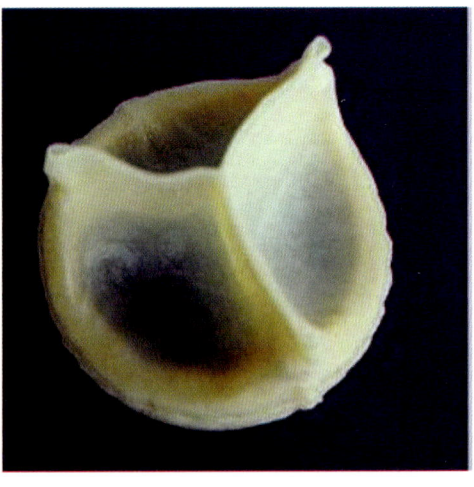

[200]

 St. Jude bileaflet mechanical valve

 Tilting disc mechanical valve

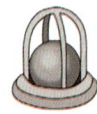 Starr-Edwards mechanical valve

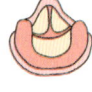 Porcine bioprosthetic valve

- < 50 yo: mechanical prosthesis if anticoagulation OK
- 50–70 yo: mechanical or bioprosthesis (patient factors)
- > 70 yo: bioprosthesis (younger if cannot anticoagulate): porcine (pig) or bovine (cow); 10- to 15-year life

PROSTHETIC HEART VALVES

Prosthetic Heart Valves[197][198]

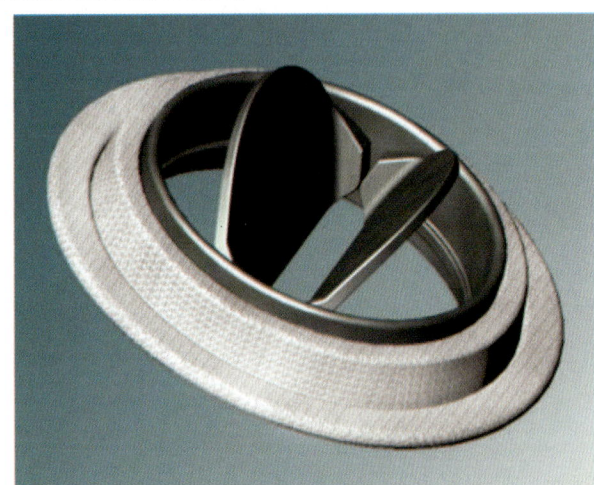

[199]

AR 15

A 60-year-old woman just underwent surgery and a mitral mechanical valve was placed last week. She is otherwise healthy and is on warfarin. Examination reveals a crisp mechanical S_1, a normal S_2, and no murmurs.

What antithrombotic medication should she take?

A. Warfarin
B. Clopidogrel and aspirin
C. Apixaban
D. Warfarin and aspirin
E. Aspirin

Answer:_____

Prosthetic Valves — Antithrombotic Tx[201]

- **Vitamin K antagonists (VKAs)**; e.g., warfarin for mechanical prosthetic valve
- **Mechanical AVR** (bileaflet or current single tilting disc): **INR 2.5**; if thromboembolic risk factors (AFib, previous thromboembolism, LV dysfunction, hypercoagulable state) or older-generation (ball-in-cage): **INR 3.0**
- **Mechanical MVR: INR 3.0**
- **Aspirin 75 mg to 100 mg** daily in addition to VKA **in all** mechanical valve prosthesis to **reduce risk of ischemic events**
- **Bioprosthetic valves**: 3–6 months **INR 2.5**

Prosthetic Valves — Sx Procedures[202][203]

- **Continue VKA anticoagulation** if **minor procedures** (dental extractions/cataract removal)
- **Stop anticoagulation 5 days prior** (no bridging) **for bileaflet mechanical AVR** and no thromboembolism risk factors having invasive/surgical procedures
- **Bridging anticoagulation** (IV UFH/subcutan LMWH) pre-op if invasive/surgical procedures with:
  1) Mechanical AVR and any thromboembolic risk factor
  2) Older-generation mechanical AVR, or
  3) Mechanical MVR
- **FFP/prothrombin complex concentrate:** emergency surgery/procedures

Prosthetic Valves — Surgery[204][205]

- **TTE/TEE/fluroscopy/gated cardiac CT** if suspect thrombosis/valve dysfunction
- **Fibrinolysis (slow-infusion)** or **emergency surgery** if **thrombosed** left-sided **mechanical prosthetic** valve with **symptoms**
- **VKA** if **thrombosed bioprosthetic** valve
- **Repeat valve replacement** for severe symptomatic prosthetic valve **stenosis**
- **High risk bioprosthetic aortic valve stenosis/regurg.** → transcatheter **valve-in-valve**
- **Surgery** for patients with mechanical heart valves with intractable **hemolysis/HF** due to severe prosthetic or paravalvular leak (high risk → catheter-based Tx)

Lecture 4

L4 Outline

- **Arrhythmias**
- **Supraventricular Arrhythmias**
- **Ventricular Arrhythmias**
- **Pacemakers**
- **Syncope**
- **Hypertrophic Cardiomyopathy (HCM)**
- **Heart Failure**
- **Acute Pericarditis**
- **Constrictive Pericarditis**
- **Restrictive Cardiomyopathy "Filet Mignon Heart"**

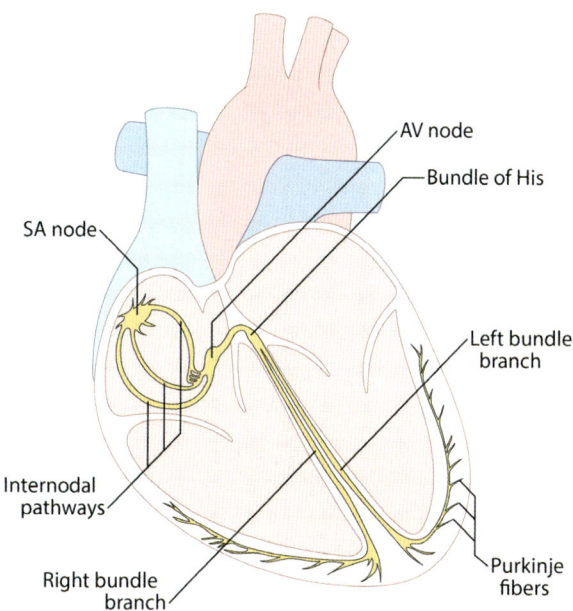

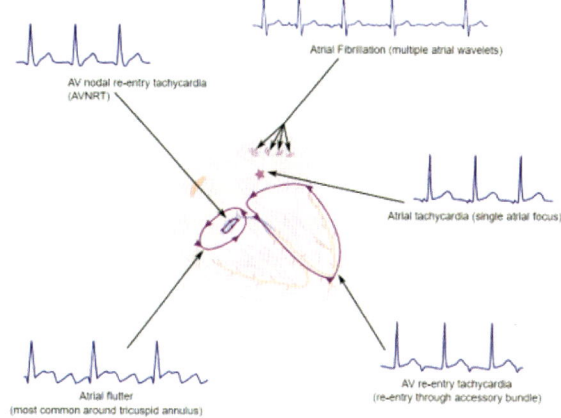

[206]

Arrhythmias — Pearls[207][208][209]

- 90% are **reentrant**; TTE to rule out structural heart disease
- **Narrow** QRS tachycardias = **supraventricular**
- Bradycardia/symptoms during **sleep**: consider **OSA**
- **Smartphone-based:** for tech-savvy patient
- **Holter monitor (24–72 hours)**: for frequent arrhythmias
- **Event recorders/External loop recorder** for symptoms likely to recur within 2–6 weeks
- **External patch recorder** for symptoms likely to recur within 2–14 days
- **Implantable cardiac monitor** for recurrent but infrequent arrhythmia (2–3 year battery)

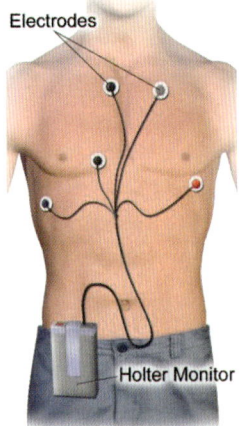

Electrodes

Holter Monitor

Holter Monitor

[210]

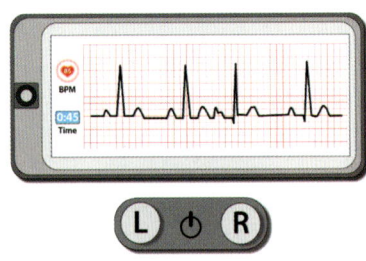

SUPRAVENTRICULAR ARRHYTHMIAS

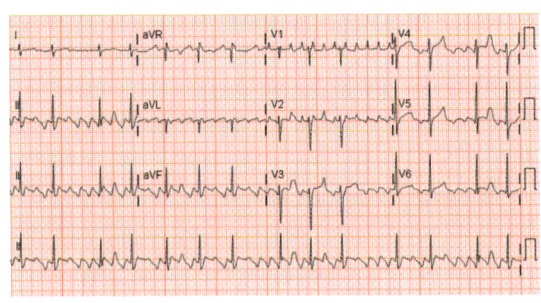

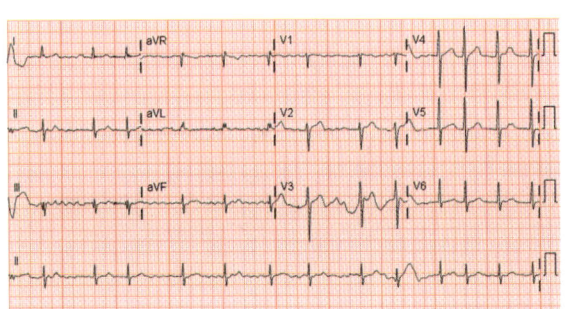

Atrial flutter

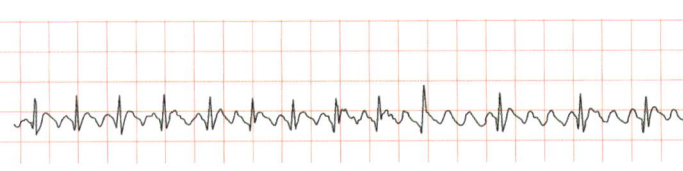

Atrial fibrillation

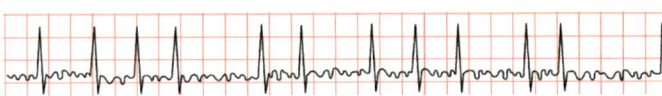

"In the supraventricular system, the people are represented by 2 separate, yet equally important arrhythmias: **Atrial flutter**, which is regular, **and atrial fibrillation**, which is highly irregular. These are their stories!!"

ATRIAL FLUTTER

AR 16

A 76-year-old female had atrial flutter 1 month ago and was cardioverted to normal sinus rhythm. She reports palpitations again, is fatigued, and cannot exercise. ECG today shows recurrent atrial flutter, ventricular rate 71 bpm.

PMH: hypertension, HFpEF, diabetes, hyperlipidemia
Meds: apixaban, metoprolol, lisinopril, metformin, rosuvastatin
PE: Irregular pulse, otherwise normal. Echo post cardioversion showed EF 55%, left atrial dilation, diastolic dysfunction

What is the most appropriate treatment?

A. Cardiac catheterization
B. Cardioversion
C. Catheter ablation
D. Do nothing.

Answer:_____

Atrial Flutter[211]

- Atria 250–300 bpm; vent. 100–150 bpm; "Sawtooth" II, III, aVF
- Typical/**Type I = cavotricuspid isthmus (CTI)-dependent** counterclockwise running **between IVC and tricuspid valve**
- **Vagal maneuvers/AV nodal blockers** — slow ventricular response; often have structural heart disease or COPD
- **Rx = same as AFib! Acute: DC cardioversion if unstable**; pharm cardioversion in hemodynamically. stable: dofetilide or IV ibutilide; **chronic:** BB, dilt, or verapamil
- Symptoms despite meds: **Catheter ablation (95% success)**

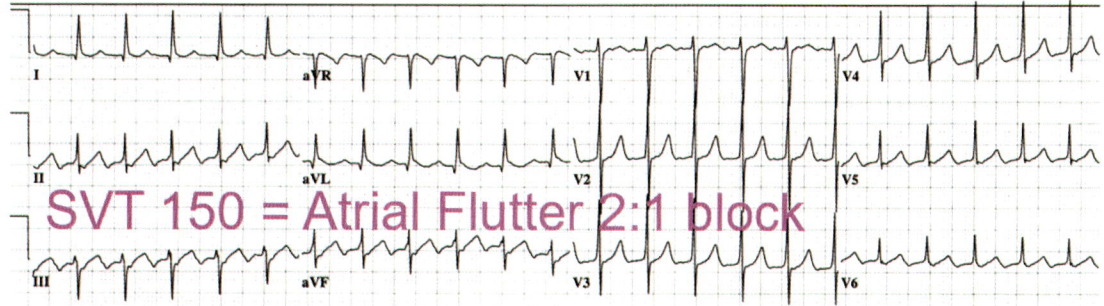

SVT 150 = Atrial Flutter 2:1 block

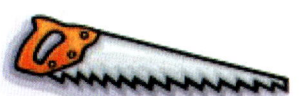

ATRIAL FIBRILLATION (AFib)

- Irregular atrial fibrillatory (f) waves
- Multiple macro reentrant circuits
- Ventricular rate 100–180 bpm

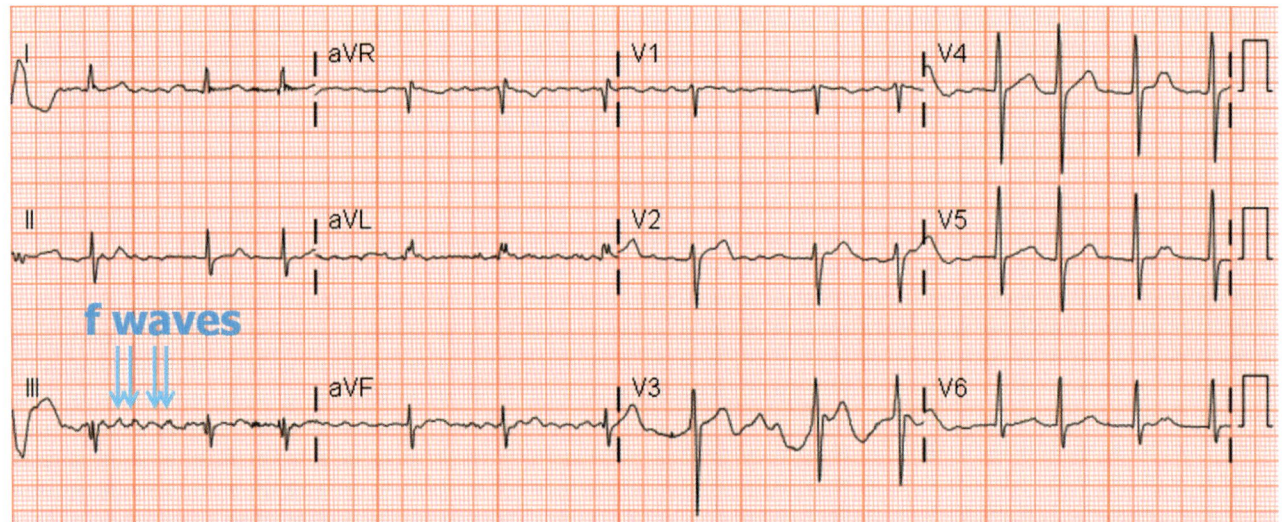

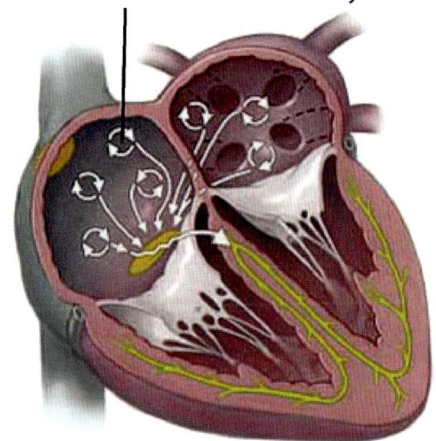

Abnormal Electrical Pathways

Atrial Fibrillation

AFib — Classification[212][213]

1) **Paroxysmal:** self-terminating, **≤ 7 days**
2) **Persistent:** continuous, **> 7 days**
3) **Long-standing persistent: > 12 months**
4) **Permanent: Continuous** and no further attempts to restore/maintain sinus rhythm
5) **Nonvalvular: Absence** of rheumatic mitral stenosis, mechanical/bioprosthetic heart valve, or mitral valve repair

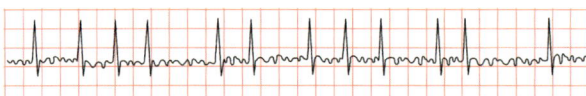

AFib — Rate Control[214][215]

Goal	Strict: 80 bpm at rest, or 110 bpm during 6-min walk; resting heart rate < 110 bpm acceptable if EF ≥ 40% and no/acceptable symptoms; weight loss
Acute AFib	IV: BBs (esmolol, metoprolol T, propranolol), non-dihydropyridine-CCBs (diltiazem, verapamil) block myocyte calcium channels, digoxin, amiodarone
Chronic AFib	BBs (atenolol, metoprolol T/S, propranolol, nadolol, carvedilol, bisoprolol), NDP-CCBs (diltiazem, verapamil), digoxin
Heart failure & AFib	HFpEF: BBs (metoprolol succinate, carvedilol) or NDP-CCBs; HFrEF: BBs, dofetilide, digoxin, amiodarone (IV to control heart rate acutely)
AFib & ACS (hemodynamically stable, no HF or bronchospasm)	IV BBs
Unstable AFib (myocardial ischemia, hypotension, HF, or inadequate rate control)	Synchronized cardioversion

AFib — Rate vs. Rhythm Control[216]
- No difference in life quality, morbidity, or mortality
- Maintain sinus rhythm in highly symptomatic patients:
  - **Cardioversion:** electrical (Hemod. Unstable); IV flecainide, IV dofetilide, IV propafenone, IV ibutilide (no structural heart disease); IV amiodarone (structural heart disease)
  - **Maintenance:** class I (flecainide, propafenone [both CI:HF]) or III (amiodarone = best drug if structural HD, sotalol*, dronedarone both CI:HF, dofetilide)

*Chronic kidney disease → increased torsades

AFib — Anticoagulation[217][218][219][220]
- **Lone AFib:** No clinical/echo findings of other cardiac/pulmonary disease, or abnormalities such as left atrial enlargement, HTN, and age < 60
  Rx: aspirin/nothing
- **Valvular AFib:** rheumatic mitral stenosis, mechanical heart valve, bioprosthetic heart valve ≤ 3 months*, mitral valve repair
  Rx: vitamin K antagonists (VKA) = warfarin (Coumadin, Jantoven)
- **Hypertrophic cardiomyopathy: Rx DOAC** 1st line (warfarin 2nd line) independent of **CHA2DS2-VASc score**
- **Nonvalvular AFib: Rx: CHA2DS2-VASc**

* bioprosthetic > 3 months Rx warfarin/DOAC

AR 17
A 67-year-old African American female patient has permanent atrial fibrillation. She is taking metoprolol succinate for rate control, lisinopril for hypertension, and metformin for T2DM. Her labs are normal, including normal renal function. She refuses to take warfarin.

What would you recommend for her anticoagulation?

A. Aspirin 25 mg + dipyridamole extended-release 200 mg/day
B. Aspirin 325 mg/day
C. Dabigatran 150 mg twice a day
D. Dabigatran 75 mg twice a day
E. Clopidogrel 75 mg/day

Answer:_____

Nonvalvular AFib CHA$_2$DS$_2$-VASc & Rx[221][222]

C	**C**HF (any history) / LVEF ≤ 40%	1
H	**H**TN (any history)	1
A$_2$	**A**ge ≥ 75	2
D	**D**M	1
S$_2$	**S**troke, TIA, or thromboembolism	2
V	**V**ascular disease (prior MI, PAD, or aortic plaque)	1
A	**A**ge 65–74	1
Sc	**S**ex **c**ategory (female)	1
	Rx	
0 men or 0–1 women	None	
1 men or 2 women	ASA 81–325 mg/day or no Rx	
≥ 2 men OR ≥ 3 women	DOAC Dabigatran, rivaroxaban, apixaban, edoxaban [preferred over warfarin except if moderate-severe MS or mechanical heart valve], **warfarin (INR 2.0–3.0), or LAA-occluding device** if can't take long term anticoagulation; **caution required if HAS-BLED ≥ 3**	

Dabigatran (Pradaxa)[182]

- **D**irect thrombin inhibitor; cannot comply with warfarin (transition at INR < 2.0)
- 150 mg bid; CrCl 15–30 mL/min: 75 mg bid; **Don't use if CrCl < 15 mL/min or on dialysis**; Idarucizumab (Praxbind) to reverse if life-threatening bleeding of urgent procedure;
  e.g., **GI bleed — transfuse packed RBCs and give idarucizumab**
- Cr initial and annually; **no need to heparin bridge**
- Inhibitors of **P**-glycoprotein (**C**larithromycin, **A**miodarone/Dronedarone, **T**icagrelor, **Ver**apamil, **K**etoconazole) → Toxic!

Rivaroxaban (Xarelto), Apixaban (Eliquis), Edoxaban (Savaysa)

- **RAEF**: **R**ivarox **(20 mg daily)** **A**pix **(5 mg bid)** **E**dox **(60 mg daily)** = **F**actor 10a inhibitors (transition at INR ≤ 2.5)
- **Rivar**oxaban: **STRONG** inhibitors of **CYP**3A4 (**N**efazodone, **P**rotease inhibitors, **K**etoconazole, **I**traconazole, **C**larithromycin; avoid with **RIVA**roxaban and P-glycoprotein → toxicity
- **CKD: CrCl < 50 mL/min:** Rivaroxaban 15 mg daily, edoxaban 30 mg daily; apixaban 2.5 mg bid (age ≥ 80 yo or body wt ≤ 60 kg/132 lbs + serum Cr ≥ 1.5 mg/dL)
- **A**ge ≥ 75/high risk for **A**nemia(GI)/**A**cting up kidneys (& dialysis) = **A**pixaban; CYP3A4 inhibitors → toxicity
- **CKD CrCl < 15 or on dialysis: coumadin or apixaban**

AR 18

A 77-year-old woman is seen for routine clinic follow-up. She is chest pain free and feels good. PMH: HTN, hyperlipidemia, CAD s/p LCx stent 3 years ago. Meds: aspirin, metoprolol, ramipril, atorvastatin.

PE: Vital signs normal. Heart sounds irregularly irregular. Remainder of physical is normal. ECG shows atrial fibrillation, average ventricular rate 72 beats per minute.

Which of the following is the most appropriate treatment?

A. Add oral anticoagulation.
B. Add clopidogrel and oral anticoagulation.
C. Add clopidogrel.
D. Stop aspirin and begin oral anticoagulation.

Answer:_____

Prevent Thromboembolism[223][224][225]

- <u>AFib/atrial flutter **≥ 48 h or unknown**</u>: 3 weeks before and 4 weeks after cardioversion (electrical/ pharmacologic)
- **<u>Hemodyn unstable</u>** <u>AFib/atrial flutter ≥ 48 h</u>: 4 weeks after cardioversion
- <u>AFib/atrial flutter < 48 h and **high risk stroke**</u>: IV heparin, LMWH, DTI or Factor 10a inhibitor ASAP before cardioversion, then per **CHA$_2$DS$_2$-VASc**
- <u>**CAD**</u>: **Recent ACS/stent (≤ 12 months) & AFib: DAPT + CHA$_2$DS$_2$-VASc anticoag (≥ 6 weeks)**
- **Stable CAD > 12 months & AFib: STOP DAPT + oral anticoagulation (CHA$_2$DS$_2$-VASc)**
- <u>Sx</u> & **NOAC**: stop

1 day — Minor	Sx/procedure; e.g., colonoscopy
2 days — Major	Sx/spinal anesthesia; e.g., kidney biopsy

Ablation for Sinus Rhythm[226][227]

- Catheter ablation → **pulmonary vein isolation**
- **Symptomatic paroxysmal AFib refractory or intolerant** to at least one class **I (flecainide, propafenone)** or **III (amiodarone, dronedarone, sotalol, dofetilide*)** antiarrhythmic when rhythm-control strategy desired (symptomatic AF and HFrEF may also benefit)
- Complications: PV stenosis/occlusion 2% (dyspnea), stroke/TIA 1% tamponade 1%; atrio-esophageal fistula (sudden-onset neurological symptoms from esophageal air embolization), AV fistula, groin hematoma, death
- <u>**CI**</u>: If cannot be anticoagulated: 2 months post procedure & indefinitely if **CHA$_2$DS$_2$-VASc ≥ 2**

*Start inpatient; CI: HCTZ, trimethoprim, ketoconazole, megestrol, verapamil, prochlorperazine, QT$_c$ long

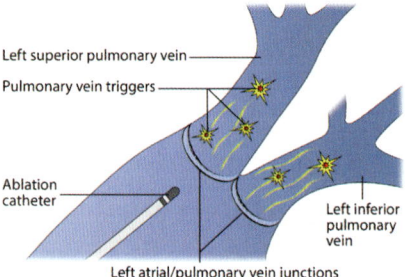

Ablation for Rate Control[228]

- AV nodal catheter ablation with permanent ventricular pacing when:
  - Medical therapy inadequate, and
  - Rhythm control not achievable
- **Improves exercise tolerance, LVEF, and quality of life**
- 6% 1-year mortality (~ to antiarrhythmic therapy)
- Continue anticoagulation if **CHA$_2$DS$_2$-VASc ≥ 2**
  - Can have brief asymptomatic AFib

VENTRICULAR ARRHYTHMIAS

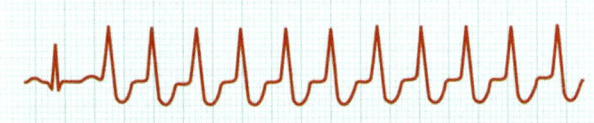

Ventricular tachycardia

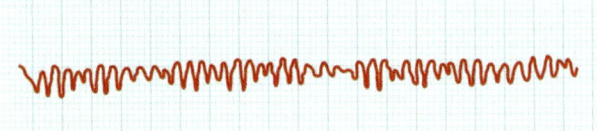

Ventricular fibrillation

Premature Ventricular Complexes (PVCs) — a.k.a. Ventricular Extrasystoles[229]

- Wide abnormal QRS
- Compensatory pause
- Rare PVCs are normal (75% of healthy persons!)
- Symptomatic/frequent monomorphic PVCs (> 10,000 in 24 hours or > 10%) — with normal heart Rx BB or NDP-C

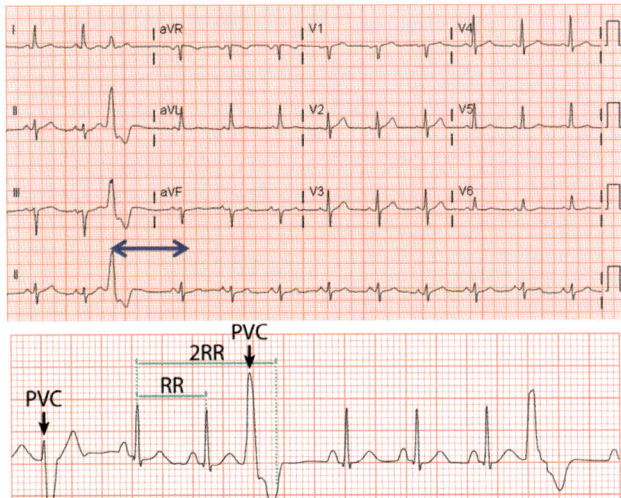

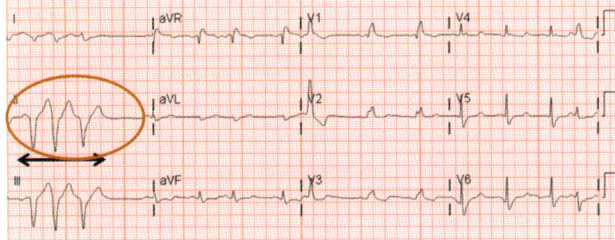

Nonsustained Ventricular Tachycardia (NSVT)[230]

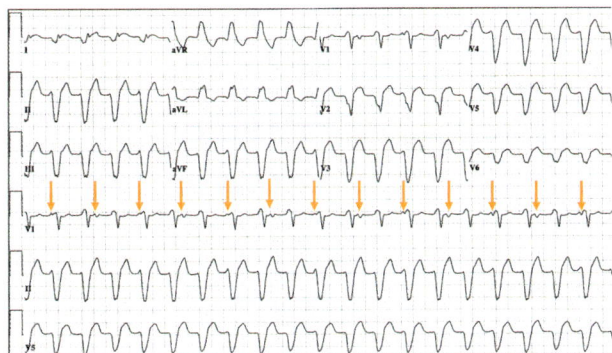

≥ 3 sequential PVCs at ≥ 100 bpm

Sustained Ventricular Tachycardia (> 30 sec)

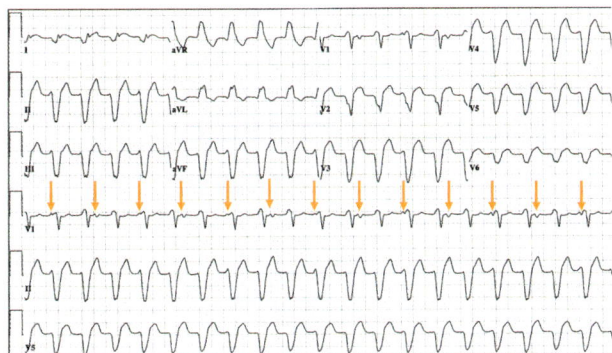

AV dissociation. This ECG negative concordance = impulse initiated in apex — must be VT.

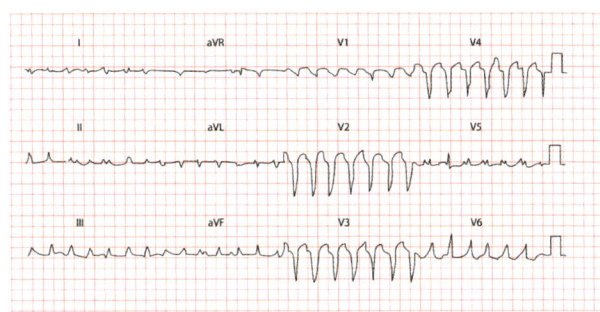

Ventricular Tachycardia (VT) — Dx

- 90% of wide-complex (QRS > 140 msec) tachycardias = VT; more Vs than As
- Associated with structural heart disease
- The wider and "uglier" the QRS, more likely VT
- AV dissociation; fusion beats; cannon *a* waves
- Shortening of QRS — if broad in sinus rhythm
- **Capture (Dressler's) beats** = a normal QRS complex identical to the sinus QRS complex, occurring during the VT at a rate faster than VT (the normal conduction system has momentarily captured control of ventricular activation from the VT focus)

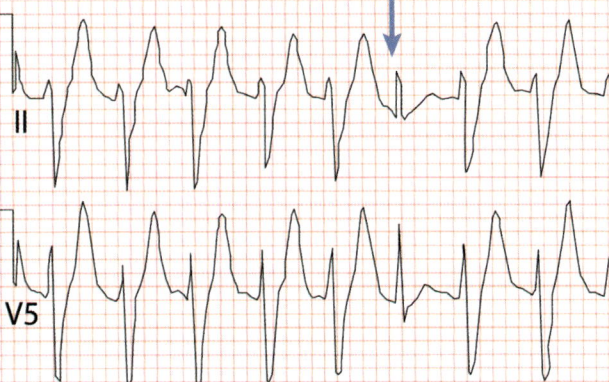

CARDIOLOGY

VT — Management
- **Unstable**
  - Synchronized cardioversion
- **Stable**
  - Correct reversible causes (electrolytes, ischemia)
  - Amiodarone 150 mg IV over 10 minutes ± infusion
  - Metoprolol 5 mg IV if VT in structurally normal heart; e.g., RVOT VT

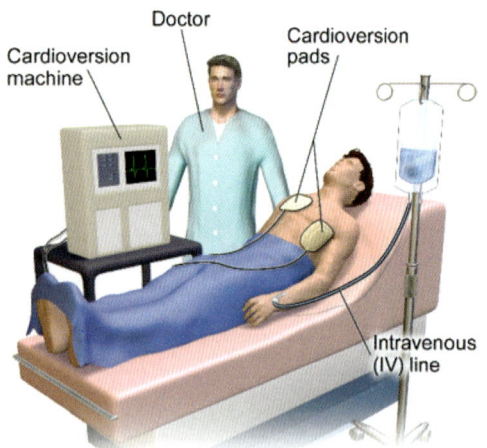

Cardioversion

[231]

VENTRICULAR FIBRILLATION (VFib)
- **Chaotic** irregular deflections of varying amplitude
- **No discernible** P waves, QRS complexes, or T waves
- Rate 150 to 500 per minute

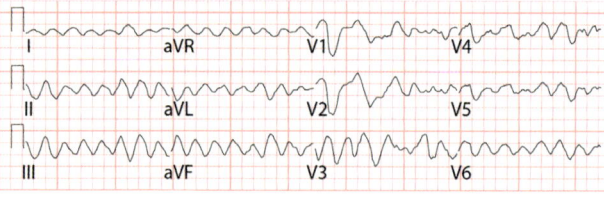

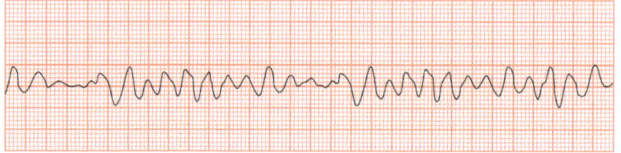

PACEMAKERS

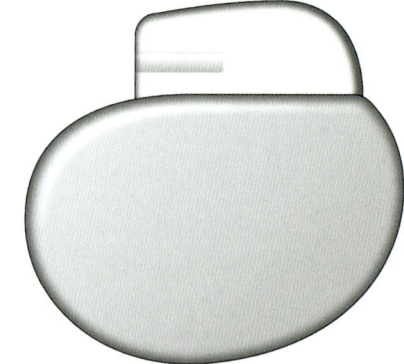

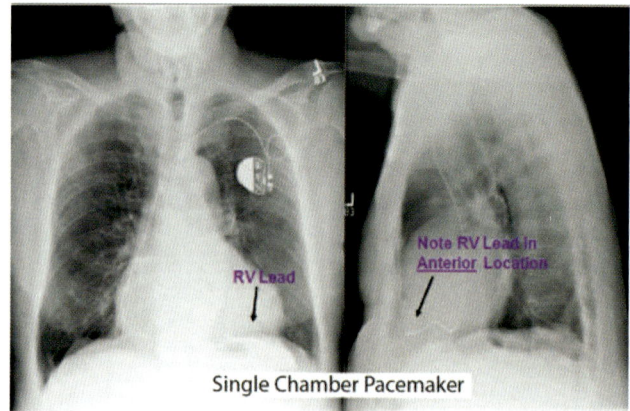

Single Chamber Pacemaker

Permanent Pacing Indications[232][233][234]

- **Symptomatic bradycardia from required med Rx, sinus node dysfunction (atrial-based pacing best), sinus pauses, chronotropic incompetence (cannot get to 80% MPHR)**
- **Symptomatic 2nd and 3rd degree AV block (dual-chamber pacing best if also have sinus node dysfunction)**, asystole ≥ 3.0 seconds or escape rate < 40 bpm
- **Symptomatic:** AFib and bradycardia, or pauses **≥ 5 seconds**
- **Syncope** and BBB with infranodal block or HV interval ≥ 70 msec at EP study
- **Asymptomatic** advanced 2nd degree and 3rd degree AV block
- **Asymptomatic alternating (bifascicular) BBB**

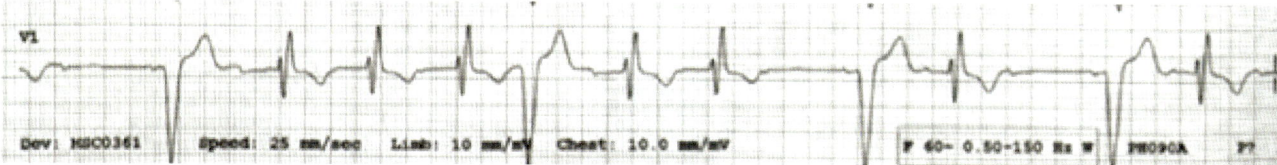

SYNCOPE

1922 vs. 2022

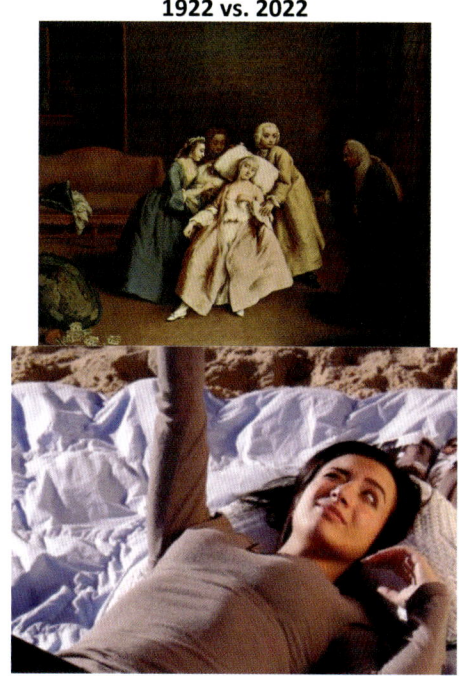

Syncope — Definitions and Causes[235][236]
- **Transient** loss of consciousness **and postural tone**
- **Cerebral** hypoperfusion; SBP ≤ 60 mmHg
- **Rapid** onset, brevity (< 30 seconds), and spontaneous recovery
- 3 main types:

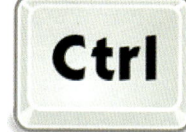 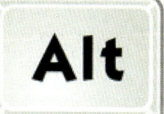 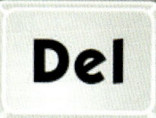

1) Neurocardiogenic (Reflex, Neurally Mediated, Vasovagal, Vasodepressor) = Most Common Cause[237]
- **Hypotension and vasodilation with absolute/relative bradycardia**
- **Prodrome**: Diaphoresis, pallor, palpitations, "tunnel vision," nausea, hyperventilation, yawning, head rotation (carotid sinus); **situational syncope (cough, micturition)**
- **Vasovagal/"common faint"**: Precipitated by **stress/pain/claustrophobia**
- **Carotid Sinus Sd**: Syncope during carotid sinus massage (asystole > 3 secs [Rx PPM], and/or ≥ 50 mmHg SBP drop); men > 40 years of age (contraindications to massage: MI/stroke within 3 months, carotid bruits)
- Rx: **Avoid triggers (prolonged standing, warm environments), incr. fluid/salt intake (sports drinks); midodrine (α-agonist) 2.5–10 mg tid if no HTN, HF, or urinary retention** (take 1st dose 30 mins after waking up before getting out of bed & last dose of day before 5 p.m. to avoid supine hypertension)

2) Orthostatic (Postural) Hypotension[238][239]

- **321** Rule! Within **3** minutes of standing, drop in SBP ≥ **2**0 (or to < 90 mmHg) or DBP ≥ **1**0 mmHg
- **Insufficient** peripheral vasoconstriction/increase HR
- **Neurogenic**: autonomic neuropathy — Parkinson's, diabetes
- **Drugs**: diuretics, vasodilators, negative chronotropes
- **Dehydration/massive hemorrhage**

Rx:
- **Water ingestion or IV bolus; incr. salt intake; hold meds**
- **Counter measure maneuvers;** e.g., leg crossing, squatting, tensing of legs/buttocks; **compression garments**
- Medications don't work!

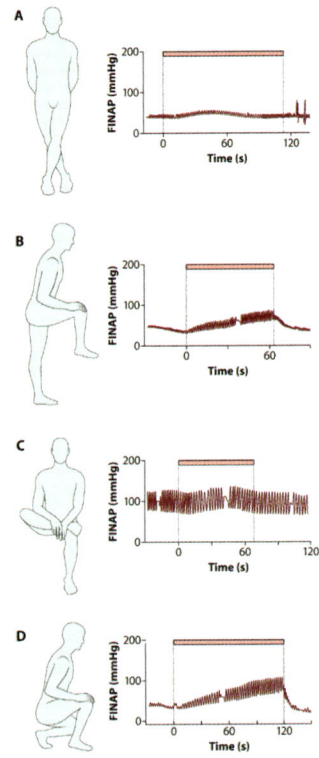

3) Cardiac (Cardiogenic) Syncope[240]

- **Bradyarrhythmia**: sinus node fibrosis, medications
- **Tachyarrhythmia**: VT, torsades de pointes
- **Hemodynamic/valvular**: AS, **PS,** MS, HCM, LA myxoma, prosthetic valve dysfunction
- Usually no prodrome; rarely palpitations, chest pain
- FHx SCD; e.g., Brugada syndrome
- Hx **HF**, low EF, or previous MI
- Exertional syncope: **AS, HCM**
- Nonexertional syncope: **massive pulmonary emboli**
- Syncope with adult congenital heart disease: **Refer to congenital heart specialist**

HYPERTROPHIC CARDIOMYOPATHY (HCM)

Hypertrophic Cardiomyopathy (HCM)[241][242]

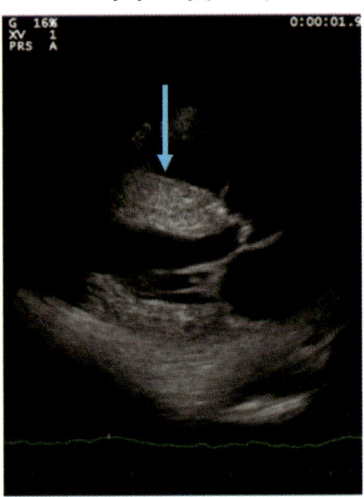

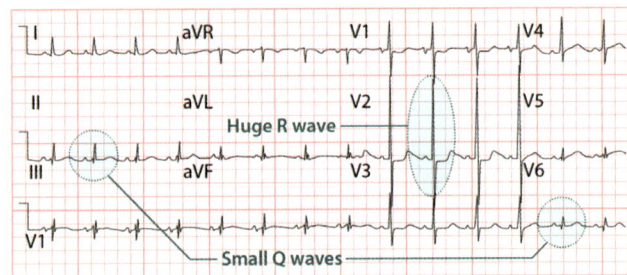

TTE — **Asymmetric septal hypertrophy, diastolic dysfn, small LV size**
Dx: LV anterior septum ≥ 1.3 cm or posterior septum ≥ 1.5 cm & severe systolic anterior mitral motion (septum-leaflet contact)
Do CMR if TTE inconclusive

Do ECG & echo on:
- **1st degree relatives**
- **Genotype-positive but phenotype-negative (< 18 years every 1–2 years, older every 3–5 years)**

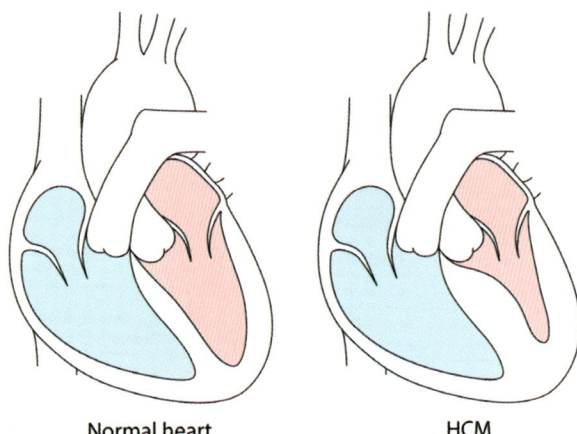

Normal heart   HCM

HCM — Tx[243][244][245]

- Autosomal dominant: Screen all 1st degree family members
- **TTE every 1–2 years** for hypertrophy, MR, EF, and obstruction; **Holter every 1–2 years** to identify those at risk for SCD
- Evidence of myocardial ischemia: **Coronary angiography/CCTA**
- **Nonvasodilating BBs** (metopr-, propran-, atenolol) or **non-dihydropyridine CCB** (verapamil, diltiazem) +/- disopyramide for angina or dyspnea; slow HR ↑ diastolic filling (vasodilators worsen obstruction!); goal resting **HR < 60 bpm**
- **Septal reduction therapy: Myectomy or Alcohol Septal Ablation** of part of ventricular septum — may reduce obstruction if severe drug refractory symptoms & **LVOT gradient ≥ 50** mmHg at rest or physiologically provoked (maneuvers or exercise TTE)
- But **risk of SCD unchanged**!!!
- **Mild-moderate recreational exercise & static/low-intensity competitive sports okay:** golf, curling, bowling, cricket

HCM — ICD[246][247][248][249]

- **Prior cardiac arrest**
- **Ventricular fibrillation (VFib)/sustained ventricular tachycardia (VT)**
- **Syncope from/hemodynamically significant (VT)**

Relative:
- **NSVT** on Holter (≥ 10 beats, ≥ 3 runs, or ≥ 200 bpm)
- **Massive LVH:** Wall thickness **≥ 30 mm**
- **Blunted BP response or hypotension** during exercise
- **Family Hx SCD** ≤ 50 years old likely due to HCM
- Systolic dysfunction **LVEF < 50%** or apical aneurysm
- Extensive **late gadolinium enhancement (fibrosis)** on CMR

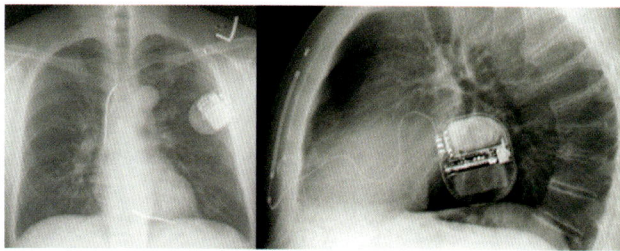

Transvenous / Subcutaneous ICD

HEART FAILURE (HF)

"Holy heart failure, Batman!"

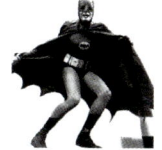

HF — Introduction[250][251][252]

- Heart failure with reduced ejection fraction (**HFrEF**):
  - EF ≤ 40%, systolic HF
- Heart failure with preserved ejection fraction (**HFpEF**):
  - EF ≥ 50, diastolic HF **Rx HTN; diurese; if AFib rate control**
- **TTE** initially (systolic/diastolic) and if change in clinical status
- Baseline natriuretic peptides and/or cardiac troponin in ADHF
- **BNP < 100 pg/mL not HF, ≥ 400 pg/mL HF likely**
- NYHA I (nl), II (slight limitation), **III (marked; mild activity)**, IV (rest); if suspicion, do sleep assessment
- 50% 4-year mortality; 40% re-admitted/dead in 1 year

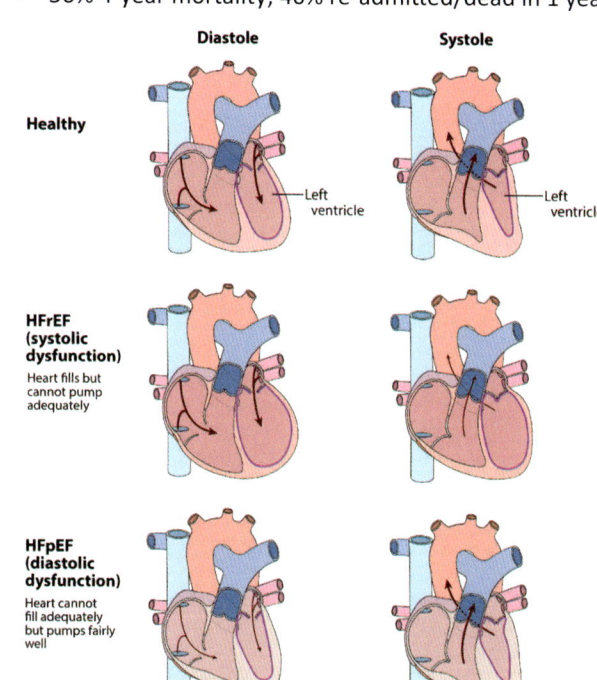

AR 19

A 59-year-old Hispanic male patient had a large anterior STEMI 1 year ago, LVEF 15%, s/p 3-V CABG. He is retired, paints, and does activities of daily living.

Meds: Carvedilol, valsartan/sacubitril, aspirin, clopidogrel, furosemide, eplerenone, and atorvastatin.

Physical: HR 70 bpm, BP 125/85 mmHg, R 16 breaths/min. CVS: S1 S2 S3. LUNGS: CTA bilateraly; extremities: < 1 mm pedal edema;
ECG: NSR 70 bpm, old anterolateral MI

Echo (1 month ago): LVEF 29%, anterolateral hypokinesis, moderately dilated LV

How would you manage the patient now?

A. No changes and repeat echo in 1 year.
B. Switch β-blocker to metoprolol tartrate.
C. Refer for ICD implantation.
D. Refer for transplant.
E. Add candesartan.

Answer:_____

HF Stages — Rx[253]

A	**High risk:** HTN, CAD, DM, cardiotoxins; e.g., doxorubicin (Adriamycin)	**AC**E inhibitors/**A**RBs (target BP < 130/80), **A**torvastatin — statins
B	**Structural heart disease:** MI, LVH, low EF, valvular HD	**B**Bs, **B**ypass: revascularization if appropriate, **B**uzz 'em! ICD in selected patients
C	**Symptoms:** dyspnea, fatigue, decreased exercise tolerance	**C**urtail edema: loop diuretics; **C**ombo hydralazine/isosorbide for African Americans NYHA III–IV, mineralo**C**orticoid: aldosterone antagonist for NYHA II–IV (**C**rCl > 30 mL/min, K+ < 5 mEq/dL), **C**RT: Cardiac resynchronization therapy (Bl-V PM)
D	**Rest** symptoms and frequent **hospital**izations	**D**onor heart (transplant), **D**obutamine: chronic inotropes and **D**rugs/Sx, **D**evices; e.g., LVAD, **D**NR, palliative care, hospice, **D**eactivation of ICD

Transplant contraindications: age > 65, DM with endorgan complications, malignancies within 5 years, kidney dysfunction, other chronic diseases that decrease survival, poor social support, noncompliance.

Meds to Prolong Survival[254]

Angiotensin-converting enzyme inhibitors (ACEIs)	First-line vasodilator therapy for HFrEF CI: **PARK**: **P**reg., **A**llergic/**A**ngioedema, **R**AS-bilat/**R**F Cr > 3.0 mg/dL, **K**+ > 5.5	Captopril, enalapril, lisinopril, benazepril, fosinopril, perindopril, quinapril, ramipril, trandolapril
Angiotensin II receptor blockers (ARBs)	Alternative in ACEI intolerant	Candesartan, valsartan (mortality benefit); irbesartan, olmesartan, eprosartan, losartan, telmisartan
Angiotensin receptor neprilysin inhibitor (ARNI)	**Replace** ACEI/ARB for symptomatic HFrEF patients (NYHA II–III); neprilysin inhibitor prevents breakdown of B-type natriuretic peptide → enhanced diuresis, natriuresis, and myocardial relaxation	Sacubitril/valsartan (Entresto): start 49/51 mg bid, target (97/103 mg bid). **Stop taking ACEI, wait 36 hours, then start PARADIGM-HF: sacubitril/ valsartan superior to enalapril (↓16% death & 20% HF hospitalizations)!**
Aldosterone antagonists	NHYA II–IV HFrEF & EF ≤ 35% on BB/ACEI (Cr < 2.5 & K+ < 5.0 mEq/L)	Spironolactone, eplerenone (both start 25 mg, target 50 mg daily)
β-Blockers (up-titrate every 2–4 weeks until HR 60 bpm or symptomatic hypotension)	All except NYHA IV (↑ EF, ↓ hospitalizations and mortality, improve remodeling)	Carvedilol (β1, β2, α1), metoprolol succinate (s for sustained release; β1), bisoprolol (β1)
Hydralazine/nitrates	African Americans with NYHA III–IV HFrEF as adjunctive therapy to ACEIs (or ARBs) and BBs; or cannot be given ACEI/ARB (drug intolerance, hypotension, chronic kidney disease)	Hydralazine, isosorbide dinitrate

Meds for Symptom Control[255][256]

Loop diuretics	Relief of dyspnea & hypoxia due to pulmonary edema/volume overload (dose greater than outpatient dose) **NB: Can add oral thiazides (metolazone, HCTZ) or IV chlorothiazide to intensify loop diuretic effect**	Furosemide, bumetanide, torsemide, ethacrynic acid
Aquaretics	V2 receptor antagonists; increase blood flow to the kidneys without increasing Na^+ and Cl^- resorption → increase in urine while retaining electrolytes	Conivaptan
Digoxin	HFrEF → decrease hospitalizations; Rx: AFib resting VR > 80 (**exercise** > 110); NSR EF ≤ 40%, NYHA II–IV on GDMT	Digitalis 0.125 mg every other day → 0.5 mg daily
Sinus node I(f) channel inhibitor/modulator	NYHA II–III HFrEF, EF ≤ 35% on GDMT (BB at max dose) and in **NSR** with **HR ≥ 70 bpm** at rest → slows heart rate → ↑ myocardial blood flow → decrease hospitalizations **(SHIFT trial)**	Ivabradine start 5 mg bid, max 7.5 mg bid. CI: AFib
Positive inotropes	Severe ventricular failure (Stage D) patients may require short-term treatment with inotropes	Dobutamine, dopamine, milrinone
IV vasodilators	**Rdn in afterload → increase stroke volume if elevated systemic vascular resistance with reasonable CO**	**Nitroprusside, nitroglycerine**
In HFrEF AVOID	**Thiazolidinediones (glitazones), most CCBs (except amlodipine, felodipine), NSAIDs, & cyclooxygenase-2 inhibitors**	**Worsen HFrEF!**

Cardiac Resynchronization Therapy (CRT)[257]

- Cardiac resynchronization therapy pacemaker (**CRT-P**) or biventricular pacing Rx: **Symptomatic HFrEF and electrical dyssynchrony**
- → Reduction in mitral regurgitation, optimization of ventricular filling and pumping efficiency
- **CRT-P** for HFrEF on GDMT with:
  - LVEF ≤ **35%** and
  - Sinus rhythm **LBBB QRS ≥ 150** msec, and
  - **NYHA II, III**, or ambulatory IV symptoms
- Cardiac resynchronization therapy **D**efibrillator (**CRT-D**) or biventricular ICD = **CRT** + IC**D**

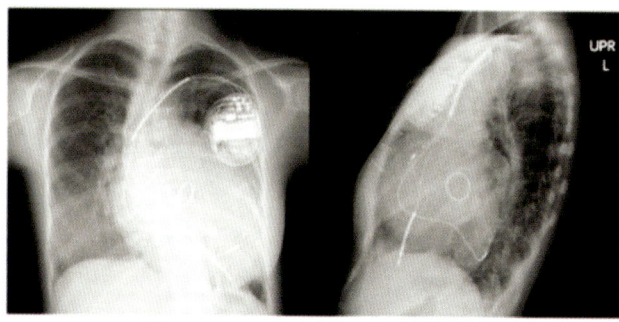

PA   Lateral

PERICARDIAL DISEASES

ACUTE PERICARDITIS

I	Diffuse concave up ST elevation, PR-segment depression (aVR = opposite)
II	ST segments normalize
III	T-wave inversion
IV	ECG normal

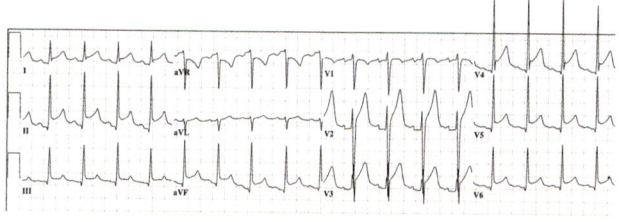

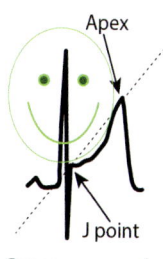

Apex

J point

Concave upward

CARDIOLOGY

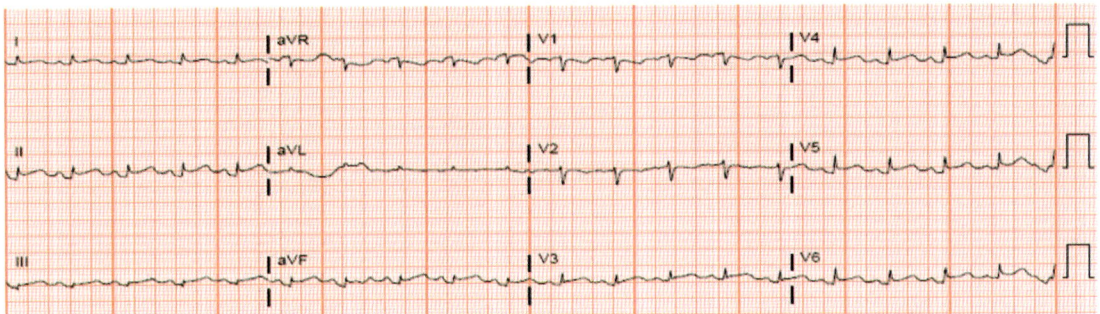

Acute Pericarditis — Diagnosis[258][259][260]

- **Viral, bacterial (TB, Lyme), autoimmune (RA, SLE), uremic, lymphoma, Dressler's, radiation, meds** (minoxidil, penicillins, clozapine), **myxedema**
- **Pleuritic chest pain** (worse with breath) & worse supine; relieved by **sitting/leaning forward**
- Fever, tachycardia
- **Friction rub, 3-component** (systolic — with ventricular contraction; diastolic — with rapid ventricular filling and atrial contraction)
- **CKMB/cTn** elevated if myocarditis
- Differentiate from acute MI — echo: **no RWMA**, sometimes effusion
- **Purulent** pericarditis — Sx drain and IV antibiotics
- **No strenuous exercise** — can trigger recurrence!

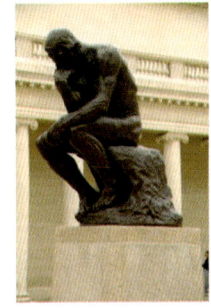

Le Penseur (The Thinker). Auguste Rodin.

Acute Pericarditis — Rx[261][262][263]

- **High-dose**
  - **ASA** for 4 weeks: 650 mg every 6 hours × 2 weeks; or
  - **NSAIDs** for 4 weeks: ibuprofen 600 mg tid, or
  - indomethacin 50 mg tid × 2 weeks
  - Taper over 2–4 weeks
- **And**
  - **Colchicine** 0.5 mg daily (if on ASA/NSAID or wt < 70 kg), bid (≥ 70 kg) for 3 months to reduce risk of recurrent pericarditis
  - Rx of choice of **recurrent pericarditis (6 months) and post-MI pericarditis (1st line: aspirin; 2nd line: add colchicine)**
  - N, V, D uncommon; < 1%: BM suppression, hepato-/myotoxicity

Avoid steroids due to higher rate of recurrent pericarditis!

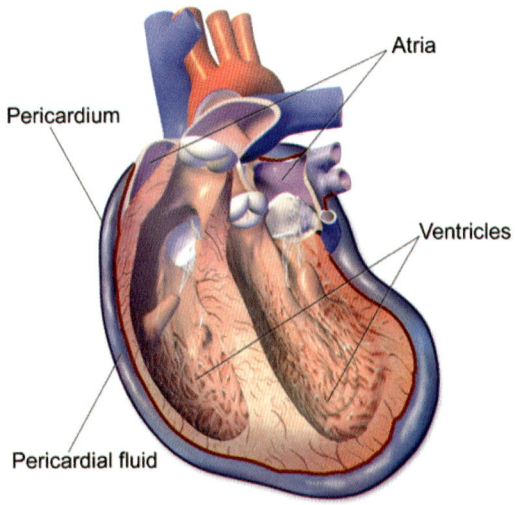

Inflammation of the Pericardium in the Heart

[264]

CONSTRICTIVE PERICARDITIS

AR 20

A 64-year-old man with a history of lymphoma S/P chemo and radiation has been to the ED multiple times complaining of dyspnea, general fatigue, and peripheral edema. Nebulizers don't help. You note elevated neck veins that increase on inspiration and a diastolic knocking sound at the left sternal border, ascites, and pedal edema.

What is the likely diagnosis?

A. Multiple pulmonary emboli
B. Atrial septal defect
C. Exacerbation of COPD
D. Constrictive pericarditis

Answer:_____

Constrictive Pericarditis

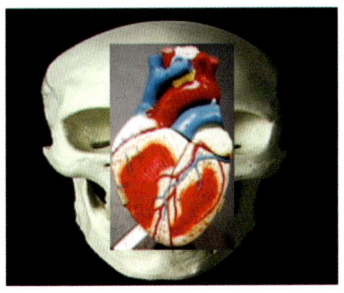

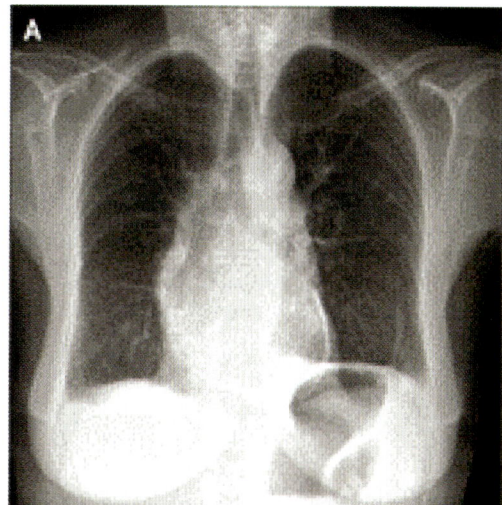

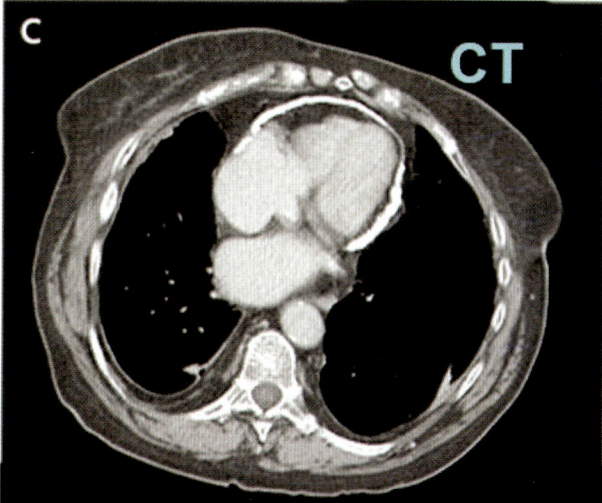

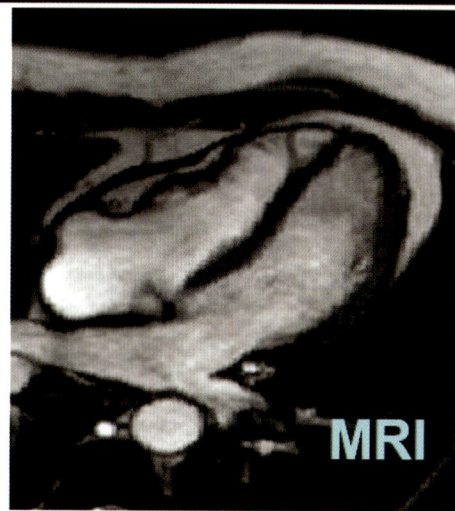

37-year-old female patient from Philippines with a history of a positive PPD

Constrictive Pericarditis — U.S.[265][266]

- **46% idiopathic** (viral); **37% prior cardiac surgery, 9% radiation, 4% TB** (developing countries), purulent infection, RA, SLE, neoplastic disease (breast and lung cancer, **lymphoma**), uremic/dialysis
- **R-HF signs** (peripheral edema, ascites, hepatomegaly); **Kussmaul sign = no fall or rise in JVP on inspiration**
- **Pericardial knock early diastole (50%)**
- Calcification of pericardium on chest x-ray (TB)
- **Thick pericardium > 4 mm (CT, MRI); atria dilated**
- **Echo: septal bounce; equalization of diastolic pressures in all chambers; reduced mitral inflow velocities with inspiration = ventricular interdependence: Overfilling of one ventricle results in reduced filling of the other**
- Pericardiectomy if NYHA II, III (mortality ~ 10%)!

RESTRICTIVE CARDIOMYOPATHY

Restrictive Cardiomyopathy "Filet Mignon Heart"[267][268]

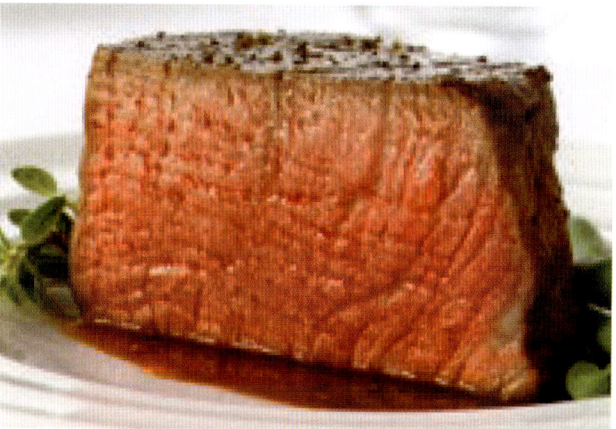

[269]

Thickened granular myocardium; diastolic dysfunction; dilated atria; *restrictive diastolic filling; normal systolic function; pulmonary HTN*

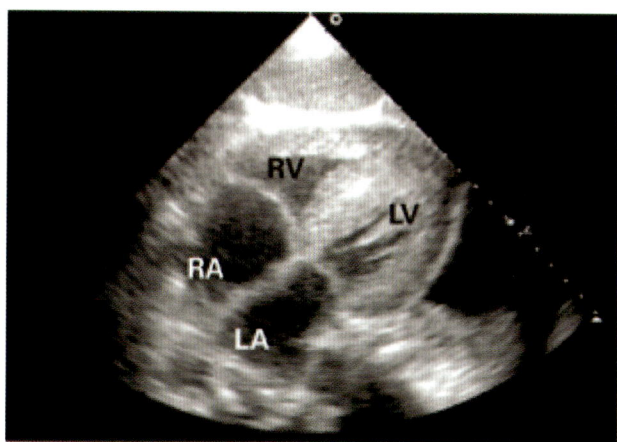

Amyloid = most common cause (Dx: MRI or Bx)

CARDIOLOGY

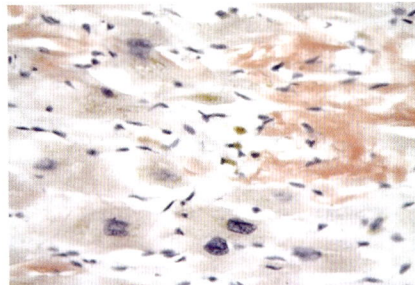

Cardiac amyloidosis (Congo red stain): amyloid (extracellular washed-out red material)

Restrictive Cardiomyopathy[270]
1) **Hypertrophic:** hypertension, AS
2) **Infiltrative:** amyloid (CI:Dig.), sarcoid (Dx: FDG PET/CMR; Rx: CS), hemochromatosis
3) **Storage:** Fabry disease (Dx: ↓ α-galactosidase)
4) **Inflammatory:** endomyocardial fibrosis (**hypereosinophilic Sd**), eosinophilic CMP (**Löffler** endocarditis), **anthra**cycline toxicity, **radiation**
5) **Idiopathic:** scleroderma, diabetes
• **R-HF signs (peripheral edema, ascites, hepatomegaly); Kussmaul sign;** (~ constrictive pericarditis!)
• **Right heart catheter: concordant rise and fall of left and right systolic pressures with respiration**
• S$_3$; **BNP high: > 400 pg/mL (> 400 ng/L)**; ECG: BBB, ventricular hypertrophy, Q waves, impaired AV conduction
• **Rx underlying condition**; diuretics; AFib: digoxin

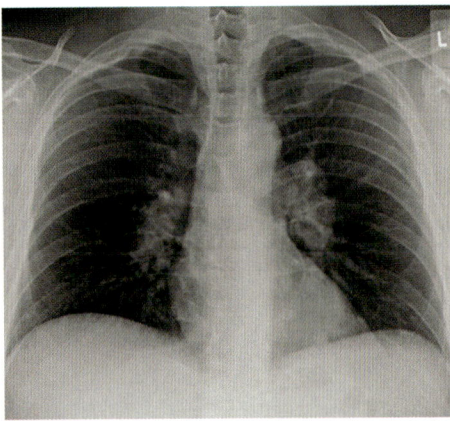

Hilar adenopathy due to sarcoidosis

Lecture 5

L5 Outline
• **Congenital Heart Disease**
• **Sudden Cardiac Death (SCD) in Young Athletes**
• **Pulmonary Heart Disease**
• **Pulmonary Hypertension (PH)**
• **The 12-Lead ECG**
• **Some Extra Exam ECGs**
• **Final Thoughts**

CONGENITAL HEART DISEASES

Congenital Heart Disease[271][272]
DROP IT Shaun White!
• **D**efect: VSD
• **R**ight ventricular hypertrophy
• **O**verriding aorta
• **P**ulmonic stenosis
• **T**etralogy of Fallot
Shaun White "the flying tomato," who won Olympic Gold in snowboarding, had surgery for tetralogy of Fallot as an infant.
• Pulmonic regurgitation common after repair
  – **QRS > 180 msec or large RV** = marker for VT/SCD in repaired tetralogy

Periodic Holter monitoring recommended as arrhythmias common.

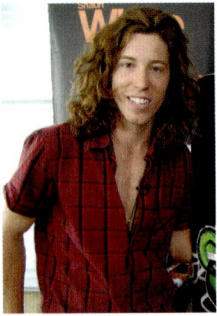

[273]

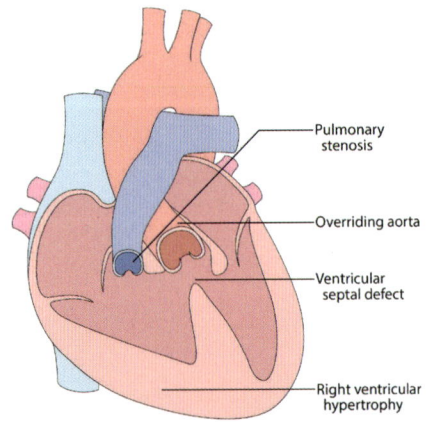

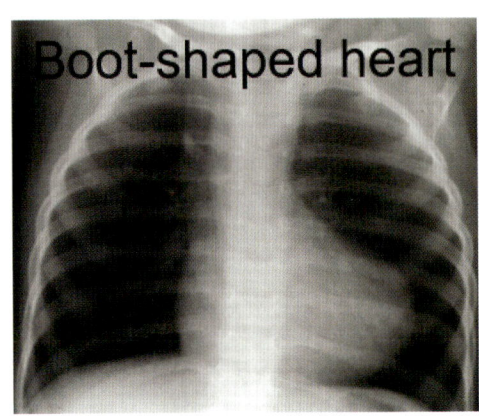

AR 21

Which of the following patients should be referred for surgery?

A. Coarctation of the aorta with heart failure
B. VSD with pulmonary hypertension
C. Anomalous left main coronary artery running between the aorta and pulmonary artery
D. ASD with a > 1.5:1 L-to-R shunt
E. All of the above

Answer:_____

Patent Foramen Ovale (PFO)[274][275]

- **30%** population, M = F, average size **5 mm**
- Asymptomatic = **Do nothing!**
- Consider closing if recurrent CVA/TIA of unknown origin (cryptogenic) despite antiplatelet Rx

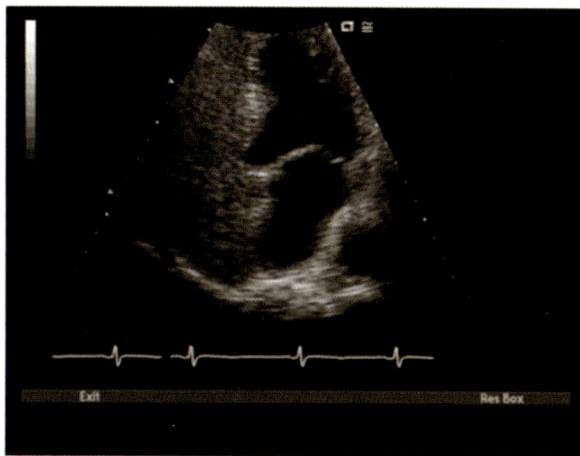

TTE with bubbles in right atrium

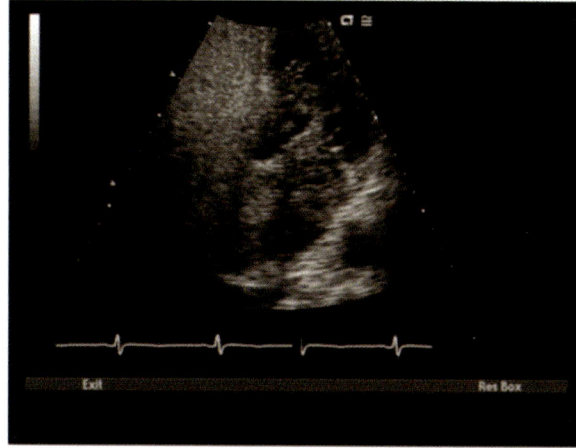

TTE depicting passage of saline contrast from RA to LA across a PFO

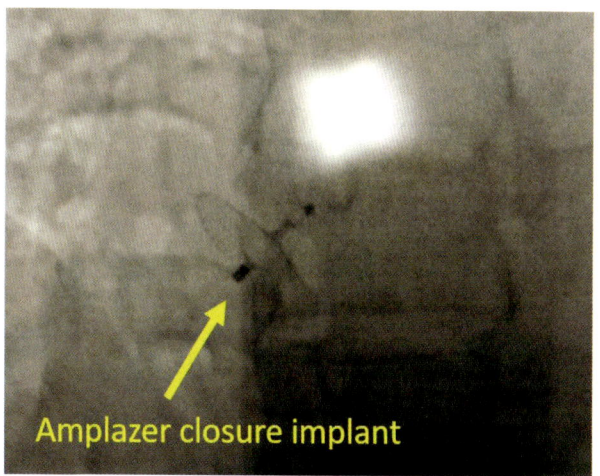

Amplazer closure implant

Patent Ductus Arteriosus (PDA)[276][277]

- Fetus: O$_2$ blood bypass lungs via FO & PDA
- LUSB: Continuous **"machinery"** murmur **under L clavicle**; bounding pulses, wide pulse pressure
- Differential cyanosis: **Blue lower/Pink upper extremities**, with pulmonary HTN (R-to-L shunt!)
- CXR: calcification of PDA, cardiomegaly, prominent central pulm a
- Surgical/Catheter closure if:
    - **LA or LV enlargement with L-to-R shunting**
    - **PA systolic pressure < 50% systemic**
    - **Pulmonary vascular resistance < 1/3 systemic**

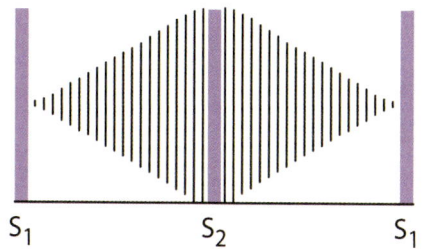

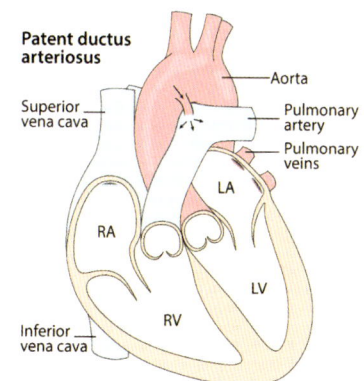

Valvular Pulmonic Stenosis[278][279][280]

- **Congenital**; **RVH**
- **PEN**: **P**S + **E**ars low set = **N**oonan Sd (autosomal dominant)
- P_2 delayed, soft/absent; JVP: prominent *a* wave
- **Ejection click** = only R-sided sound that becomes **softer in inspiration**: RVH → thickened RV doesn't distend normally during inspiration → pulm v. partially opened when RV contracts → v. excursion less → ejection click softer + earlier
- **Moderate-severe PS (peak gradient > 36 mmHg /peak velocity > 3 m/s) with HF symptoms, cyanosis from interatrial R-to-L communication, and/or exercise intolerance: Balloon valvuloplasty;** dysplastic valve, moderate coexisting pulmonic regurgitation, small annulus, severe sub-/supravalvular stenosis: Surgical pulmonary valve replacement

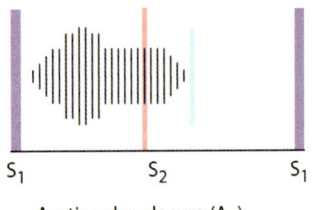

- Aortic valve closure (A_2)
- Pulmonic valve closure (P_2)

S_1 S_2 S_1

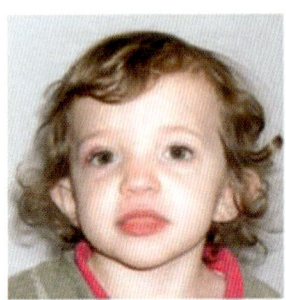

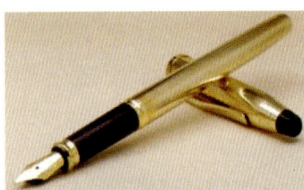

[281]

Ventricular Septal Defect (VSD) — a.k.a. Very Small Dudes!!![282]

- Most **common** congenital HD in children
- Commonest 80% = **membranous**, a.k.a. perimembranous
- Majority close spontaneously
- **Harsh holosystolic murmur** — L → R shunt throughout systole (increases with handgrip); **palpable thrill**
- Small asymptomatic uncomplicated VSD = periodic observation
- <u>Sx closure if:</u>
  - **LV volume overload and Qp:Qs > 1.5:1 (large shunt)**
  - **PA systolic pressure < 50% systemic**
  - **Pulmonary vascular resistance < 1/3 systemic**
  - **Valvular disruption (AI = supracristal), or**
  - **Hx endocarditis**

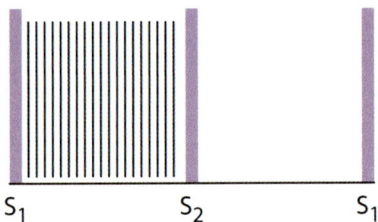

S_1 S_2 S_1

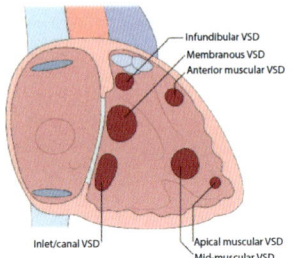

Anomalous Coronary Artery[283][284]

- Myocardial ischemia, ventricular dysfunction, VT or VFib, and sudden death
- **Exertional chest pain**, dyspnea, palpitations, syncope, or cardiac arrest
- Dx: **Coronary angiography, CT, MRI**
- Sx: **(1) Anomalous coronary artery from left or right sinus with symptoms or ischemia; or (2) Anomalous left coronary artery from the PA; (3) Anomalous right coronary artery from PA with symptoms**

A.

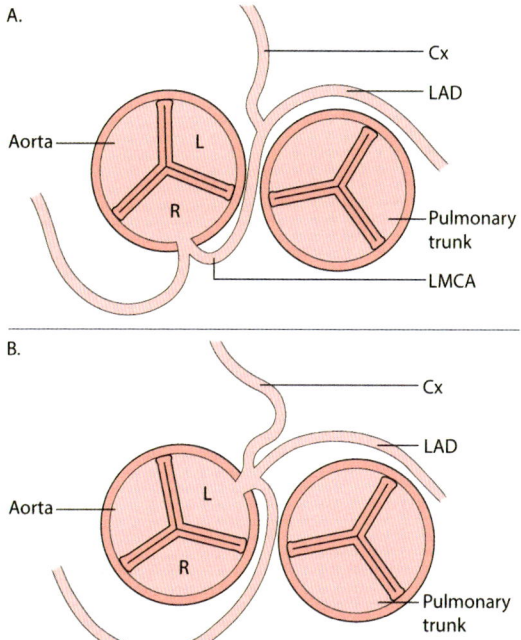

A. A left coronary artery arising from the right sinus of Valsalva
B. A right coronary artery arising from the left sinus of Valsalva

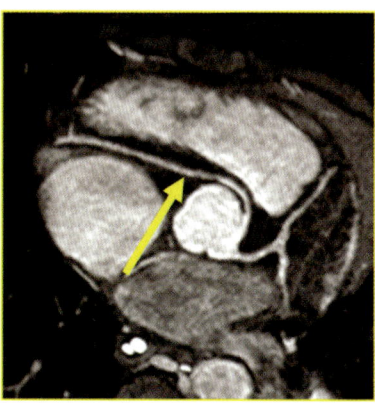

Anomalous RCA from left coronary sinus with interarterial course

SUDDEN DEATH IN EXERCISING YOUNG PEOPLE

Sudden Cardiac Death (SCD)* in Young Athletes

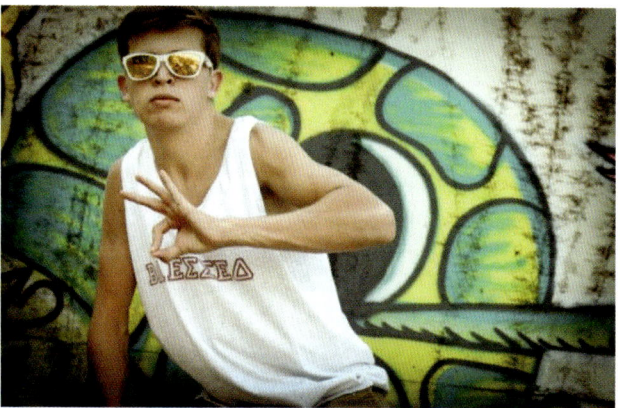

* Unexpected circulatory arrest, usually due to a cardiac arrhythmia, within 1 hour of onset of symptoms

AR 22

Conditions associated with sudden cardiac death in exercising young people include:

A. Hypertrophic cardiomyopathy
B. Congenital coronary artery anomalies
C. Long QT syndrome
D. Brugada syndrome
E. All of the above

Answer:_____

SCD in Young Athletes (Most AD)[286][287]
- **Inherited/Acquired cardiomyopathies**
  - Hypertrophic cardiomyopathy **(No. 1 in U.S.)**
  - Arrhythmogenic right ventricular cardiomyopathy
  - Myocarditis/Dilated CMP
- **Congenital coronary artery anomalies (No. 2 in U.S.)**
- **Electrical disorders and channelopathies**
  - Long-QT Sd/Short-QT Sd
  - Brugada Sd
  - Wolff-Parkinson-White Sd
  - Catecholaminergic polymorphic ventricular tachycardia
  - Commotio cordis (mechano-electric syndrome)
- **Valve and aortic disorders**
  - Bicuspid aortic valve/Aortic rupture/Marfan Sd/ Coarctation of the aorta
  - Pulmonic stenosis

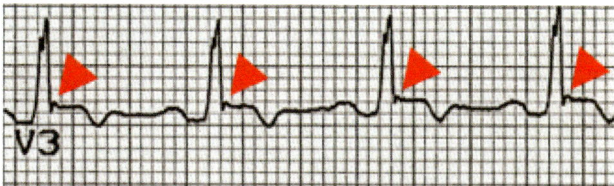

The Epsilon wave of arrhythmogenic right ventricular cardiomyopathy

CARDIOLOGY

PULMONARY HEART DISEASE

COR PULMONALE

Cor Pulmonale[288]
- Altered structure/function of the **right ventricle** from **chronic lung disease**
- Often changes in left heart function
- COPD, interstitial lung disease, pulmonary embolism, acute respiratory distress syndrome
- **Chronic slowly progressive course**, with acute exacerbations
- Former heavy smoker, dyspneic at rest, cyanotic, neck vein distention, and lower extremity edema

EISENMENGER SYNDROME

Eisenmenger Syndrome[289][290]
- **Large** unrepaired **L**-to-**R** shunt (high pressure and flow: **VSD***, AVSD, PDA) →
- Severe pulmonary HTN → pulmonary arteriolar remodeling:
  - Pulmonary vascular resistance > systemic → shunt now **R**-to-**L**
- **Cyanosis**, clubbing, left parasternal impulse (RVH) and increased P$_2$ (pulmonary HTN)
- **Iron deficiency anemia common: Rx short-term iron**
- CXR: Enlarged central pulmonary arteries with decreased pulmonary vascularity

***Most common cause**

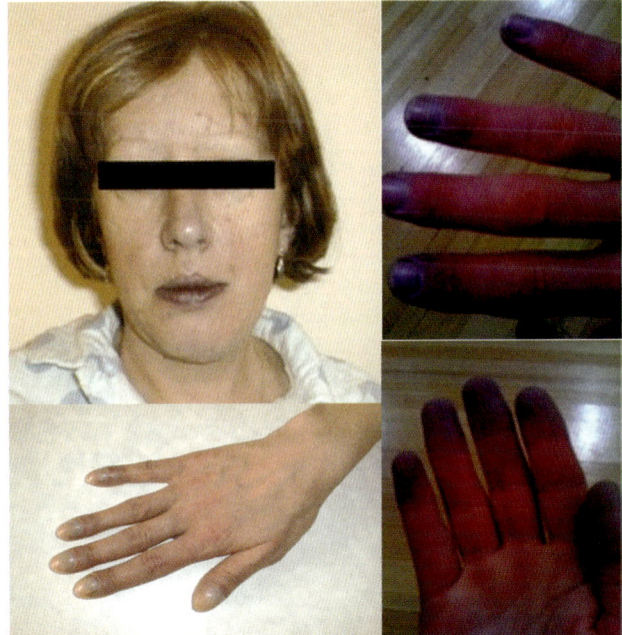

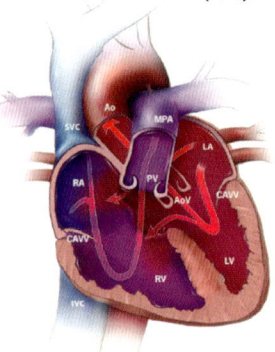

Atrioventricular Septal Defect (AVSD)

RA Right Atrium	SVC Superior Vena Cava	CAVV Common Atrioventricular Valve
RV Right Ventricle	IVC Inferior Vena Cava	PV Pulmonary Valve
LA Left Atrium	MPA Main Pulmonary Artery	AoV Aortic Valve
LV Left Ventricle	Ao Aorta	

Rx: Heart-Lung Transplant

PULMONARY HYPERTENSION

Pulmonary Hypertension (PH)[291]
Dyspnea on exertion
RH Cath: Resting mean pulmonary artery pressure ≥ 25 mmHg, pulmonary vascular resistance of > 3 Wood units (240 dynes-sec/cm^5), with normal PCWP.

WHO PH Classification[292]
1) **Pulmonary arterial hypertension** — idiopathic, CT diseases
2) PH from **L heart disease** — S or D dysfn **(Abn echo, elevated PCWP)**
3) PH from **lung diseases** and/or hypoxia — COPD, ILD, OSA **(Abn PFTs or polysomnography)**
4) **Chronic thromboembolic** PH **(highest risk/ worst prognosis)** **(Abn VQ scan/CTPA)** — **Rx riociguat & embolectomy**
5) PH with **unclear/multiple** mechanisms — sarcoidosis
- Oxygen to maintain saturation > 90%
- **Loop diuretics and spironolactone** good if R-HF

Pulmonary Arterial Hypertension (Drug Induced, Heritable, Idiopathic)[293][294][295]
- **Young women, refractory**, death in 5–10 years
- **Reactive** to vasodilator = nitric oxide or IV epoprostenol = fall in mean PAP of ≥ 10 mmHg to ≤ 40 mmHg, with unchanged/↑ cardiac output
  Rx: **CCBs** (nifedipine, diltiazem, amlodipine)
- **Unreactive** Rx: **1st line ambrisentan plus tadalafil (AMBITION trial)**
- **Endothelin receptor antagonists** (ambrisentan, bosentan, macitentan); **PDE5 inhibitors** (sildenafil, tadalafil, vardenafil); **guanylate cyclase stimulators** (riociguat); **prostacyclin analogues** (epoprostenol, iloprost, treprostinil, beraprost — **more advanced fn class III, IV**); **prostacyclin receptor (IP) agonists** (selexipag)
- All get **warfarin** to reduce risk of **in situ thrombus**
- **Heart-Lung transplant**

THE 12-LEAD ECG

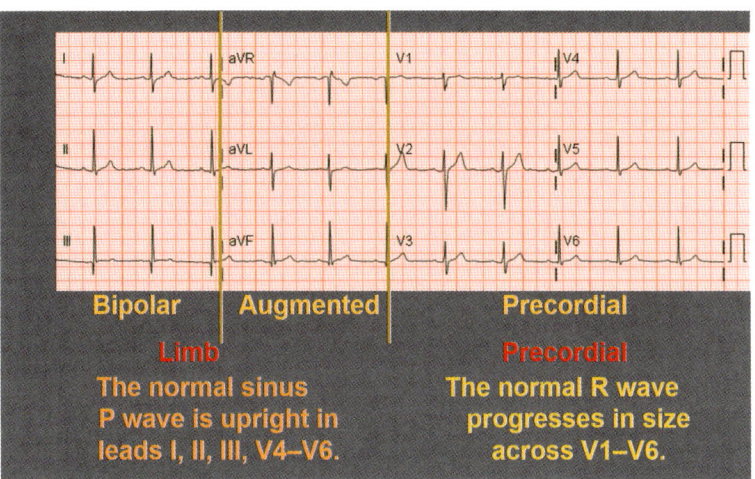

Bipolar   **Augmented**   **Precordial**

Limb   **Precordial**

The normal sinus P wave is upright in leads I, II, III, V4–V6.

The normal R wave progresses in size across V1–V6.

Premature Atrial Complexes (PACs)
- Premature = early
- Atrial = from atria
- P-wave morphology different
- PR ≥ 0.12 sec
- Rare PACs are normal

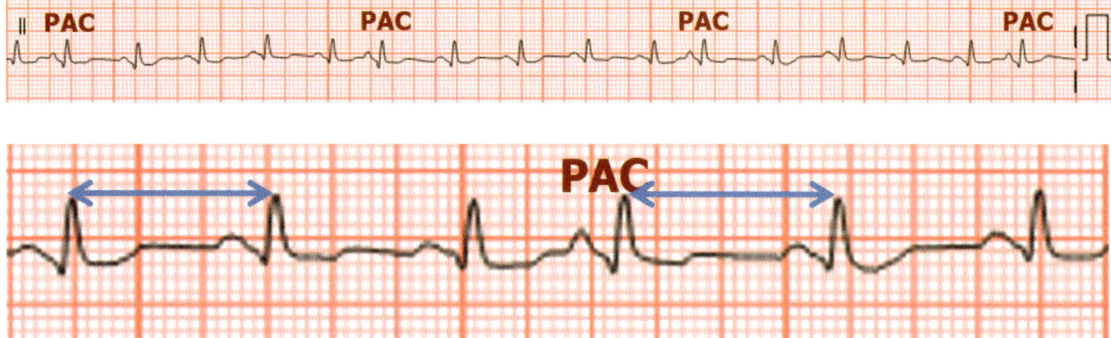

Focal Atrial Tachycardia[296]
- Discrete P waves (rate 100–200 bpm) and typically an **isoelectric** segment between P waves; long RP
- Rx: hemodynamically
  - **Stable**: IV β-blockers, diltiazem, or verapamil
  - **Unstable**: synchronized cardioversion
  - Refer for **catheter ablation**

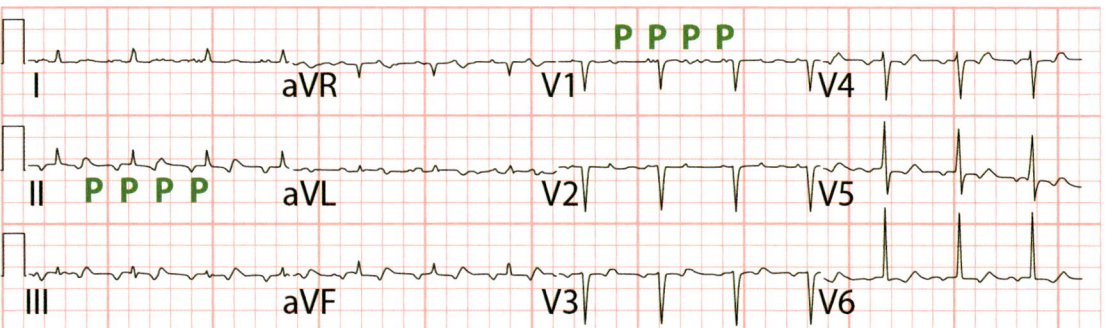

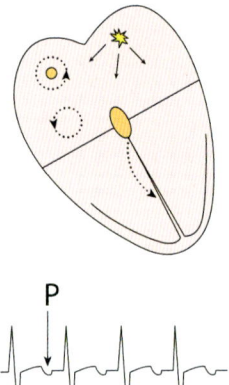

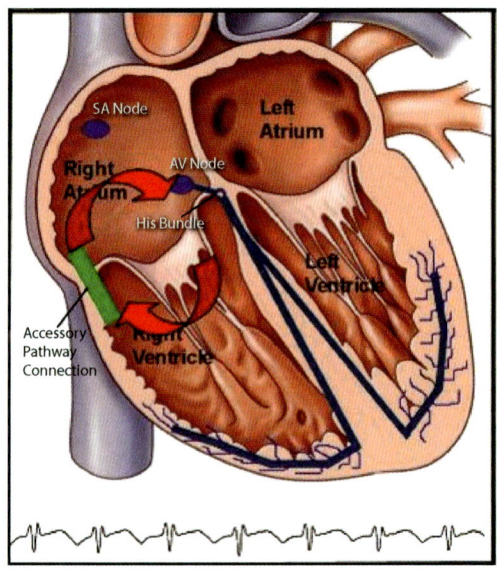

Supraventricular Tachycardia — Narrow Complex[297]
- Vagal maneuvers or IV Adenosine will terminate AVNRT (**slows down your game!**) and AVRT (orthodromic)

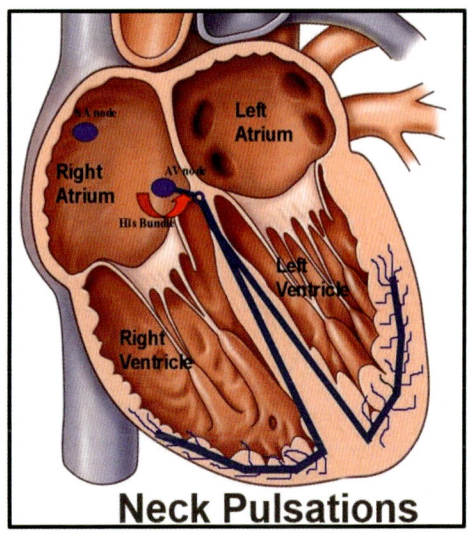

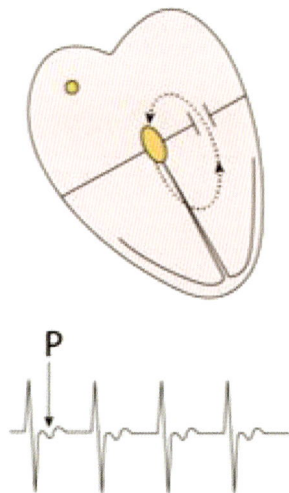

AV reentrant tachycardia with an accessory pathway

Stable: (1) vagal man, (2) adenosine
Unstable: synchronized cardioversion

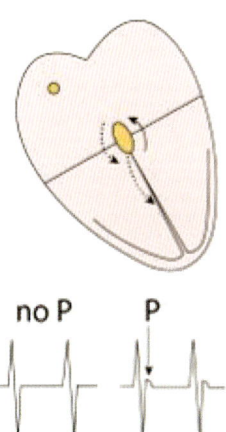

AV nodal reentrant tachycardia (typical)

AVNRT (Slows Down Your Game!) "Slow-Fast"[298]

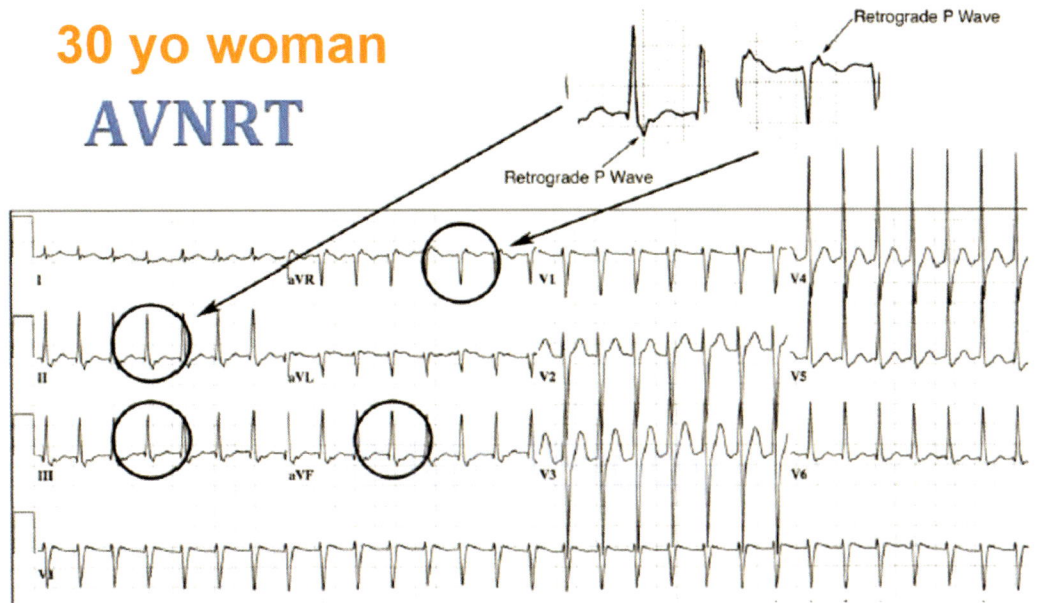

Short RP: *The retrograde P wave is at the terminal portion of the QRS complex (c/w AVRT the P wave is a notching within the ST-/T-wave segment).* **Rx: β-blockers, diltiazem, or verapamil and/or ablate slow-pathway.**

1° AV Block

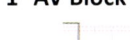
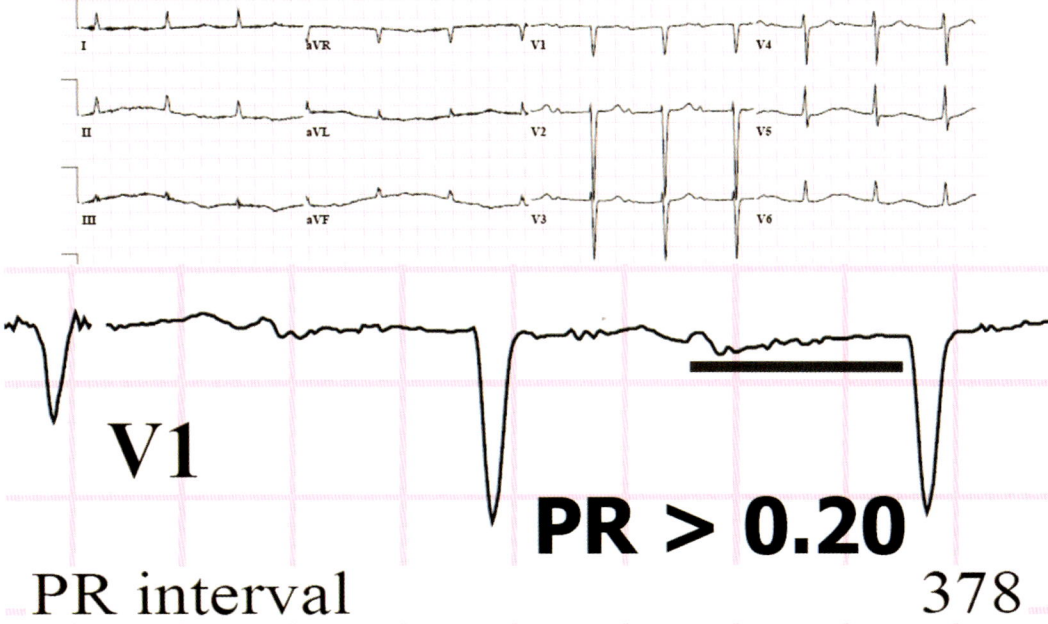

Normal PR Interval = 0.12–0.20 sec

2° AV Block Type 1 (Wenckebach)
- Dropped QRS complexes **with progressive PR prolongation**
- **Group beating** of QRS complexes: Always one more P wave than QRS complexes
- Often associated with meds (digitalis, CCB, BB)
- Tx: Symptomatic bradycardia only

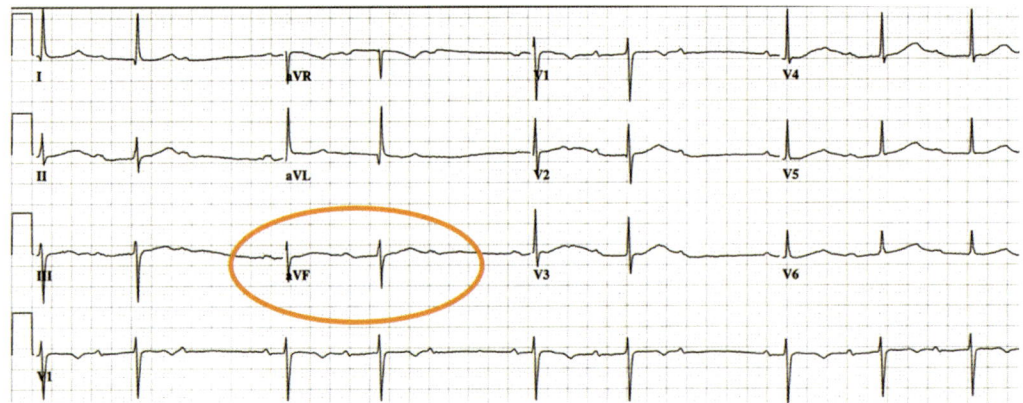

2° AV Block Type 2[299]
- Dropped QRS complexes **without progressive PR prolongation**
- **Atropine: No affect or paradoxically worsens!**
- More likely to progress to 3° AV block
- Tx: Permanent PM for symptomatic patients

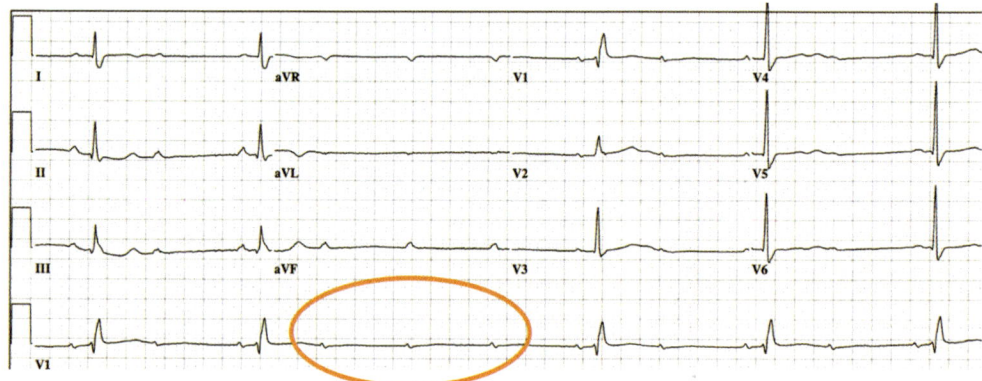

3° AV Block = Complete Heart Block
- No communication between atria and ventricles
- Slow narrow (junctional) or wide (ventricular) escape rhythm
- Tx: permanent pacemaker

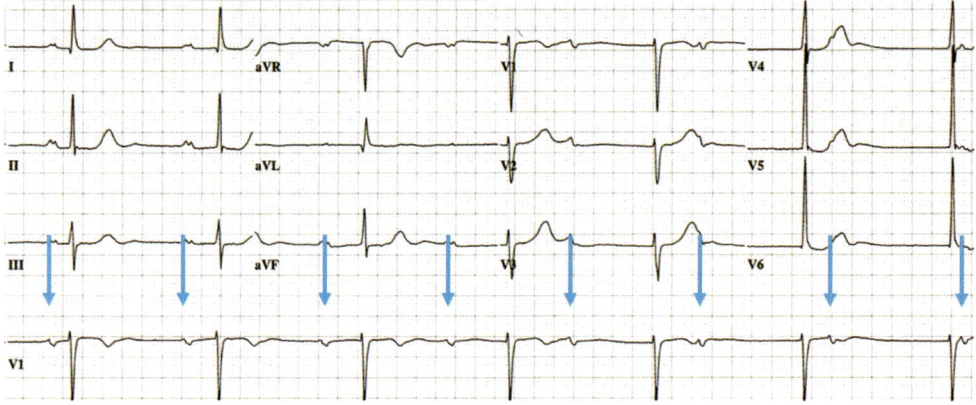

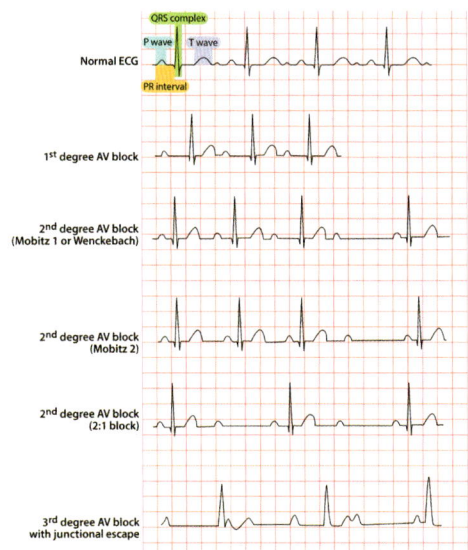

Bundle-Branch Block (BBB)

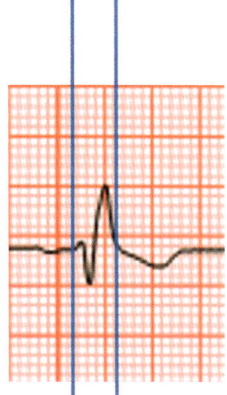

- One ventricle depolarizes later than other
- "**BBB**" rhymes with **3** QRS ≥ 0.12 sec (**3 × mm squares**)

QRS

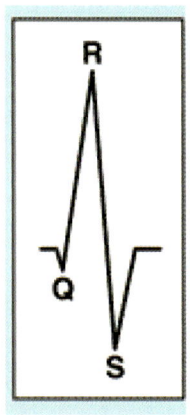

QRS = depolarization of ventricular myocardium
- Duration
  - Normal: < 0.10 sec
  - **Increased: ≥ 0.10 sec**

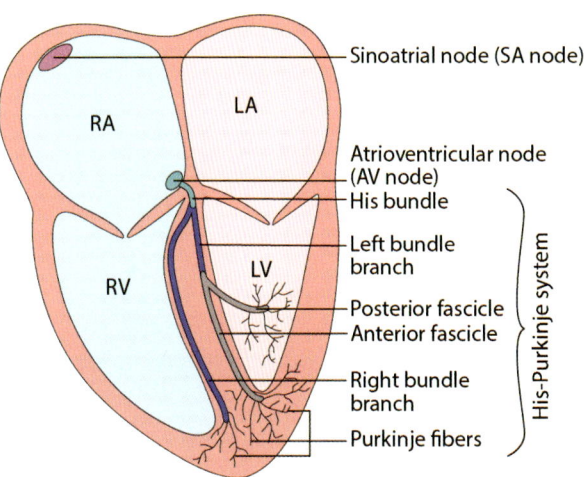

Right Bundle-Branch Block[300]

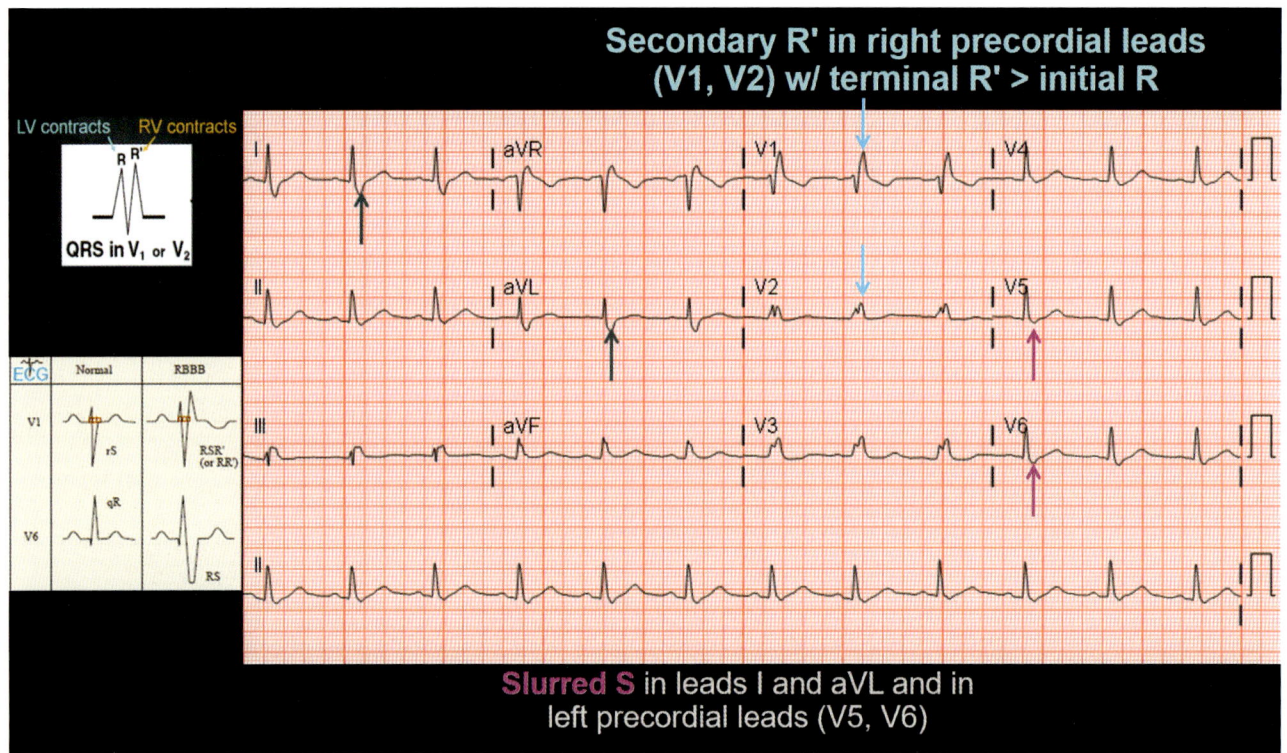

Incomplete RBBB: QRS 110–119 ms
QRS ≥ 120 ms

Left Bundle-Branch Block[301]

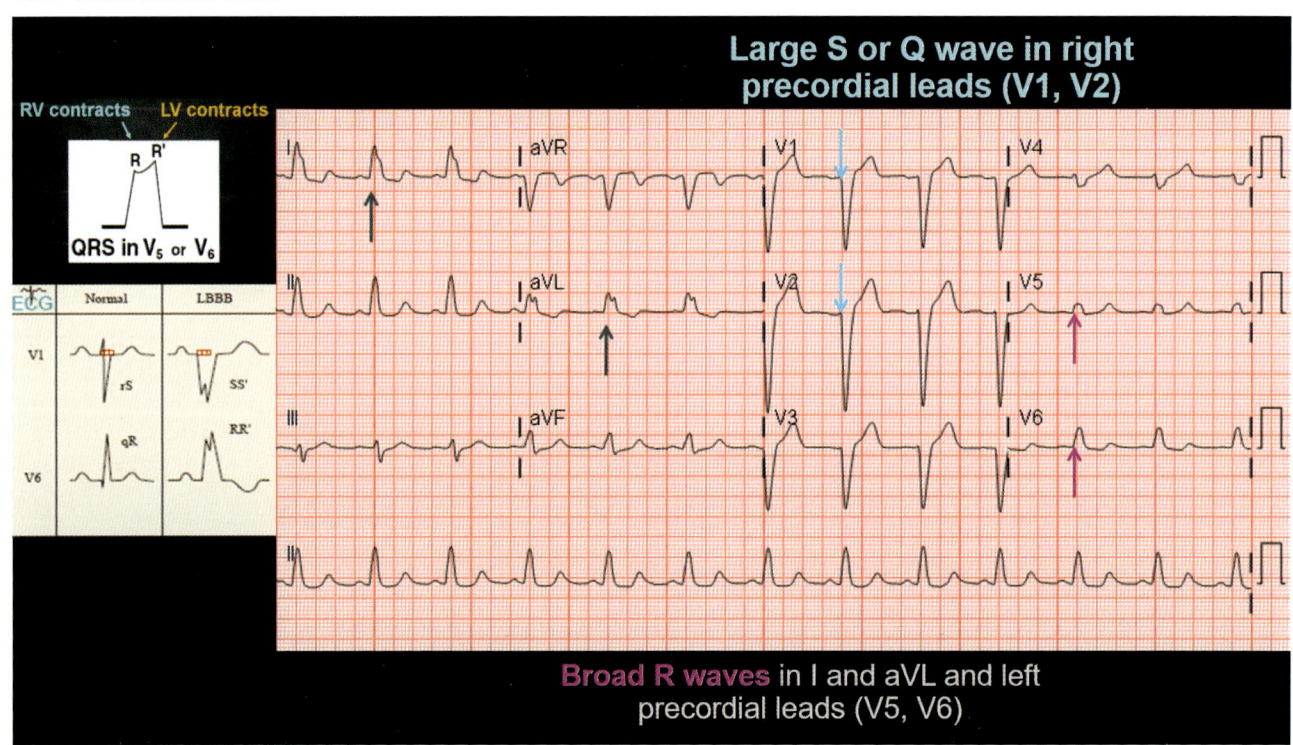

Incomplete LBBB: QRS 110–119 ms
QRS ≥ 120 ms

Ventricular Paced

- Pacemaker
- Lead tip in right ventricle

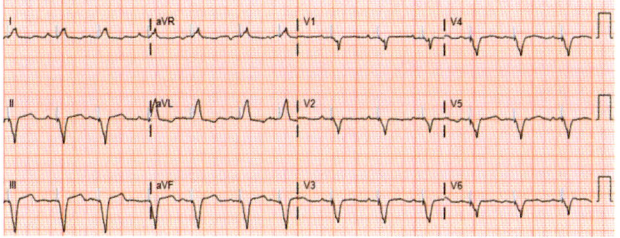

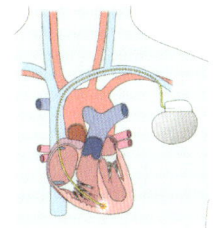

QT Interval[302][303][304][305]

- Normal QT: < 50% RR interval
- QT_c = **QT c**orrected for HR
- **Short**
  - **≤ 0.34 sec**
- **Long**
  - **≥ 470 msec (males), ≥ 480 msec (females)**
  - If on drug **QT_c > 500 msec** or
  - **Increases > 60 msec or > 15%** — Stop it!
  - LQTS patient: **Avoid** QT-prolonging meds!

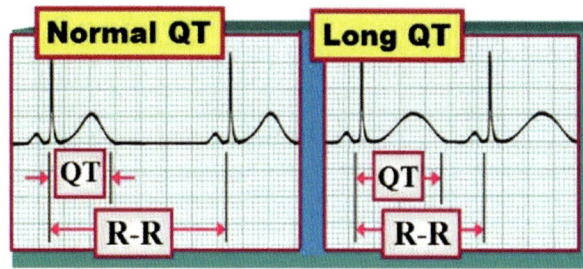

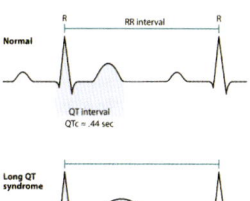

Long QT_c

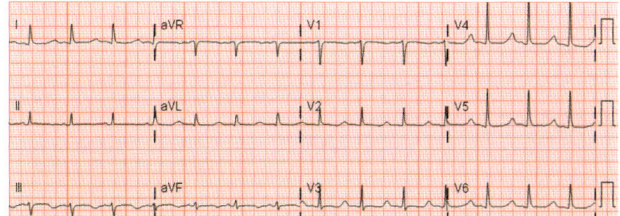

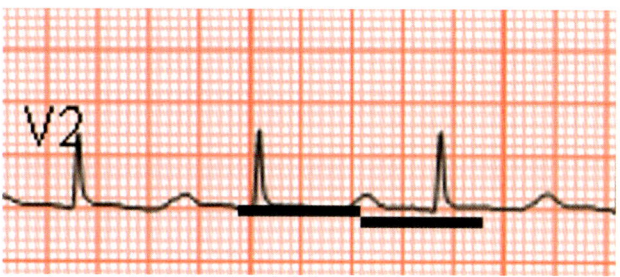

Prolong QT_c: PA ADMITS @ HQ[306]

- **P**rocainamide, **P**henothiazines
- **A**zoles (e.g., ketoconazole)
- **A**miodarone
- **D**ofetilide, **D**roperidol, **D**isopyramide
- **M**acrolides (e.g., erythromycin)
- **I**butilide
- **T**ricyclic ADs
- **S**otalol @
- **H**aloperidol, **H**ypo Ca-Mg-Pot-Thyroid-Thermia
- **Q**uinidine, **Q**uinolones (e.g., ciprofloxacin)

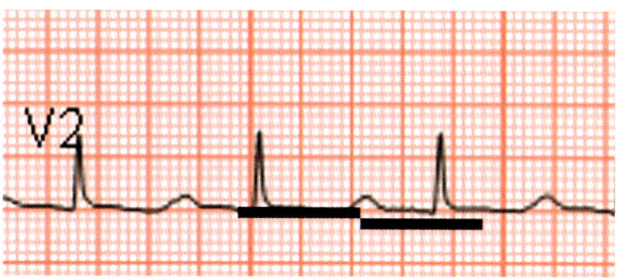

Long QT_c → Torsades de pointes[307]

- Polymorphic ventricular tachycardia with alternating amplitude and polarity
- Rx: IV $MgSO_4$ (to Mg ≥ 2 mmol/L) and/or K (to K ≥ 4 mmol/L) then increase heart rate: pacing or isoproterenol

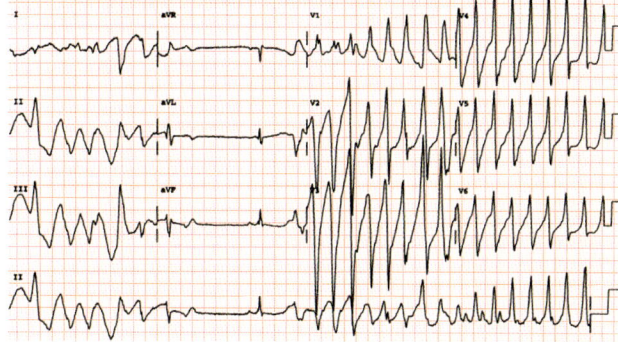

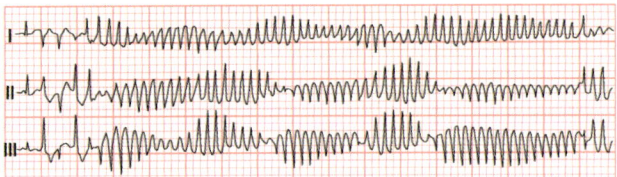

Early after depolarizations

Left Axis Deviation (−30° to −90°)
1) **Left ventricular hypertrophy**
2) **Inferior wall myocardial infarction**
3) Left anterior **fascicular block**
4) **Wolff-Parkinson-White syndrome** (R-pathway)
5) Emphysema & obesity (normal variant)

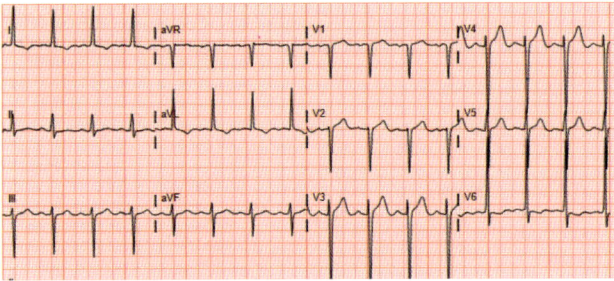

Right Axis Deviation (+90° to −90°)[308]
1) **Right ventricular hypertrophy & strain** (acute/chronic)
2) **Lateral wall myocardial infarction**
3) **Left posterior fascicular block**
4) Ostium secundum **atrial septal defect**
5) **Wolff-Parkinson-White syndrome** (L-pathway)
6) Normal in children or tall, thin adults

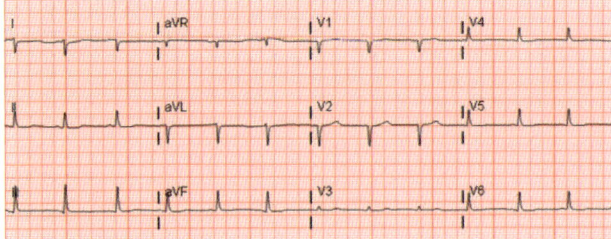

Right Atrial Enlargement
• RA depol directed anteriorly:
  – **Positive (up) portion of P wave in V1 ≥ 1.5 mm tall**
  – **P wave amplitude > 2.5 mm tall in II or III**

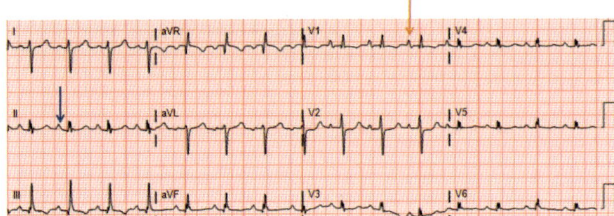

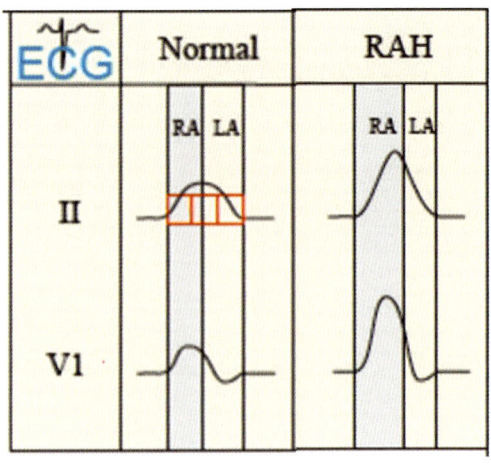

Left Atrial Enlargement
• LA depol → posteriorly:
  – **Negative (down) portion of P wave in V1 ≥ 1 mm depth**
  – **P wave duration > 0.12 sec in leads II or III**

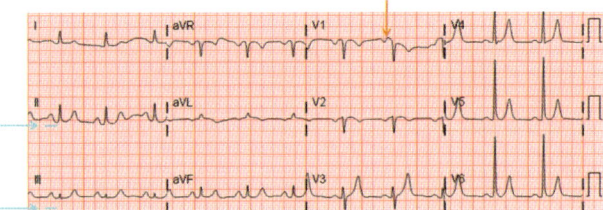

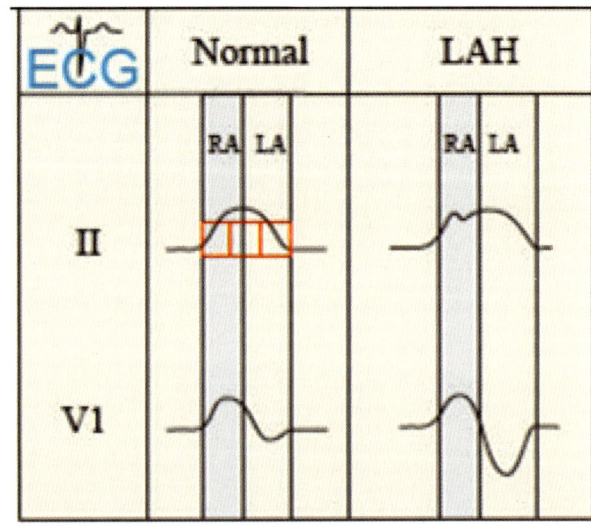

AR 23

This ECG shows electrical changes consistent with left ventricular hypertrophy.

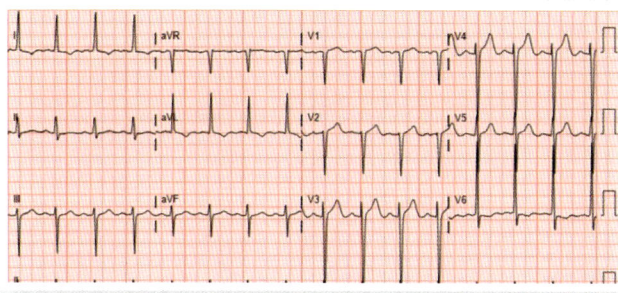

A. True
B. False

Answer:_____

Left Ventricular Hypertrophy (LVH)[309][310]

- Left ventricle wall **thick** and LV located under V3–V6 and I, aVL electrodes →
- Taller R waves in V3–V6 and I, aVL
- R aVL ≥ **11** mm
  - Specific   L1
    - (Sokolow-**L**yon)
- R aVL + S V3 > 28 mm males (> 20 mm females)
  - Sensitive (Cornell)
- S V1 + R V5/V6 ≥ 35 mm (SL)

(ECG diagram — Normal vs LVH: V1 shows rS; V6 shows qR. LVH shows Large S and Large R.)

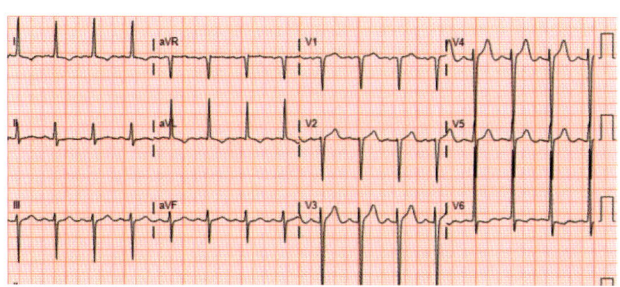

55-year-old Caucasian male with hypertension

Right Ventricular Hypertrophy (RVH)

- **Right ventricle wall <u>thick</u> and right ventricle under V1–V2 electrodes →**
- **Taller R waves in V1–V2**
- **R/S in V1 > 1**
- **R** in V1 > **7** mm
- R V1 + S V5/V6 ≥ **11** mm
- <u>The **7/11** Rule!</u>

(ECG diagram — Normal vs RVH: V1 shows rS normal, Large R with S and Q variable in RVH; V6 shows qR normal, RS in RVH.)

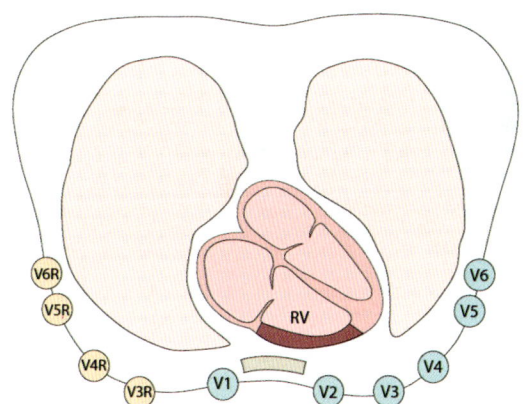

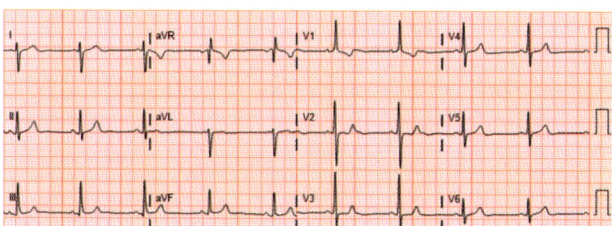

26-year-old Hispanic female with pulmonary arterial hypertension

SOME EXTRA EXAM ECGs

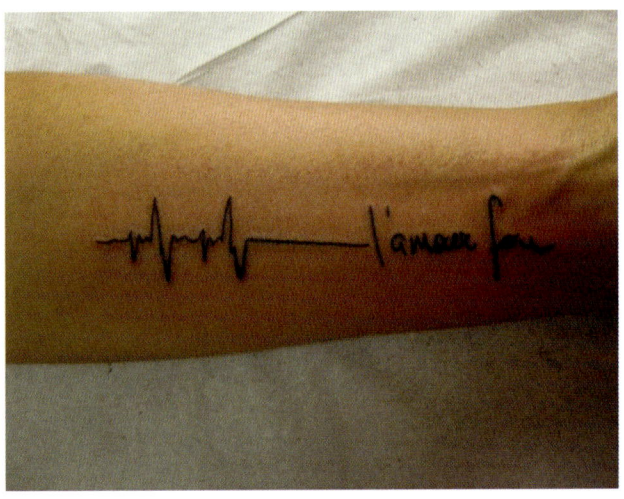

AR 24

A 19-year-old presents with 2 episodes of palpitations while playing basketball. He feels fine now.

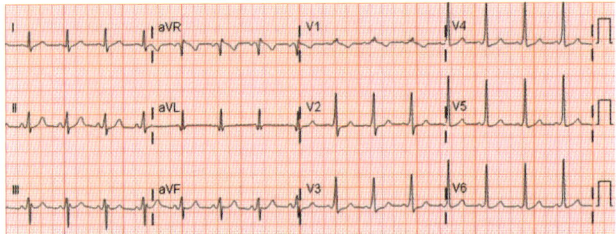

His ECG is consistent with:

A. Acute STEMI
B. Wolff-Parkinson-White pattern
C. Anomalous coronary artery
D. Long-QT syndrome

Answer:_____

Wolff-Parkinson-White Pattern (Preexcitation)

- Short PR interval, < 120 msec
- Delta wave, slurring of initial QRS
- Wide QRS, > 120 msec
- Narrow/Wide tachycardias

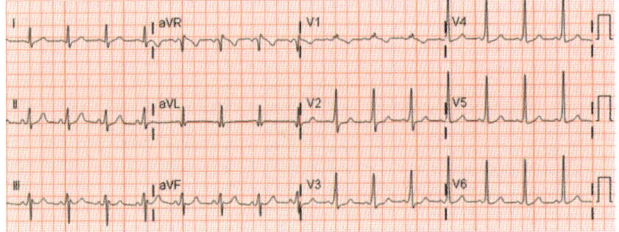

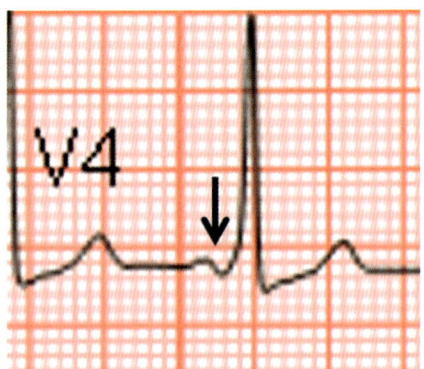

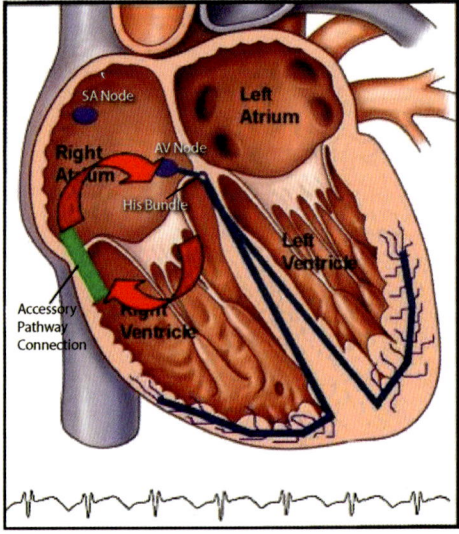

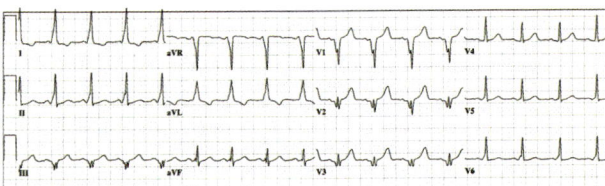

Wolff-Parkinson-White Sd and AFib

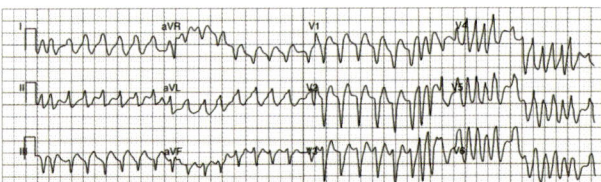

Men > women; L-sided pathways = most common

WPW Syndrome (Symptomatic Tachycardia) — Management[311][312]

- **Ablation (95%+ success)**: Symptomatic arrhythmias or AFib (risk)
- **W**PW + **H**emodyn stable AFib: IV **I**butilide, **P**rocainamide, or **A**miodarone (**WHIP-A** IT!!!)* **AVN blockers (e.g., atenolol, verapamil) contraindicated in WPW + AFib!**
- **Ic drugs (flecainide, propafenone)** if structurally nl heart (**amio** if abnormal) with AVRT and/or preexcited AFib **not candidates for, or refuse ablation**: slow conduction velocity & refractory period in accessory pathway
- Asymptomatic and abrupt **loss of conduction** over accessory pathway during **exercise testing** or intermittent loss on **ECG/Holter = low risk**
- **Ebstein anomaly:** septal leaflet apical

AR 25

A 22-year-old ESRD presents after missing dialysis for 2 weeks.

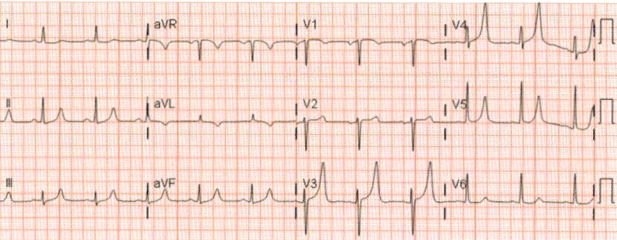

His ECG is consistent with:

A. Long-QT syndrome
B. Wolff-Parkinson-White pattern
C. Hyperkalemia
D. Brugada syndrome

Answer:_____

Hyperkalemia

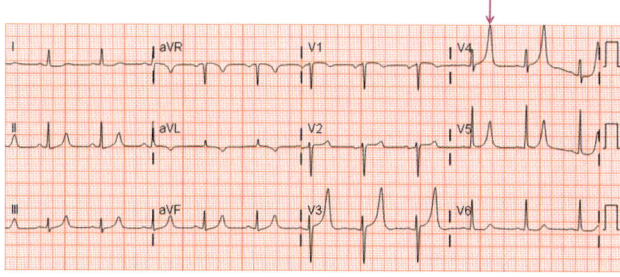

K > 5.5 mEq/L Peaked T waves
K > 6.5 Long PR segment, flattening/widening/loss of P wave
K > 7.0 Long QRS/sine wave, AV block, sinus BC/slow AFib
K > 9.0 AVP: Asystole, **V**Fib, **PEA**

Moderate Hyperkalemia

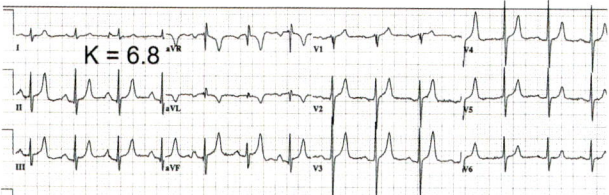

Severe Hyperkalemia

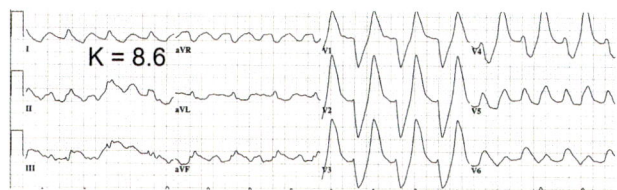

Preparticipation Sports — Dx?

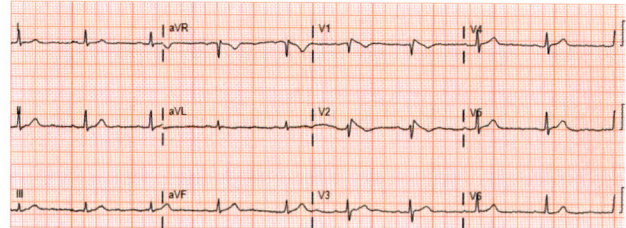

This 18-year-old Caucasian male presents for preparticipation screening for Rice University football; Hx and physical are normal.

Brugada Syndrome — AD, Male[313][314][315][316]

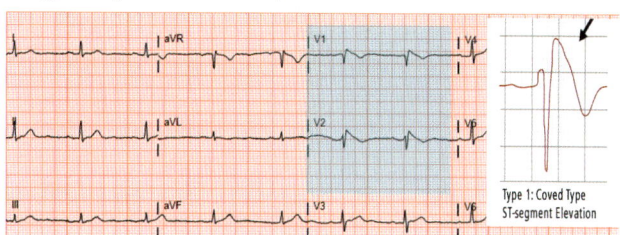

Type I: "Coved" J-point elevation ≥ 2 mm (0.2 mV), down-sloping ST elevation, T-wave inversion ≥ 2 right precordial leads (V1–V3)*
Loss of function *SCN5A* gene.
Rx BB; **if syncope, SCD, VT → ICD**
Spontaneously, by fever, or after challenge with IV Na channel blockers (ajmaline, flecainide)

We will not stand by as evil EXAMS wipe out billions of innocent lives.
Peter Quill, a.k.a. STARLORD &

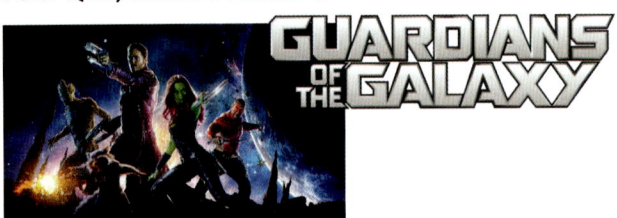

Final Thoughts

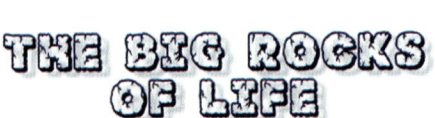 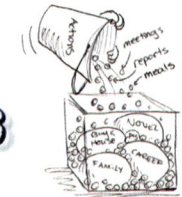

Be the change that you wish to see in the world.
Fate rarely calls upon us at a moment of our choosing!
Fortitudine Vincimus: "By Endurance We Conquer"
To give anything less than your best is to sacrifice the gift.
Try not. Do or do not. There is no try.

物极必反

Seems to me that when I die these words will be written on my stone …
Story of my life
There are two wolves who are always fighting. One is darkness and despair.
The other is light and hope. The question is … which wolf wins?
The one you feed.

Thank you
Guardians of the Medical Galaxy
If you **enjoyed** my presentation, I would be <u>honored</u> to receive a **sweet feedback score** on your evaluation of me!
Go Forth
And CRUSH YOUR MEDICAL EXAMS!
Dr. STARLORD

AUDIENCE RESPONSE ANSWERS

Audience Response 1
B. Coarctation of the aorta

AR 2
B. An exercise test with imaging (nuclear or echo)

AR 3
D. Cardiac tamponade

AR 4
B. Widely split second heart sound

AR 5
C. Atrial septal defect

AR 6
C. Urgent coronary angiography

AR 7
B. Full-dose reteplase (rPA), then transfer to PCI-capable hospital.

AR 8
B. Papillary muscle rupture/severe MR

AR 9
E. Ranolazine

AR 10
D. Moderate-intensity statin

AR 11
D. MRI of the lumbar spine

AR 12
B. Urgent invasive angiography

AR 13
A. True

AR 14
B. Refer for mitral valve repair/replacement.

AR 15
D. Warfarin and aspirin

AR 16
C. Catheter ablation

AR 17
C. Dabigatran 150 mg twice a day

AR 18
D. Stop aspirin and begin oral anticoagulation.

AR 19
C. Refer for ICD implantation.

AR 20
D. Constrictive pericarditis

AR 21
E. All of the above

AR 22
E. All of the above

AR 23
A. True

AR 24
B. Wolff-Parkinson-White pattern

AR 25
C. Hyperkalemia

ENDNOTES

[1]   Neon Tommy

[2]   J. Heuser

[3]   Npatchett, CC BY-SA 4.0 <https://creativecommons.org/licenses/by-sa/4.0>, via Wikimedia Commons

[4]   Circulation. 2015;131:1884–1931.

[5]   Johannes Nielsen [CC BY 2.0 (https://creativecommons.org/licenses/by/2.0)], via Wikimedia Commons

[6]   Drickey [CC BY-SA 2.5 (https://creativecommons.org/licenses/by-sa/2.5)], via Wikimedia Commons

[7]   Patrick J. Lynch, medical illustrator [CC BY 2.5 (https://creativecommons.org/licenses/by/2.5)]

[8]   2019 AHA/ACC/HRS Focused Update of the 2014 AHA/ACC/HRS Guideline for the Management of Patients With Atrial Fibrillation: Circulation. 2019 Jul 9;140(2):e125-e151. doi: 10.1161/CIR.0000000000000665. Epub 2019 Jan 28.

[9]   2018 AHA/ACC Guideline for the Management of Adults With Congenital Heart Disease: Circulation. 2019 Apr 2;139(14):e637-e697. doi: 10.1161/CIR.0000000000000602.

[10] Eur J Echocardiogr. 2008 Jan; 9(1):60–62.

[11] JAMA 1997;277:564-71

[12] Source: Bobjelly55

[13] Patrick J. Lynch,CC BY 2.5 <https://creativecommons.org/licenses/by/2.5>, via Wikimedia Commons

[14] Am Soc Echocardiogr. 2013; 26(9):921–964.

[15] http://bjcardio.co.uk/files/uploads/2012/03/fig1_howe_pg46.png

[16] J Am Soc Echocardiogr. 2013; 26(9):921–964.

[17] J Am Soc Echocardiogr. 2013; 26:443–456.

[18] Circulation. 2021 Oct 28:CIR0000000000001029. doi: 10.1161/CIR.0000000000001029.

[19] Circulation 2014;130:350-79.

[20] Int J Cardiol. 2007;116:285-99.

[21] Circulation. 2013 Aug 20;128(8):873-934.

[22] J Am Coll Cardiol. 2009; 53:2201-29.

[23] J Am Coll Cardiol. 2014; 63(4):380–406.

[24] J Am Coll Cardiol. 2014; 63(4):380–406.

[25] By Joseph Caballero, U.S. Navy [Public domain], via Wikimedia Commons

[26] Patrick J. Lynch, [CC BY-SA 3.0 (https://creativecommons.org/licenses/by-sa/3.0)], via Wikimedia Commons

[27] Circulation. 2013; 128:436–472.

[28] Global Journal of Health Science. 2012; 4(1):65–93.

[29] Journal of Cardiothoracic Surgery. 2010;5:108.

[30] Circulation. 2021 Oct 28:CIR0000000000001029. doi: 10.1161/CIR.0000000000001029.

[31] Circulation. 2010; 122:631–641.

[32] Front Physiol. 2014; 5:291.

[33] N Engl J Med 2008; 358:1336–45.

[34] J Am Coll Cardiol. October 2017 DOI: 10.1016/j.jacc.2017.10.053

[35] J Thorac Imaging. 2014; 29(6):318–330.

[36] Rofo 2014; 186:661-9.

[37] www.scientificanimations.com [CC BY-SA 4.0 (https://creativecommons.org/licenses/by-sa/4.0)]

[38] Eur Heart J. 2015; 36:2921–2964.

[39] J Am Coll Cardiol Intv. 2009; 2(8):705–717.

[40] Sarah Zucca [CC BY-SA 2.0 (https://creativecommons.org/licenses/by-sa/2.0)], via Wikimedia Commons

[41] http://mynotes4usmle.tumblr.com/post/36458617946/splitting-of-second-heart-sound-s2-physiological#.VHDvBIvF9ws

[42] 2018 AHA/ACC Guideline for the Management of Adults With Congenital Heart Disease: Circulation. 2019 Apr 2;139(14):e637-e697. doi: 10.1161/CIR.0000000000000602. PMID: 30586768

[43] http://circulation.or.kr/info/case/200909/fig2.gif

[44] Cleve Clin J Med. 2013; 80(10):638-44.

[45] By Pöllö [CC BY 3.0 (http://creativecommons.org/licenses/by/3.0)], via Wikimedia Commons

[46] https://www.myupchar.com/en, CC BY-SA 4.0 <https://creativecommons.org/licenses/by-sa/4.0>, via Wikimedia Commons

[47] J Am Coll Cardiol. 2014;63(18):1815–1822.

[48] Lancet. 2004; 364(9438):937–952.

[49] Am Heart J. 2013;166:622-8.

[50] J Am Coll Cardiol. 2017;69(1):73–82.

[51] Circulation. 2019 Sep 10;140(11):e596-e646

[52] Circulation. 2021 Oct 28:CIR0000000000001029. doi: 10.1161/CIR.0000000000001029.

[53] Lilly LS. Pathophysiology of Heart Disease. 2010 Nov.

[54] Lilly LS. Pathophysiology of Heart Disease. 2010 Nov.

[55] Circulation. 2013; 127:529–555.

[56] J Am Coll Cardiol 2012;60:96-105.

[57] Circulation. 2011; 124:2350–2354.

[58] Circulation. 2014; 130(25):2354–2394.

[59] Eur Heart J. 2021 Apr 7;42(14):1289-1367.

[60] Gage Skidmore [CC BY-SA 2.0 (https://creativecommons.org/licenses/by-sa/2.0)], via Wikimedia Commons Peter Ko [CC BY 3.0 (http://creativecommons.org/licenses/by/3.0)], via Wikimedia Commons Ewen [CC BY 2.0 (http://creativecommons.org/licenses/by/2.0)], via Wikimedia Commons By Scott Mecum [CC BY 2.0 (http://creativecommons.org/licenses/by/2.0)], via Wikimedia Commons Mingle Media TV [CC BY-SA 2.0 (https://creativecommons.org/licenses/by-sa/2.0)], via Wikimedia Commons karina3094 [CC BY-SA 2.0 (https://creativecommons.org/licenses/by-sa/2.0)], via Wikimedia Commons

[61] JAMA. 2000; 284(7):835–842.

[62] Emerg Med J. 2008; 25(2):122

[63] JAMA. 2000; 284(7):835–842.

[64] Circulation. 2014; 130(25):2354–2394.

[65] Circulation. 2014; 130(25):2354–2394.

[66] European Heart Journal 2016; 37:267–315.

[67] Eur Heart J. 2011;32:2945-53.

[68] N Engl J Med 2015;372:1791-800.

[69] Circulation. 2021 Oct 28:CIR0000000000001029. doi: 10.1161/CIR.0000000000001029.

[70] Circulation. 2014; 130(25):2354–2394.

[71] Circulation 2016; 134(10):e123–55.

[72] Circulation. 2014; 130(25): 2354–2394

[73] Circulation. 2014; 130(25):2354–2394.

[74] European Heart Journal 2016; 37:267–315.

[75] By Fir0002 CC-BY-SA-3.0 (http://creativecommons.org/licenses/by-sa/3.0/)], via Wikimedia Commons

[76] Circulation. 2014; 130(25):2354–2394.

[77] Front Neurol Neurosci. 2015; 37:51–61.

[78] Circulation. 2014; 130(25):2354–2394.

[79] Valerie Everett (CC-SA 3.0)
Radspunk CC BY-SA 4.0-3.0-2.5-2.0-1.0 (https://creativecommons.org/licenses/by-sa/4.0-3.0-2.5-2.0-1.0)], via Wikimedia Commons

[80] Circulation. 2013; 127:529–555.

[81] European Heart Journal 2016; 37:267–315.

[82] Source: JHeuser

[83] Circulation. 2013; 127:529–555.

[84] European Heart Journal 2016; 37:267–315.

[85] Circulation. 2013; 127:529–555.

[86] Vasc Health Risk Manag. 2015; 11:93–106

[87] Circulation. 2013; 127:529–555.

[88] Circulation. 2013; 127:529–555.

[89] Circulation. 2013; 127:529–555.

[90] Stroke. 2018;49(3):e46-e110

[91] Circulation. 2013; 127:529–555.

[92] Circulation. 2013; 127:529–555.

[93] Circulation. 2014; 130:2354–2394.

[94] Vasc Health Risk Manag. 2013; 9:321–331.

[95] Circulation. 2013; 127:529–555.

[96] Circulation. 2013; 127:529–555.

[97] Circulation. 2018;137:e578–e622. DOI: 10.1161/CIR.0000000000000560

[98] By Patrick J. Lynch [CC BY 2.5 (http://creativecommons.org/licenses/by/2.5)], via Wikimedia Commons

[99] J Am Coll Cardiol. October 2017 DOI: 10.1016/j.jacc.2017.10.053

[100] J Am Coll Cardiol. October 2017 DOI: 10.1016/j.jacc.2017.10.053

[101] Circulation. 2016; 133:1715-1727.

[102] J Am Coll Cardiol. 2013; 61:1318–1368.

[103] n28ive1 [CC BY 2.0 (http://creativecommons.org/licenses/by/2.0)], via Wikimedia Commons

[104] J Am Coll Cardiol. 2013; 61(12):1318–1368.

[105] J Am Coll Cardiol. October 2017 DOI: 10.1016/j.jacc.2017.10.053

[106] Circulation. 2014; 130:1749–1767.

[107] Circulation. 2014; 130:1749–1767.

[108] Hypertension. 2015; 65:1372–407.

[109] J Am Coll Cardiol. 2018;71(19):2199-2269.

[110] Circulation. 2018 May 17. pii: CIR.0000000000000574. doi: 10.1161/CIR.0000000000000574.

[111] Circulation. 2019 Sep 10;140(11):e596-e646

[112] Circulation. 2014; 130:1749–1767.

[113] Circulation. 2019 Sep 10;140(11):e596-e646

[114] Circulation. 2014; 130:1749–1767.

[115] Curr Cardiol Rep. 2016;18(1):1.

[116] Circulation. 2014; 130(24):2215–45

[117] N Engl J Med. 2009;360(3):213–224.

[118] Circulation. 2016; 134(10):e123–55

[119] Circulation. 2016;134:e156-e178.

[120] Circulation. 2014;130:399–409

[121] NEJM 2016;374:1511-20.

[122] Circulation. 2012;126:3097–3137.

[123] Source: Blausen.com staff

[124] Phil Denton. CC-SA-20 https://creativecommons.org/licenses/by-sa/2.0/

[125] Circulation. 2014; 129:S1–45.

[126] J Am Coll Cardiol. 2016;68(1):92–125.

[127] 2018 AHA/ACC/AACVPR/AAPA/ABC/ACPM/ADA/AGS/APhA/ASPC/NLA/PCNA Guideline on the Management of Blood Cholesterol

Circulation. 2019 Jun 18;139(25):e1046-e1081. doi: 10.1161/CIR.0000000000000624. Epub 2018 Nov 10.

[128] http://tools.acc.org/ASCVD-Risk-Estimator/

[129] 2018 AHA/ACC/AACVPR/AAPA/ABC/ACPM/ADA/AGS/APhA/ASPC/NLA/PCNA Guideline on the Management of Blood Cholesterol

Circulation. 2019 Jun 18;139(25):e1046-e1081. doi: 10.1161/CIR.0000000000000624. Epub 2018 Nov 10.

[130] Circulation. 2013; 127:1425–1443.

[131] Circulation. 2017;135(12):e686–e725.

[132] Circulation. 2017;135(12):e686–e725.

[133] Circulation. 2017;135(12):e686–e725.

[134] Blausen.com staff (2014). "Medical gallery of Blausen Medical 2014". WikiJournal of Medicine 1 (2). DOI:10.15347/wjm/2014.010. ISSN 2002-4436. [CC BY 3.0 (http://creativecommons.org/licenses/by/3.0)], via Wikimedia Commons

[135] Circulation. 2017;135(12):e686–e725.

[136] J Am Coll Cardiol. 2018;71(19):2199-2269.

[137] By Jim Winstead [CC BY 2.0 (http://creativecommons.org/licenses/by/2.0)], via Wikimedia Commons

[138] Circulation. 2017;135(12):e686–e725.

[139] Circulation. 2017;135(12):e686–e725.

[140] https://www.scientificanimations.com, CC BY-SA 4.0 <https://creativecommons.org/licenses/by-sa/4.0>, via Wikimedia Commons

[141] Circulation. 2017;135(12):e686–e725.

[142] NEJM 2012; 366: 2198-206.

[143] Circulation. 2013; 127:529–555.

[144] J Am Coll Cardiol. October 2017 DOI: 10.1016/j.jacc.2017.10.053

[145] Blausen.com staff (2014). "Medical gallery of Blausen Medical 2014". WikiJournal of Medicine 1 (2). DOI:10.15347/wjm/2014.010. ISSN 2002-4436., CC BY 3.0 <https://creativecommons.org/licenses/by/3.0>, via Wikimedia Commons

[146] Circulation. 2011; 124:e54–e130.

[147] Circulation. 2011; 124:e54–e130.

[148] J Am Coll Cardiol. 2018;71(19):2199-2269.

[149] N Engl J Med 2010; 363:11–23.

[150] Stroke. 2015; 46:3020–35.

[151] Blausen.com staff (2014). "Medical gallery of Blausen Medical 2014". WikiJournal of Medicine 1 (2). DOI:10.15347/wjm/2014.010. ISSN 2002-4436., CC BY 3.0 <https://creativecommons.org/licenses/by/3.0>, via Wikimedia Commons

[152] scientificanimations.com, CC BY 4.0 <https://creativecommons.org/licenses/by/3.0>, via Wikimedia Commons

[153] By Blausen Medical Communications, Inc. [CC BY 3.0 (http://creativecommons.org/licenses/by/3.0)], via Wikimedia Commons

[154] N Engl J Med. 2016;374(21):2065–2074.

[155] Stroke. 2013;44(3):870–947.

[156] Circulation. 2016; 133: 680–686.

[157] Anesth Analg. 2010;111(2):279–315.

[158] J Am Coll Cardiol. 2016;68(5):502–516.

[159] Eur Heart J. 2011;32(24):3147–3197.

[160] Am J Cardiol 2011;107:1227–234.

[161] Circulation. 2021 Oct 28:CIR0000000000001029. doi: 10.1161/CIR.0000000000001029.

[162] Circulation. 2013; 127:1425–1443.

[163] Hertzer NR, CC BY-SA 4.0 <https://creativecommons.org/licenses/by-sa/4.0>, via Wikimedia Commons

[164] Fortschr Röntgenstr 2014; 186: 337–347.

[165] J Vasc Interv Radiol 2010; 21:1632–1655.

[166] http://www.uspreventiveservicestaskforce.org/Page/Topic/recommendation-summary/abdominal-aortic-aneurysm-screening

[167] N Engl J Med. 2013; 368:1425–1433.

[168] Heart. 2015;101:250-2.

[169] Circulation. 2021 Feb 2;143(5):e35-e71.

[170] Popculturegeek via Flickr, CC-SA 2.0

[171] Source: Randy Robertson

[172] Circulation. 2017;135(25):e1159–e1195.

[173] Circulation. 2021 Feb 2;143(5):e35-e71.

[174] BruceBlaus [CC BY-SA 4.0 (https://creativecommons.org/licenses/by-sa/4.0)], from Wikimedia Commons

[175] Circulation. 2010; 121:458–477.

[176] Circulation. 2021 Feb 2;143(5):e35-e71.

[177] By Steven Fruitsmaak CC BY 3.0 (http://creativecommons.org/licenses/by/3.0)], via Wikimedia Commons

[178] Circulation. 2017;135(25):e1159-e1195.

[179] Circulation. 2021 Feb 2;143(5):e35-e71.

[180] Stif Komar, CC BY-SA 3.0 <https://creativecommons.org/licenses/by-sa/3.0>, via Wikimedia Commons

[181] J Atheroscler Thromb. 2019 Aug 3. doi: 10.5551/jat.49239. [Epub ahead of print] Disappearance of Angiodysplasia Following Transcatheter Aortic Valve Implantation in a Patient with Heyde's Syndrome: A Case Report and Review of the Literature.

[182] Circulation. 2021 Feb 2;143(5):e35-e71.

[183] J Postgrad Med. 2008; 54(2):163–165.

[184] Ciernik M, CC BY-SA 4.0 <https://creativecommons.org/licenses/by-sa/4.0>, via Wikimedia Commons

[185] Circulation. 2017;135(25):e1159–e1195.

[186] N Engl J Med. 2004;351:1539-46.

[187] Circulation. 2021 Feb 2;143(5):e35-e71.

[188] Circulation. 2017;135(25):e1159-e1195.

[189] . J Am Soc Echocardiogr 2001;14:676-81.

[190] Circulation. 2021 Feb 2;143(5):e35-e71.

[191] Source: Blausen Medical Communications, Inc.

[192] J Am Coll Cardiol 2014; 63:e57–185.

[193] J Am Coll Cardiol. 2017 Oct 17. pii: S0735–1097(17)39677–8.

[194] Circulation. 2017;135(25):e1159–e1195.

[195] Circulation. 2021 Feb 2;143(5):e35-e71.

[196] Source: J. Heuser

[197] Circulation. 2017;135(25):e1159–e1195.

[198] Circulation. 2021 Feb 2;143(5):e35-e71.

[199] Source: Stif Komar

[200] Source: Robertolyra

[201] Circulation. 2017;135(25):e1159–e1195.

[202] Circulation. 2017;135(25):e1159–e1195.

[203] Circulation. 2021 Feb 2;143(5):e35-e71.

[204] Circulation. 2017;135(25):e1159–e1195.

[205] Circulation. 2021 Feb 2;143(5):e35-e71.

[206] CardioNetworks: Drj, CC BY-SA 3.0 <https://creativecommons.org/licenses/by-sa/3.0>, via Wikimedia Commons

[207] J Am Coll Cardiol. 2018 Nov 6. pii: S0735-1097(18)38985-X. doi: 10.1016/j.jacc.2018.10.044. [Epub ahead of print]

[208] Heart. 2010; 96(20):1611–1616.

[209] Prog Cardiovasc Dis. 2013;56:203-10

[210] BruceBlaus, CC BY-SA 4.0 <https://creativecommons.org/licenses/by-sa/4.0>, via Wikimedia Commons

[211] Circulation. 2016; 133(14):e506–574.

[212] Circulation. 2016; 133(14):e506–74.

[213] Circulation. 2014; 130:2071–2104.

[214] Circulation. 2016;133(14):e506–74.

[215] Circulation. 2014;130:2071–2104.

[216] Circulation. 2014; 130:2071–2104.

[217] Circulation. 2014; 130:2071–2104.

[218] Eur Heart J. 2014;35:2733-79.

[219] Circulation. 2020 Dec 22;142(25):e533-e557. doi: 10.1161/CIR.0000000000000938.

[220] Circulation. 2021 Feb 2;143(5):e35-e71.

[221] 2019 AHA/ACC/HRS Focused Update of the 2014 AHA/ACC/HRS Guideline for the Management of Patients With Atrial Fibrillation: Circulation. 2019 Jul 9;140(2):e125-e151. doi: 10.1161/CIR.0000000000000665. Epub 2019 Jan 28.

[222] J Am Coll Cardiol. 2015;65:2614-2623.

[223] Circulation. 2014; 130:2071–2104.

[224] Hematol Oncol Clin North Am 2016; 30(5):1073–1084. 2019 AHA/ACC/HRS Focused Update of the 2014 AHA/ACC/HRS Guideline for the Management of Patients With Atrial Fibrillation: Circulation. 2019 Jul 9;140(2):e125-e151. doi: 10.1161/CIR.0000000000000665. Epub 2019 Jan 28.

[225] Circulation 2013; 128:721-8.

[226] Circulation. 2014; 130:2071–2104.

[227] N Engl J Med 2018; 378:417-427

[228] Circulation. 2014; 130:2071–2104.

[229] JACC October 2017 DOI: 0.1016/j.jacc.2017.10.053

[230] Eur Heart J. 2004;25(13):1093-9.

[231] Blausen.com staff (2014). "Medical gallery of Blausen Medical 2014". WikiJournal of Medicine 1 (2). DOI:10.15347/wjm/2014.010. ISSN 2002-4436., CC BY 3.0 <https://creativecommons.org/licenses/by/3.0>, via Wikimedia Commons

[232] J Am Coll Cardiol. 2018 Nov 6. pii: S0735-1097(18)38985-X. doi: 10.1016/j.jacc.2018.10.044. [Epub ahead of print]

[233] Circulation. 2012; 126:1784–1800.

[234] Pacing Clin Electrophysiol. 2012; 35(2):223–226.

[235] Circulation. 2017;136(5):e60–e122.

[236] Circulation. 2013; 127(12):1330–1339.

[237] Circulation. 2017;136(5):e60–e122.

[238] Circulation. 2017;136(5):e60–e122.

[239] J Intern Med. 2015; 277(1):69 – 82.

[240] Circulation. 2017;136(5):e60–e122.

[241] Prog Cardiovasc Dis. 2014 Jul–Aug;57(1):91–99.

[242] Circulation. 2020 Dec 22;142(25):e533-e557. doi: 10.1161/CIR.0000000000000938.

[243] Circulation. 2011; 124:2761–2796.

[244] Eur Heart J. 2014; 35: 2733–79.

[245] Circulation. 2020 Dec 22;142(25):e533-e557. doi: 10.1161/CIR.0000000000000938.

[246] JACC October 2017 DOI: 0.1016/j.jacc.2017.10.053

[247] Circulation. 2011; 124:2761–2796.

[248] J Am Coll Cardiol. 2015; 66: 2362-2371

[249] Circulation. 2020 Dec 22;142(25):e533-e557. doi: 10.1161/CIR.0000000000000938.

[250] Circulation. 2017;136(6):e137–e161.

[251] Eur J Heart Fail 2016 18(8) 891–975.

[252] NEJM 2016:375:1868-1877.

[253] Circulation. 2017;136(6):e137–e161.

[254] Circulation. 2017;136(6):e137–e161.

[255] Circulation. 2017;136(6):e137-e161.

[256] Lancet. 2010;376:875-885.

[257] Circulation. 2017;136(6):e137–e161.

[258] Circulation. 2013; 127:529–555.

[259] European Heart Journal. 2015; 36:2921–2964.

[260] Circulation. 2021 Oct 28:CIR0000000000001029. doi: 10.1161/CIR.0000000000001029.

[261] Circulation. 2013; 127:529–555.

[262] Eur Heart J. 2015; 36:2921–2964.

[263] J Am Coll Cardiol 2020;75:76-92

[264] BruceBlaus, CC BY-SA 4.0 <https://creativecommons.org/licenses/by-sa/4.0>, via Wikimedia Commons

[265] J Am Coll Cardiol. 2004; 43(8):1445–1452.

[266] J Am Coll Cardiol Img. 2011; 4(6):567–575

[267] www.cardiachealth.org/amyloid-disease-heart

[268] Circulation. 2015;132:1525–27.

[269] Source: Jason Lam

[270] Heart. 2016; 102(2):100–106.

[271] Radiology. 2008; 246(1):328–9.

[272] Cardiol Clin. 2015;33:531-41..

[273] By Veronica Belmont [CC BY-SA 2.0 (https://creativecommons.org/licenses/by-sa/2.0)], via Wikimedia Commons

[274] Clin Med Res. Dec 2007; 5(4):218–226.

[275] Circulation. 2016; 133:337–340.

[276] Circulation. 2015; 131:1884–1931.

2018 AHA/ACC Guideline for the Management of Adults With Congenital Heart Disease: Circulation. 2019 Apr 2;139(14):e637-e697. doi: 10.1161/CIR.0000000000000602. PMID: 30586768

[277] https://pediatricheartspecialists.com/heart-education/15-congenital-heart-defects/172-patent-ductus-arteriosus

[278] Circulation. 2015; 131:1884–1931.

[279] Am J Med Genet A. 2010; 152A(8):1960–1966.

[280] Habermann TM (ed.) Mayo Clinic Internal Medicine Review. Mayo Clinic Scientific Press, 2006.

[281] Source: Edesaintjores

[282] Circulation. 2015; 131:1884–1931.

[283] 2018 AHA/ACC Guideline for the Management of Adults With Congenital Heart Disease: Circulation. 2019 Apr 2;139(14):e637-e697. doi: 10.1161/CIR.0000000000000602. PMID: 30586768

[284] Pediatr Cardiol. 2012 Mar;33(3):434–438.

[285] Source: Jamie Buchsbaum

[286] JACC October 2017 DOI: 0.1016/j.jacc.2017.10.053

[287] European Heart Journal. 2015; 36: 2793–2867.

[288] J Am Coll Cardiol. 2013 Sep 17;62(12):1112–1113.

[289] Circulation. 2015; 131:1884–1931.

[290] Int J Cardiol 2011;151:307-12.

[291] J Am Coll Cardiol 2009; 54:S55–66.

[292] Circulation. 2018;137:e578–e622.DOI: 10.1161/ CIR.0000000000000560

[293] European Heart Journal. 2016; 37:67–119.

[294] Circulation. 2018;137:e578–e622. DOI: 10.1161/ CIR.0000000000000560

[295] N Engl J Med. 2015;373:834-843.

[296] Circulation. 2016; 133(14):e506–74.

[297] Circulation. 2016; 133(14):e506–74.

[298] Circulation. 2016;133(14):e506–74.

[299] J Am Coll Cardiol. 2008;51:e1-62.

[300] 2019 AHA/ACC/HRS Focused Update of the 2014 AHA/ ACC/HRS Guideline for the Management of Patients With Atrial Fibrillation: Circulation. 2019 Jul 9;140(2):e125-e151. doi: 10.1161/CIR.0000000000000665. Epub 2019 Jan 28.

[301] 2019 AHA/ACC/HRS Focused Update of the 2014 AHA/ ACC/HRS Guideline for the Management of Patients With Atrial Fibrillation: Circulation. 2019 Jul 9;140(2):e125-e151. doi: 10.1161/CIR.0000000000000665. Epub 2019 Jan 28.

[302] JACC October 2017 DOI: 0.1016/j.jacc.2017.10.053

[303] Circulation. 2010;121(8):1047–1060.

[304] Circulation. 2014; 129: 1524–9.

[305] European Heart Journal. 2015;36:2793–2867.

[306] Br J Clin Pharmacol. 2010; 70(1): 16–23.

[307] JACC October 2017 DOI: 0.1016/j.jacc.2017.10.053

[308] Circulation. 1979; 60(1):12–21.

[309] Sokolow M and Lyon TP. Am Heart J. 1949; 37:161–186.

[310] Casael PN, et al. JACC. 1985; 6(3):572–580.

[311] Circulation. 2016; 133(14):e506–74.

[312] Circulation. 2014; 130:2071–2104.

[313] JACC October 2017 DOI: 0.1016/j.jacc.2017.10.053

[314] European Heart Journal. 2015; 36: 2793–2867.

[315] Heart Rhythm 2016; 13:1274–1282.

[316] http://cdn.agilitycms.com/canadian-journal-of-diagnosis/ Images/Articles/2013/06-June2013/CaseoftheMonth/ Figure-2.gif

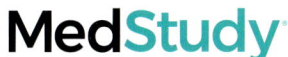

INTERNAL MEDICINE REVIEW

Dermatology

Presented by

Aaron J. Calderon, MD

TABLE OF CONTENTS

Why Some Topic Names Are Not Printed in This Section

At MedStudy, we do all we can to optimize your self-testing and learning.

In this section, the speaker has chosen to introduce topics with an Audience Response question to help you learn. In the syllabus, we've intentionally "hidden" some topic names that would give away the answers—so you can self-test more effectively. Where we've done this, instead of the topic name, you'll see an empty teal band or some extra space, but you can still find the topic on the page using the Table of Contents.

Dermatology Overview
- 3% of examination
- **Wide** number of topics
- Be thorough with the *Internal Medicine Core*
- Highlighted in **yellow**!

What Will We Be Covering?
- Common Skin Problems
- Mouth Findings
- Cutaneous Drug Reactions
- Inflammatory Skin Disorders
- Skin Infections
- Cutaneous Malignancies
- Blistering Lesions
- Round/Annular Lesions
- Pigment Changes
- Conditions Associated with Systemic Disease

COMMON SKIN PROBLEMS

Audience Response 1

A 26-year-old female with asthma presents with numerous rough, weeping, pruritic, erythematous patches in the antecubital and popliteal fossas.

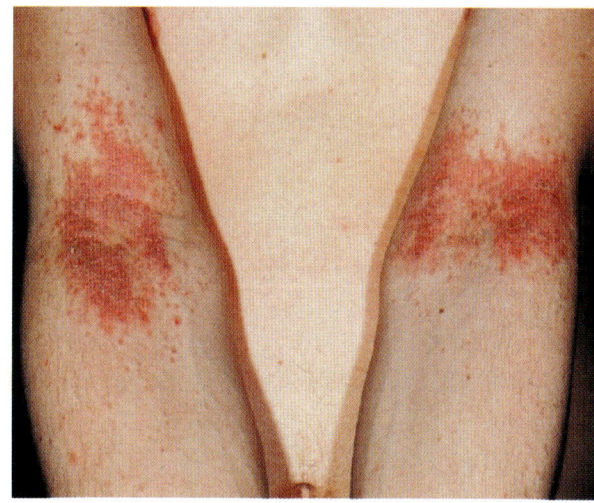

[1]

What is the preferred treatment for her condition?

A. Oral antihistamines
B. Topical tacrolimus
C. Oral azathioprine
D. Topical antifungal
E. Topical corticosteroids

Answer:_____

ATOPIC DERMATITIS (AD)

Atopic Dermatitis (AD; Eczema, Atopic Eczema)
- Eczema comes from the Greek word that means "to boil over"
- Acute eczema appears "wet," while chronic eczema appears dry and the skin thickened (lichenified)

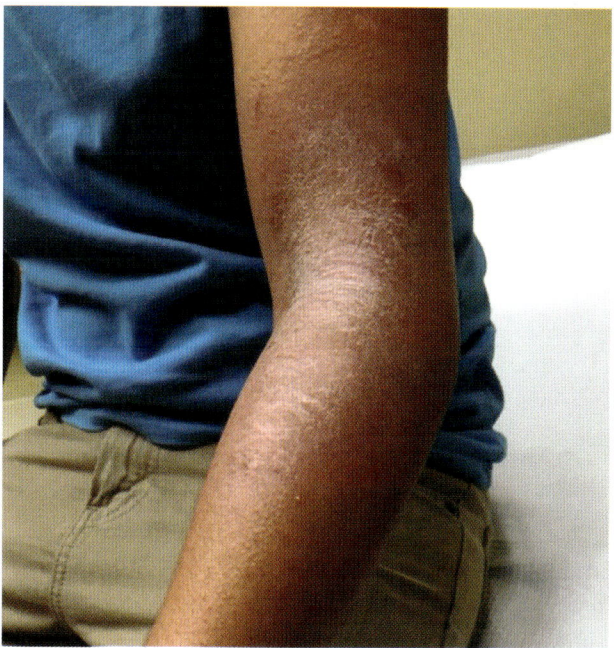

AD
- Begins in childhood
- Very pruritic
- Chronic
- Relapsing and remitting
- **Flexural distribution**
  - Antecubital fossa
  - Popliteal fossa
  - Wrists
- Asthma and allergies
- Persons with atopy have a strong overall Th2 diathesis

AD — Maintenance
- **Skin hygiene**
  - Tub soaks or showers < 10 minutes
  - Moisturize within 3 minutes
  - Ointment-based emollients best
    - Petroleum jelly is cheap and effective
    - Discourage lotions and oils
  - Gentle cleansers (i.e., nonsoap)
- **Avoid irritants**
  - Wool, fragrances, excessive hand washing
  - Heat, stress

AD — Treatment
- **Topical corticosteroids**
  - Mainstay Rx for acute flares
  - Use lowest effective dose
  - Use only low potency on face
- **Topical immunomodulators**
  - Calcineurin inhibitors (tacrolimus, pimecrolimus)
  - Topical crisaborole (phosphodiesterase-4 inhibitor)
- **Systemic immunomodulators/Light therapy**
  - Methotrexate, mycophenolate mofetil
  - Cyclosporine, azathioprine
  - Dupilumab (IL-4)

DERMATOLOGY

SEBORRHEIC DERMATITIS

AR 2

This 37-year-old man has not responded to adequate seborrheic dermatitis therapy.

What is the next step in management?

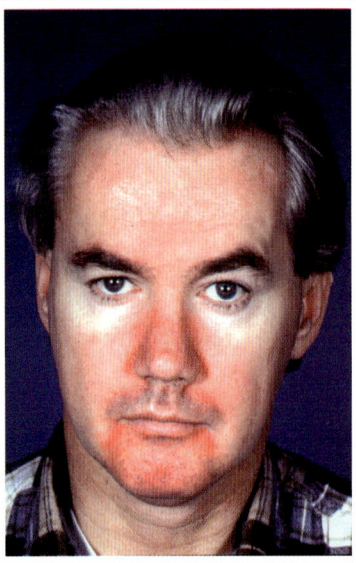

A. Genetic testing
B. Skin biopsy
C. CT chest/abdomen/pelvis
D. Check for HIV.
E. Start oral corticosteroids.

Answer: _____

Seborrheic Dermatitis
- Common, chronic inflammatory condition
- **Greasy, yellow scale ± erythema**
- Typical sebaceous locations
- Remits and relapses
- *Malassezia furfur* yeast thought to play an etiologic role
- More severe in **HIV**
- Higher prevalence in **Parkinson's**

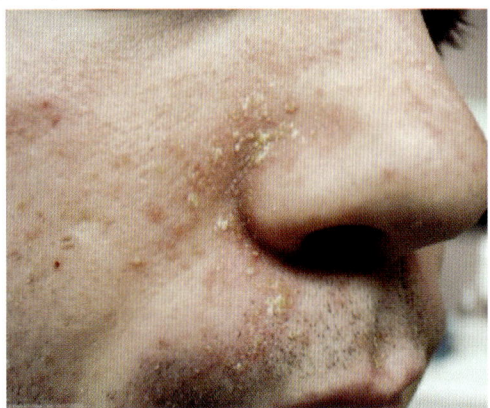

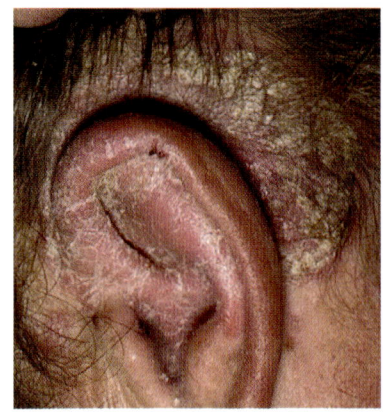

- **Distribution**
  - Scalp
  - Eyebrows
  - Conchal bowls
  - Nasolabial folds
  - Chest
  - Axilla
  - Groin

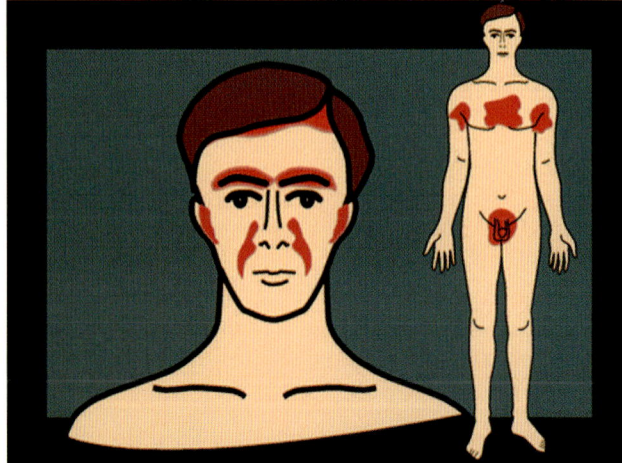

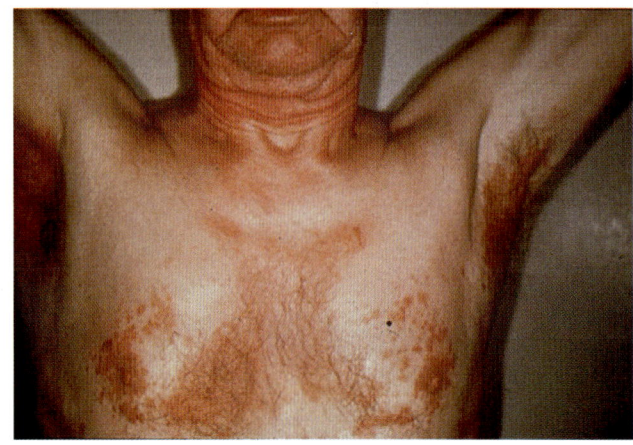

- Treatment
  - Topicals (ketoconazole, selenium sulfide, zinc pyrithione)
    - Shampoos
    - Creams, foams
  - Topical steroids (low potency); not recommended as maintenance
  - Topical immunomodulators
    - Pimecrolimus and tacrolimus

AR 3

What is the most likely cause of this patient's rash?

A. Poison ivy
B. Penicillin allergy
C. Atopic dermatitis
D. Viral exanthem
E. Seborrheic dermatitis

Answer:_____

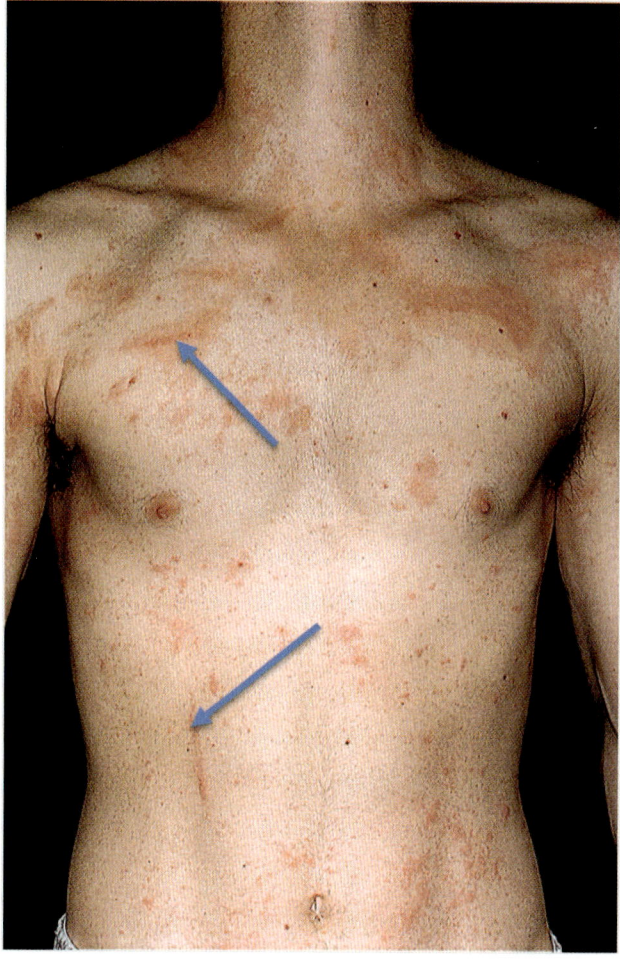

Contact Dermatitis
- **Irritant** (80%)
  - Direct chemical damage (soap, detergent, hair dyes)
  - No previous exposure necessary
  - Occurs immediately after contact
- **Allergic**
  - Latex gloves, nickel, poison ivy/oak, neomycin
  - **Delayed Type 4 hypersensitivity response** (10 days +)
  - Sensitization (before exposure) required
  - 1–2 days if 2nd or subsequent exposures
  - Patch testing is gold standard for diagnosis

Patch Testing

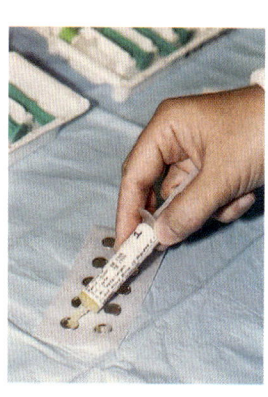
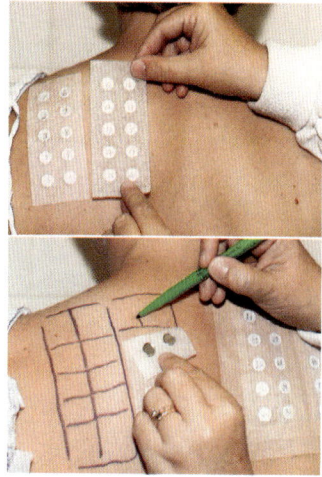

Contact Dermatitis

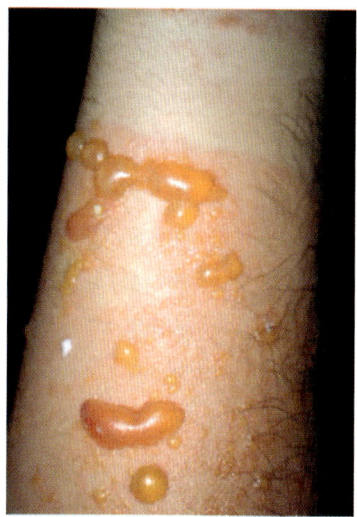

DERMATOLOGY

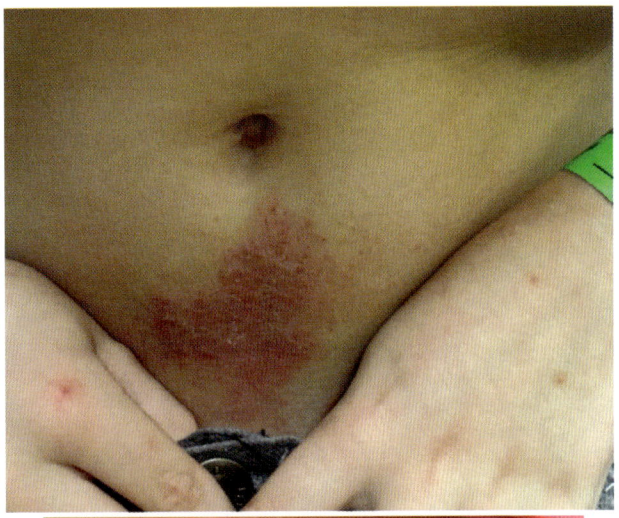

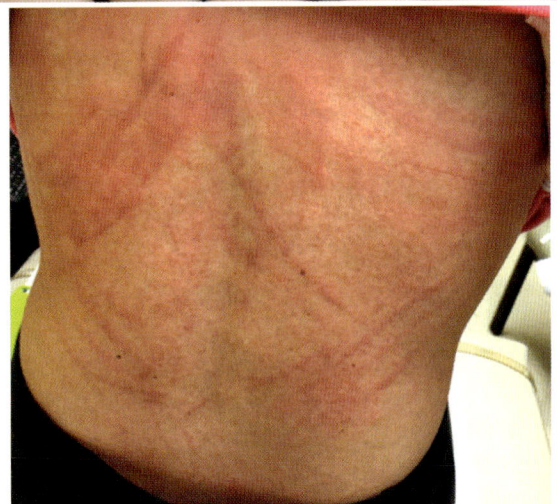

Contact Dermatitis — Treatment
- Treatment similar for both (irritant/allergic)
- Identify and remove offending irritant/allergen
- Topical corticosteroids
- Systemic corticosteroids for severe cases
- Aluminum acetate soaks (antiseptic, drying agent)
  - Good for weeping lesions
- Keep affected areas dry

ACNE AND ROSACEA

AR 4

The treatment of choice for this patient's comedonal acne is:

A. Oral tetracycline
B. Isotretinoin
C. Spironolactone
D. Hydrocortisone 2.5% cream
E. Topical retinoid

Answer:_____

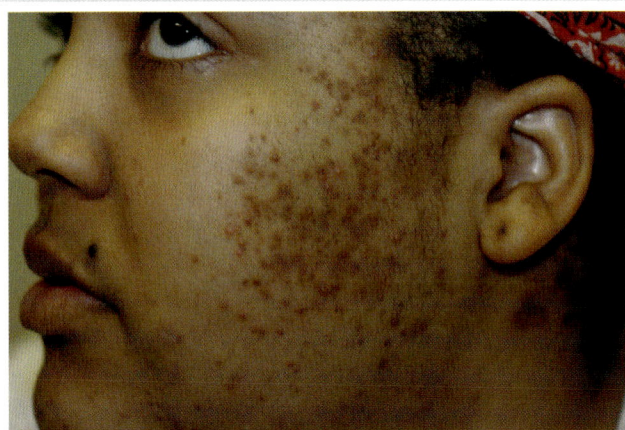

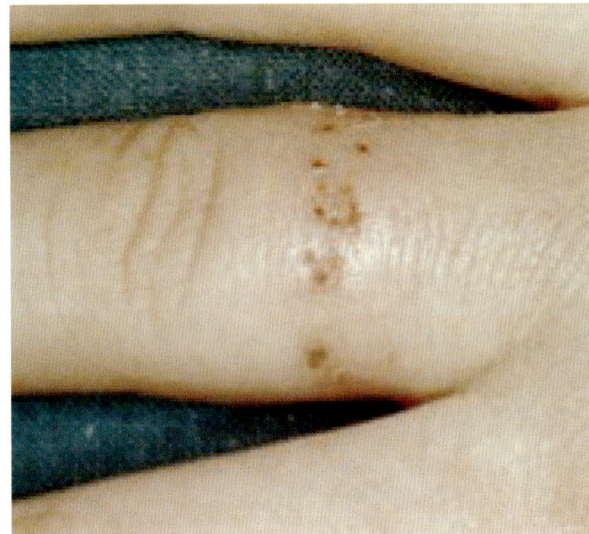

AR 5

Which are potential side effects of this oral medication used for severe nodulocystic acne?

A. Pancreatitis
B. Idiopathic intracranial hypertension
C. Hepatotoxicity
D. Choices B and C
E. All of the above

Answer:_____

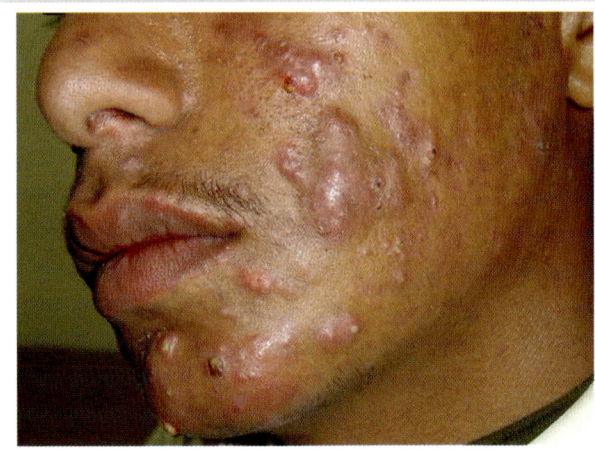

Acne Vulgaris

- Affects 85% of adolescents
- 12% of women continue to get lesions through their 40s
- Predisposing factor is hyperresponsiveness to androgens (e.g., polycystic ovary syndrome)
- **Main types:**
  - **Comedonal** (noninflammatory)
    - Occlusion of follicles
  - **Inflammatory** (papulopustular)
    - Directed against *Cutibacterium acnes* (previously known as *Propionibacterium acnes*), excess sebum around hair follicle, follicular plugging
  - **Severe nodulocystic** (know isotretinoin)

Acne

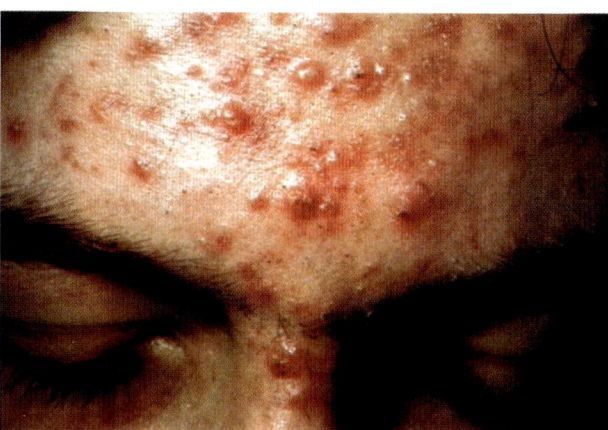

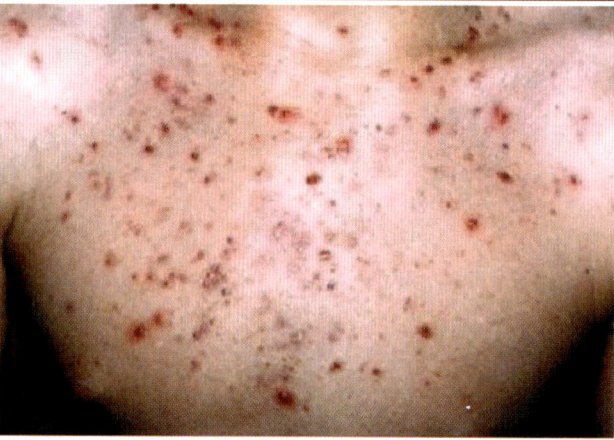

Acne Therapy

- **Comedonal** (noninflammatory)
  - Topical retinoid (e.g., tretinoin, adapalene)
- **Mild inflammatory** (papules and pustules)
  - Topical antibiotic (e.g., clindamycin or erythromycin)
  - Benzoyl peroxide
  - Combination decreases resistance
- **Moderate/Severe inflammatory**
  - Oral antibiotics (e.g., tetracyclines); < 4 months
- **Severe nodulocystic**
  - Isotretinoin (systemic retinoid)
  - Hormonal
    - OCP (increases steroid-binding globulins), spironolactone (antagonizes androgen receptors)

Isotretinoin

- **Teratogen** — contraindicated in pregnancy
- iPLEDGE enrollment required
- Serious side effects include:
  - Hypertriglyceridemia and pancreatitis
  - Arthralgia/Skeletal abnormalities
  - Hearing; night visual loss
  - Idiopathic intracranial hypertension (IIH; formerly known as pseudotumor cerebri); especially with **tetracycline**
  - Hepatotoxicity

Acne — Pregnancy

- Topical
  - Retinoids
    - **Contraindicated in pregnancy**
  - Benzoyl peroxide — prevents resistance in *C. acnes*
  - Topical antibiotics
    - Clindamycin and erythromycin safe in pregnancy
  - Salicylic acid
  - Azelaic acid
    - Safest in pregnancy

AR 6

A 40-year-old thin woman comes to the office complaining of worsening acne on her central face. She had acne as a child but that resolved. She also complains of facial flushing associated with spicy foods, hot liquids, or alcohol intake.

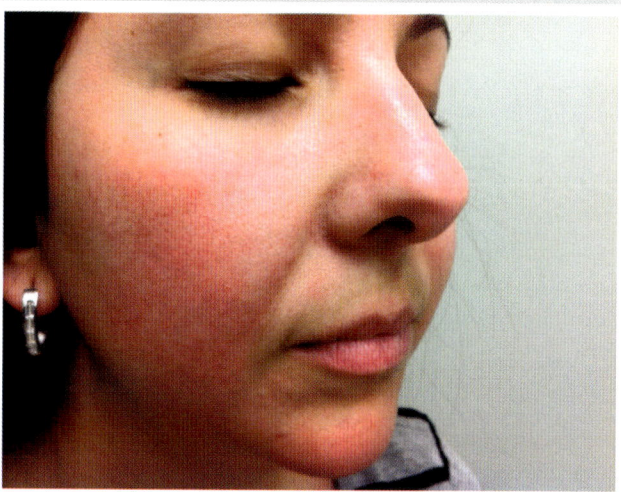

What would you recommend for this patient?

A. Topical steroids
B. Topical metronidazole
C. Pheochromocytoma evaluation
D. Carcinoid workup
E. SLE workup

Answer:_____

DERMATOLOGY

Acne Rosacea

- Fair-skinned, middle-aged patients ("adult acne")
- More common in women; worse in men
- Central face involved
- **2 main types:**
  1) Vascular (erythematotelangiectatic)
  2) Inflammatory (papulopustular)
- **No comedones**
  - Associated with flushing (spicy foods, alcohol)
  - Associated with:
    - Demodex folliculorum — likely exacerbating factor
    - Medication induced — steroids, niacin

Erythrotelangiectatic Rosacea (Vascular)

- Early: recurrent blush
- Later: persistent central facial erythema and telangiectasias

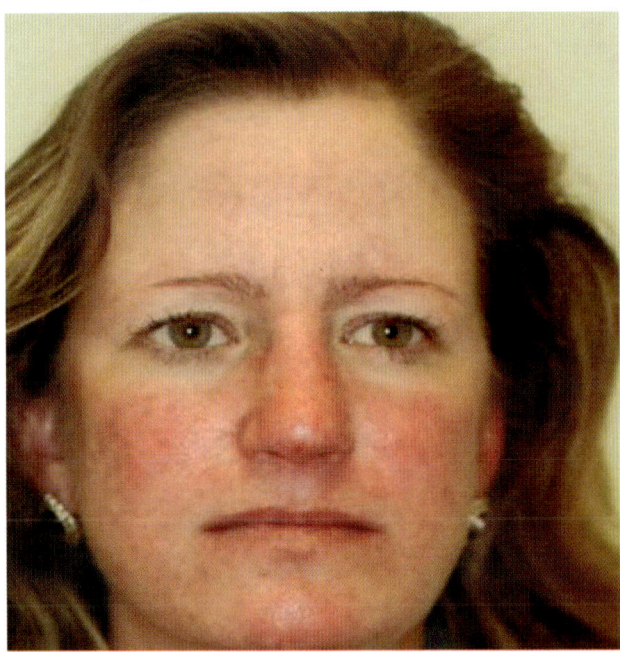

Papulopustular Rosacea (Inflammatory)

- Papules, pustules, nodules
- **No comedones**
- Facial erythema

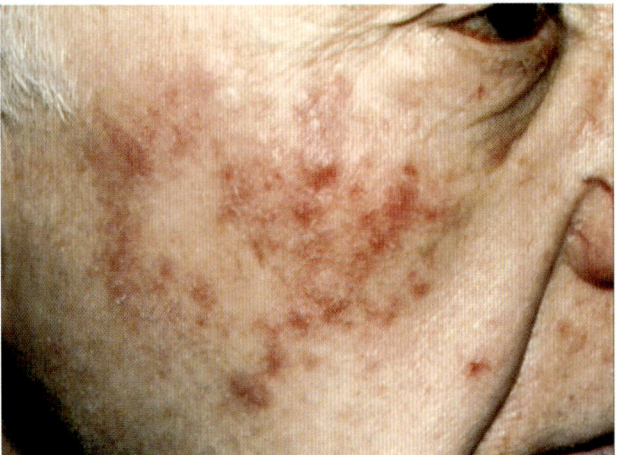

Phymatous Rosacea

- Occurs nearly exclusively in men
- Thickening of skin, irregular surface nodularity
- Involving nose (most common), chin, forehead, cheeks, ears

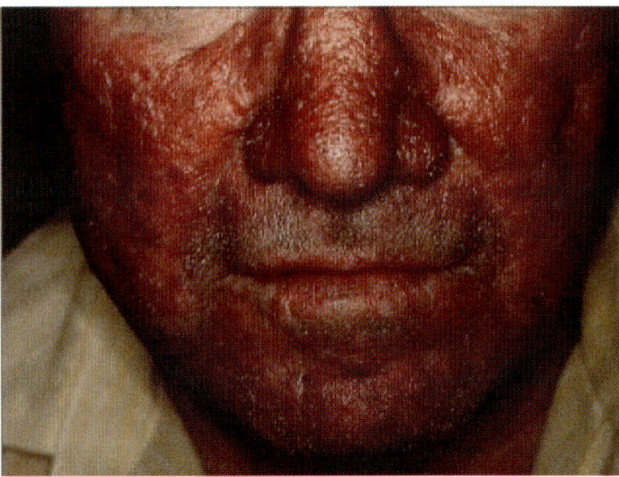

Ocular Rosacea

- Sx
  - Burning, stinging, dryness, itching, conjunctivitis
- Involvement in 50% of patients with rosacea
- Warrants ophthalmology consultation

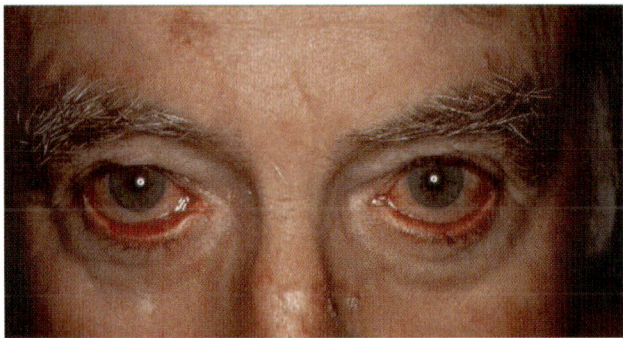

Treatments

- Avoid triggers (sun, EtOH, caffeine, spicy foods)
- Topical
  - **Brimonidine**
  - **Metronidazole cream/gel**
  - Azelaic acid
  - Sodium sulfacetamide
  - Topical ivermectin (Soolantra)
- Oral
  - Tetracyclines — most common
    - Doxycycline and minocycline
- Isotretinoin
- Avoid topical steroids; sun protection
- Surgical/Laser correction for rhinophyma

HIDRADENITIS SUPPURATIVA

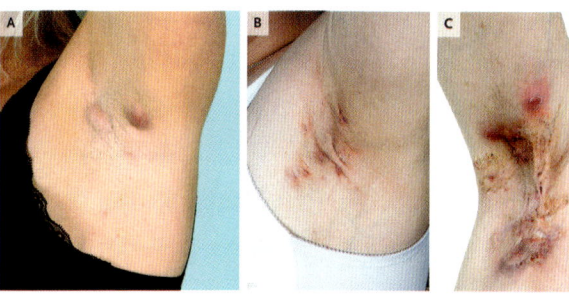

[2]

- Chronic recurrent **inflammatory** condition affecting skin containing apocrine glands
  - Axillae, anogenital region, inframammary
- Recurrent abscess/inflammatory nodules in the same location should increase clinical suspicion
- Significant scar formation and sinus tracts
- Associated with **smoking** and obesity

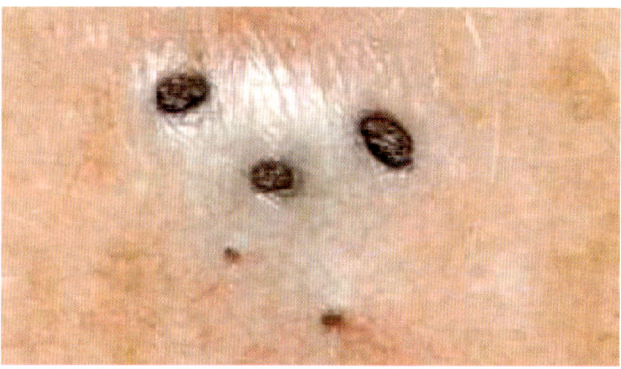

- Treatment
  - **Smoking cessation and weight loss**
  - I&D only if immediate relief is required
  - Topical antibiotic (clindamycin)
  - Oral antibiotic (tetracycline, clindamycin + rifampin)
  - Intralesional steroids
  - Biologics
    - Adalimumab
  - Surgical removal of affected area in severe/refractory cases

AR 7

Your patient presents with the following finding and states that he unsuccessfully tried to scrape it off.

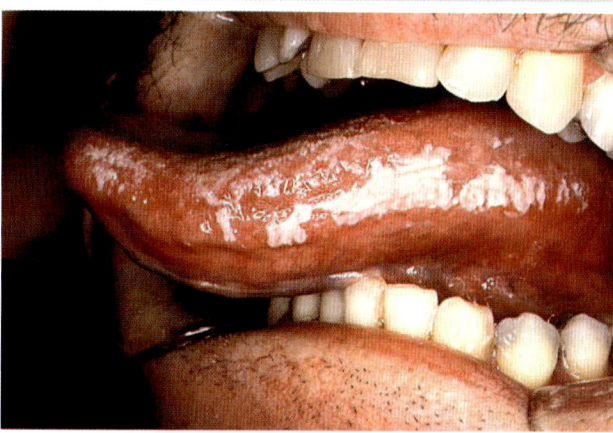

What is the best next step for this patient?

A. Refer to ENT for immediate biopsy.
B. Serologic testing for herpesvirus 8
C. HIV testing
D. Nystatin swish and swallow until resolved
E. Refer to GI for upper endoscopy.
F. Reassurance — no further testing

Answer:_____

Oral Hairy Leukoplakia

- Clinical
  - Adherent white plaques on the lateral tongue
  - Most commonly seen in patients with **HIV**
  - **Caused by EBV in the superficial epithelium**
  - Not a premalignant lesion
  - In contrast to *Candida*, **it cannot be scraped off**
  - No treatment usually necessary
  - HAART therapy
  - Antivirals if cosmetic concern

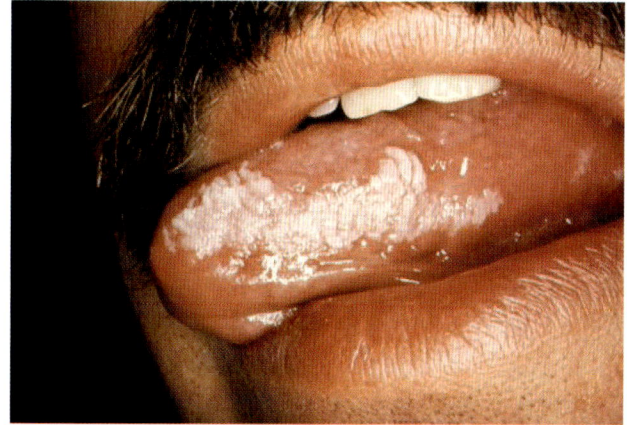

AR 8

Your patient presents with the following physical exam findings and states that her tongue feels like it is burning.

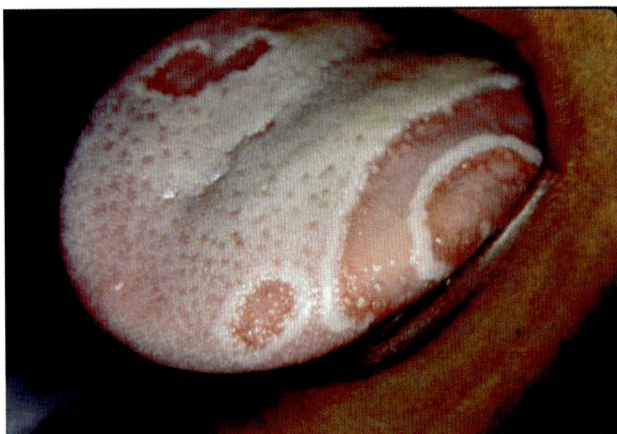

What is the best next step for this patient?

A. Reassurance
B. Smoking cessation
C. Refer to GI for possible Crohn disease.
D. Antibacterial mouth wash
E. Nystatin swish and spit
F. Refer to ENT for immediate biopsy.

Answer:_____

Geographic Tongue (Benign Migratory Glossitis)
- Clinical
  - Well-demarcated, red patches on the dorsal tongue with white periphery
  - Resembles a map — lesions can change in a matter of hours
  - Associated with **psoriasis and reactive arthritis**
  - No therapy needed

AR 9

A 52-year-old patient with ESRD presents with woody, indurated plaques on the legs.

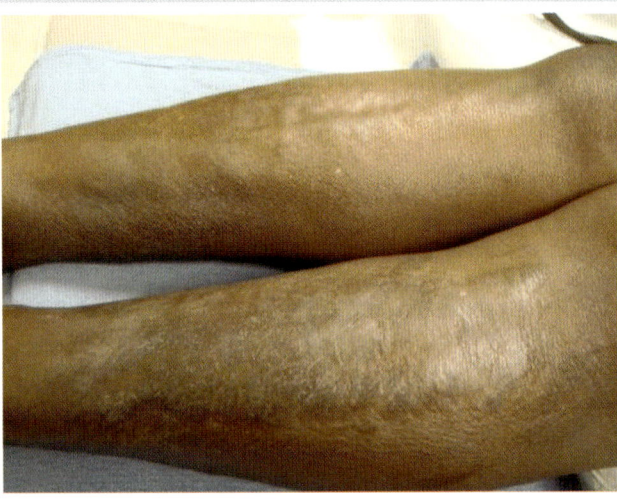

[3]

What likely triggered this condition?

A. Gadolinium during an imaging study
B. An abundance of glycosaminoglycans
C. An autoimmune condition with positive anti-Scl-70 antibodies
D. A strep infection in the deep tissues of the leg

Answer:_____

- Fibrosing disease similar to scleroderma
  - Face typically spared
- Associated with **gadolinium**
  - Primarily Group I agents
- Typically occurs in patients with ESRD or GFR < 30
- No proven therapy (transplant?)
- Prevention is key
  - **Do not give gadolinium to patient with GFR < 30**
  - **Hemodialysis**

AR 10

A 62-year-old woman was started on carbamazepine 2 weeks ago. Yesterday morning, she awoke with red and raw painful skin lesions. Many areas have blisters and sloughed off skin.

Her lesions cover at least 30% of her body. She went to the emergency department where she was also found to have mouth sores and a fever of 102.7°F (39.3°C), BP 100/60, HR 117. She has no lymphadenopathy. Her LFTs and eosinophil count are normal.

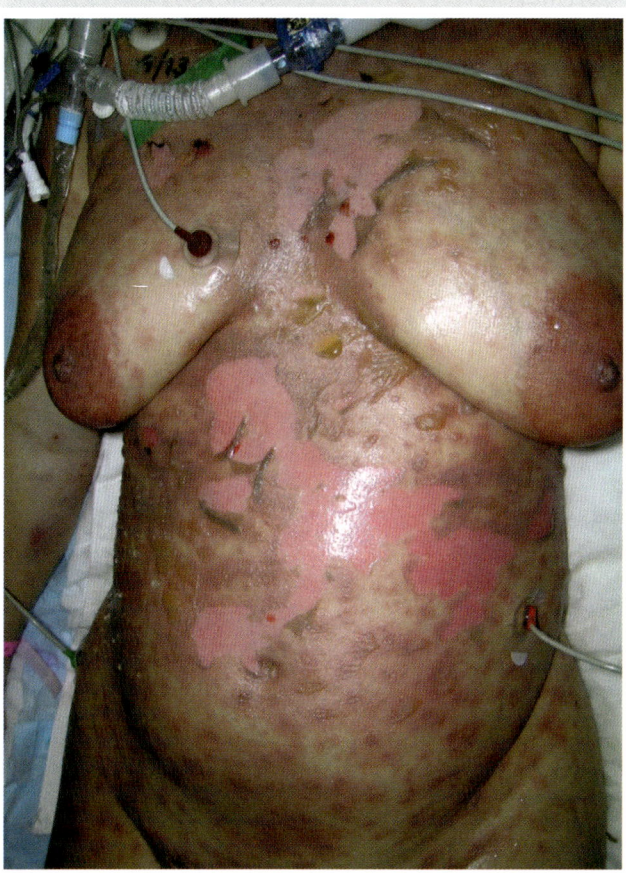

What is the patient's most likely diagnosis?

A. Erythema multiforme
B. Stevens-Johnson syndrome
C. Toxic epidermal necrolysis
D. DRESS syndrome
E. Dermatitis herpetiformis

Answer:_____

AR 11
This eruption is most often associated with which virus?

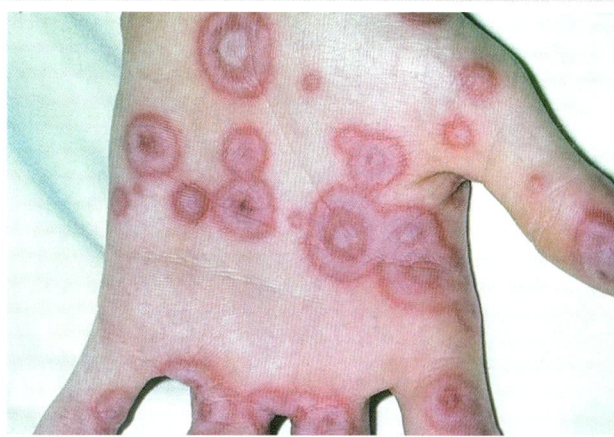

A. Epstein-Barr
B. Cytomegalovirus
C. Herpes simplex
D. Varicella zoster
E. HIV

Answer:_____

Toxic Epidermal Necrolysis (TEN)
- Medical emergency
- Mortality rate ~ 25–40%
- **Stop offending drug**
- 90% due to drug
  - Sulfa
  - Allopurinol
  - NSAIDs
  - Antiseizure medications
- ICU; burn unit
- > 30% body surface area (BSA) + mucosal involvement
- **Cyclosporine**; steroids/IVIG?

Stevens-Johnson Syndrome (SJS) and Toxic Epidermal Necrolysis (TEN)
- SJS < 10% BSA
- TEN > 30% BSA
- **SCORTEN score**
  - Age > 40
  - BSA
  - Elevation of HR, urea
  - Decreased bicarb, glucose
  - Malignancy
- Mortality: infection/water loss/electrolyte imbalances

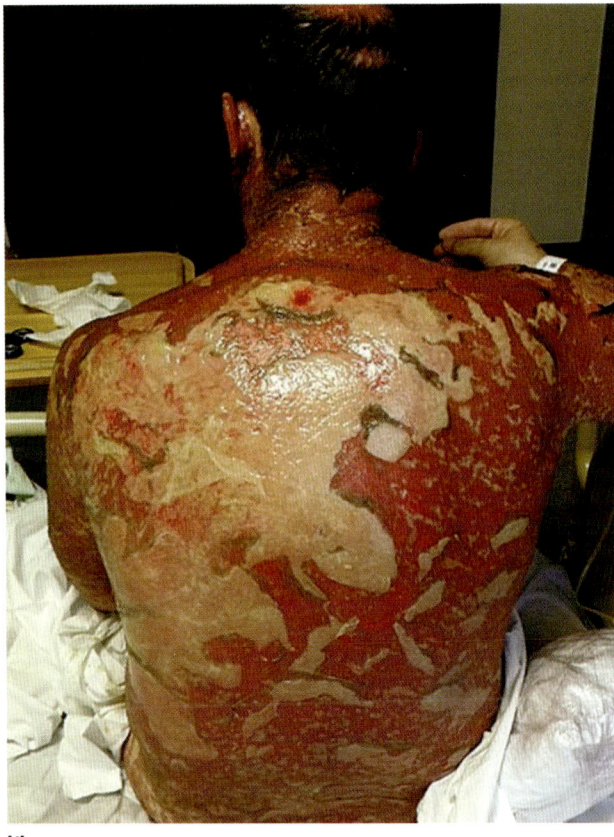

[4]

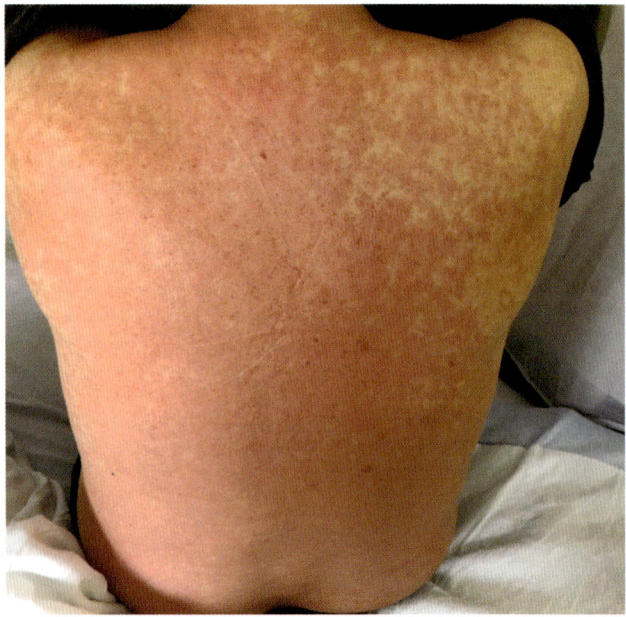

- Major culprits
  - **Antiseizure medications**
  - **Allopurinol**
  - Sulfonamides
  - Minocycline, vancomycin, dapsone, HIV drugs
- Treatment
  - Withdrawal of drugs
  - Corticosteroids for several weeks to months!
    - Relapse can occur when dose is tapered
    - Alternative treatment is a 7-day course of cyclosporine followed by a taper

ERYTHEMA MULTIFORME (EM)
- Acute, target lesions pathognomonic
- Often self-limiting (muco-) cutaneous disorder
- Systemic steroids for severe mucosal involvement
- Infections
  - **HSV** most common cause
  - Often recurrent; may benefit from suppression
  - *Mycoplasma pneumoniae*
  - Only treat active infection
- Drugs (< 10%)
  - Sulfonamides, antiseizure medications, penicillins,
  - NSAIDs, allopurinol

DRUG REACTION WITH EOSINOPHILIA AND SYSTEMIC SYMPTOMS (DRESS)
- Clinical
  - Develops **2–8 weeks after drug** is started
  - Cutaneous findings
    - Morbilliform eruption; mucosal involvement uncommon
    - **Edema of face** is hallmark of DRESS
  - Visceral involvement
    - **Hepatitis** → can become fulminant and fatal
    - Myocarditis, interstitial pneumonitis, interstitial nephritis, thyroiditis
  - Fever
  - **Eosinophilia** (absent in up to 20% of cases)
  - **Atypical lymphocytes common**

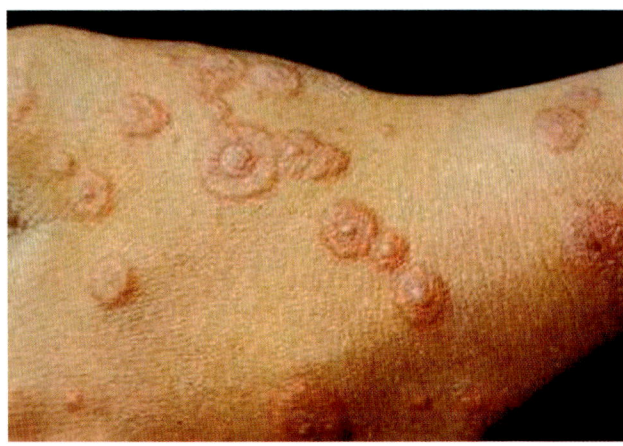

INFLAMMATORY SKIN DISORDERS

AR 12

Which of the following is not a common trigger of psoriasis?

A. Lithium
B. Strep infection
C. β-Blocker
D. Steroid taper
E. Aspirin

Answer:_____

PSORIASIS

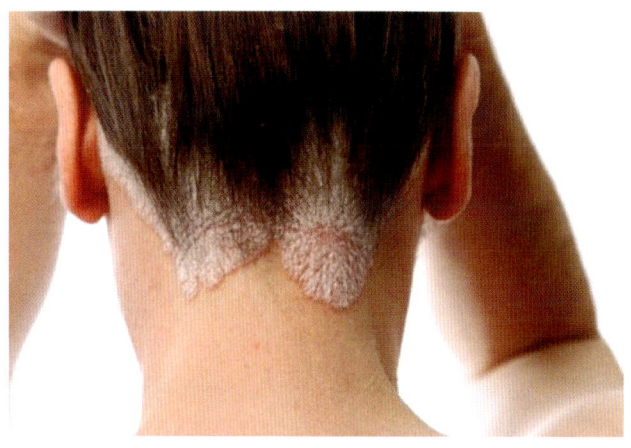

Plaque Psoriasis
- Most common type
- Well-demarcated, erythematous plaques with scale
- Extensor surfaces, scalp, gluteal cleft
- May be exacerbated by β-blockers, lithium, and antimalarials

Psoriasis
- Guttate (gutta means "raindrop")
  - **Strep infection** can be inciting factor

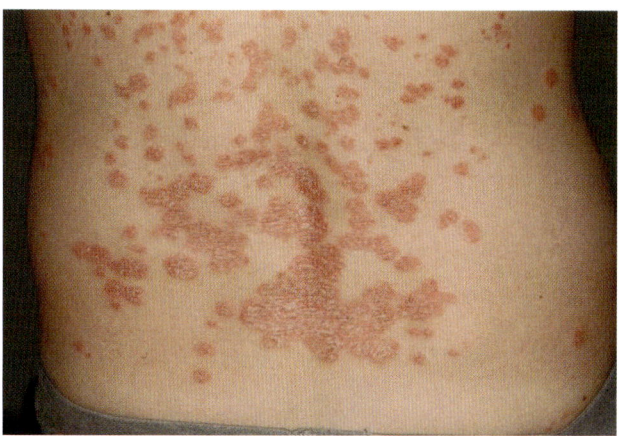

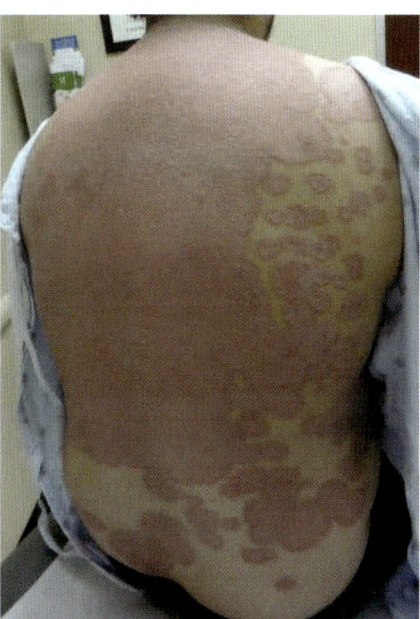

- Pustular/Palmoplantar
- Erythrodermic psoriasis

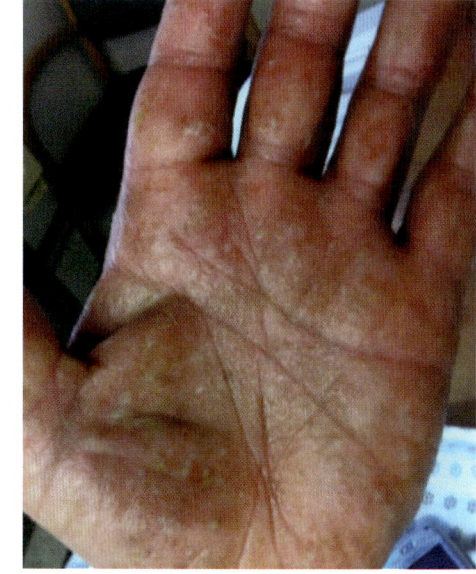

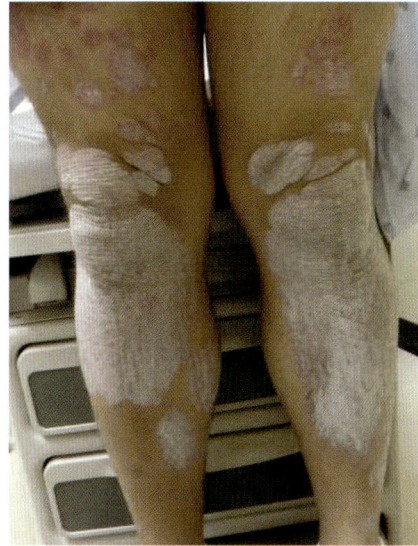

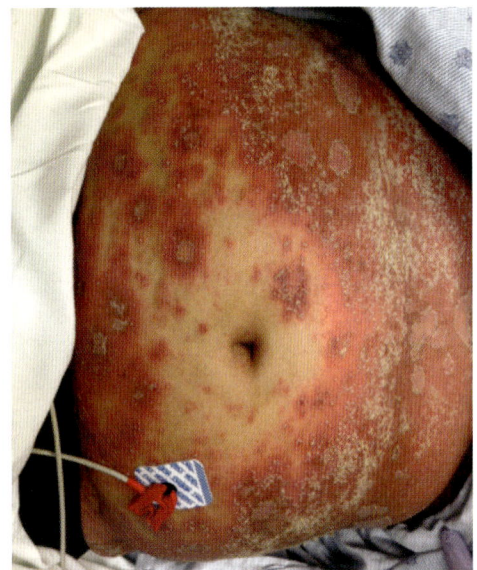

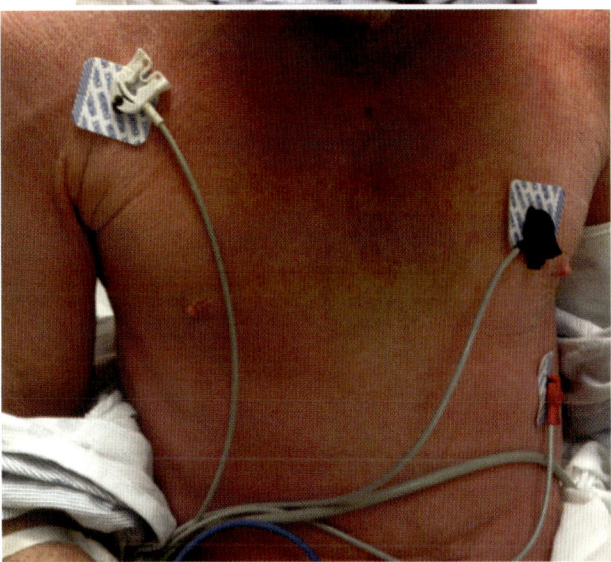

Plaque Psoriasis — Treatment
- **Topical for mild-to-moderate disease**
  - Emollients
  - Corticosteroids (1st line)
  - Can also use vitamin D analogues, calcineurin inhibitors
- **Add phototherapy for moderate-to-severe disease**
  - NBUVB, PUVA
  - No immunosuppression; but does not treat arthritis
- **Recalcitrant disease**
  - Methotrexate, cyclosporine, biologics, apremilast

SCLERODERMA

AR 13
Which antibody is most closely associated with limited sclerosis as well as digital ischemia and pulmonary hypertension?

A. Anticentromere
B. Anti-Smith
C. Anti-Scl-70 (antitopoisomerase I)
D. Anti-Jo
E. Antinuclear antibody

Answer:_____

Scleroderma
- Raynaud phenomenon
- Limited disease
  - CREST
  - Anticentromere (specific)
- Diffuse disease
  - Anti-Scl-70 (antitopoisomerase I)
  - Multiorgan involvement

- Nail changes
  - Oil spots (most specific)
  - Pitting
  - Onycholysis
  - Changes are associated with greater risk of psoriatic arthritis

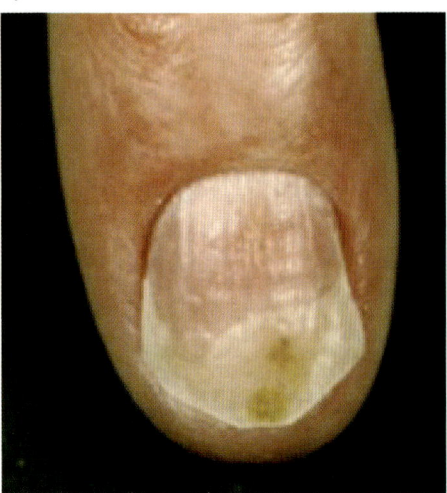

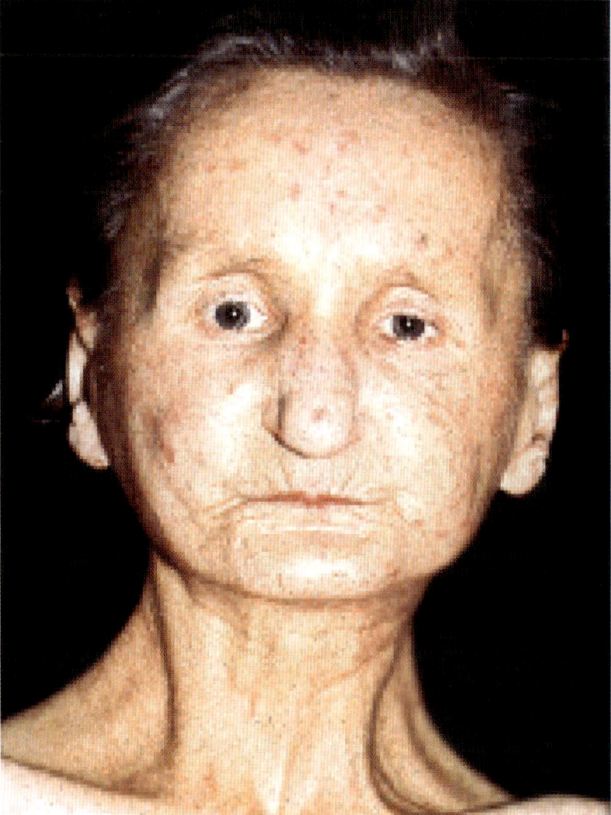

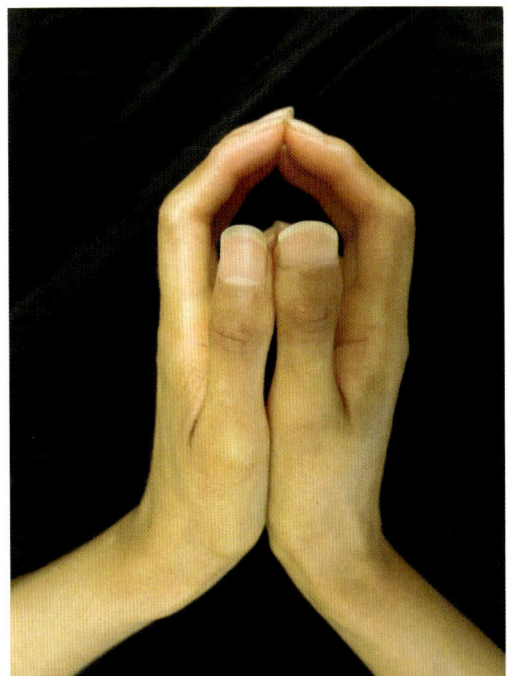

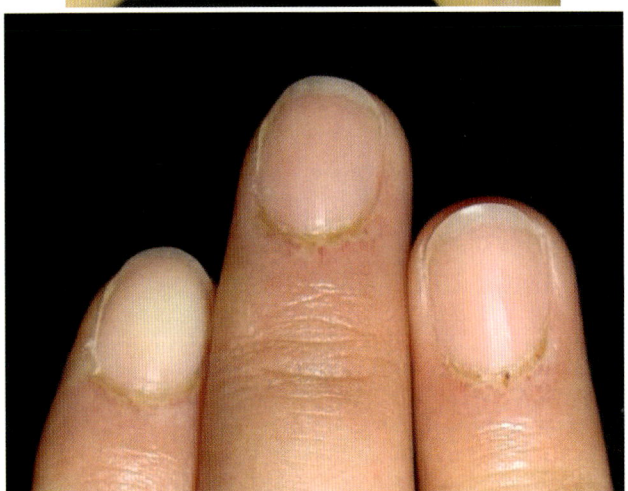

[5]

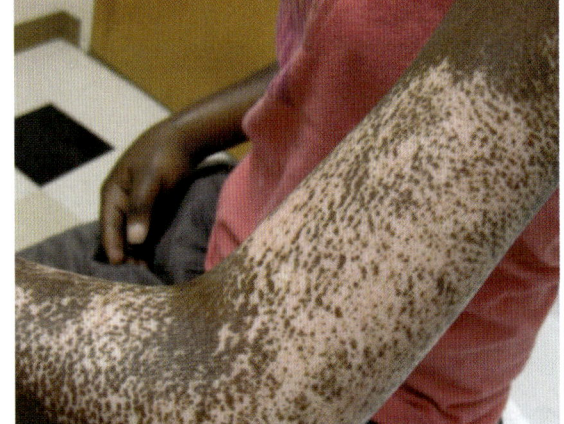

SARCOIDOSIS

AR 14

Which of the following evaluations should be performed in a newly diagnosed sarcoidosis patient?

A. ECG
B. Ophthalmology evaluation
C. Chest x-ray
D. Pulmonary function tests
E. All of the above

Answer:_____

AR 15

A 30-year-old female presents acutely with fever, polyarthralgias, and painful anterior pretibial nodules. Her CXR reveals bilateral hilar adenopathy.

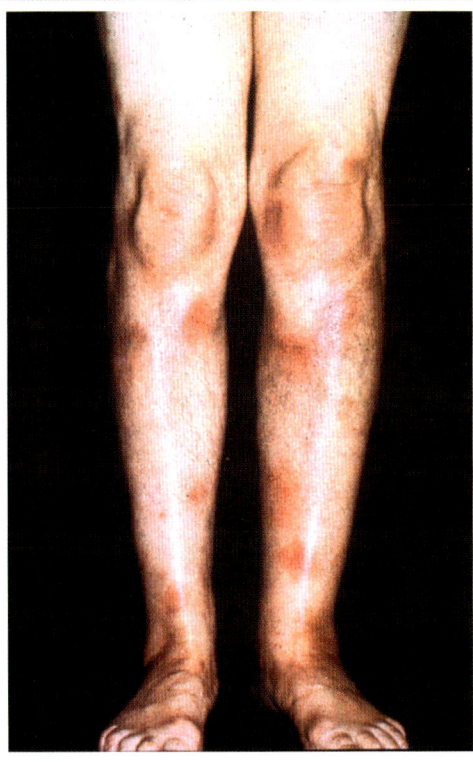

What is the most likely diagnosis?

A. Sweet syndrome
B. Löfgren syndrome
C. Lymphoma
D. Streptococcal infection
E. SLE

Answer:_____

- Acute form of sarcoidosis
- Manifests as erythema nodosum, bilateral hilar adenopathy, fever, and arthralgias
- **Excellent prognosis**; resolves in months to years

Cutaneous Sarcoidosis — Lupus Pernio

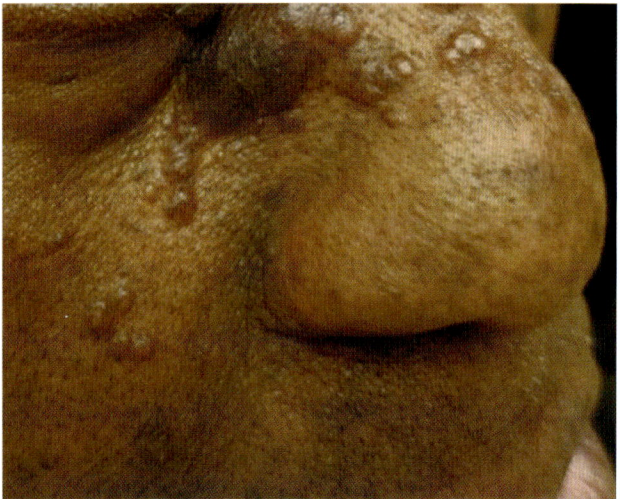

[6]

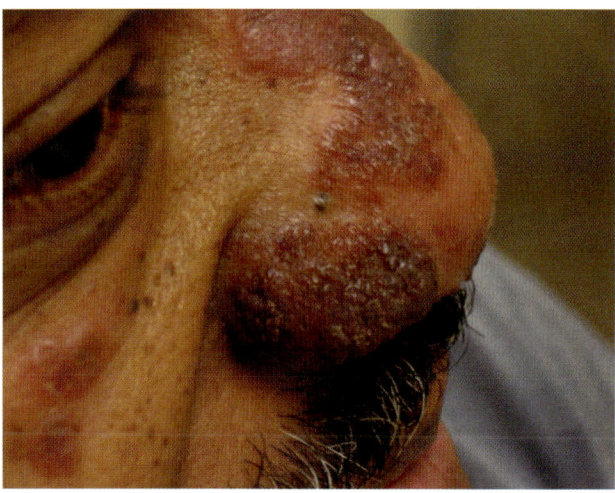

- Clinical
  - Lesions found mostly on head, neck, and back
    - Pink, brown, violaceous papules, plaques, or nodules
    - Within scars
  - Erythema nodosum

ERYTHEMA NODOSUM
- **Differential diagnosis**
  - Idiopathic
  - Streptococcal infection
  - Sarcoidosis
  - TB/Fungal infections
  - HRT, OCP, antibiotics
  - Pregnancy
  - Inflammatory bowel disease
  - Behçet disease
  - Lymphoma

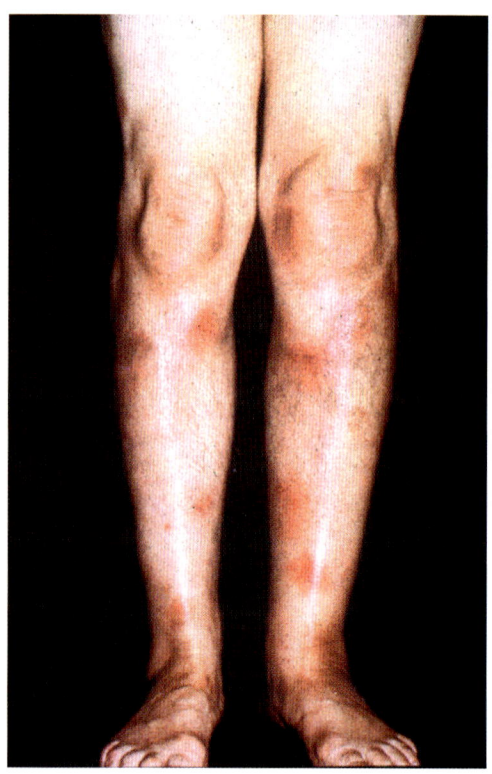

- **Treatment**
  - Supportive care
  - NSAIDs or potassium iodide
  - Systemic steroids
  - Biopsy not needed if typical presentation

SYSTEMIC LUPUS ERYTHEMATOSUS (SLE)
- Malar rash with **sparing of the nasolabial folds**, erythema of proximal nail folds
- Malar rash erythema persists longer than rosacea
- Patients with discoid lupus have < 10% chance of developing systemic lupus
- Sunscreen can help prevent flares

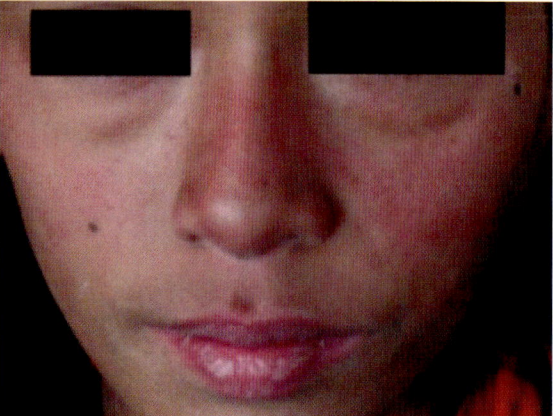

[7]

Discoid Lupus

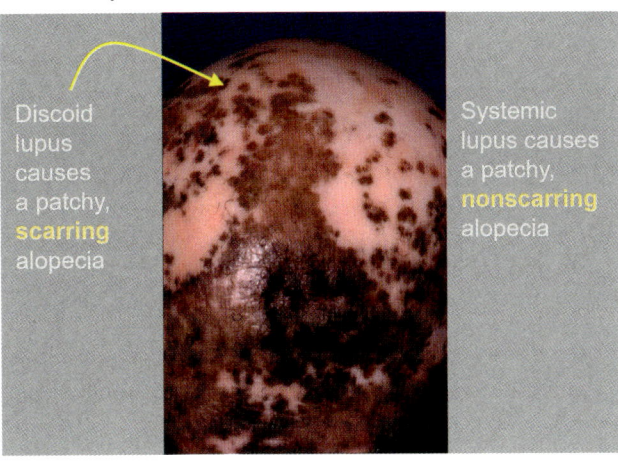

Discoid lupus causes a patchy, **scarring** alopecia

Systemic lupus causes a patchy, **nonscarring** alopecia

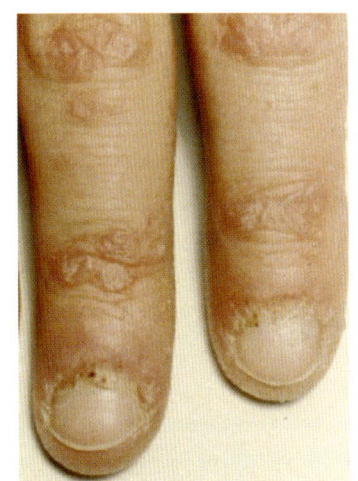

[8]

DERMATOMYOSITIS

AR 16

What further studies should you strongly consider in a 52-year-old patient with dermatomyositis?

A. Blood sugar and hemoglobin A1c
B. Antistreptolysin O titer
C. Zinc levels
D. Interferon-γ release assay
E. Cancer screening

Answer:_____

Dermatomyositis
- Progressive symmetrical proximal muscle weakness
- Elevated muscle enzymes
- Muscle biopsy consistent with myositis
- Abnormal electromyogram
- Pathognomonic cutaneous disease
    - **Heliotrope rash** (periorbital)
    - **Gottron papules** (bony prominence of hands/fingers)
- Strong association with **malignancy**
    - All: age-appropriate cancer screening
    - High-risk (p155/140, NXP2 antibodies)

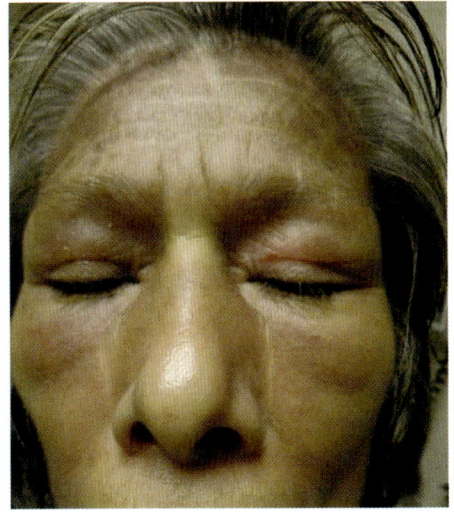

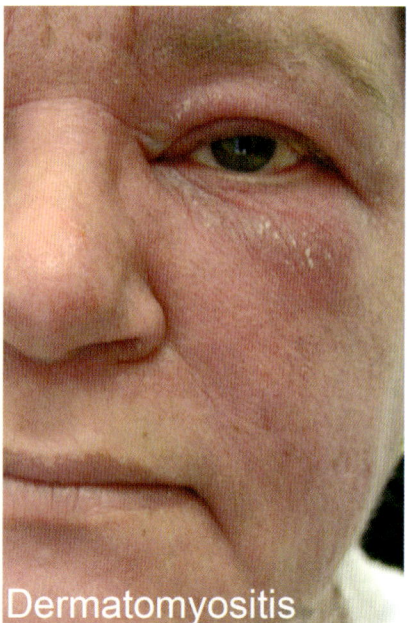
Dermatomyositis

[9]

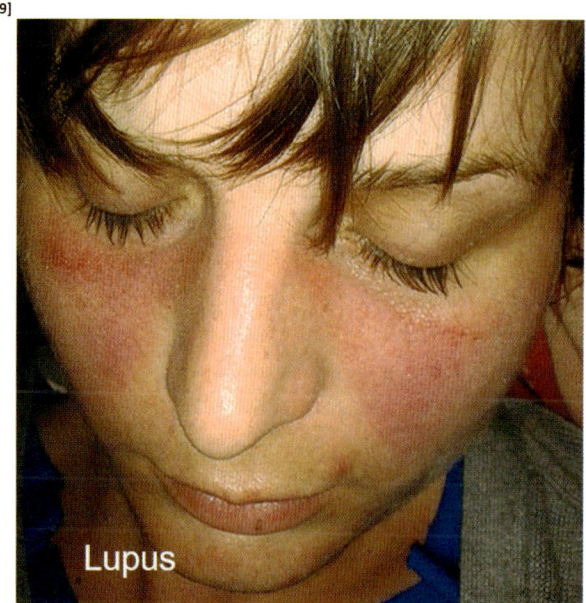
Lupus

[10]

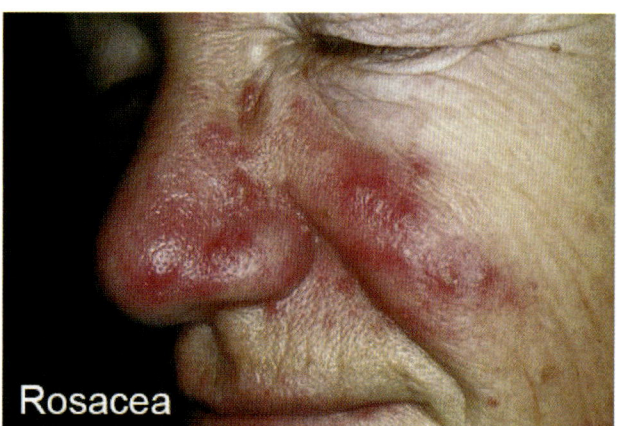
Rosacea

REACTIVE ARTHRITIS

- Clinical
  - Reactive process
    - Typically 1–4 weeks after GU or GI infection
  - Most common cutaneous findings
    - Oral or genital ulcers
    - Keratoderma blenorrhagicum on palms and soles
    - Can also have balanitis circinata
  - "Can't see, can't pee, can't climb a tree" = (< 1/3 of patients)

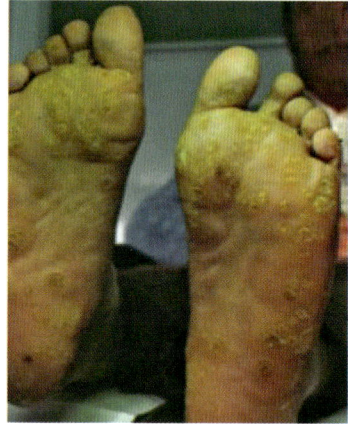

AR 17

A 55-year-old man developed a pustule that turned into a painful ulcer. The ulcer is deep, has an inflamed border that overhangs the ulcer, and has a violaceous hue. After appropriate testing, no bacteria or fungus was found. He was in good general health except for severe rheumatoid arthritis.

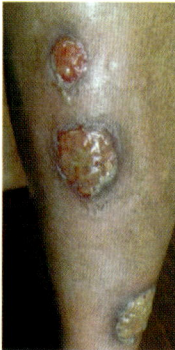

AR 17A

The most likely diagnosis is:

A. Pyoderma gangrenosum
B. "Flesh-eating bacteria"
C. Osteomyelitis
D. Brown recluse bite
E. Vasculitis

Answer:_____

Pyoderma Gangrenosum

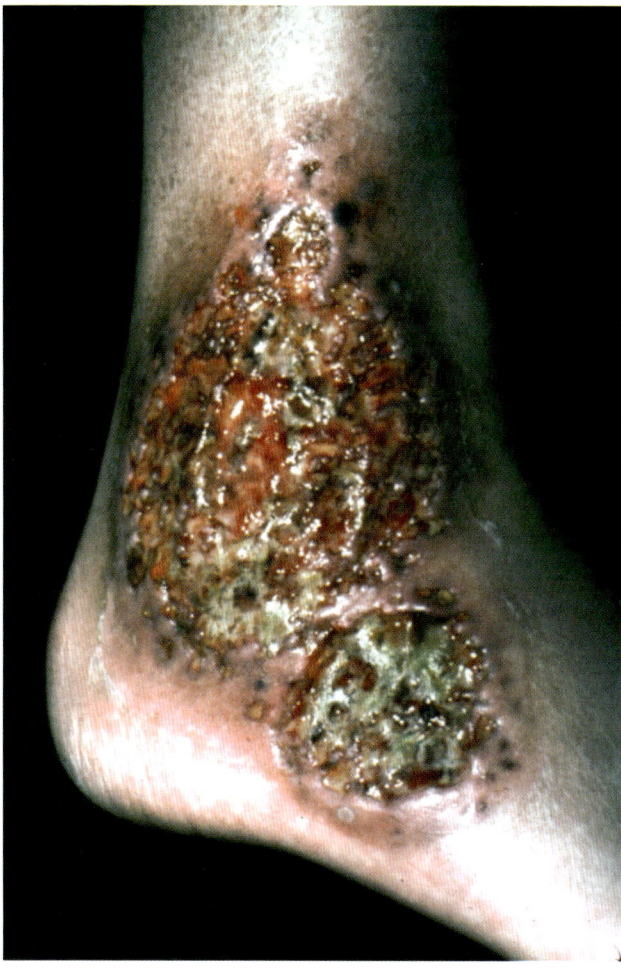

- Diagnosis of exclusion; often associated with an underlying disease, but can be idiopathic; commonly on the leg
  - **Inflammatory bowel disease**
  - Inflammatory arthritis
  - Hematologic malignancy or disorder
- **25% demonstrate pathergy**
- **Biopsy is not diagnostic**
  - Rules out other causes
  - Cultures are negative
- Treat underlying disease
- If idiopathic — systemic steroids/immunosuppressants

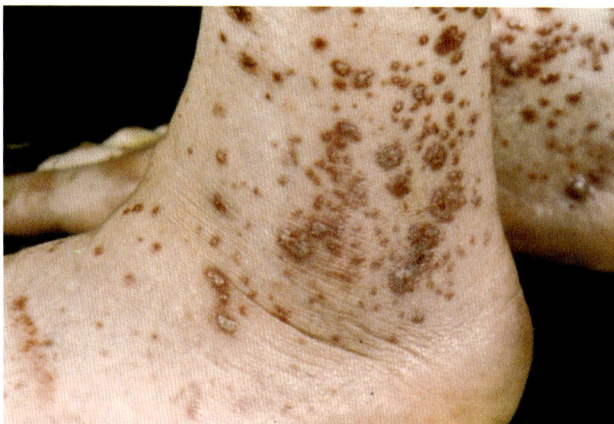

Vasculitis — Palpable Purpura

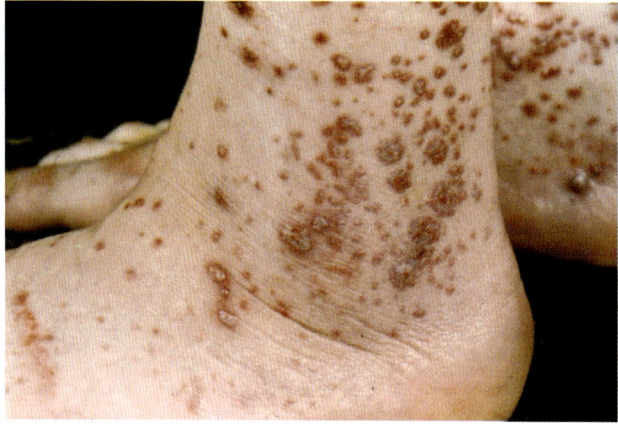

IgA vasculitis may have associated arthritis and abdominal pain accompanied by renal or bowel vasculitis.

Leukocytoclastic Vasculitis

- Palpable, nonblanching purpuric papules
- Involvement of small vessels
- Causes: 50% idiopathic, bacterial, viral (hepatitis B/C), neoplastic (SPEP), autoimmune
- If **widespread, consider IgA vasculitis**
- GI, neurologic, or renal symptoms should increase concern for systemic disease
- Biopsy ± direct immunofluorescence

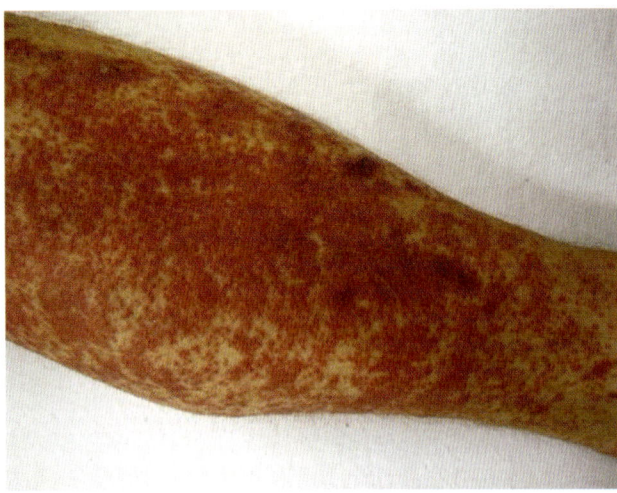

AR 19

A 65-year-old alcoholic man who lives alone presents with longstanding history of a scaly and erythematous rash on his extremities, groin, and buttocks.

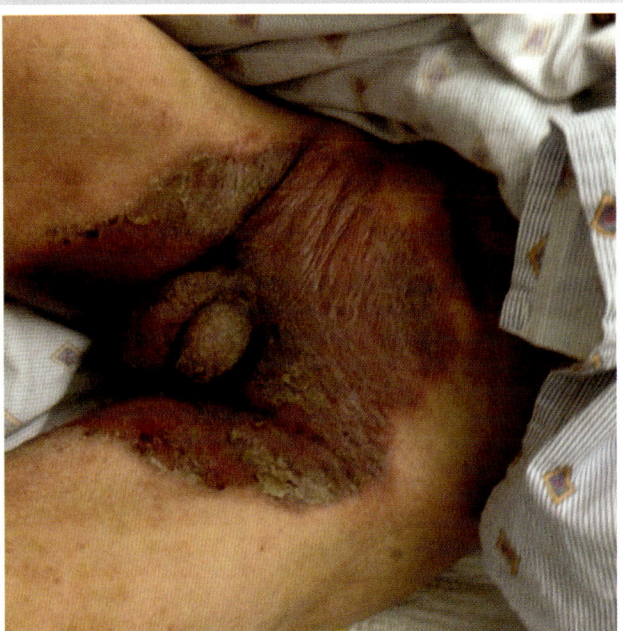

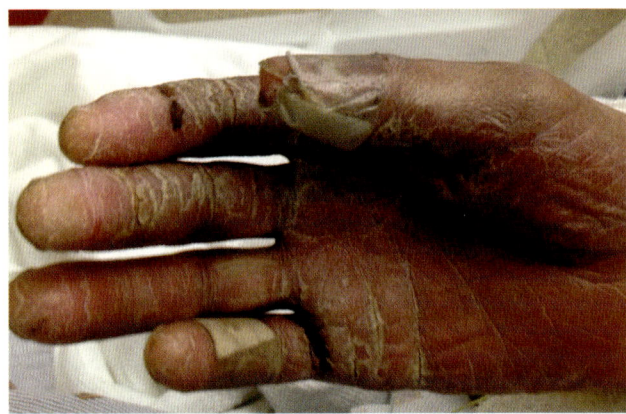

What is your diagnosis?

A. Psoriasis
B. Pellagra (niacin deficiency)
C. Eczema
D. Acrodermatitis enteropathica (zinc deficiency)
E. Decubitus ulcer and venous stasis

Answer:_____

- Alcoholics, older adults, eating disorders, malabsorption
- Favors acral and periorificial sites
- Plasma zinc levels generally reliable; may be suppressed in inflammatory states

SKIN INFECTIONS

AR 20

A 50-year-old woman with poorly controlled diabetes is admitted to the hospital for cellulitis manifested by fever and a red, painful lower extremity. 2 hours later, the nurse wakes you up to say that the infection has spread rapidly despite appropriate antibiotics and is 50% bigger than it was and more painful.

What is the best next step?

A. Add clindamycin to her antibiotic regimen.
B. Order a CT or MRI scan of the leg.
C. Order a plain film to look for gas.
D. Obtain a surgical consultation.
E. Ask the nurse not to call you anymore so you can get some sleep.

Answer:_____

Necrotizing Fasciitis (NF)

- A surgical emergency
- Most important is to obtain surgical consultation
- **Imaging and lab studies should not delay surgical evaluation**
- Deep infection can spread very quickly along fascial planes
- Pain often out of proportion to appearance of the infection
- **Type 1:** polymicrobial, older, or immunocompromised
- **Type 2:** group A strep, any age, even healthy

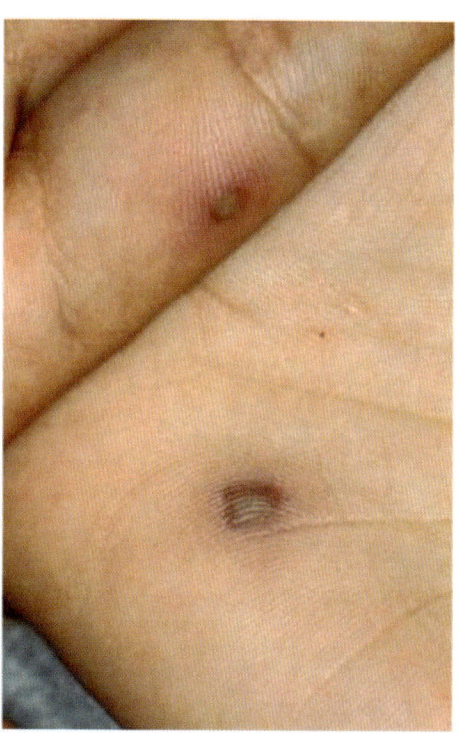

- **Hemorrhagic petechiae/pustules often around joints**
- Fever, arthralgias ± asymmetric arthritis
- Cultures of lesions are usually negative
- Can culture initial site of infection for better yield

AR 21

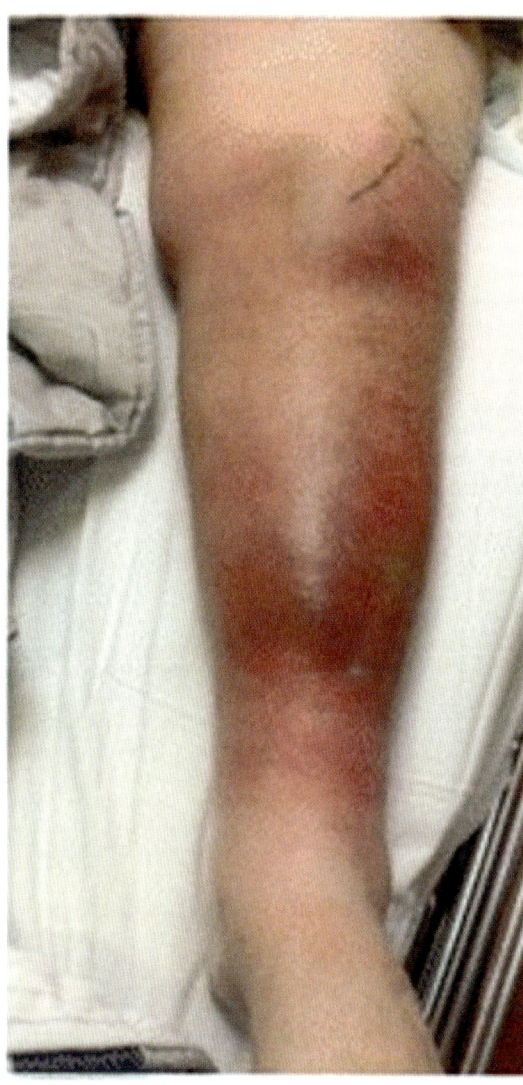

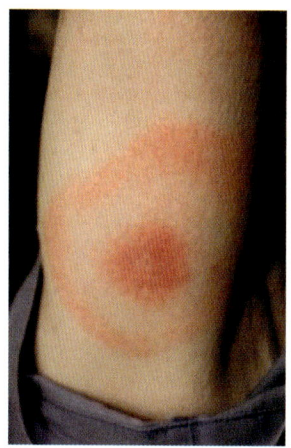

A 23-year-old woman comes to your office after spending a week hiking in Maine. She complains of flu-like symptoms and has this rash.

What is the most likely diagnosis?

A. Rocky Mountain spotted fever
B. Lyme disease
C. Ehrlichiosis
D. Spider bite
E. Erythema nodosum

Answer:_____

What Is Your Diagnosis?

A 28-year-old man presents to your office with joint pains and malaise. You incidentally notice this lesion on his hands.

DERMATOLOGY

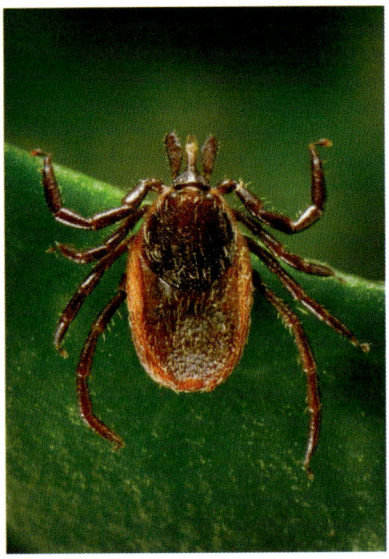

- *Borrelia burgdorferi*
- *Ixodes* spp. tick
- **Erythema (chronicum) migrans**
  - Bull's-eye; 80%
- Northeast, Great Lakes, Northern California
- Serology not needed
- Rx
  - Doxycycline
  - Amoxicillin
  - Cefuroxime

CONDYLOMA ACUMINATUM

- Skin-colored to pink to brown cauliflower papules or plaques in anogenital area
- Caused by HPV
  - Mostly **HPV-6 and HPV-11 (90%)**
  - Can be associated with oncogenic **HPV Types 16, 18, and 31**

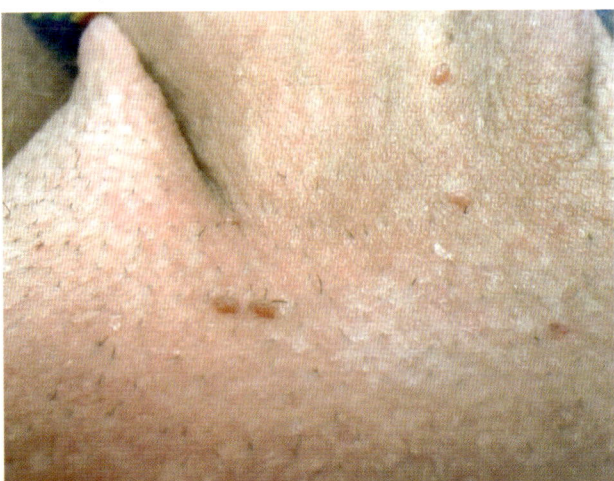

[11]

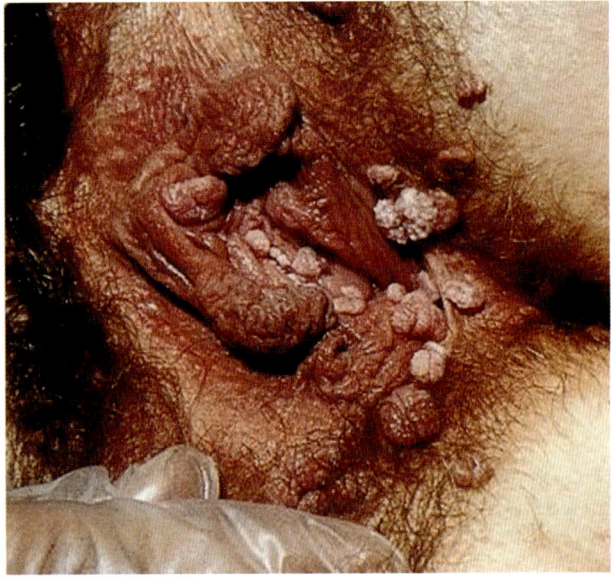

[12]

SYPHILIS

AR 22

A 33-year-old man presents with pink macules on the palms and soles. RPR and VDRL are both positive.

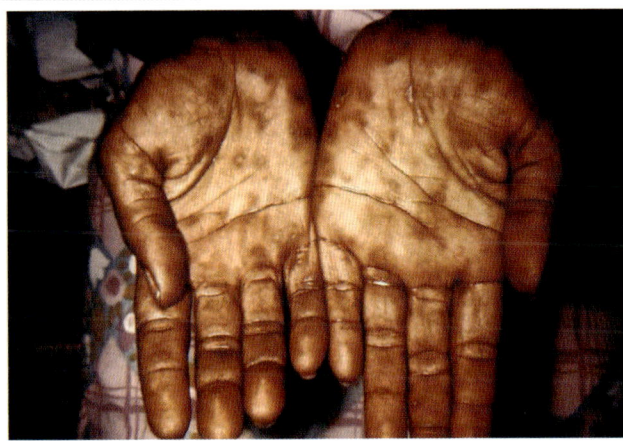

What stage of syphilis does this patient have?

A. Primary
B. Secondary
C. Latent
D. Tertiary
E. Quaternary

Answer:_____

Primary Syphilis

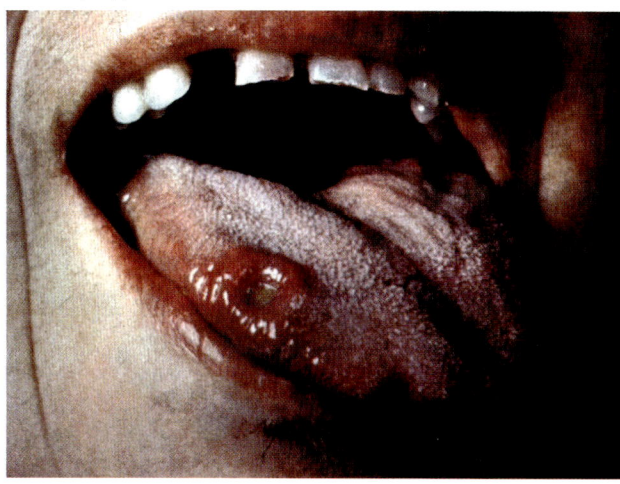

Condylomata Lata — Secondary Syphilis

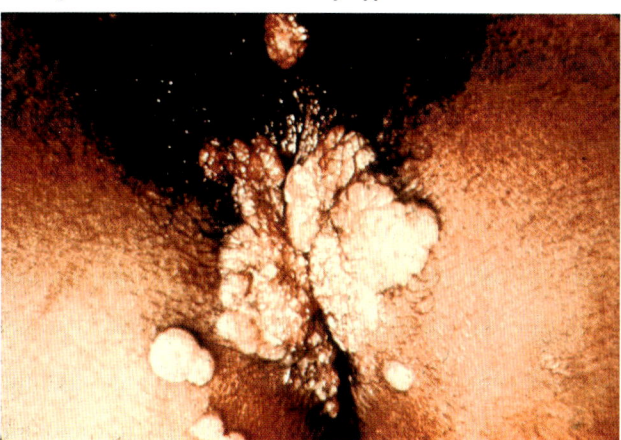

Tertiary Syphilis — Gumma

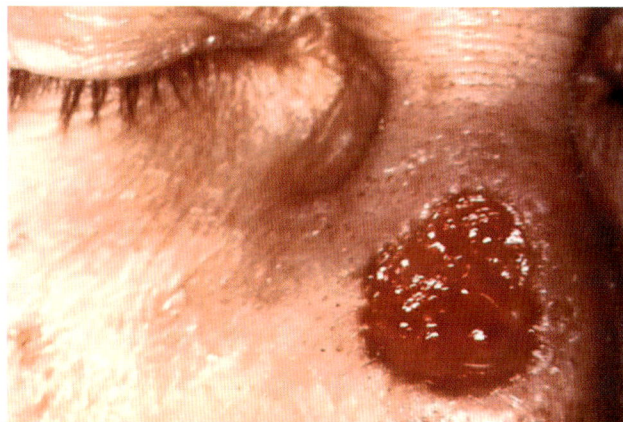

Syphilis (*Treponema pallidum*)
- **Primary**
  - Painless chancre (genitals, mouth)
  - Rx: benzathine PCN G 2.4 M units IM
- **Secondary**
  - All have positive serologies
  - "Palms and soles" rash; condylomata lata
- **Latent**
  - Positive serologies; asymptomatic
- **Tertiary**
  - CNS and cardiac involvement
  - Most have gummas

HERPES ZOSTER (SHINGLES)

AR 23

A 62-year-old man with diabetes presents to the office with unilateral, painful, grouped vesicles on an erythematous base. He also has a lesion on the tip of his nose.

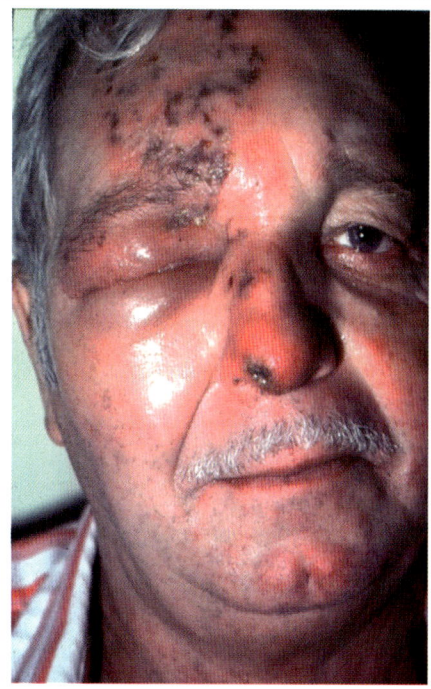

In addition to antiviral therapy, what is the best next step?

A. High-dose oral steroids
B. Gabapentin for pain
C. Herpes zoster vaccine
D. Ophthalmology consult
E. Steroid eye drops

Answer:_____

Herpes Zoster (Shingles)

- Highly contagious until **all** lesions have crusted

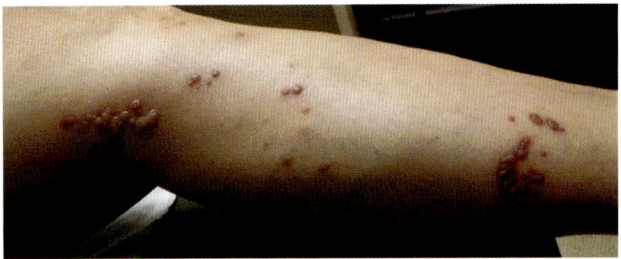

- Reactivation of latent varicella-zoster virus
- Older, immunocompromised patients
- Grouped vesicles within dermatome(s) with focal pain
  - HZ ophthalmicus can lead to **vision loss (Hutchinson sign)**
  - **Ramsay Hunt syndrome**
- Treatment
  - Acyclovir, valacyclovir, or famciclovir for 7 days
  - Most effective within **72 hours**
  - **Steroids typically not used**
- Other
  - **Postherpetic neuralgia** (TCAs, gabapentin, pregabalin)
  - Candidates over 50 years of age should be offered **zoster vaccine**

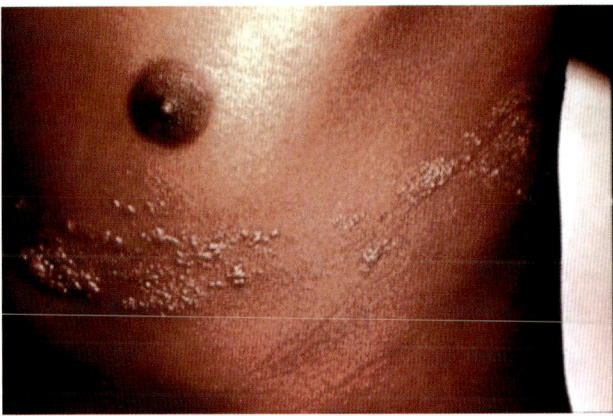

HERPES SIMPLEX VIRUS

Herpes Simplex Virus (HSV 1 or 2)

- Grouped vesicles on an erythematous base
  - Oral/genital common
- Primary infection can be mild or severe; systemic symptoms
- Persists in sensory ganglia; recurs often on lips (prodrome)
- **Dx:** PCR or DFA (direct fluorescent ab); Tzanck smear not typically used anymore
- **Rx:** for primary infection if severe; can use oral antivirals with prodrome

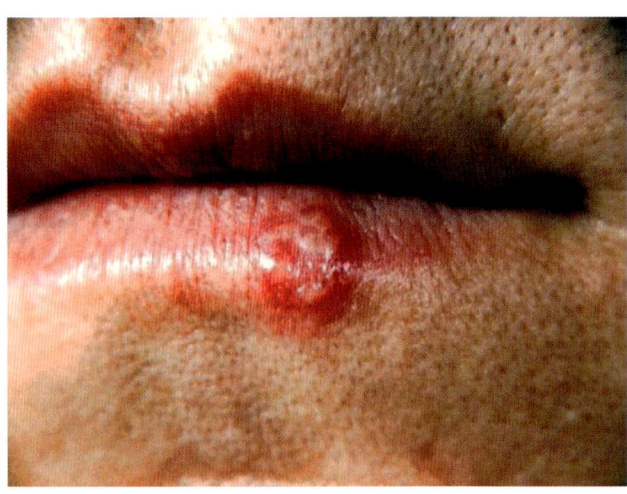

HSV — Herpetic Whitlow

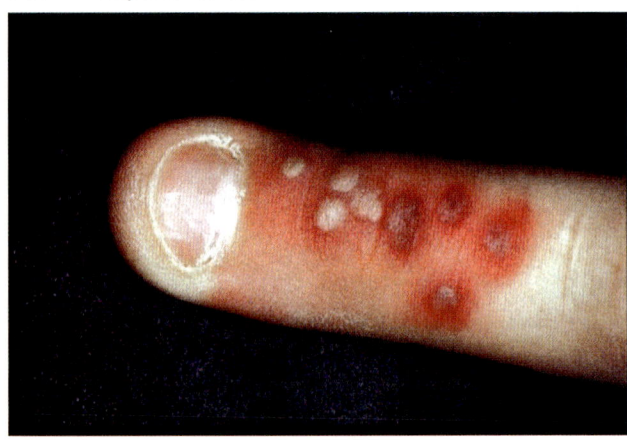

DERMATOPHYTOSIS

AR 24

A 28-year-old schoolteacher presents with scaly patches of alopecia. Culture confirms tinea capitis.

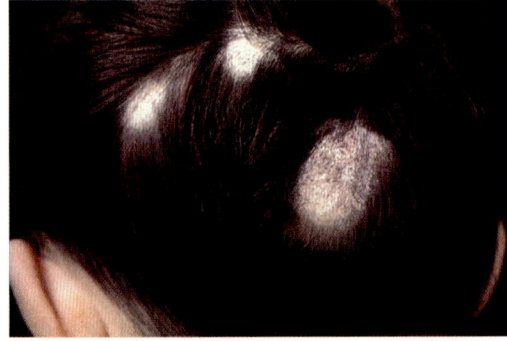

The treatment of choice is:

A. Terbinafine cream
B. Ketoconazole cream
C. Griseofulvin by mouth
D. Selenium sulfide shampoo
E. Ciclopirox gel

Answer:_____

AR 25

A 30-year-old male comes to see you for a second opinion regarding treatment of his onychomycosis. He was told to take terbinafine for 12 weeks but has concerns about liver toxicity. He has multiple thickened toenails with yellowish, periungual debris.

What is the next best step?

A. Tell him to "man up" and not worry about it.
B. Tell him he can take it for 6 weeks instead.
C. Obtain and send a nail clipping sample to the lab.
D. Prescribe topical terbinafine instead.
E. Prescribe oral ketoconazole instead.

Answer:_____

Tinea Unguium (Onychomycosis)

- **Up to 50% of patients with suspected onychomycosis do not have a fungal infection; given the potential toxicity of terbinafine, confirmation of the diagnosis is warranted**

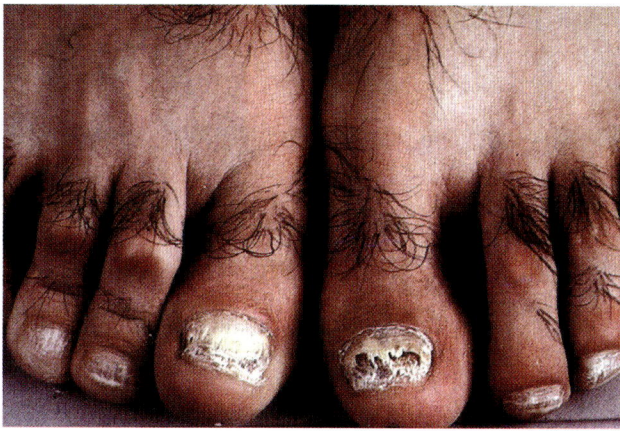

Dermatophytosis

- Clinical
  - **Tinea corporis**
  - Tinea pedis/unguium
  - Tinea nigra
  - Tinea profunda
  - Tinea barbae
  - Tinea incognito

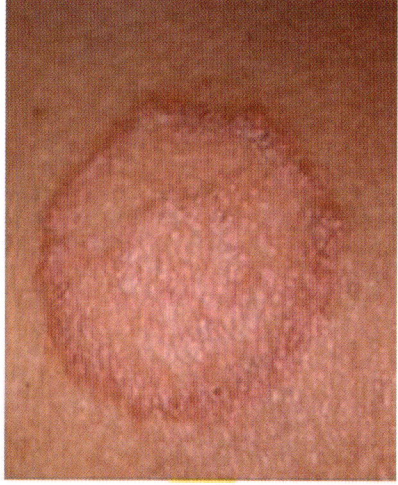

- Clinical
  - Tinea corporis
  - **Tinea pedis/unguium**
  - Tinea nigra
  - Tinea profunda
  - Tinea barbae
  - Tinea incognito

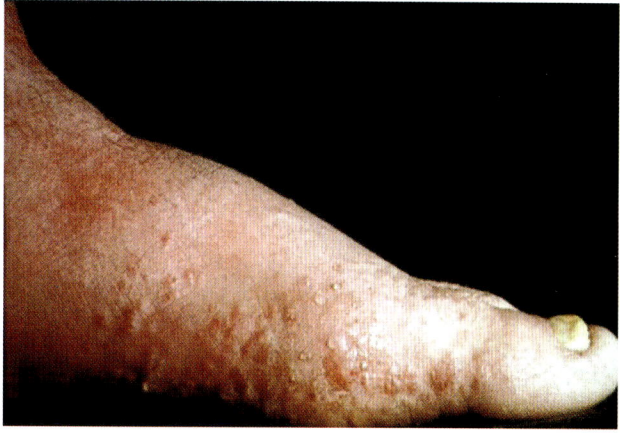

Tinea — Treatment

- Topicals
  - Ketoconazole, ciclopirox, terbinafine
- Systemics
  - Terbinafine for corporis/profunda/unguium/barbae
  - Griseofulvin or terbinafine for tinea capitis
  - ± Burow solution soaks for tinea pedis
  - **Ketoconazole no longer** given systemically given risk of fulminant hepatitic failure

Tinea Versicolor

- Caused by a **yeast, *Malassezia furfur*,** not a dermatophyte
- Hypo- or hyperpigmented lesions
- "Spaghetti and meatballs" on KOH
- Treatment: selenium sulfide shampoo, topical ketoconazole, oral fluconazole or itraconazole

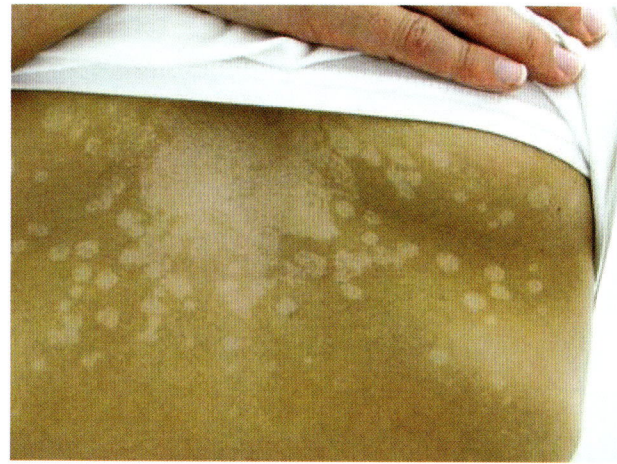

AR 26

A 70-year-old nursing home patient is sent to the emergency department for 3 weeks for severe, intense pruritus all over his body. Other tenants have had similar symptoms. Small papules are present on finger web spaces and wrist. Microscopic exam confirmed the diagnosis.

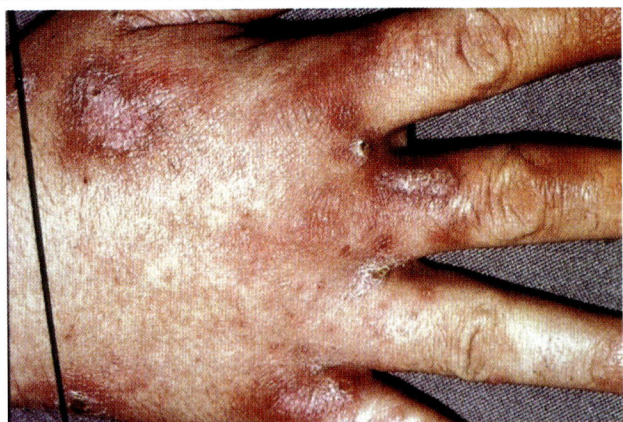

What is the best recommended treatment?

A. Topical steroid
B. Antihistamine
C. Topical ivermectin
D. Lindane 1% lotion
E. Permethrin 5% cream

Answer:_____

- Mite — transmitted person to person
- Intense, unexplained itching; hypersensitivity
- Institutionalized at higher risk
- **Dx:** mites, feces, or eggs under microscope
- **Rx:** permethrin 5%; repeat 1 week later
- Oral ivermectin can also be used
- Crusted scabies (Norwegian): Use combination therapy

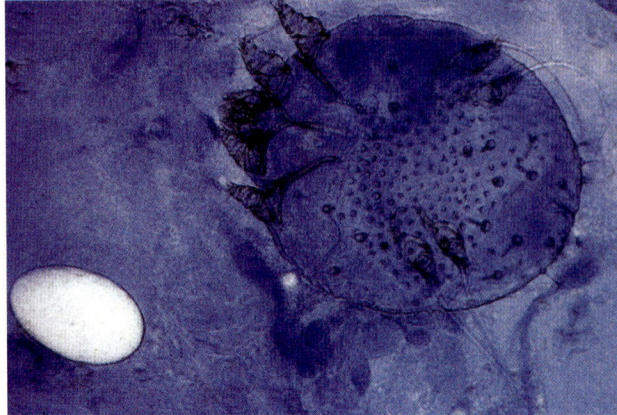

MELANOMA

AR 27

Which of the following is most important in determining the prognosis of a patient with melanoma?

A. Location of the melanoma
B. Depth of the melanoma
C. Presence or absence of ulceration
D. Duration of the melanoma
E. Surface size of the melanoma

Answer:_____

Melanoma

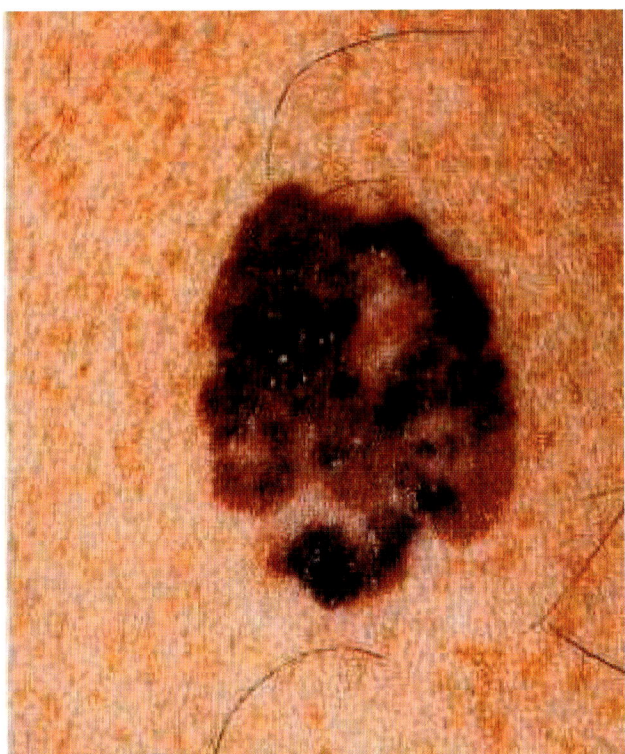

- **A** – **A**symmetry
- **B** – **B**orders are irregular
- **C** – **C**olor variation
- **D** – **D**iameter > 6 mm is suspicious
- **E** – **E**levation or **E**volution over time

Melanoma — Prognosis
- **Depth**
  - < 0.76 mm → 99% five-year survival
  - > 3.6 mm → < 50% five-year survival
- Age
  - Best if < 50 years of age
- Location
  - Best if on trunk

Melanoma — Treatment[13]

- Wide local excision
- ± **Sentinel lymph node dissection** depending on staging
- Immunotherapy

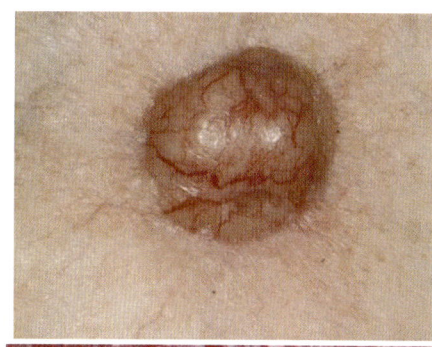

Surgical Margin Recommendations for Primary Cutaneous Melanoma	
Tumor Thickness	**Surgical Margin**
In situ	0.5–1.0 cm
≤ 1.0 mm	1.0 cm
> 1.0–2.0 mm	1.0–2.0 cm
> 2.0 mm	2.0 cm

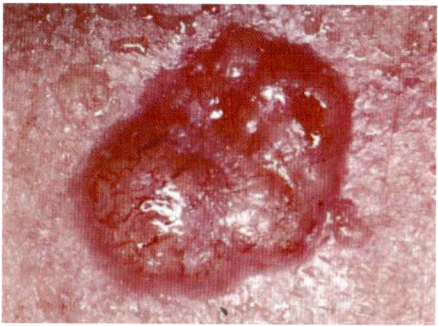

- Acral Melanoma
  - **Dark-skinned individuals** tend to get acral melanomas
  - **Hutchinson sign** is indicative of melanoma (in contrast to benign melanonychia)

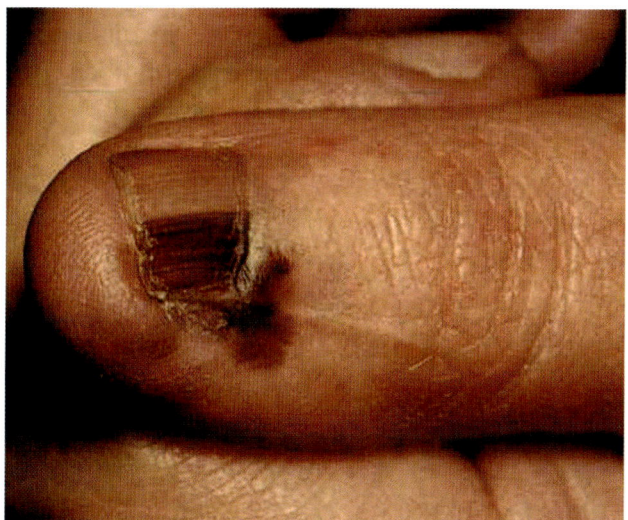

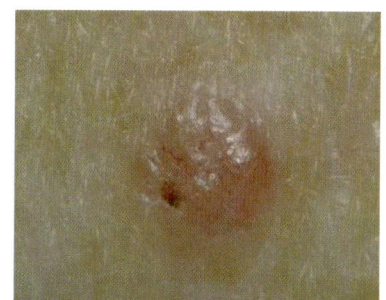

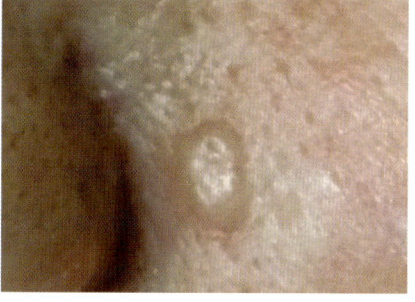

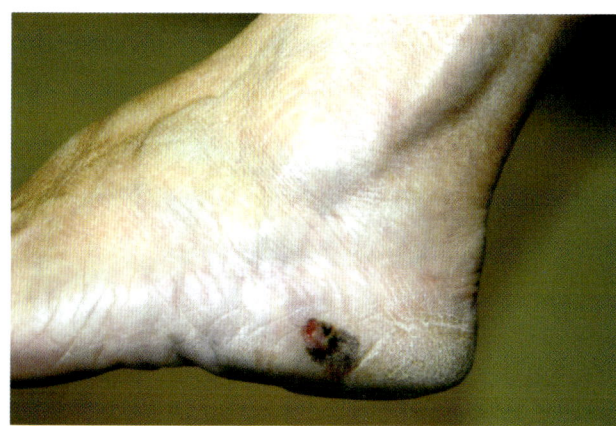

- Treatment
  - Depends on subtype of BCC
    - Wide local excision
    - Electrodessication and curettage
    - Topical chemotherapy
    - Mohs micrographic surgery

BASAL CELL CARCINOMA

Basal Cell Carcinoma
- Most commonly on the face, head, and neck
- Rarely metastasize but are locally destructive — **mets rate is < 0.1%**
- Pearly and/or pigmented papules or plaques, often with arborizing vessels and central ulceration

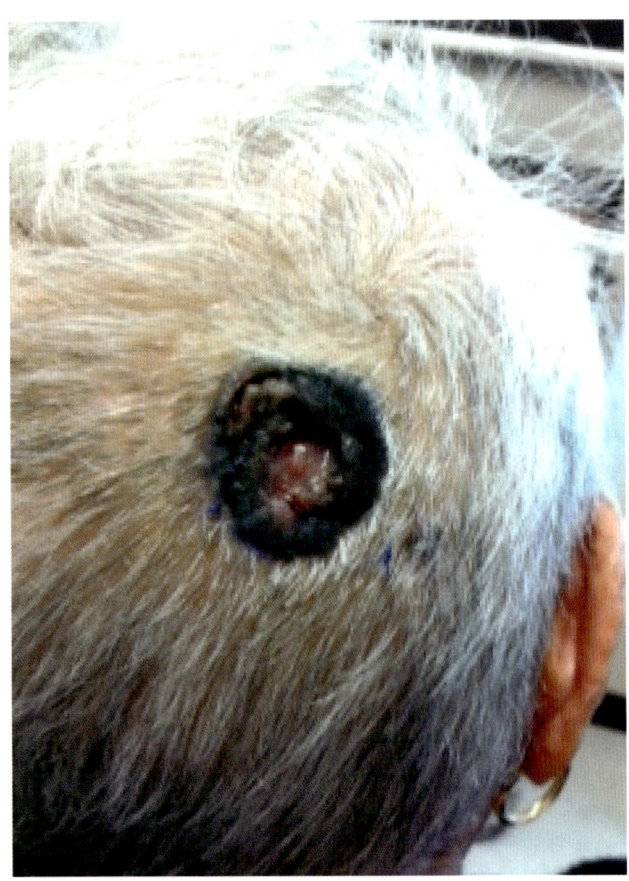

SQUAMOUS CELL CARCINOMA

- 2nd most common skin cancer
- Indurated pink, keratotic, and scaly macules, papules, ulcers
- Mets rate of 0.3–5%
- Mets more common from:
  - Lesions on ear and lip or in chronic ulcers
  - Lesions from inflammation/scars
- **Most common cancer after solid organ transplant**

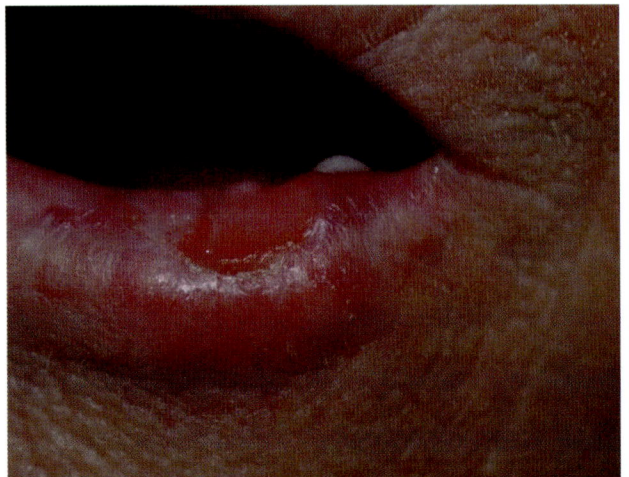

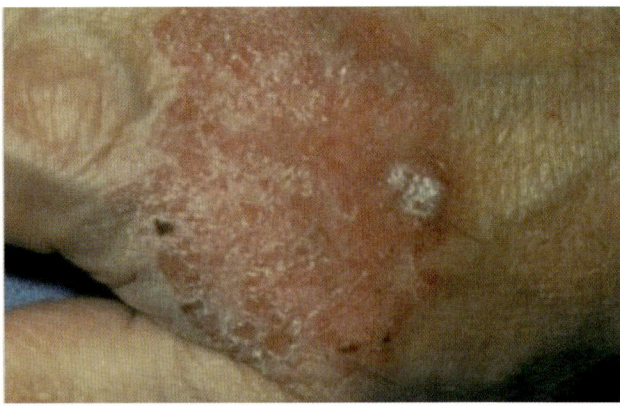

ACTINIC KERATOSIS

- White-to-yellow scale on an erythematous base presenting on sun-exposed areas
- 10–20% can progress to SCC over a 10-year period
- Can present as cutaneous horns (always biopsy), pigmented, atrophic, or actinic cheilitis

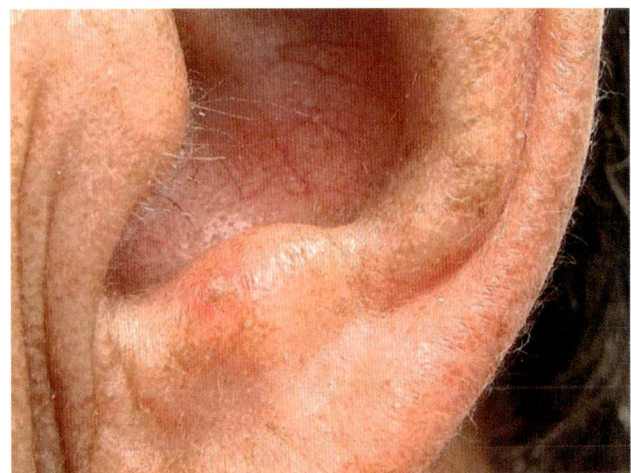

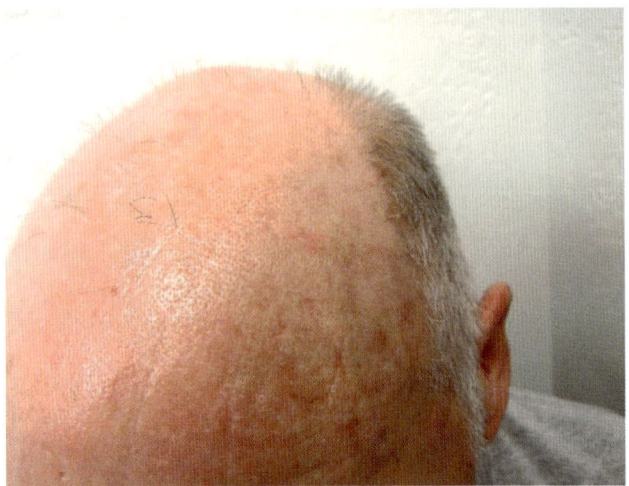

[14]

BLISTERING LESIONS

Bullous Pemphigoid
- Large tense bullae (intact)
- Nikolsky sign negative
- Mucosal involvement uncommon
- Older adult

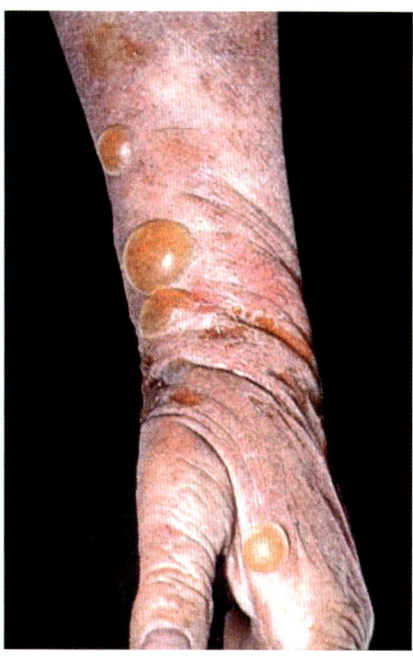

AR 28
A 72-year-old woman is seen for worsening blistering skin lesions. She has no history of hepatitis C or celiac disease and is on no medications. On exam, there are tense blisters on her lower extremities. Nikolsky sign is negative. She has no mucosal involvement.

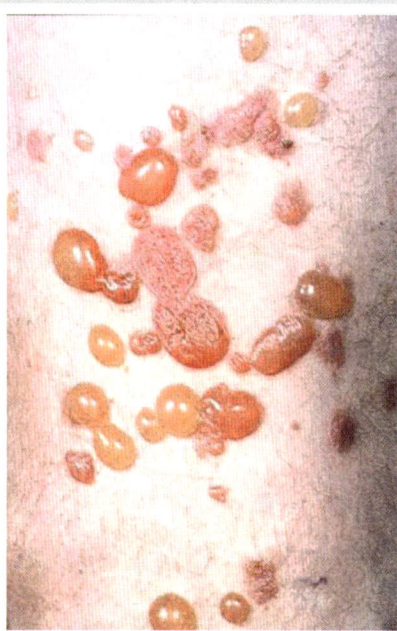

What is the most likely diagnosis?

A. Porphyria cutanea tarda
B. Erythema multiforme
C. Pemphigus vulgaris
D. Dermatitis herpetiformis
E. Bullous pemphigoid

Answer:_____

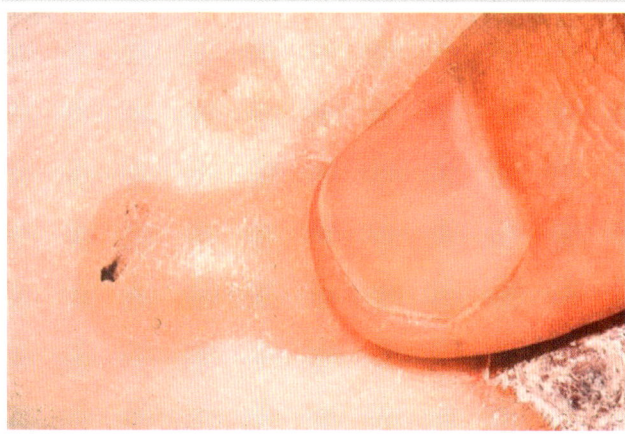

Pemphigus Vulgaris
- Fragile blisters (denuded)
- Nikolsky sign positive
- Mucosal involvement common
- Middle age

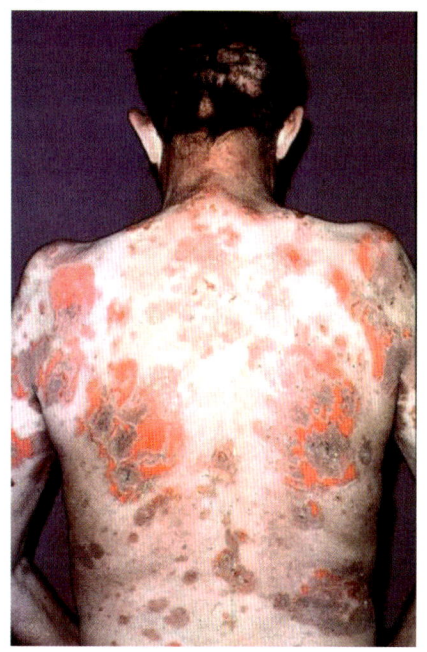

DERMATOLOGY

Bullous Pemphigoid
- Antibodies to **basement membrane** (tense and deep)

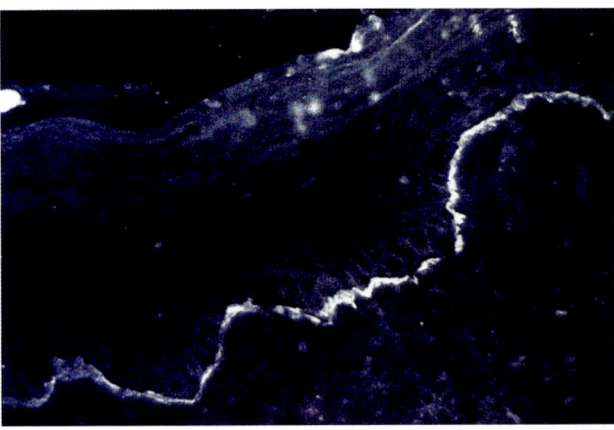

Pemphigus Vulgaris
- Intraepidermal antibodies against **desmosome** (fragile and superficial)

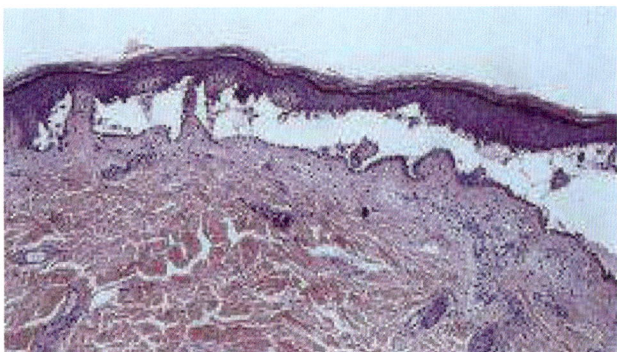

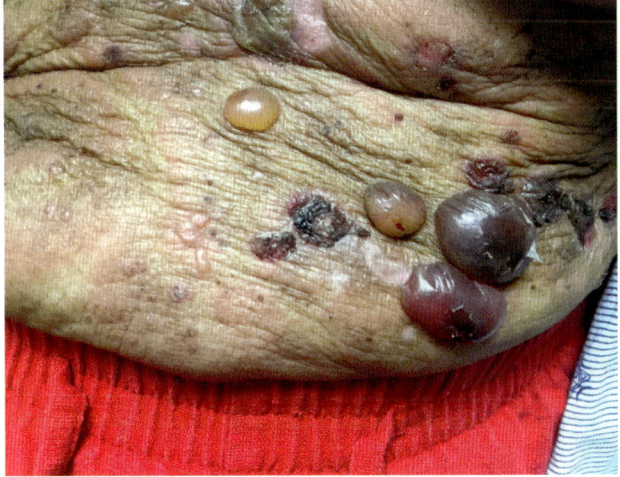

DERMATITIS HERPETIFORMIS
- Extremely itchy, symmetric, grouped vesicles most frequently located on extensor surfaces
- Vesicles often broken
- All patients have **celiac disease** (may be asymptomatic)
- **IgA** deposition in dermal papillary tips
- **Gluten-free diet** treats DH and celiac disease
- **Dapsone** will treat DH but not celiac disease
  - Check for G6PD first if at risk

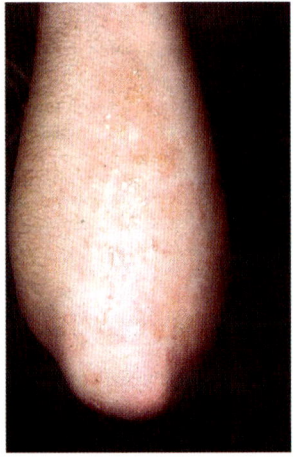
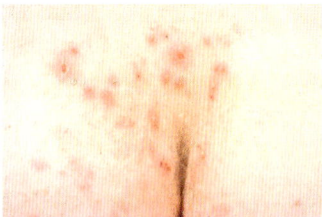
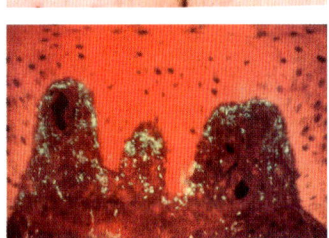

PORPHYRIA CUTANEA TARDA
- Deficiency of heme synthetic enzyme uroporphyrinogen decarboxylase
- **Dx:** ↑↑ Urinary copro- and uroporphyrins
- Build-up of phototoxic porphyrins in the skin
- Blisters on sun-exposed skin
- Associated with HIV and **hepatitis C**
- Hypertrichosis
- **Rx:** serial phlebotomy or hydroxychloroquine
  - HCV Rx if positive

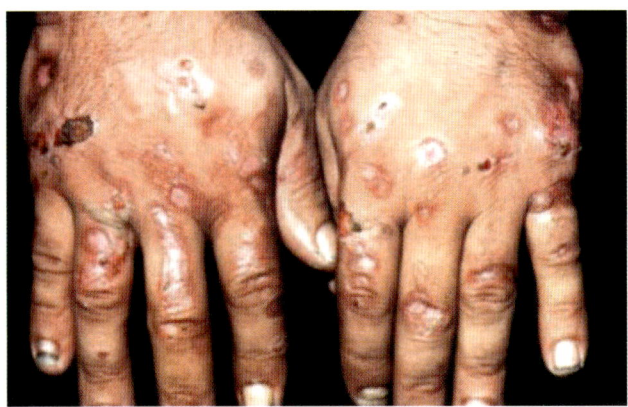

ROUND / ANNULAR LESIONS

Diagnosis?

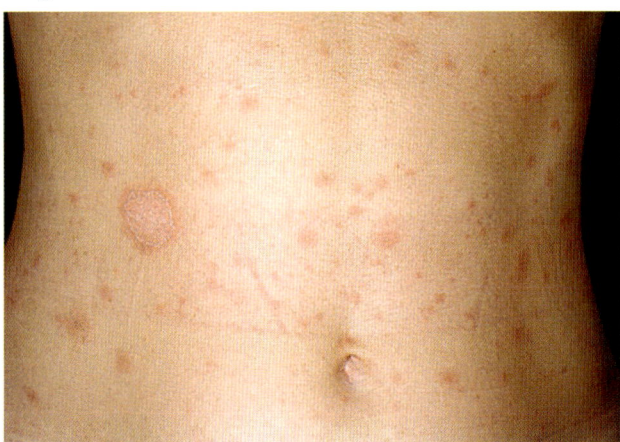

- Fine scaling papules and plaques with **collarette of scale**
  - Trunk and proximal extremities
  - Asymptomatic or mild pruritus
  - Unlike syphilis, spares palms/soles; **consider RPR**
- Oval, follow skin lines of cleavage ("Christmas Tree")
- **Herald patch** appears 1–2 weeks before generalized rash
- Resolves spontaneously
- Low-potency steroid if pruritic

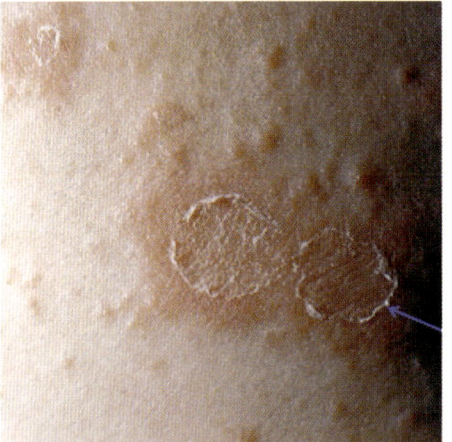

PIGMENT CHANGES

Seborrheic Keratoses
- Brown, white, black, inflamed, flat or **stuck on** papules
- Eruptive SKs reported in pregnancy, inflammatory conditions, and rarely a malignancy called sign of **Leser-Trélat**, which is associated with GI or breast cancers or lymphoma

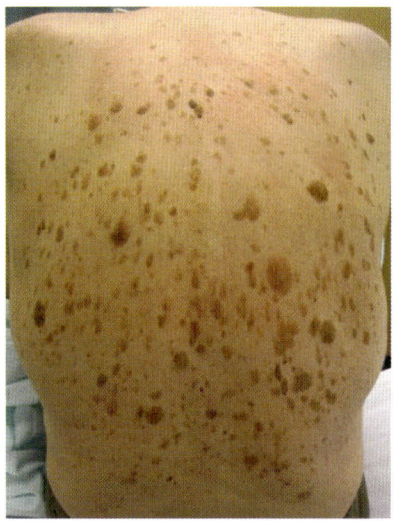

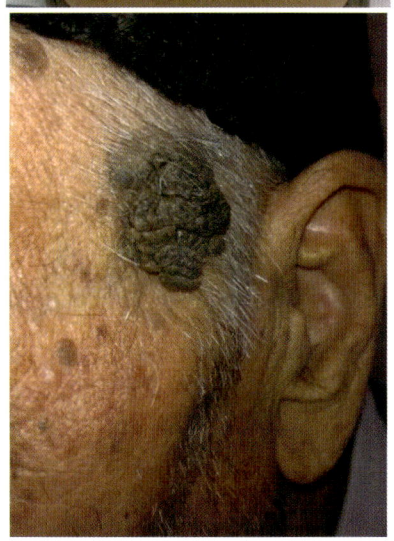

AR 29

A 72-year-old woman with a history of ESRD and secondary hyperparathyroidism presents with painful, violaceous, symmetric lesions on the legs that then developed into nonhealing necrotic ulcers.

Labs: Ca^{2+} 10.0, Phos 8.1, BUN 82, Cr 5.3.

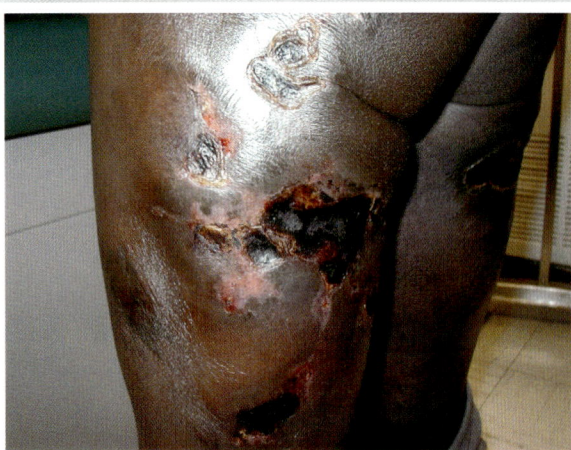

The most likely diagnosis is:

A. Nephrogenic systemic fibrosis
B. Calciphylaxis
C. Pyoderma gangrenosum
D. Necrotizing fasciitis
E. Multiple bites from a brown recluse spider gone rogue

Answer:_____

- Most commonly seen in **ESRD** patients
- Associated with **secondary hyperparathyroidism**
  - Ca^{2+} × **Phos product** > 55–70
- Medial calcification of **arterial** wall with intimal proliferation → ischemia and tissue necrosis
- Painful, symmetric, violaceous nodules → ulcerate
  - Areas of greatest adiposity (thighs, buttocks, abd)
- Poor prognosis, especially proximal lesions
- **Rx**
  - Wound care
  - Lower Ca^{2+} × Phos product
  - Sodium thiosulfate
  - Discontinue contributing medications (warfarin)

Audience Response 1
E. Topical corticosteroids

AR 2
D. Check for HIV.

AR 3
A. Poison ivy

AR 4
E. Topical retinoid

AR 5
E. All of the above

AR 6
B. Topical metronidazole

AR 7
C. HIV testing

AR 8
A. Reassurance

AR 9
A. Gadolinium during an imaging study

AR 10
C. Toxic epidermal necrolysis

AR 11
C. Herpes simplex

AR 12
E. Aspirin

AR 13
A. Anticentromere

AR 14
E. All of the above

AR 15
B. Löfgren syndrome

AR 16
E. Cancer screening

AR 17A
A. Pyoderma gangrenosum

AR 17B
B. Debridement

AR 18
D. IgA vasculitis

AR 19
D. Acrodermatitis enteropathica (zinc deficiency)

AR 20
D. Obtain a surgical consultation.

AR 21
B. Lyme disease

AR 22
B. Secondary

AR 23
D. Ophthalmology consult

AR 24
C. Griseofulvin by mouth

AR 25
C. Obtain and send a nail clipping sample to the lab.

AR 26
E. Permethrin 5% cream

AR 27
B. Depth of the melanoma

AR 28
E. Bullous pemphigoid

AR 29
B. Calciphylaxis

ENDNOTES

[1]   Kimberly Salkey, MD.

[2]   Jemec GB. Clinical practice. Hidradenitis suppurativa. *NEJM.* 2012;366:158–164.

[3]   Brent Kelly, MD

[4]   Jay2Base [CC BY-SA 4.0 (https://creativecommons.org/licenses/by-sa/4.0)], from Wikimedia Commons

[5]   Photos courtesy of Natalie Wright, MD and Ruth Ann Vleugels,MD

[6]   Courtesy of Natalie Wright

[7]   CNX OpenStax [CC BY 4.0 (https://creativecommons.org/licenses/by/4.0)], via Wikimedia Commons

[8]   Kimberly Salkey, MD

[9]   Elizabeth M Dugan, Adam M Huber, Frederick W Miller, Lisa G Rider [CC BY-SA 3.0 (https://creativecommons.org/licenses/by-sa/3.0)], via Wikimedia Commons

[10]   Doktorinternet [CC BY-SA 4.0 (https://creativecommons.org/licenses/by-sa/4.0)], from Wikimedia Commons

[11]   Rrreewww [CC BY-SA 3.0 (https://creativecommons.org/licenses/by-sa/3.0)], via Wikimedia Commons

[12]   SOA-AIDS Amsterdam [CC-BY-SA-3.0 (http://creativecommons.org/licenses/by-sa/3.0/)], via Wikimedia Commons

[13]   *Journal of the American Academy of Dermatology: Guidelines of care for the management of primary cutaneous melanoma.* January, 2019; Vol. 80, Issue 1, 208–250.

[14]   Future FamDoc [CC BY-SA 4.0 (https://creativecommons.org/licenses/by-sa/4.0)], from Wikimedia Commons

MedStudy®

INTERNAL MEDICINE REVIEW

Endocrinology

Presented by

Brandy A. Panunti, MD

TABLE OF CONTENTS

Why We Moved Some Slide Information to the Audience Response Answers Page

At MedStudy, we do all we can to optimize your self-testing and learning.

In this presentation, the speaker will give some extra information after their AR questions to help explain the correct and incorrect answers. To keep from interfering with your self-testing, we've moved that explanatory text to the Audience Response Answers page(s) at the end of the section.

Be assured, all the content on the slides is in your syllabus—so you can focus on the teaching instead of taking detailed notes.

Why Some Topic Names Are Not Printed in This Section

At MedStudy, we do all we can to optimize your self-testing and learning.

In this section, the speaker has chosen to introduce topics with an Audience Response question to help you learn. In the syllabus, we've intentionally "hidden" some topic names that would give away the answers—so you can self-test more effectively. Where we've done this, instead of the topic name, you'll see an empty teal band or some extra space, but you can still find the topic on the page using the Table of Contents.

We Will Be Covering:
- General Principles
- Pituitary Disease
- Thyroid Disease
- Adrenal Disease
- Hormones of Reproduction
- Dyslipidemia
- Diabetes Review
- Calcium Disorders
- Multiple Endocrine Neoplasia (MEN)

GENERAL PRINCIPLES

Audience Response 1

A 33-year-old obese woman with fatigue and inability to lose weight comes in for evaluation. She questions if she has cortisol excess.

She does have diabetes and is on metformin but does not have HTN.

Exam: BMI 38 kg/m^2; BP 130/80 mmHg

Central obesity, pale striae

Labs:

TSH normal

HbA1c 6.6%

Which of the following is the best screening test for cortisol excess?

A. Random cortisol
B. ACTH-stimulated cortisol
C. 8 a.m. cortisol after dexamethasone
D. 8 a.m. free cortisol

Answer:_____

Endocrinology Basics
- If you wish to test for **hypo**secretion of a hormone, try to stimulate it
  - ACTH stimulation to rule out AI
- If you wish to test for **hyper**secretion of a hormone, try to suppress it.
  - DST rule out cortisol excess
- Random hormone levels are **generally** not helpful
- The term **"primary"** refers to the gland itself
  - **Primary** hypothyroidism = underactive thyroid
- The term **"secondary"** refers to whatever controls the gland (master)
  - **Secondary** hypothyroidism = pituitary insufficiency
- The term **"tertiary"** refers to something that controls whatever it is that controls the gland (supreme)
  - **Tertiary** hypothyroidism = hypothalamic insufficiency
    - Not used clinically

POSTERIOR PITUITARY GLAND

Pituitary Gland
- Master gland
  - Hormonal deficiencies
    - **Secondary** AI, hypogonadism, hypothyroidism
- 2 parts:
  1) Posterior
  2) Anterior

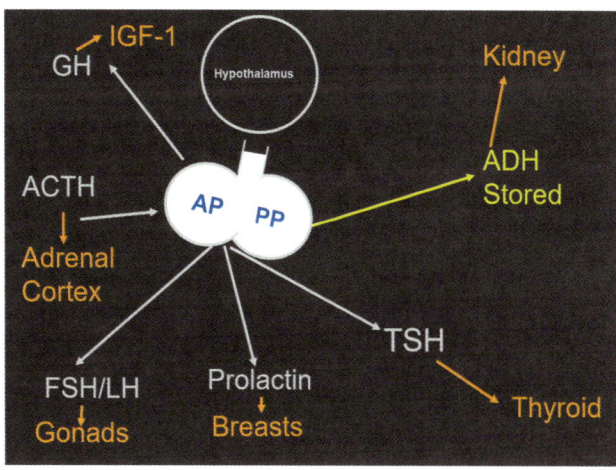

Posterior Pituitary Gland
- Stores and releases ADH (vasopressin) and oxytocin
- **ADH** = antidiuretic hormone
  - "Water hormone"
  - Regulated by serum osmolality
  - Controls urine concentration … and thirst
- Deficiency = central diabetes insipidus
  - Suspect if polyuria (> 2.5 L/day)
  - Confirmation: water deprivation test

Diabetes Insipidus
1) Central
   - Pituitary surgery, trauma, sarcoid
     - Treatment = desmopressin (DDAVP)
2) Nephrogenic
   - Lithium, hypercalcemia
     - Treatment = diuretics

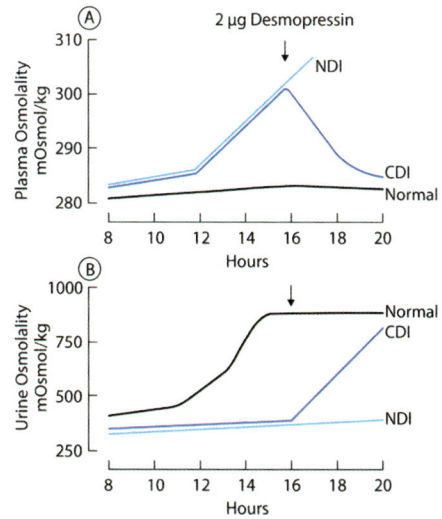

Water deprivation test

ANTERIOR PITUITARY GLAND

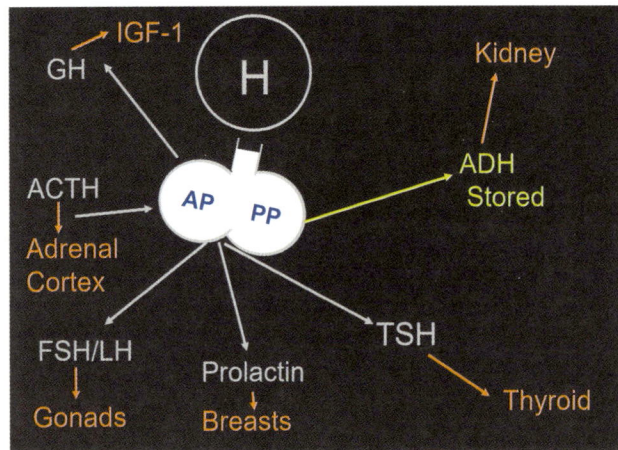

1) Adrenocorticotropic hormone (ACTH)
2) Thyroid-stimulating hormone (TSH)
3) Luteinizing hormone (LH)
4) Follicle-stimulating hormone (FSH)
5) Growth hormone (GH)
6) Prolactin (PRL)
• Lose 1st what you need least!
  – Sex and growth hormones ...

Empty Sella Syndrome
• Incidentally found
  – Squished pituitary by CSF → all hormones intact 90% of the time!!
• Usually seen in **multiparous** women
• **Ignore if all systems are functioning**

PITUITARY TUMORS

AR 2

A 24-year-old woman is found to have an incidental 7-mm pituitary adenoma in an otherwise normal MRI; you originally ordered a brain MRI because she was complaining of worsening headache.

She is on OCPs with regular periods

BMI = 31 kg/m²

BP = 120/77 mmHg

HR 70 bpm

Normal TSH and CMP

Which of the following is the best next step in this patient's care?

A. Check an FT₄.
B. Check all anterior pituitary hormones for hyper- and hyposecretion.
C. Reassurance
D. Neurosurgical evaluation
E. Check prolactin and IGF-1; screen for cortisol excess.

Answer:_____

Pituitary Tumors
• Often found incidentally
• Size dictates evaluations
  – < 1 cm, ask: Hypersecretion?
  – prolactin, cortisol, and GH excess ...
  – > 1 cm, ask:
    • Hypersecretion?
    • Hyposecretion?
    • Visual field deficits?

Prolactinoma
• Most common secreting pituitary tumor
• ↑ PRL → ↓ secretion of GnRH → ↓ LH/FSH and their target organ functions
  – ♀ **Amenorrhea**, **galactorrhea**, infertility; **micro**adenomas
  – ♂ **Impotence and hypogonadism**; **macro**adenomas

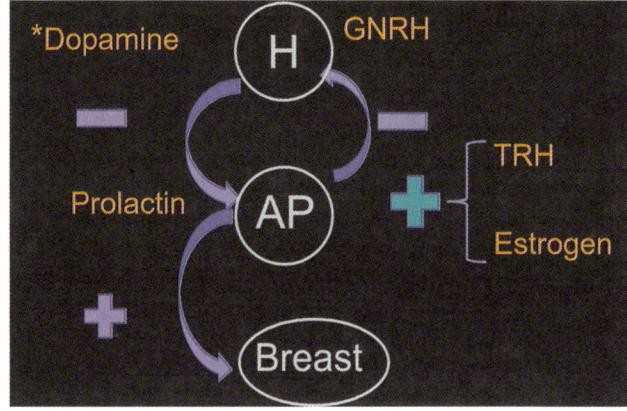

Prolactinoma — Treatment
• **Drug therapy first** for macroadenomas and symptomatic microadenomas
  – Dopamine agonists: cabergoline preferred
• Transsphenoidal resection when meds are ineffective or not tolerated — **rare**
• **Caution oral contraceptives** in macroadenomas → estrogen ↑ size

Hyperprolactinemia
• Rx related
  – Phenothiazines
  – Risperidone
  – Butyrophenones
  – SSRIs
  – Tricyclics
  – Opiates
  – Verapamil
  – Metoclopramide
• Prolactinoma
• **Primary hypothyroidism** } Check TSH and β-hCG
• Pregnancy
• **Chronic kidney disease**
• Chest trauma or nipple stimulation

PRL level roughly correlates with tumor size

Normal = < 20 ng/mL
> 100 ng/mL usually due to adenoma

AR 3

A 52-year-old male complaining of headache and fatigue × 2 years:

No PMH

+ ROS: Snoring, hypersomnolence, exertional pain in knees and ankles, paresthesias, and pain in R hand that wakes him from sleep

BMI = 31 kg/m^2

BP = 165/94 mmHg

Coarse hair and skin on face; laterally displaced PMI

Normal TSH and CMP

HbA1c 8.6%

Screening colonoscopy: polyps

Which of the following is the best next step in this patient's care?

A. Check TSH with an FT$_4$.
B. Check serum growth hormone.
C. Order a polysomnogram.
D. Start metformin 500 mg bid.
E. Check random serum IGF-1.

Answer:_____

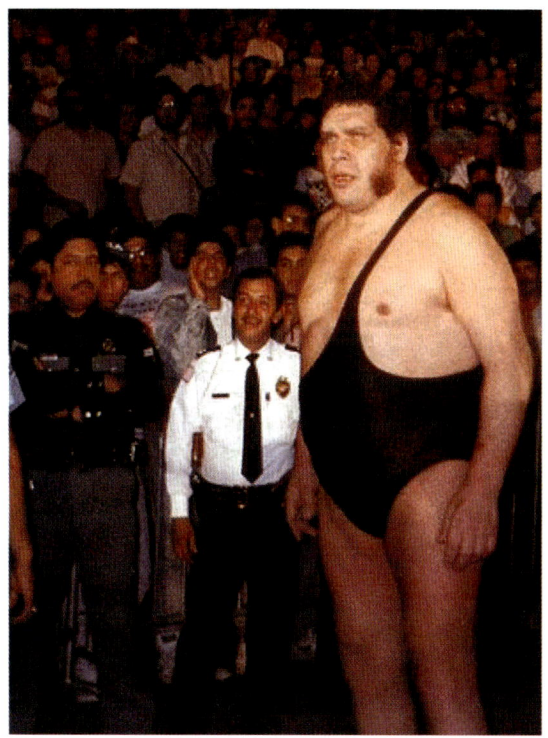

[1]

Acromegaly

- Classification based on age
  - Kids: ↑ GH → gigantism
  - Adults: ↑ GH → acromegaly
- Classic findings
  - Enlarging hands and feet ("rings" or "shoes")
  - Frontal bossing
  - Deepening voice
  - Coarse facial features
  - Excessive sweating and body odor
  - Progressive jaw malocclusion

Acromegaly Diagnosis

- Screening: IGF-1
- Confirm with 75-g glucose tolerance test
- GH fails to be suppressed with hyperglycemia

  If you wish to test for **hyper**secretion of a hormone, try to suppress it

- Surgery for all!
- Look for:
  - Heart failure (echo for all)
  - Adenomatous colon polyps (C-scope for all)
  - OSA (sleep evaluation for all)

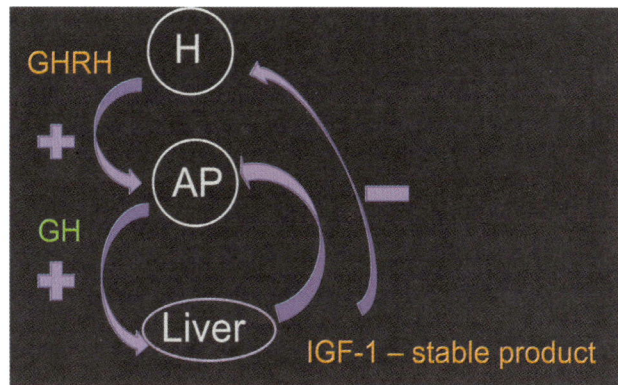

Pituitary Apoplexy

- Endocrine emergency: recognize and treat
- Tumor outgrows blood supply or bleeds into preexisting tumor
  - Nonfunctional macroadenomas
- Usual presentation
  - **Severe headache**
  - Nausea and vomiting
  - Visual field defects
  - Altered consciousness
- Imaging: CT
- Emergent treatment: glucocorticoids
- Neurosurgical emergency

THYROID GLAND

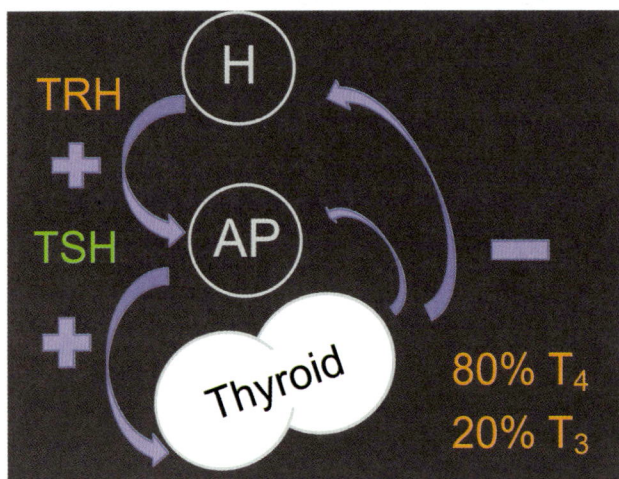

TRH +
TSH +
Thyroid
H
AP
—
80% T$_4$
20% T$_3$

Thyroid Basics
- TSH is always the best screening test
- Do not be fooled ... Never need reverse T$_3$, T$_4$:T$_3$ ratios ...
- ↓ TSH = **hyper**thyroidism
- ↑ TSH = **hypo**thyroidism
- Order both TSH and FT$_4$ when suspect for **secondary** (pituitary) disease

Thyroid Rules
- TSH and FT$_4$ are inverse except:
  - Both low (low/nl) = pituitary disease = euthyroid sick syndrome
  - Both high = pituitary disease = resistance

EUTHYROID SICK SYNDROME
- Self-preservation
  - Sick body cannot convert T$_4$ to T$_3$
  - Instead T$_4$ → "reverse T$_3$" (rT$_3$)
- Usual labs
  - **Low**-normal TSH
  - **Low**-normal FT$_4$
  - **Low** FT$_3$
  - High **rT3** (not usually measured)
- Thyroid is not the problem
  - **Never check TFTs in the very sick unless you suspect thyroid storm or myxedema coma!**

HYPOTHYROIDISM

Hypothyroidism — Causes
- **Chronic autoimmune** (Hashimoto's; 20% population)
- Others
  - Postpartum (autoimmune)
    - Can treat with selenium
  - Postsurgical
  - **Painful thyroiditis**
  - Medication induced
    - Lithium, amiodarone
  - Post I-131

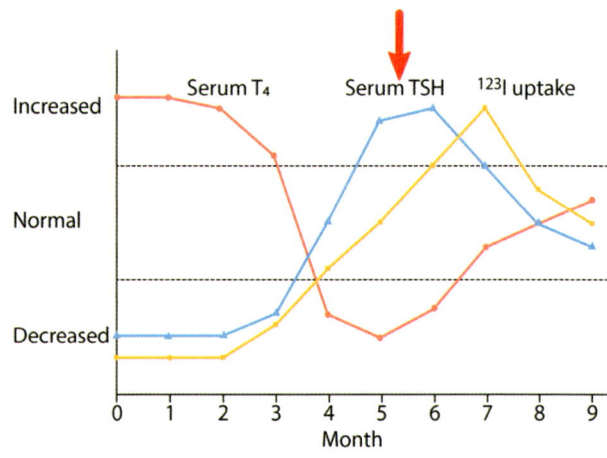

Serum T$_4$ · Serum TSH · ^{123}I uptake · Increased · Normal · Decreased · Month

Hypothyroidism
- Symptoms: nonspecific
- Signs: delayed reflexes, bradycardia, galactorrhea
- Labs: **hyperlipidemia**, **hyponatremia**, normocytic **anemia**, hyperprolactinemia

Primary Hypothyroidism
- Labs: ↑ TSH
  - FT$_4$ would be low if checked
- Antithyroid antibodies??
  - Not needed, but if checked likely +++
  - Thyroid peroxidase
- Treat all with overt hypothyroidism: ↑ TSH and low free T$_4$
- Treat all with ↑ TSH and normal free T$_4$ if **TSH > 10 mU/L, goiter, pregnant** (subclinical hypothyroidism)
- No imaging needed
  - Unless thyroid nodule palpated on exam

Hypothyroidism — Treatment
- T$_4$ (levothyroxine [L-T$_4$])
  - Cardiac disease, start **low** and go **slow**
  - 1.6 µg/kg of body weight/day
  - Allow 6 weeks after dose change
- T$_3$ (liothyronine [Armour Thyroid])
  - Rarely used to treat hypothyroidism
  - Offers no real advantage to traditional L-T$_4$
- Exogenous hyperthyroidism
  - AFib and bone loss

Myxedema Coma
- Medical emergency
- Clinical diagnosis (no TSH level predicts myxedema coma)
  - ↓ MS, ↓ temp, ↓ heart rate
- Mortality 30–40% and related to degree of hypothermia
- Initiate empiric Rx
  - Hypothyroidism
    - IV T$_4$
  - Adrenal insufficiency
  - Coincident
  - Infection
  - Passive warming

AR 4

A 60-year-old woman with chronic hypothyroidism comes in for evaluation of weight loss and palpitations. She stopped estrogen-based HRT about 3 months ago.

Meds: levothyroxine 175 mcg; calcium 1,200 mg

Exam: HR 104 bpm

Mild tremor, no goiter

Labs:

TSH = < 0.01 uIU/mL

Free T4 = 2.6 ng/dL

Which of the following is the best next step in her management?

A. Thyroid uptake scan
B. Restart her estrogen replacement therapy.
C. Decrease her dose of L-thyroxine.
D. Check thyroid peroxisome antibodies.
E. Advise her to take her thyroid medication 1 hour after her calcium supplements.

Answer:_____

Learning Point

- Starting or stopping any estrogen therapy will change the dosage of thyroid hormone needed
  - Start ERT (OCP, HRT, pregnancy) → ↑ TBG → need more L-T$_4$
  - Stop ERT → ↓ TBG → need less L-T$_4$

HYPERTHYROIDISM

- Graves disease
  - Most common cause
  - Younger
  - Autoimmune (+TSI, +TrAB)
- Postpartum thyroiditis (autoimmune, within 1 year of delivery)
- Painful thyroiditis
- Toxic multinodular goiter
  - Older
- Exogenous
- Medication induced
  - Contrast, amiodarone

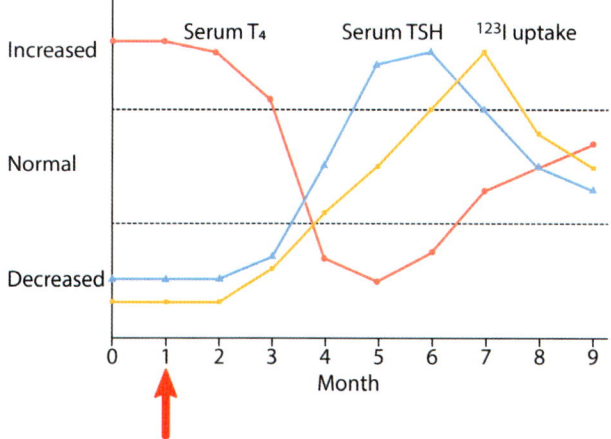

Clues to Diagnosis

- **Graves'**
  - Bruit and Graves orbitopathy (GO)
- **Postpartum** thyroiditis
  - Within 1 year of delivery
- **Painful** thyroiditis
  - Sed rate
  - Recent URI
- **Toxic multinodular goiter**
  - Recent contrast
- **Exogenous**
  - Overweight nurse
  - Thyroglobulin level (low)

Hyperthyroidism

- Symptoms — increased metabolism
  - Weight loss, palpitations, diarrhea, anxiety
  - New-onset breast tenderness (gynecomastia → increased SHBG)
- Signs — lid lag, AFib, tremor, goiter
- Labs — hypercalcemia, increased alkaline phosphatase (ALP)
- Labs: ↓ TSH
  - Elevated free T$_4$ and/or free T$_3$
- Thyroid-stimulating antibodies?
  - Not needed, but if checked likely +++ in Graves'
  - Can check if cannot do scan (pregnant, recent contrast)
- Imaging helps determine etiology
  - Thyroid scan and uptake

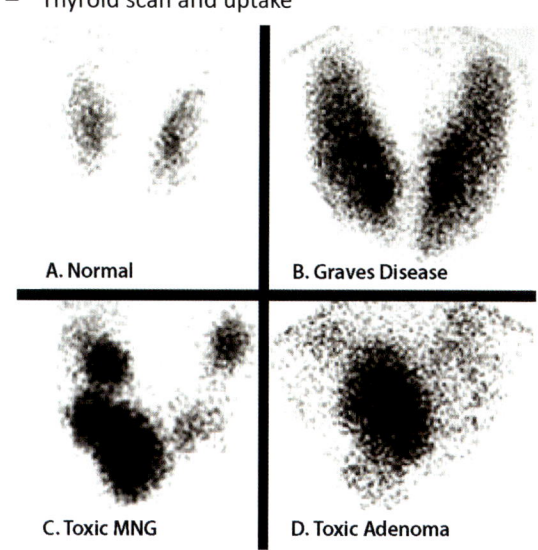

A. Normal   B. Graves Disease

C. Toxic MNG   D. Toxic Adenoma

[2]

Never order for a woman who might be pregnant or is nursing

No uptake in all thyroiditis and exogenous

Graves' — Treatment

- **β-Blockers**
  - Treat symptoms
  - Propranolol will block $T_4 \rightarrow T_3$
- **Methimazole**
  - 30% will go into remission with 1–2 years of therapy
  - PTU (black box warning)
    - Used only 1st trimester, storm
- **I-131 therapy**
  - Can worsen GO (so can smoking!!)
- **Surgery**

Hyperthyroidism Treatment

- **Postpartum** thyroiditis
  - Within 1 year of delivery
    - β-Blockers if needed
- **Painful** thyroiditis
  - Sed rate
  - NSAIDs and/or steroids
- Toxic multinodular goiter
  - I-131 therapy

Thyroid Storm

- Medical emergency
  - Mortality is high
- Clinical diagnosis
  - ↓ MS, fever, tachycardia
- Initiate empiric Rx
  - Hyperthyroidism
    - PTU
      - New + will block $T_4 \rightarrow T_3$
    - Iodide
      - Preformed + will block $T_4 \rightarrow T_3$
  - Glucocorticoids
    - AI+ will block $T_4 \rightarrow T_3$
  - β-Blockers
    - Symptoms + will block $T_4 \rightarrow T_3$
  - Supportive + antibiotics

PREGNANCY AND THYROID

- Hypothyroidism
  - Thyroid hormone requirements increase by 30–50%
  - TFTs q 4–6 weeks; goal TSH < 2.5 uIU/mL (IQ)
- Hyperthyroidism
  - Goal is a normal free T_4
    - Not TSH
  - Graves' generally gets better
  - Drug of choice PTU (1st trimester)

AR 5

A 32-year-old woman:

Pain in the RUQ and fever × 2 days

Jaundice

Dx: ascending cholangitis → ICU

HR of 65 bpm × 2 days

TSH = 0.20 uIU/mL (0.5–5.0)

FT_4 = 0.6 ng/dL (0.7–1.8)

You are consulted for recommendations on the need for further evaluation and institution of thyroid replacement.

Which of the following is the best next step in patient care?

A. Order an MRI of the pituitary.
B. Start levothyroxine 100 mcg PO daily.
C. Start levothyroxine 50 mcg IV daily.
D. Reassure the consulting physician.
E. Order a thyroid uptake scan.

Answer:_____

AR 6

A 49-year-old man with 4 months of:

Cold intolerance, easy fatigue, depression, weight gain, constipation

History of pituitary surgery 5 years ago for a nonfunctional tumor but did not require therapy after

TSH = 0.5 uIU/mL (0.5–4.0)

Free T_4 = 0.6 ng/dL (0.7–1.8)

Which of the following is the most likely diagnosis?

A. Chronic autoimmune thyroiditis
B. Secondary hypothyroidism
C. Hyperthyroidism
D. Euthyroid sick syndrome
E. No thyroid disease

Answer:_____

THYROID NODULES AND CANCER

Thyroid Nodules[3]

- Nodules are extremely common!
  - > 1 cm in 50–65% on autopsy
  - Palpable in 5% of individuals
- Thyroid cancer is **not** common
  - < 10% of nodules are malignant
  - Screening for thyroid nodules is not recommended

Thyroid Malignancy — Risk Factors
- **Prior neck irradiation**
- **Family history**
- **Ultrasound characteristics**
  - Solid + microcalcifications, irregular margins, tall > wide
- Dysphagia or dysphonia
- Age < 20 years or > 70 years
- Fixed, hard, lymphadenopathy +
- High TSH
- PET + (focal uptake 40% risk)
  - vs. diffuse uptake = Hashimoto's

Palpable Nodule Evaluation
1) Check TSH
   - Low → RAI uptake for toxic nodule/MNG
   - Normal or elevated → thyroid U/S
2) Thyroid U/S
3) Possible FNA
   - Depending on size + U/S characteristics
     - Microcalcifications, irregular boarders, solid, hypoechoic, tall > wide
   - Risk of malignancy
     - Focal PET+, prior radiation
- Surgical indications
  - Abnormal FNA
  - Significant growth over time
  - Compressive symptoms
- **Note:** Workup of incidentally found thyroid nodules on imaging is the same as nodules found on exam

AR 7

You evaluate a 44-year-old woman with anxiety, weight loss, mild tremor, and tachycardia. She has a nontender goiter.

Free T_4 = 2.0 ng/dL (0.9–1.8)

TSH = 0.1 uIU/mL (0.5–5.0)

Nuclear scan: homogeneous pattern

Uptake 59% (↑)

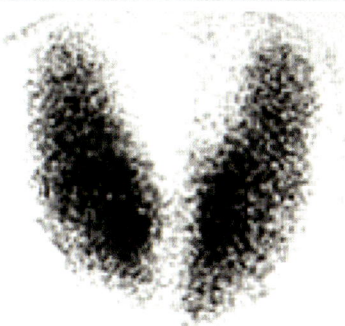

Which of the following is the most likely diagnosis?

A. Graves disease
B. Subacute thyroiditis
C. Silent thyroiditis
D. Exogenous T_4
E. Toxic multinodular goiter

Answer:_____

ADRENAL GLAND

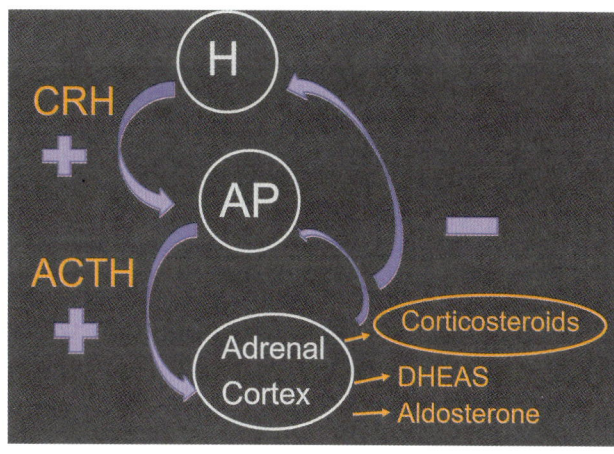

Adrenal Basics
- The adrenal cortex makes 3 big hormones
  - **Cortisol**
  - Main regulator: ACTH
  - **Aldosterone**
    - Main regulator: renin system
    - ACTH influences
  - **Androgens** → DHEAS
    - ACTH influences
- The adrenal medulla makes
  - Metanephrines (adrenaline)
    - Not under ACTH influence

CUSHING SYNDROME
- Cortisol excess
  - Proximal muscle weakness
  - Easy bruisability
  - Cervicodorsal fat pad
  - Supraclavicular fat pads
  - Moon facies
  - Plethora
  - Central obesity
  - Thin arms and legs

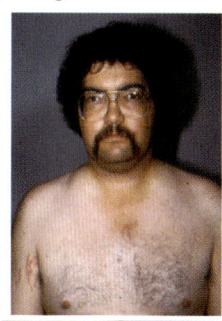

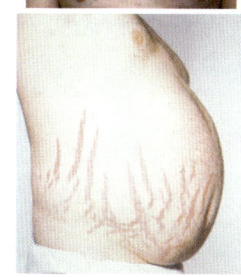

Etiologies of Cushing Syndrome
- Exogenous glucocorticoids
  - Iatrogenic
  - Most common
- Endogenous hypercortisolism
  - ACTH-dependent
    - Pituitary (Cushing disease)
      - Most common
    - Ectopic
  - ACTH-independent
    - Adrenal

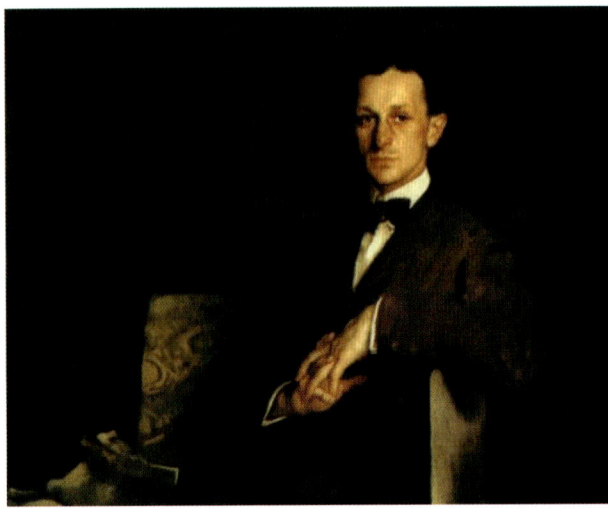

Cushing's — Diagnostic Workup
- Screen → Confirm → Localize
- Screen
  1) 24-hour urine free cortisol;
     Pitfall: depression, alcoholism, false+
  2) 1-mg overnight dexamethasone suppression test;
     Pitfall: estrogen increases CBG, false+
  3) Late-night salivary cortisol;
     Pitfall: shift workers??
- Confirm abnormal test
- Measure ACTH levels to dictate imaging
  1) Plasma ACTH level **low**:
     - CT adrenals
  2) Plasma ACTH level is **not** low (inappropriately normal or high):
     - Pituitary MRI
     - If MRI neg, choices:
       - CT chest, abd
       - IPSS

AR 8

A 22-year-old Caucasian female:

MVA: broken thumb

Lost consciousness during cast placement

BP 75/palp; HR 130 bpm

BP 100/64 with saline infusion; HR 80 bpm

Temp 98.7°F (37.0°C)

Thin and tan

Skin vitiligo

Other medical conditions: hypothyroidism and celiac disease

Labs:

Na^+ = 134 mmol/L (↓)

K^+ = 5.6 mEq/L

BUN = 42 mg/dL

Creat = 0.7 mg/dL

Glu = 61 mg/dL

TSH = 2.4 uIU/mL

Head CT = normal

Which of the following is the most appropriate next step in patient care?

A. Hydrocortisone
B. Hydrocortisone + fludrocortisone; order an ACTH stimulation test.
C. Dexamethasone; order an ACTH stimulation test.

Answer:_____

Adrenal Insufficiency
- Primary
  - Adrenal failure
  - **High ACTH**
- Secondary
  - Pituitary failure (chronic exogenous GC)
  - **Low ACTH**
- Weakness and fatigue
- Anorexia and abdominal pain
- Hypercalcemia
- When AI presents acutely, it is an endocrine emergency

Primary Adrenal Insufficiency
- Addison disease
  - Autoimmune
  - High ACTH
    - Hyperpigmentation
  - Lose aldosterone production
    - Hyponatremia
    - Hyperkalemia
    - High renin
    - Supplement with fludrocortisone (Florinef)
- Dx: **ACTH stimulation** test
  - Cortisol fails to increase > 18–20 µg/dL
  - Can be done anytime of the day
- Rx
  - Acute: dexamethasone or hydrocortisone
  - Chronic: glucocorticoid + mineralocorticoid

Secondary Adrenal Insufficiency
- Chronic **exogenous** glucocorticoids
- Pituitary disease
  - Low ACTH
    - No hyperpigmentation
  - No loss of aldosterone production (renin-angiotensin system is intact)
    - So **K⁺ is normal**
- Dx
  - **ACTH stimulation** test
  - Cortisol fails to increase > 18–20 μg/dL
    - False — test if recent secondary AI Dx as adrenals have not had time to atrophy
- MRI pituitary may be needed
- Rx
  - Acute: dexamethasone or hydrocortisone
  - Chronic: glucocorticoid

Autoimmune Diseases Run Together
- **Schmidt syndrome**
  - Primary adrenal insufficiency + hypothyroidism + T1DM
- You must replace cortisol prior to giving thyroid replacement
  - Can precipitate AI

HYPERALDOSTERONISM

AR 9
53-year-old with poorly controlled HTN on 5 BP meds:

Exam: normal BMI; no bruits

Labs:

Na⁺ = 142 mEq/L (nl)

K⁺ = 3.5 mEq/L (low-nl)

HCO₃⁻ = 30 mEq/L (high-nl)

Creat = 1.0 mg/dL

What is the best next step in this patient's management?

A. Renal angiogram
B. Random cortisol level
C. Check serum renin and aldosterone levels.
D. CT of the adrenals

Answer:_____

1° Hyperaldosteronism
- Causes
  - Single adrenal adenoma
  - Bilateral adrenal hyperplasia
- Key features
  - Hypertension
  - Hypokalemia (can be normal)
  - Metabolic alkalosis

1° Hyperaldosteronism — Dx
Screen → Confirm → Localize
1) Screen
   - Check simultaneous levels of plasma aldosterone and renin
     - PAC elevated, PRA suppressed → elevated ratio
2) Confirm with high salt load
3) Image the adrenals
4) Possible adrenal venous sampling
5) Surgery vs. medical management (aldosterone antagonist)

1° Hyperaldosteronism — Tx
1) **Adenoma** → surgical resection*
   - K⁺ returns to normal in > 90%
   - Hypertension normalizes in 2/3, improves in other 1/3
2) **Adrenal hyperplasia** → medical therapy with aldosterone antagonist (spironolactone or eplerenone)

*Medical therapy is an option for select patients with adenoma

PHEOCHROMOCYTOMA

AR 10
A 46-year-old woman with a pheo is scheduled for resection.

What is the best initial method for managing her blood pressure pre-op?

A. Propranolol
B. HCTZ
C. Metoprolol
D. Terazosin
E. Lisinopril

Answer:_____

Pheochromocytoma
- Rare disorder in practice
  - Common on boards
- Clinical presentation
  - Hypertension in > 90%, episodic or sustained
  - Episodes of sweating, palpitations, headache, nausea, pallor, anxiety

Pheochromocytoma — Dx
Screen:
Plasma metanephrines (high pretest probability)
Urine metanephrines (low pretest probability)

Confirm:
Clonidine suppression

Localize:
Abdominal CT or MRI

Pheo Rules
- Not all the same …
  - Some bilateral
  - Some malignant
  - Some extraadrenal ("paraganglioma")
    - Increased malignant potential (30%)
  - Some asymptomatic
- Consider genetic screening
  - *RET*, VHL, NF1
- Always α-block
  - **Never β-block first**

ADRENAL INCIDENTALOMA

AR 11

A 63-year-old man was having abdominal pain, and you suspected kidney stones. It was negative for stones, but imaging showed a 2-cm left adrenal adenoma.

He does not have HTN or diabetes.

BMI = 26 kg/m^2

BP = 120/77 mmHg; HR 80 bpm

Normal TSH and CMP

Which of the following is the best next step in this patient's care?

A. Check a 1-mg overnight DST and urine metanephrines.
B. Check a 1-mg overnight DST, urine metanephrines, and renin-to-aldosterone ratio.
C. Reassurance
D. Surgery evaluation
E. Check a 24-hour urine free cortisol and 17 ketosteroids.

Answer:_____

Adrenal Incidentaloma
- A mass, larger than 1 cm, discovered by accident on an imaging study
- Increasing incidence with ↑ imaging studies (seen on 4% of abdominal CT scans!)
- 2 questions:
  1) Functional?
  2) Cancer?
     - Size, patient history, imaging characteristics

Incidentaloma — Functional Status
- ~ 10% of incidentalomas secrete hormones

  1) Rule out pheo → everyone!!  Scariest

  2) Rule out Cushing's → 1-mg DST everyone! 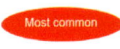 Most common

  3) Consider test for hyperaldosteronism
     - Hypertensive
     - Hypokalemic

Adrenal Incidentaloma — Tx
- Repeat CT in 6–12 months
- Repeat hormone testing
- Surgery
  - Unilateral and > 4–6 cm
  - Mass increases in size
  - Functional (pheo, cortisol)

AR 12

A 60-year-old man presents with a 30-lb weight gain over the past 2–3 years, HTN, abdominal striae, and a compression Fx.

1-mg dexamethasone suppression test:

8 a.m. cortisol = 8 μg/dL (normal < 1.8 μg/dL)

24-hour urine free cortisol = 420 μg (normal < 200 μg)

ACTH = 60 pg/mL (normal 9–52)

Which of the following is the most likely cause of the cortisol excess?

A. Pituitary adenoma
B. Adrenal adenoma
C. Ectopic ACTH
D. Surreptitious prednisone use

Answer:_____

HORMONES OF REPRODUCTION

FEMALES

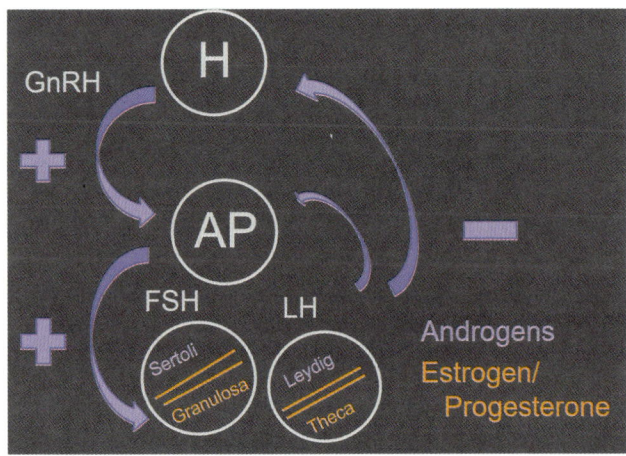

AR 13

A 36-year-old woman with amenorrhea for 4 months is interested in fertility.

Exam:

Thin, white fluid expressed from each breast

Labs:

Prolactin level: 40 ng/mL (1.4–14.2)

β-hCG is negative, TSH is normal

Imaging:

MRI shows 6-mm pituitary mass

Which of the following is the best next step in management?

A. Refer her to a neurosurgeon for resection of a prolactinoma.
B. Start cabergoline.
C. Observation, recheck prolactin level in 6–12 months.

Answer:_____

Secondary Amenorrhea
- Absence of menstruation for 3 cycles or 6 consecutive months
  - Test all women for **pregnancy**
- Consider
  - Premature ovarian failure (↑ FSH)
  - Polycystic ovary syndrome (metabolic abnormalities and androgen excess)
  - Hypothalamic amenorrhea (low FSH, low BMI)
  - Androgen excess
  - Prolactin excess
  - Primary hypothyroidism (↑ PRL and lower levels of LH and FSH)

Lab Evaluation
- Screen first with pregnancy test, FSH, TSH, and prolactin level
- If normal → progesterone challenge
  - Withdrawal bleeding → estrogen is present
    - Chronic anovulation
    - PCOS most common
  - No withdrawal bleeding → low estrogen level
    - MRI pituitary (inappropriately normal)
    - DDx: hypothalamic amenorrhea, pituitary tumor

PCOS
- Most common etiology of hirsutism with oligomenorrhea
- Diagnosis requires **2** of the following
  - Ovulatory dysfunction (amenorrhea, oligomenorrhea)
  - Laboratory or clinical evidence of hyperandrogenism
  - Ultrasonographic evidence of polycystic ovaries
    +
  - Rule out other causes
    - DHEAS (adrenal tumor)
    - Testosterone (ovarian tumor)
    - 17-OH progesterone (CAH)
    - Cortisol excess

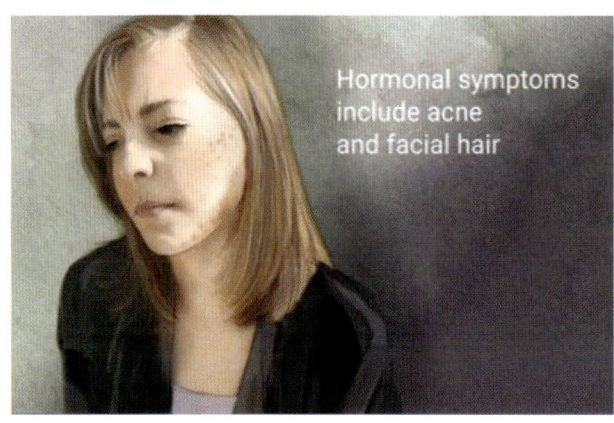

Hormonal symptoms include acne and facial hair

Premature Ovarian Failure
- Occurs before 40 years of age (average is 52 years of age)
  - ↑↑↑ FSH
- Karyotype for Turner's
- Treatment
  - Estrogen to prevent osteoporosis

MALES

Hypogonadism in Men
- Symptoms
  - Poor libido, hot flashes, decreased motivation, erectile dysfunction, gynecomastia, decreased morning erections
- Diagnosis
  - Measure 8 a.m. serum total testosterone
    - A low level on **2** occasions supports diagnosis

Labs
- If testosterone low
  - Measure LH, FSH, prolactin levels
  - ↑ LH and FSH → primary testicular failure
    - Younger, small testes → Klinefelter syndrome
  - Normal or ↓ LH and FSH → secondary hypogonadism
    - Look for chronic opioid use and/or glucocorticoid use
    - Measure prolactin
    - Iron studies (hemochromatosis)
    - Consider pituitary MRI
    - ? Screen for obstructive sleep apnea

Think Anabolic Steroids
- Seek care for infertility, gynecomastia
- Look for muscular hypertrophy, acne, testicular atrophy
- ↓ LH and FSH levels
- Variable testosterone levels
- Difficult to treat … very sophisticated regimens

GENDER TERMINOLOGY

Gender Terminology
- Transgender — people who have been assigned either male or female, yet self-identify as opposite of, neither, or somewhere along the male-female spectrum
- Gender dysphoria — distress or discomfort that occurs if gender identity and anatomic sex are not completely congruent
  - A psychiatric diagnosis in DSM-5
  - Push for a medical Dx of gender incongruence
- Not related to sexual orientation
  - Sexual attraction

DYSLIPIDEMIA

Lipid Basics
- Lipid facts are hard to remember
  - Very little day-to-day impact
- LDL = TC − HDL − (TG/5)
  - If TG > 400 mg/dL, then LDL is inaccurate
    - Measure direct LDL
- Statins are indicated for most high-risk patients (CHD, T2DM)

LDL Stuff
- Provides cholesterol for the synthesis of hormones
- Lp(a) as an independent risk factor for coronary heart disease and stroke
  - Targeted treatment does not modify risk
- LDL receptors are up-regulated, leading to lower LDL levels
  - When dietary cholesterol or saturated fats are low
  - By estrogen
  - By thyroxine
  - By the "statins" (HMG-CoA reductase inhibitors)
  - By a decrease in bile acid uptake from the intestines (as with bile acid resins)

HDL Stuff
- HDL is good
  - Raise with exercise, alcohol, diet, niacin
- **Scavenges** the unesterified cholesterol
- Low HDL → low levels of apo A-1
  - Hypoalphalipoproteinemia
  - Premature CAD
- No good data to solely target low HDL levels from an outcomes (boards) standpoint

SCREENING

Lipid Screening
- Starting at 20 years of age (familial dyslipidemia and secondary causes)
  - Assess major ASCVD risk factors q 4–6 years
    - Lipids (TC, LDL, HDL, TG)
    - Blood pressure
    - DM
    - Smoking status
- Starting at 40 years of age
  - Calculate 10-year ASCVD risk to determine next step
- Do **not** measure lipoprotein(a), apolipoprotein B, or homocysteine levels
  - Treatment has no impact on mortality

ASCVD Risk Factors
- Major risk factor: LDL
- Risk equivalent: DM, PAD, CVA, AAA
- Non-LDL risk factors:
  - Age: ♂ ≥ 45 and ♀ ≥ 55
  - FH **premature** CHD in 1st degree relative
    - < 55 ♂ and < 65 ♀
  - Current cigarette smoking
  - Hypertension (≥ 140/90 mmHg or on Rx)
  - HDL 40 mg/dL (HDL ≥ 60 = −1 RF)

Why Treat Dyslipidemia (Statins)?
- 1° prevention is beneficial for reducing CV morbidity and mortality
  - Without CHD
  - Preventing first event
- 2° prevention trials have shown the largest benefits in mortality and CV events

Statin Principles
- The higher the CV risk, the greater the benefit with statin therapy
- The higher the dose of statin, the greater the benefit
- The higher the dose of statin, the higher the risk of harm
- On boards, always the right treatment answer for those with high CV risk even if LDL is not very high

AR 15

A 47-year-old healthy man has the following lipid values after a 6-month program of diet and exercise:

TC = 230 mg/dL

LDL = 175 mg/dL

HDL = 45 mg/dL

TG = 320 mg/dL

His AHA 10-year risk estimate is 4%.

In addition to continued diet and exercise, which of the following would you recommend?

A. Initiate statin therapy with goal LDL < 160 mg/dL.
B. Initiate statin therapy with goal LDL < 130 mg/dL.
C. Initiate fenofibric acid therapy with a goal TG < 150 mg/dL.
D. Start niacin.
E. No additional treatment

Answer:_____

ACC / AHA 2019 Guidelines[4]
*   Emphasis on treatment with statin medications based on level of risk for ASCVD
*   Removes emphasis on LDL goals
    –   "Treat to target"
*   Identifies 4 target groups that should receive statins

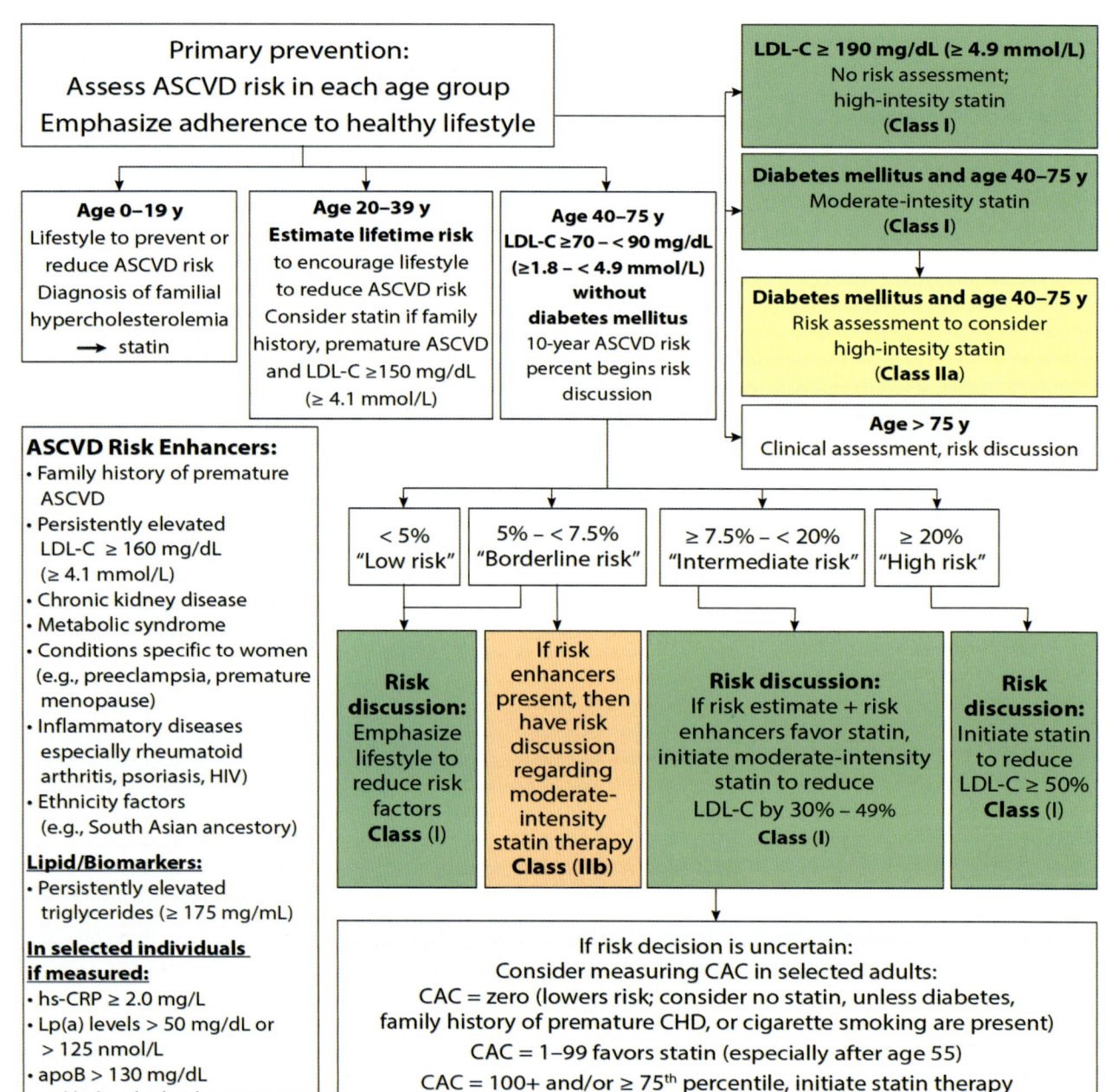

Primary prevention:
Assess ASCVD risk in each age group
Emphasize adherence to healthy lifestyle

LDL-C ≥ 190 mg/dL (≥ 4.9 mmol/L)
No risk assessment;
high-intesity statin
(Class I)

Diabetes mellitus and age 40–75 y
Moderate-intesity statin
(Class I)

Diabetes mellitus and age 40–75 y
Risk assessment to consider
high-intesity statin
(Class IIa)

Age > 75 y
Clinical assessment, risk discussion

Age 0–19 y
Lifestyle to prevent or
reduce ASCVD risk
Diagnosis of familial
hypercholesterolemia
⟶ statin

Age 20–39 y
Estimate lifetime risk
to encourage lifestyle
to reduce ASCVD risk
Consider statin if family
history, premature ASCVD
and LDL-C ≥150 mg/dL
(≥ 4.1 mmol/L)

Age 40–75 y
LDL-C ≥70 – < 90 mg/dL
(≥1.8 – < 4.9 mmol/L)
without
diabetes mellitus
10-year ASCVD risk
percent begins risk
discussion

ASCVD Risk Enhancers:
• Family history of premature
  ASCVD
• Persistently elevated
  LDL-C ≥ 160 mg/dL
  (≥ 4.1 mmol/L)
• Chronic kidney disease
• Metabolic syndrome
• Conditions specific to women
  (e.g., preeclampsia, premature
  menopause)
• Inflammatory diseases
  especially rheumatoid
  arthritis, psoriasis, HIV)
• Ethnicity factors
  (e.g., South Asian ancestry)

Lipid/Biomarkers:
• Persistently elevated
  triglycerides (≥ 175 mg/mL)

In selected individuals
if measured:
• hs-CRP ≥ 2.0 mg/L
• Lp(a) levels > 50 mg/dL or
  > 125 nmol/L
• apoB > 130 mg/dL
• Ankle-brachial index (ABI) < 0.9

< 5%
"Low risk"

5% – < 7.5%
"Borderline risk"

≥ 7.5% – < 20%
"Intermediate risk"

≥ 20%
"High risk"

Risk discussion:
Emphasize
lifestyle to
reduce risk
factors
Class (I)

If risk
enhancers
present, then
have risk
discussion
regarding
moderate-
intensity
statin therapy
Class (IIb)

Risk discussion:
If risk estimate + risk
enhancers favor statin,
initiate moderate-intensity
statin to reduce
LDL-C by 30% – 49%
Class (I)

Risk discussion:
Initiate statin
to reduce
LDL-C ≥ 50%
Class (I)

If risk decision is uncertain:
Consider measuring CAC in selected adults:
CAC = zero (lowers risk; consider no statin, unless diabetes,
family history of premature CHD, or cigarette smoking are present)
CAC = 1–99 favors statin (especially after age 55)
CAC = 100+ and/or ≥ 75th percentile, initiate statin therapy

Primary Prevention

> ### LDL-C ≥ 190 mg/dL (≥ 4.9 mmol/L)
> No risk assessment;
> high-intesity statin
> **(Class I)**

> ### Diabetes mellitus and age 40–75 y
> Moderate-intesity statin
> **(Class I)**

> ### Diabetes mellitus and age 40–75 y
> Risk assessment to consider
> high-intesity statin
> **(Class IIa)**

> ### Age > 75 y
> Clinical assessment, risk discussion

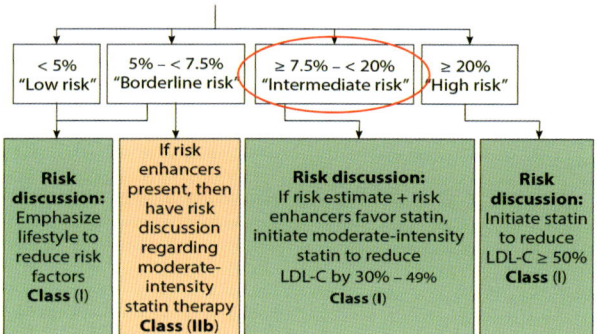

< 5% "Low risk"	5% – < 7.5% "Borderline risk"	≥ 7.5% – < 20% "Intermediate risk"	≥ 20% "High risk"
Risk discussion: Emphasize lifestyle to reduce risk factors **Class** (I)	**If risk enhancers present**, then have risk discussion regarding moderate-intensity statin therapy **Class** (IIb)	**Risk discussion:** If risk estimate + risk enhancers favor statin, initiate moderate-intensity statin to reduce LDL-C by 30% – 49% **Class** (I)	**Risk discussion:** Initiate statin to reduce LDL-C ≥ 50% **Class** (I)

4 Major Statin Benefit Groups[5]
1) Known ASCVD
2) Diabetics
   – 40–75 years of age
   – LDL ≥ 70 mg/dL
3) LDL ≥ 190 mg/dL
   – Rule out secondary causes
4) No ASCVD or DM
   – 40–75 years of age
   – LDL 70–189 mg/dL
   – 10-year ASCVD risk ≥ 7.5%
• Clinical atherosclerotic cardiovascular disease:
   – Acute coronary syndrome
   – MI
   – Stable or unstable angina
   – CVA or TIA
   – PAD or coronary revascularization

AR 16
A 73-year-old obese woman with diabetes has the following lipid values:

LDL = 98 mg/dL

HDL = 39 mg/dL

TG = 470 mg/dL

In addition to lifestyle modifications, which of the following would you recommend?

A. Initiate fibrate to target triglycerides.
B. Follow her lipid panel and initiate statin therapy only if her LDL rises above 100 mg/dL.
C. Initiate moderate-intensity statin therapy without a specific LDL goal.
D. Niacin

Answer:_____

Intensity of Statin Therapy

Low	Moderate (↓ LDL 30–50%)	High (↓ LDL > 50%)
Simvastatin 10 mg Pravastatin 20 mg Lovastatin 20 mg	Simvastatin 20–40 mg Pravastatin 40–80 mg Lovastatin 40 mg Atorvastatin 10–20 mg Rosuvastatin 5–10 mg	Atorvastatin 40–80 mg Rosuvastatin 20–40 mg

High-Intensity Statin Therapy (LDL ↓ ≥ 50%)
1) All ASCVD patients
2) LDL ≥ 190 mg/dL (unless > 75 years of age)
3) DM Type 1 or 2, 40–75 years of age with 10-year ASCVD risk ≥ 7.5%
• For super high CAD risk or super high LDL levels

Moderate-Intensity Statin Therapy (LDL ↓ 30–49%)
1) DM Type 1 or 2, 40–75 years of age with 10-year ASCVD risk < 7.5%
2) Primary prevention, 40–75 years of age with 10-year ASCVD risk ≥ 7.5%*

*May consider high-intensity therapy in these individuals

DM is a CAD "Risk Equivalent"

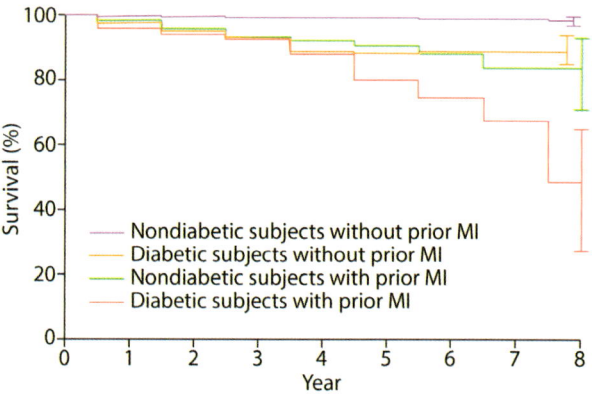

[6]

TREATMENT STRATEGIES

Dyslipidemia Treatment
- Therapeutic lifestyle modifications first!
  - Diet
    - Total fat < 30% daily calories (< 7% saturated)
    - Trans & polyunsaturated fats are bad (margarines)
    - Monounsaturated fats are better (olive oil)
  - Exercise
  - Smoking cessation
  - Maintenance of normal BMI
- No longer sole therapy for those that are in a statin benefit group

Dyslipidemia Treatment — Drugs
- **Statins**
- **Everything else**
  - Inhibitors of cholesterol absorption
  - Fibric acid derivatives
  - Niacin
  - Bile acid resins
  - PCSK9 inhibitors
  - Omega-3 fatty acids (fish oil)
    - Never the right first-line therapy in a statin benefit group

Statins — Benefits
- ↓ Mortality in 1° and 2° prevention
  - All cause
  - CV
- ↓ Myocardial Infarction
- ↓ Stroke
- ↓ Revascularization procedures

Statins — Complications
- Liver enzymes elevations (< 1.5%/5 years)
  - Usually minor and reversible
- Muscle problems
  - Myalgias (2–11%)
  - Myositis (0.5%)
  - Rhabdomyolysis (< 0.1%)
- DM: Excess 0.1% cases/year at low dose
  - 0.3% cases/year at high dose

Statin Drug Interactions
- Statins do not combine well with:
  - Fibrates
    - Avoid gemfibrozil
  - Azole antifungals
  - Macrolides (especially clarithromycin)
  - Diltiazem and verapamil
  - Grapefruit juice
  - Fetuses!
    - Avoid in women < 40

Statins — Monitoring
- FDA recommends checking liver enzymes only when indicated by clinical signs of hepatitis
- ACC/AHA recommends against routine monitoring of liver enzymes or CK levels
- No increase in routine screen for DM is recommended

AR 17
Statins have RCTs showing CV benefit for which of the following?

A. Dialysis patients
B. Diabetics without CAD
C. Age > 80 years
D. All of the above

Answer:_____

Ezetimibe
- Inhibits intestinal cholesterol absorption
- Reduces LDL alone or in combination with statins
- AE: myopathy; hepatic dysfunction

AR 18
A 45-year-old healthy man has a routine check of his lipids:

TC = 198 mg/dL

LDL = 125 mg/dL

HDL = 35 mg/dL

TG = 460 mg/dL

His ACC/AHA 10-year risk is 4%.

Which of the following is the best next step?

A. Counsel on diet and exercise
B. Fenofibric acid
C. Cholestyramine
D. Ezetimibe
E. Niacin therapy

Answer:_____

Fibrates
- **Decrease TG and raise HDL** (small effect on LDL)
- Gemfibrozil is the only fibrate with demonstrated CV benefit (Helsinki Heart, VA-HIT)
  - Gemfibrozil vs. placebo
- Fenofibrate, while more effective for reducing TG and less statin interaction, did not show benefit in RCTs (ACCORD trial, 2010) for 2° prevention
- Myopathy risk alone and especially when gemfibrozil + statins

Niacin
- Favorable effect on all lipids, especially **raising HDL** and lowering triglycerides
  - Lowers Lp(a) — but not a reason to treat on boards
- Side effects: flushing (80%), abdominal pain, myalgias
  - Aspirin 30 minutes prior can help
- Adverse effects: hyperglycemia, hyperuricemia, hypotension, hepatitis

Bile Acid Sequestrants
- Block reabsorption of bile acids, lowering LDL levels
- LRC trial: Cholestyramine reduced CVD events in primary prevention for men
- Safe for use in combination with statins
- Colesevelam lowers A1c by 0.5%
- Caution: May significantly elevate TG levels

PCSK9 Inhibitors

- PCSK9 is an enzyme produced in the liver
- It binds to the LDL receptor which leads to a receptor # reduction and higher LDL cholesterol levels
- Monoclonal antibodies (PCSK9 inhibitors) bind free PCSK9 → interferes with the binding to the LDL receptor → higher receptor # → lowers plasma LDL concentrations
- Lowers LDL as much as 70%
- Generally considered 3rd line for familial hypercholesterolemia and secondary prevention (if statin + ezetimibe do not achieve LDL targets)

AR 19

A healthy 32-year-old woman comes in for a routine checkup. She is a nonsmoker and has no family history of heart disease or DM. She exercises and eats a heart-healthy diet.

TC = 285 mg/dL

LDL = 210 mg/dL

HDL = 35 mg/dL

TG = 180 mg/dL

What is the most appropriate next step in management?

A. Moderate-intensity statin therapy
B. High-intensity statin therapy
C. Fish oil
D. Therapeutic lifestyle changes and monitor
E. Metabolic panel, TSH, and urinalysis and urine hCG

Answer:_____

Secondary Dyslipidemia

- Do not forget!
  - ↑↑↑ LDL
    - Hypothyroidism
    - Pregnancy
    - Obstructive liver disease
    - Nephrotic syndrome
    - Poorly controlled DM

Statin Therapy — Areas of Uncertainty

- 1° Prevention
  - < 40 years of age
  - 40–75 years of age with low ASCVD risk
- 2° Prevention
  - Advanced HF and ESRD patients
- Overall
  - Women, > 75 years of age, minorities

DIABETES MELLITUS (DM)

CLASSIFICATION

Classification of Diabetes[7]

- Type 1 DM
  - β-Cell destruction
- Type 2 DM
  - Insulin resistance
  - Progressive insulin secretory defect
- Diseases of the exocrine pancreas
  - CFRD
- Drug- or chemical-induced
- Gestational diabetes mellitus (GDM)
- MODY = maturity-onset diabetes of the young
  - Hereditary autosomal dominant (+++FH)
  - GAD−
  - Treatment is determined by the specific mutation
    - Some do not need medication, some respond to sulfonylureas
- LADA = latent autoimmune diabetes of adulthood
  - Thin adults
  - > 40 years of age
  - GAD+
  - Initially on orals (Type 1.5)

AR 20

A 36-year-old woman is concerned about developing diabetes, as her mother was diagnosed with Type 2 DM at the same age. She is asymptomatic. She does not smoke.

BP 134/75 mmHg; Wt 190 lbs; Ht 5'3"

BMI = 34 kg/m^2

What is the best screening method?

A. Fasting glucose
B. Anti-islet cell antibodies
C. Random blood sugar
D. No screening is indicated

Answer:_____

ADA Guidelines

- All adults starting at 45 years of age
- Screen earlier if BMI > 25 kg/m^2 **(or ≥ 23 kg/m2 in Asian Americans)** and > 1 risk factor
  - HTN
  - 1° relative with DM
  - Gestational DM
  - Physical inactivity
  - PCOS
  - HDL < 35 mg/dL
  - High-risk ethnicity
  - Vascular disease
  - Impaired glucose tolerance (IGT)
- **Repeat screen every 3 years if normal**

DIAGNOSIS AND SCREENING

Diagnosis of Type 2 DM
- Random glucose ≥ 200 mg/dL with symptoms of DM (polyuria, polydipsia, polyphagia, weight loss)
- Fasting plasma glucose ≥ 126 mg/dL × **2**
- Glucose ≥ 200 mg/dL on 2-hour OGTT
- HbA1c ≥ 6.5% × **2**

AR 21

A 56-year-old with T2DM comes in for a follow-up 2 weeks after emergent vascular surgery. His post-op course was complicated. He was transfused 3 units of packed RBCs.

He reports fasting BG of 100 mg/dL. Pre-lunch, pre-dinner, and pre-bed blood sugars are in the 250–300 mg/dL range.

Regimen: glargine 30 units daily

His CBC is normal.

HbA1c is 5.8%

POCT in your office: 271 mg/dL after breakfast

Which of the following is the best next step in management of his DM?

A. Add prandial insulin to his regimen.
B. He is at goal for his A1c; no change in therapy.
C. He is below goal for his A1c; decrease his long-acting insulin.
D. Check for nocturnal hypoglycemia.

Answer:_____

PREDIABETES
- Impaired glucose
  - Fasting = 100–125 mg/dL
  - OGTT = 140–199 mg/dL
  - HbA1c = 5.7–6.4%
- 6× risk of overt T2DM!
  - At risk for microvascular and cardiovascular disease

AR 22

Which of the following is the best way to prevent progression to overt DM?

A. Intensive diet and exercise
B. Pioglitazone
C. Metformin therapy
D. Acarbose

Answer:_____

Prediabetes — ADA Recs[8]

- 7% weight loss

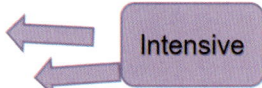

- Exercise 150 min/week

- Metformin "may be considered" if high risk
- Monitor A1c yearly
- Screen for and treat modifiable risk factors for CVD

TREATMENT

Diabetes Treatments

Sulfonylureas & Meglitinides	
glipizide	Glucotrol
glimepiride	Amaryl
glyburide	DiaBeta, Glycron, Glynase, Micronase
repaglinide	Prandin
nateglinide	Starlix
Biguanides	
metformin	Fortamet, Glucophage, Glumetza, Riomet
α-Glucosidase Inhibitors	
acarbose	Precose
miglitol	Glyset
Thiazolidinediones	
rosiglitazone	Avandia
pioglitazone	Actos

Dipeptidyl Peptidase-4 Inhibitors	
sitagliptin	Januvia
saxagliptin	Onglyza
sitagliptin + simvastatin	Juvisync
GLP-1 Analogs	
exenatide	Bydureon, Byetta
liraglutide semaglutide dulaglutide	Saxenda, Victoza, Tanzeum, Trulicity
Amylin Analog	
pramlintide	Symlin
SGLT-2 Inhibitors	
canagliflozin	Invokana
dapagliflozin	Farxiga
empagliflozin	Jardiance

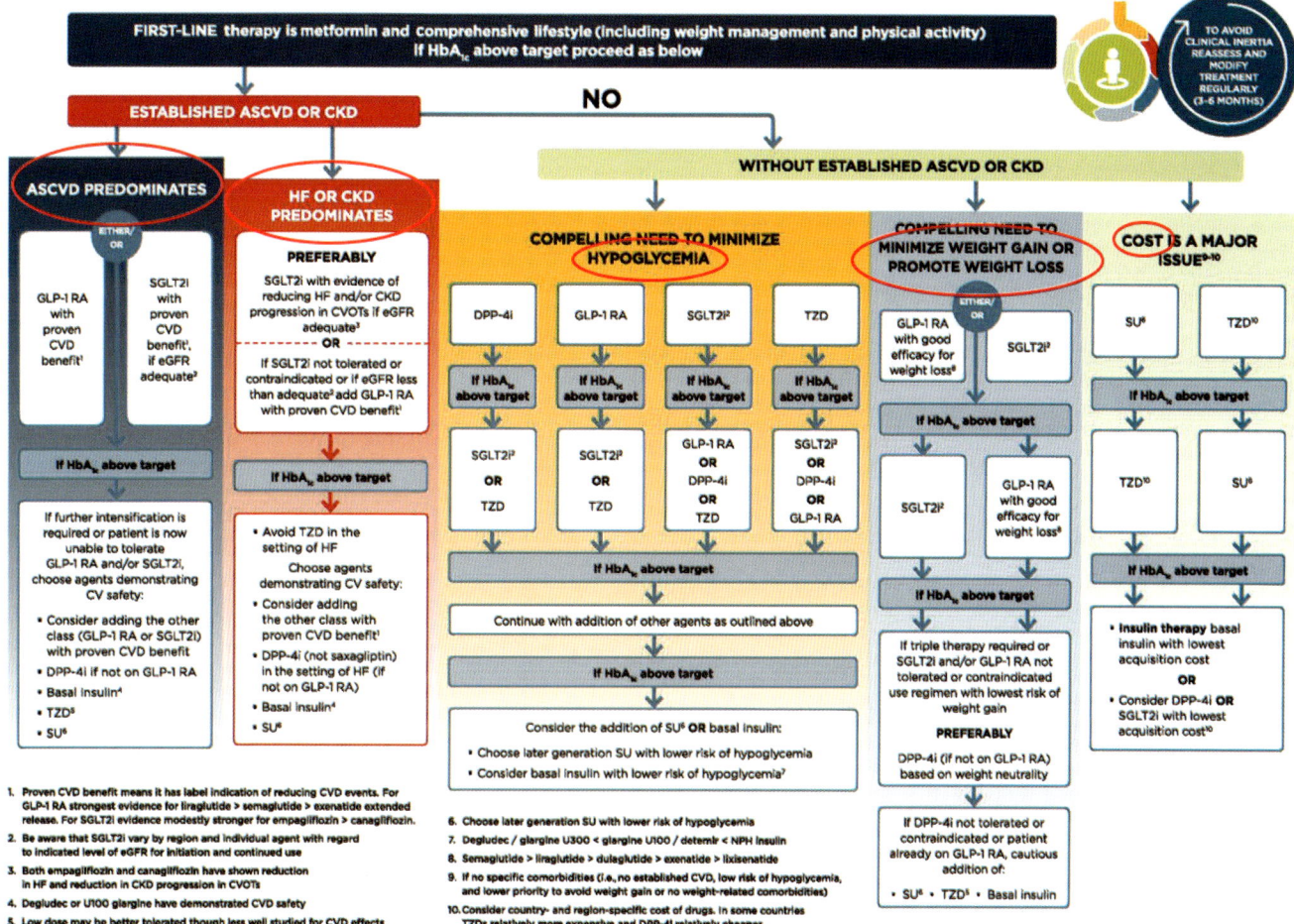

FIRST-LINE therapy is metformin and comprehensive lifestyle (including weight management and physical activity) if HbA₁c above target proceed as below

ESTABLISHED ASCVD OR CKD **NO**

ASCVD PREDOMINATES

EITHER/OR

GLP-1 RA with proven CVD benefit[1]

SGLT2i with proven CVD benefit[1], if eGFR adequate[2]

If HbA₁c above target

If further intensification is required or patient is now unable to tolerate GLP-1 RA and/or SGLT2i, choose agents demonstrating CV safety:
- Consider adding the other class (GLP-1 RA or SGLT2i) with proven CVD benefit
- DPP-4i if not on GLP-1 RA
- Basal insulin[4]
- TZD[5]
- SU[6]

HF OR CKD PREDOMINATES

PREFERABLY
SGLT2i with evidence of reducing HF and/or CKD progression in CVOTs if eGFR adequate[3]

OR

If SGLT2i not tolerated or contraindicated or if eGFR less than adequate[3] add GLP-1 RA with proven CVD benefit[1]

If HbA₁c above target

- Avoid TZD in the setting of HF
  Choose agents demonstrating CV safety:
- Consider adding the other class with proven CVD benefit[1]
- DPP-4i (not saxagliptin) in the setting of HF (if not on GLP-1 RA)
- Basal insulin[4]
- SU[6]

WITHOUT ESTABLISHED ASCVD OR CKD

COMPELLING NEED TO MINIMIZE HYPOGLYCEMIA

| DPP-4i | GLP-1 RA | SGLT2i[2] | TZD |

If HbA₁c above target / If HbA₁c above target / If HbA₁c above target / If HbA₁c above target

SGLT2i[2] OR TZD | SGLT2i[2] OR TZD | GLP-1 RA OR DPP-4i OR TZD | SGLT2i[2] OR DPP-4i OR GLP-1 RA

If HbA₁c above target

Continue with addition of other agents as outlined above

If HbA₁c above target

Consider the addition of SU[6] OR basal insulin:
- Choose later generation SU with lower risk of hypoglycemia
- Consider basal insulin with lower risk of hypoglycemia[7]

COMPELLING NEED TO MINIMIZE WEIGHT GAIN OR PROMOTE WEIGHT LOSS

EITHER/OR

GLP-1 RA with good efficacy for weight loss[8] | SGLT2i[2]

If HbA₁c above target

SGLT2i[2] | GLP-1 RA with good efficacy for weight loss[8]

If HbA₁c above target

If triple therapy required or SGLT2i and/or GLP-1 RA not tolerated or contraindicated use regimen with lowest risk of weight gain

PREFERABLY
DPP-4i (if not on GLP-1 RA) based on weight neutrality

If DPP-4i not tolerated or contraindicated or patient already on GLP-1 RA, cautious addition of:
- SU[6] • TZD[5] • Basal insulin

COST IS A MAJOR ISSUE[9-10]

| SU[6] | TZD[10] |

If HbA₁c above target

| TZD[10] | SU[6] |

If HbA₁c above target

- Insulin therapy basal insulin with lowest acquisition cost

OR

- Consider DPP-4i OR SGLT2i with lowest acquisition cost[10]

TO AVOID CLINICAL INERTIA REASSESS AND MODIFY TREATMENT REGULARLY (3-6 MONTHS)

1. Proven CVD benefit means it has label indication of reducing CVD events. For GLP-1 RA strongest evidence for liraglutide > semaglutide > exenatide extended release. For SGLT2i evidence modestly stronger for empagliflozin > canagliflozin.
2. Be aware that SGLT2i vary by region and individual agent with regard to indicated level of eGFR for initiation and continued use
3. Both empagliflozin and canagliflozin have shown reduction in HF and reduction in CKD progression in CVOTs
4. Degludec or U100 glargine have demonstrated CVD safety
5. Low dose may be better tolerated though less well studied for CVD effects
6. Choose later generation SU with lower risk of hypoglycemia
7. Degludec / glargine U300 < glargine U100 / detemir < NPH insulin
8. Semaglutide > liraglutide > dulaglutide > exenatide > lixisenatide
9. If no specific comorbidities (i.e., no established CVD, low risk of hypoglycemia, and lower priority to avoid weight gain or no weight-related comorbidities)
10. Consider country- and region-specific cost of drugs. In some countries TZDs relatively more expensive and DPP-4i relatively cheaper

Efficacy-Lowering A1c

Efficacy Lowering A1c	
MET	1–2%
Sulfonylureas	1–2%
TZDs	0.5–1.4%
Acarbose	0.5–0.8%
Meglitinide	0.5–2%
Exenatide	0.5–1% ($2,800)
Sitagliptin	0.5–0.8% ($1,700)
Pramlintide	0.2–0.5% ($2,556)

AR 23

At a routine visit, a 66-year-old is diagnosed with T2DM. She has no complaints and her exam is normal except for a BMI of 30 kg/m².

FBG = 230 mg/dL

HbA1c = 7.9%

She has normal renal and thyroid function

In addition to therapeutic lifestyle changes, what would you recommend to improve her blood sugar control?

A. Pioglitazone
B. Glyburide
C. Metformin
D. Insulin
E. Cinnamon

Answer:_____

AR 24

Which of the following is associated with metformin therapy?

A. Weight gain
B. Hypoglycemia
C. Increase in MI
D. Birth defects
E. None of the above

Answer:_____

Metformin
- In February 2012, USPSTF named metformin the preferred initial drug for diabetes
  - Weight loss of about 2–3 kg (4.4–6.6 lbs)!
  - UKPDS long-term follow-up: ↓ MI, ↓ mortality, and ↓ DM-related endpoints
  - Little hypoglycemia
  - Cheap
  - Effective

Metformin vs. Sulfonylureas[9]
- Retrospective cohort study of 253,690 veterans initiating therapy with either sulfonylurea or metformin looking at rates of cardiovascular disease (CVD) events
- **CVD events were 15% higher with glipizide and 26% higher with glyburide when compared to metformin therapy**

Metformin — Downsides
- GI side effects are common
  - Decreased when taken with food
- Long-term use may cause what vitamin deficiency?
$$B_{12}$$

Metformin — Contraindications?
- Significant kidney disease
  - OK if eGFR > 45 mL/minute/1.73 m^2
- Decompensated heart failure
- Radiographic dye studies
  - Hold for 1 day prior and 2 days after
- Serious illness (liver disease, sepsis, surgery)

Sulfonylureas
- **Mechanism:** secretagogues
- Reduce HbA1c by about 1–1.5%
- Poor choice
  - Weight gain
  - Hypoglycemia

Dipeptidyl Peptidase-4 (DPP-4) Inhibitors
- Examples: sitagliptin, saxagliptin, and linagliptin
- **Mechanism:** oral drugs that potentiate insulin secretion and inhibit glucagon production
- Lowers HbA1c by 0.7% with once-daily pill
- Weight neutral
- No hypoglycemia
- Very expensive!

GLP-1 Agonists
- Examples: exenatide, liraglutide, semaglutide, dulaglutide
- Mechanism
  - Promotes satiety
  - Slows down gastric emptying
  - Glucose-mediated insulin release
  - Decreased glucagon
- **Benefits**
  - Lower A1c by 0.8–1.2%
  - Cause significant weight loss (~ 3 kg [6.6 lbs])
  - Low risk for hypoglycemia
- **Downsides**
  - Injectable
  - Very expensive!
  - Medullary thyroid cancer
  - Pancreatitis

SGLT-2 Inhibitors
- Oral drugs that inhibit sodium glucose cotransporter (SGLT-2) in proximal tubules of kidney, inducing glucosuria
- Downsides
  - Expense
  - UTI/Yeast infections
  - **DKA in euglycemic T2DM**

Target HbA1c
- There is uncertainty as to the optimal target for HbA1c levels
- Younger patients with new-onset DM may benefit from tighter control early on (goal ~ 6.5%)
  - "Metabolic memory"
- Older patients reasonably controlled to goal of 7–7.5%
- As low as can safely be achieved
  - Avoid hypoglycemia

AR 25

Based on <u>ADA 2019 recommendations</u>, what blood pressure in diabetes should prompt a medication start?

A. > 120/80 mmHg
B. > 130/80 mmHg
C. > 140/90 mmHg

Answer:_____

Standards of Care in Diabetes
- Hemoglobin A1c < 7%
- Blood pressure < 140/90 mmHg
  - Use ACE inhibitor or ARB
- Statin use driven by risk, **not** LDL
  - Known ASCVD
  - 40–75 years of age
- Spot urine albumin yearly
  - If > 30 mg/g begin ACE inhibitor or ARB

- Eye examination yearly
  - Refer to ophthalmologist at time of diagnosis
- Foot exam every visit (high-risk patients)
- Smoking cessation
- Aspirin

AR 26

A 40-year-old has lost 8 pounds and complains of increased thirst for the past month. She also has a vaginal yeast infection.

BMI = 32 kg/m^2

Random blood glucose this a.m. = 380 mg/dL

HbA1c = 11.9%

What is the best initial therapy for her diabetes?

A. Metformin
B. Glipizide
C. Insulin
D. Pioglitazone

Answer:_____

"Basal-Bolus" Insulin

- Most physiologic regimen
  - "Basal" — unrelated to food intake (50%)
    - Never hold in T1DM ... even if NPO
  - "Bolus" — caloric intake (50%)
    - OK to hold if NPO
- Total daily dose = 40 units
  - 1/2 basal (e.g., glargine)
  - 1/2 bolus (e.g., lispro) split into thirds to be given prandially
  - 20 U glargine daily + 6 U lispro premeal

Physiologic Insulin Dosing

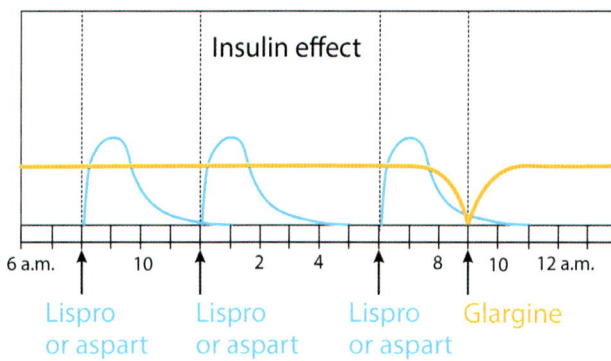

[10]

AR 27

Three months after starting glargine and slowly increasing the dose, your 64-year-old patient has the following blood sugar diary:

	Fasting	**PM**	**HS**
Day 1	130 mg/dL	250 mg/dL	280 mg/dL
Day 2	118 mg/dL	300 mg/dL	270 mg/dL

BMI 34

Meds

Metformin = 2,000 mg daily

Glargine = 30 U daily

HbA1c = 8.2%

Creatinine = 1.2 mg/dL

Which of the following do you recommend?

A. Increase metformin.
B. Add sulfonylurea.
C. Add premeal insulin.
D. Add pioglitazone.

Answer:_____

HbA1c Target

- < 7%, if ...
  - Younger
  - Shorter duration of DM
- 7–8%, if ...
  - History of severe hypoglycemia
  - Limited life expectancy
  - Advanced complications
  - Extensive comorbidities
  - Long-standing DM and low A1c has been difficult to attain even with best efforts

Treatment — Bottom Line

- T1DM = insulin
- T2DM = Metformin for everyone who can take it, except ...
  - Severe hyperglycemia and/or lots of symptoms = insulin
  - Kidney disease
- Lenient target for certain groups

Remember the Comorbidities

- T2DM
  - OSA
  - Fatty liver
  - Hypogonadism (men)
  - Hearing loss
  - Depression
- T1DM
  - Celiac screen (up to 15%)
  - Thyroid disease screen every 2 years

AR 28

A 40-year-old with T1DM is admitted to the ICU because of sepsis.

Weight is 80 kg

Outpatient insulin regimen

Glargine 20 U daily

Lispro 6 U premeals

He is on the ventilator and is receiving IV antibiotics and pressors.

Which of the following would be the optimal insulin regimen while he is in the ICU?

A. Continuous insulin infusion to keep blood glucoses 100–140 mg/dL
B. Continuous insulin infusion to keep blood glucoses 140–180 mg/dL
C. 1/2 home glargine dose plus a sliding scale
D. Sliding scale insulin

Answer:_____

Diabetes Care for Hospitalized Patients

- Intensive insulin therapy (80–110 mg/dL) → no ↓ mortality
- Glucose goals → 140–180 mg/dL
- Do not use regular insulin "sliding scale" as sole means to control glucose
- Use basal insulin in all patients requiring insulin
  - Add mealtime insulin as needed to control glucose
- **Avoid hypoglycemia**

AR 29

A 46-year-old woman with T2DM, HTN, morbid obesity (BMI 43 kg/m^2), and hyperlipidemia has an HbA1c of 9.6%.

Meds:

Metformin = 1 g bid

Glargine = 80 U bid

Aspart = 40 U tid

Liraglutide

What would you recommend as a next step in therapy?

A. Increase glargine insulin to 200 units daily.
B. Insulin pump
C. Pancreatic islet cell transplant
D. Referral for metabolic surgery

Answer:_____

BARIATRIC SURGERY FOR DM

When Should We Consider Bariatric Surgery for DM?

Bariatric Surgery

- Metabolic surgery **should be recommended** as an option to treat Type 2 diabetes in adults with
  - BMI ≥ 40 kg/m^2 (BMI ≥ 37.5 kg/m^2 in Asian Americans)
  - BMI 35.0–39.9 kg/m^2 (32.5–37.4 kg/m^2 in Asian Americans) who do not achieve durable weight loss and improvement in comorbidities (including hyperglycemia) with reasonable nonsurgical methods
- Metabolic surgery **may be considered** for adults with Type 2 diabetes and
  - BMI 30.0–34.9 kg/m^2 (27.5–32.4 kg/m^2 in Asian Americans) who do not achieve durable weight loss and improvement in comorbidities (including hyperglycemia) with reasonable nonsurgical methods

American Diabetes Association. *Diabetes Care*. 2019.

Bariatric Surgery for DM — Upsides[11]

- Bariatric surgery results in
  - Sustained weight loss out to at least 3 years
  - Remission of DM in 40–95%
  - Improved blood pressure
  - Improved LDL cholesterol
  - Low 30-day mortality (0.28%)

Bariatric Surgery — Downsides

- GI side effects
- Initial cost
- Vitamin and mineral deficiencies
- Osteoporosis
- Hypoglycemia
  - Difficult to treat

HYPOGLYCEMIA IN PATIENTS WITHOUT DIABETES

AR 30

A 24-year-old with presumed hypoglycemia is evaluated during an episode. She has diaphoresis, vocal slurring, and confusion that resolve with IV glucose.

Laboratory values drawn during the episode:

Glucose 32 mg/dL

Elevated C-peptide level

Elevated insulin level

She lives with her parents. Her mother has Type 2 diabetes.

Which is the recommended diagnostic approach?

A. Octreotide scan
B. Pancreas MRI
C. Pituitary CT
D. Serum calcium level
E. Sulfonylurea screen

Answer:_____

Hypoglycemia in Patients Without Diabetes
- Whipple triad
  1) Symptoms of hypoglycemia
  2) Associated low plasma glucose levels (< 50 mg/dL)
  3) Resolution of symptoms after glucose given
- Lab evaluation:
  - Glucose paired with a C-peptide
  - Glucose paired with an insulin level
  - Sulfonylurea screen

Hypoglycemia Evaluation
- Is it endogenous?
  - Inappropriately normal or elevated C-peptide and insulin
  - If yes, screen for surreptitious sulfonylurea use
  - If sulfonylurea screen negative, proceed with imaging
- **Never image without an established diagnosis**

DDx of Nondiabetic Fasting Hypoglycemia
- Surreptitious oral hypoglycemic use (our case)
  - Serum C-peptide, insulin levels are inappropriately normal or ↑
  - Assess with screen for sulfonylurea and meglitinide metabolites
- Surreptitious use of insulin
  - Insulin is normal or ↑
  - **Low serum C-peptide levels**
- Substrate deficiency
  - Low serum C-peptide and insulin levels
  - **++Ketosis**
  - Causes → starvation, hepatic failure, sepsis, alcoholism, hypoadrenalism

HYPERCALCEMIA

AR 31

A healthy 36-year-old woman is noted to have a high calcium on routine labs. Her mother has a history of high calcium and underwent parathyroidectomy but continues to have high calcium levels. The patient takes a multivitamin daily.

Labs:

Calcium = 11.2 mg/dL

Creatinine = 0.9 mg/dL

Serum PTH = 60 pg/mL (normal 10–60 pg/mL)

What is the best next step in management?

A. Discontinue her multivitamin and recheck calcium level in 3 months.
B. Check PTH-related protein level.
C. Check 24-hour urine calcium and creatinine.
D. Refer for a ^{99m}Tc sestamibi scintigraphy.
E. Refer to ENT surgeon for parathyroidectomy.

Answer:_____

Hypercalcemia — Diagnostic Approach
1) Confirm elevation in calcium by repeat test
2) Measure Ca^{2+} and PTH simultaneously
   - PTH mediated
   - Non–PTH mediated

BONE / CALCIUM DISORDERS

Calcium Metabolism

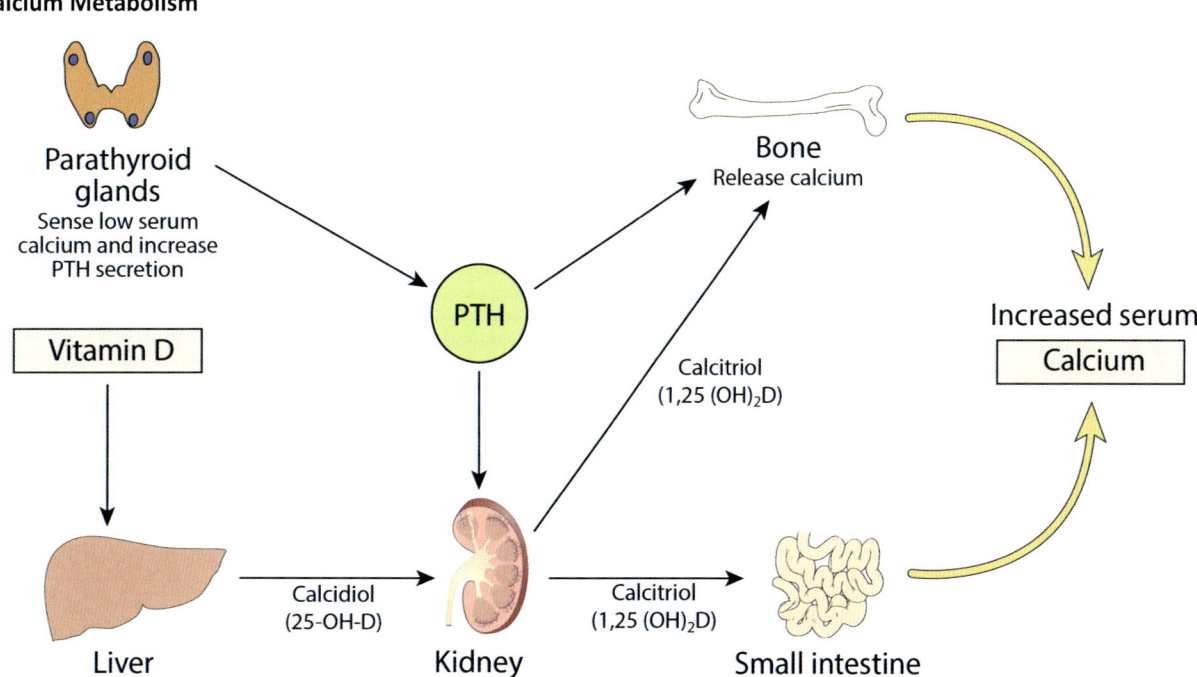

Hypercalcemia — PTH Mediated
1) Primary hyperparathyroidism
   - 80% single adenoma
2) Familial hypocalciuric hypercalcemia (FHH)
   - AD … low urine calcium, no complications
   - **24-hour urine calcium for all**
3) 3° Hyperparathyroidism
   - ESRD or renal transplant
4) Lithium and HCTZ

1° Hyperparathyroidism
- Most often seen in women > 50 years of age
- Hyperplasia seen in MEN1 and MEN2A
  - Think if young
- Biochemical diagnosis!
  - Serum Ca^{2+} is elevated
  - PTH is normal to high
  - Urine Ca excretion is not low
    - Rule out FHH on all

1° Hyperparathyroidism — Who Gets Surgery?
- All symptomatic patients → parathyroidectomy
- NIH Consensus Panel (2013) suggests surgery if any of the following are present:
  1) Calcium level > 1.0 ng/dL above upper limit of normal
  2) Creatinine clearance < 60 mL/min
     - Presence of nephrolithiasis or nephrocalcinosis by radiograph, ultrasound, or CT
     - 24-hour urine for calcium > 400 mg/day
  3) Osteoporosis
     - Vertebral fracture by imaging
  4) < 50 years of age

Hypercalcemia — Non-PTH Mediated
- Malignancy
  - PTHrP
- Multiple myeloma
  - Hypercalcemia + anemia + AKI
- Granulomatous disorders
  - ↑ 1,25-$(OH)_2$-vitamin D (sarcoidosis and TB) and B-cell lymphoma
- Milk-alkali syndrome
  - Hypercalcemia + alkalosis + AKI
- Vitamin D intoxication
  - ↑ vitamin D
- Thyrotoxicosis and adrenal insufficiency
  - Low TSH or suboptimal ACTH stimulation
- Immobilization

Hypercalcemia — Clinical Manifestations
- Mild hypercalcemia (< 11.5 ng/dL): usually asymptomatic
- **Calcium > 11.5** ng/dL
  - Polyuria (nephrogenic DI)
  - Dyspepsia (↑ gastrin secretion)
  - Bone demineralization
  - Psychiatric symptoms (depression, confusion)
  - Kidney stones
- **Calcium > 14** ng/dL
  - Lethargy; coma

Hypercalcemia — Acute Treatment
- Acute treatment depends on level of abnormality and severity of symptoms
  1) Fluids
     - Hypercalcemia induces nephrogenic DI
  2) Calcitonin
     - Calciuresis
  3) Bisphosphonates
     - 48–72 hours
  4) Steroids if 1,25 mediated
  5) Mobilization
  6) Hemodialysis

HYPOCALCEMIA

Hypocalcemia — Causes
- Hypoparathyroidism (usually from surgical destruction of the glands)
- Vitamin D deficiency
  - Think bariatric, celiac
- Loop diuretics
- Low Ca^{2+} intake
  - Eating disorders, alcoholism

Hypocalcemia — Signs and Symptoms
- Paresthesias, carpopedal spasms, tetany
- Trousseau and Chvostek signs
- **Life-threatening**
  - Laryngospasm
  - Cardiac arrhythmias
    - QT prolongation
- Treat with IV calcium

Osteomalacia "Bad Bones"
- Not all fragility fractures are due to osteoporosis
- Metabolic bone disease → failure of organic matrix of bone to mineralize (↓ vitamin D)
  - Suspect in nursing home residents; "tea and toast" diet; no sunlight
  - Labs → ↓ calcium, ↓ phosphorus, **↑ serum alkaline phosphatase**
- Look for underlying conditions affecting vitamin D availability or metabolism
  - Celiac disease, liver, kidney disease

PAGET DISEASE
- Focal disorder of bone remodeling
  - Accelerated rates of bone turnover, disruption of normal bone architecture
- Usually asymptomatic
  - Results in isolated ↑ of alkaline phosphatase
- Confirm diagnosis on bone scan
  - Follow-up x-rays of areas that localize
- Treat?
  - Symptomatic
  - Skull, long bone, and vertebral involvement
  - High alkaline phosphatase
- Can justify treatment of all (good data)
  - Zoledronic acid

MULTIPLE ENDOCRINE NEOPLASIA (MEN)
- Autosomal dominant with varying expression

Multiple Endocrine Neoplasia Syndromes	
Type	Clinical
MEN1	Primary hyperparathyroidism Pituitary adenomas Pancreatic islet cell tumors
MEN2A	Primary hyperparathyroidism Medullary thyroid cancer Pheochromocytoma
MEN2B	Medullary thyroid cancer Pheochromocytoma Developmental abnormalities*
* Marfanoid body type, skeletal deformations, mucosal neuromas (especially lips and tongue ["blubbery lips"])	

Multiple Endocrine Neoplasia (MEN)
- MEN1
  - Hyperparathyroidism most common manifestation
  - Prolactinoma is the most common pituitary tumor
  - Suspect
    - High prolactin and a high calcium
    - +FH Peptic ulcer disease (gastrinoma)
- MEN2A and 2B
  - Defect of the RET protooncogene
  - Medullary thyroid cancer occurs in almost all
    - ± prophylactic thyroidectomy
  - Screen all for pheochromocytoma (50%)
  - 2A → hyperparathyroidism
  - 2B → mucosal neuromas

HIGH-YIELD PEARLS

- Random hormone levels are rarely useful
- Rare endocrine diseases are common on the boards
- Never image without a diagnosis!
- Autoimmune diseases run together
- Statin is always the right choice for those with CVD risk

AUDIENCE RESPONSE ANSWERS AND EXPLANATORY INFORMATION

Audience Response 1
C. 8 a.m. cortisol after dexamethasone
A.   Random cortisol (not ever helpful for cortisol excess)
B.   ACTH-stimulated cortisol (for adrenal insufficiency)
C.   8 a.m. cortisol after dexamethasone
D.   8 a.m. cortisol (for adrenal insufficiency ... > 12 unlikely and < 3 likely)
- Other choices:
  - 24-hour urine free cortisol
  - Midnight salivary cortisol

AR 2
E. Check prolactin and IGF-1; screen for cortisol excess.
A.   Check an FT_4 (only if suspected TSHoma)
B.   Check all anterior pituitary hormones for hyper- and hyposecretion (only if > 1 cm)
C.   Reassurance (only if nonfunctional)
D.   Neurosurgical evaluation (only if Cushing's, TSHoma, acromegaly)
E.   Check prolactin and IGF-1; screen for cortisol excess for all incidental pituitary microadenomas.

AR 3
E. Check random serum IGF-1.
A.   Check TSH with an FT_4 (no reasons to suspect secondary hypothyroidism).
B.   Check serum growth hormone (too pulsatile).
C.   Order a polysomnogram (good idea, but no Dx).
D.   Start metformin 500 mg bid (good idea, but no Dx).
E.   Check random serum IGF-1 (Diagnosis = acromegaly).

AR 4
C. Decrease her dose of L-thyroxine.
A.   Thyroid uptake scan (endogenous)
B.   Restart her estrogen replacement therapy.
C.   Decrease her dose of L-thyroxine.
D.   Check thyroid peroxisome antibodies (not helpful).
E.   Advise her to take her thyroid medication 1 hour after her calcium supplements (consider if the TSH is elevated on a weight-based dose of T_4).

AR 5
D. Reassure the consulting physician.
A.   Order an MRI of the pituitary (not the right context).
B.   Start levothyroxine 100 mcg PO daily (not hypothyroid).
C.   Start levothyroxine 50 mcg IV daily (not hypothyroid).
D.   Reassure the consulting physician (sick euthyroid).
E.   Order a thyroid uptake scan (only in hyperthyroidism).
- Only check a TSH in those critically ill if coma or storm suspected; otherwise, labs will be confusing.

AR 6
B. Secondary hypothyroidism
A.   Chronic autoimmune thyroiditis (high TSH)
B.   Secondary hypothyroidism
C.   Hyperthyroidism (low TSH, high T_4, clinically hyperthyroid)
D.   Euthyroid sick syndrome (not sick!)
E.   No thyroid disease

AR 7
A. Graves disease
A. Graves disease (high uptake)
B.   Subacute thyroiditis (painful, low uptake)
C.   Silent thyroiditis (low uptake)
D.   Exogenous T_4 (no goiter, low thyroglobulin, low uptake)
E.   Toxic multinodular goiter (heterogenous pattern)

AR 8
C. Dexamethasone; order an ACTH stimulation test.
A.   Hydrocortisone (will not give an answer)
B.   Hydrocortisone + fludrocortisone; order an ACTH stimulation test. (HC will interfere with assay.)
C.   Dexamethasone; order an ACTH stimulation test.

AR 9
C. Check serum renin and aldosterone levels.
A.   Renal angiogram (only if proven renin mediated)
B.   Random cortisol level (rarely useful)
C.   Check serum renin and aldosterone levels.
D.   CT of the adrenals (only if confirmed pheo, ACTH independent cortisol excess, or aldosterone excess)

• Never image without a diagnosis!

AR 10
D. Terazosin
A.   Propranolol (precipitate hypertensive crisis)
B.   HCTZ (patients are dry)
C.   Metoprolol (precipitate crisis)
D.   Terazosin (gold standard is α)
E.   Lisinopril

AR 11
A. Check a 1-mg overnight DST and urine metanephrines.
A.   Check a 1-mg overnight DST and urine metanephrines (for all!).
B.   Check a 1-mg overnight DST, urine metanephrines, and renin-to-aldosterone ratio (only if HTN and/or hypokalemia).
C.   Reassurance (always needs a hormonal evaluation)
D.   Surgery evaluation (only if functional or larger > 4 cm)
E.   Check a 24-hour urine free cortisol and 17 ketosteroids (only if adrenal cortical carcinoma suspected).

AR 12
A. Pituitary adenoma
A.   Pituitary adenoma (high ACTH)
B.   Adrenal adenoma (low ACTH)
C.   Ectopic ACTH (higher ACTH, not the most common, rapid onset of symptoms)
D.   Surreptitious prednisone use (low ACTH and cortisol unless using hydrocortisone)

AR 13
B. Start cabergoline.
A.   Refer her to a neurosurgeon for resection of a prolactinoma (medically managed).
B.   Start cabergoline.
C.   Observation, recheck prolactin level in 6–12 months (only consider if she is not interested in fertility, she is not bothered by galactorrhea, and she is agreeable to starting OCPs for bone health and QOL).

AR 14
B. Gender dysphoria
A.   Gay/Lesbian (heterosexual)
B.   Gender dysphoria (DSM-5)
C.   Gender identity disorder (DSM-4)
D.   Bipolar

AR 15
E. No additional treatment
A.   Initiate statin therapy with goal LDL < 160 mg/dL (not a statin benefit).
B.   Initiate statin therapy with goal LDL < 130 mg/dL (not a statin benefit).
C.   Initiate fenofibric acid therapy with a goal TG < 150 mg/dL (will decrease triglycerides, no outcomes data).
D.   Start niacin (will increase HDL but no outcomes data).
E.   No additional treatment

AR 16
C. Initiate moderate-intensity statin therapy without a specific LDL goal.
A.   Initiate fibrate to target triglycerides (not first line).
B.   Follow her lipid panel and initiate statin therapy only if her LDL rises above 100 mg/dL (no longer "treat to target").
C.   Initiate moderate-intensity statin therapy without a specific LDL goal (statin benefit group).
D.   Niacin (not first line)

• Don't be tricked in targeting very high triglycerides or very low HDL in statin benefit groups.

AR 17
B. Diabetics without CAD
A.   Dialysis patients (no data on CV benefit)
B.   Diabetics without CAD (ABSOLUTELY)
C.   Age > 80 years (no data in those > 75 years old)
D.   All of the above

AR 18
A. Counsel on diet and exercise
A.   Counsel on diet and exercise (risk < 7.5%)
B.   Fenofibric acid
C.   Cholestyramine (will worsen triglycerides)
D.   Ezetimibe
E.   Niacin therapy

AR 19
E. Metabolic panel, TSH, and urinalysis and urine hCG
A.   Moderate-intensity statin therapy
B.   High-intensity statin therapy
C.   Fish oil
D.   Therapeutic lifestyle changes and monitor
E.   Metabolic panel, TSH, and urinalysis and urine hCG

AR 20
A. Fasting glucose
A.   Fasting glucose
B.   Anti-islet cell antibodies
C.   Random blood sugar
D.   No screening is indicated.
In practice, HbA1c would also be ok …
About 20% of patients screened with the HbA1c have false-negative tests.

AR 21
A. Add prandial insulin to his regimen.
A.   Add prandial insulin to his regimen.
B.   He is at goal for his A1c; no change in therapy (can't believe HbA1c with recent transfusion).
C.   He is below goal for his A1c; decrease his long-acting insulin.
D.   Check for nocturnal hypoglycemia.

AR 22
A. Intensive diet and exercise
A. Intensive diet and exercise
B.   Pioglitazone
C.   Metformin therapy
D.   Acarbose

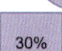

> 50%

30%

AR 23
C. Metformin
A.   Pioglitazone (worry about bone health)
B.   Glyburide (worry about hypoglycemia)
C.   Metformin (first line)
D.   Insulin (weight gain)
E.   Cinnamon

AR 24
E. None of the above

AR 25
C. > 140/90 mmHg

AR 26
C. Insulin
A.   Metformin
B.   Glipizide
C.   Insulin (for symptomatic hyperglycemia)
D.   Pioglitazone

AR 27
C. Add premeal insulin.
A.   Increase metformin (max. effective dose 2,000 mg/day).
B.   Add sulfonylurea (caution in CAD).
C.   Add premeal insulin (address prandial excursions).
D.   Add pioglitazone (caution with low BMD).

•   **Other options could be GLP-1 agonists, DPP-4 inhibitors, or SGLT-2 inhibitors**

AR 28
B. Continuous insulin infusion to keep blood glucoses 140–180 mg/dL
A.   Continuous insulin infusion to keep blood glucoses 100–140 mg/dL (increases risk of hypoglycemia and no decrease in mortality)
B.   Continuous insulin infusion to keep blood glucoses 140–180 mg/dL
C.   1/2 home glargine dose plus a sliding scale (too low of a basal + sliding scale increases risk for hypo and hyperglycemia)
D.   Sliding scale insulin (need basal even if NPO)

AR 29
D. Referral for metabolic surgery
A.   Increase glargine insulin to 200 units daily (won't achieve goal).
B.   Insulin pump (needs pump assessment first and if opted for would use concentrated insulin)
C.   Pancreatic islet cell transplant (would only consider if T1DM or chronic pancreatitis)
D.   Referral for metabolic surgery (BMI > 40 kg/m²)

AR 30
E. Sulfonylurea screen
A.   Octreotide scan
B.   Pancreas MRI
C.   Pituitary CT
D.   Serum calcium level
E.   Sulfonylurea screen (looks just like an insulinoma on labs)
Never image without a diagnosis!!!

AR 31
C. Check 24-hour urine calcium and creatinine.
A.   Discontinue her multivitamin and recheck calcium level in 3 months (PTH would be low).
B.   Check PTH-related protein level (PTH would be low).
C.   Check 24-hour urine calcium and creatinine (rule out FHH).
D.   Refer for a ⁹⁹ᵐTc sestamibi scintigraphy (not needed for diagnosis).
E.   Refer to ENT surgeon for parathyroidectomy (have not excluded FHH).

ENDNOTES

[1]   John McKeon [CC BY-SA 2.0 (https://creativecommons.org/licenses/by-sa/2.0)], via Wikimedia Commons

[2]   fitsweb.uchc.edu/student/selectives/Luzietti/Thyroid_diagnostics.htm

[3]   Popoveniyc G. and Jonklaas J. Thyroid Nodules. *Med Clin N Am*. 2012 March; 96 (2): 329–349.

[4]   circ.ahajournals.org/content/early/2013/11/11/01.cir.0000437738.63853.7a

[5]   circ.ahajournals.org/content/early/2013/11/11/01.cir.0000437738.63853.7a

[6]   *N Eng J Med*. 1998;339:229–234.

[7]   American Diabetes Association. Classification and diagnosis of diabetes. *Diabetes Care*. 2017

[8]   American Diabetes Association. Prevention or Delay of Type 2 Diabetes. *Diabetes Care*. 2017.

[9]   Roumie CL, et al. *Ann Intern Med*. 2012;157:601–610.

[10]   DeWitt DE and Hirsch IB JAMA 2003 May 7;289:2254–2264.

[11]   Gloy VL, et al. BMJ. 2013 October 22;347:f5934.

MedStudy

INTERNAL MEDICINE REVIEW

Gastroenterology

Presented by

Vijay R. Pottathil, MD, MME

Why We Moved Some Slide Information to the Audience Response Answers Page

At MedStudy, we do all we can to optimize your self-testing and learning.

In this presentation, the speaker will give some extra information after their AR questions to help explain the correct and incorrect answers. To keep from interfering with your self-testing, we've moved that explanatory text to the Audience Response Answers page(s) at the end of the section.

Be assured, all the content on the slides is in your syllabus—so you can focus on the teaching instead of taking detailed notes.

Why Some Topic Names Are Not Printed in This Section

At MedStudy, we do all we can to optimize your self-testing and learning.

In this section, the speaker has chosen to introduce topics with an Audience Response question to help you learn. In the syllabus, we've intentionally "hidden" some topic names that would give away the answers—so you can self-test more effectively. Where we've done this, instead of the topic name, you'll see an empty teal band or some extra space, but you can still find the topic on the page using the Table of Contents.

Gastroenterology Topics (Part 1)
- Esophagus
- The Stomach
  - Peptic Ulcer Disease
  - Postgastrectomy Syndromes
- Inflammatory Bowel Disease
- Diarrhea and Malabsorption
- Constipation
- Irritable Bowel Syndrome
- Diverticular Disease and Lower GI Bleed

Gastroenterology Topics (Part 2)
- Intestinal Ischemia
- GI Tract Surgical Issues
- Pancreas
- Biliary System
- Liver
  - Viral Hepatitis, Autoimmune Hepatitis, DILI, and NAFLD
  - Cirrhosis / Ascites
  - Hereditary Liver Disease
  - Liver Disease During Pregnancy
  - Liver transplant
- Nutrition

DYSPHAGIA
- Swallowing that does not proceed appropriately for any reason
- History can aid in diagnosis (solids, liquids)
- Differentiate from **odynophagia**
- 3 types
  1) Transfer (oropharyngeal): CVA, Parkinson's, ALS
  2) Anatomic/Structural: Schatzki ring, esophageal cancer
  3) Motility: failure of peristalsis and/or failure of LES relaxation

Dysphagia — By History
- Coughing/Aspiration/Gagging: transfer (oropharyngeal)
- Solids **and** liquids: motility/neurologic
- Intermittent solid food **only**: Schatzki ring
- Progressive/Solids, **then** liquids: stricture or cancer

Causes and Symptoms of Dysphagia			
Disease	**Main Problem**	**Symptoms Are ...**	**Symptoms Precipitated by ...**
Schatzki ring	Anatomic	Intermittent	Solids
Stricture	Anatomic	Progressive	Solids, **then** liquids
Cancer	Anatomic	Progressive	Solids, **then** liquids
Achalasia	Motility/Neurologic	Longstanding	Solids **and** liquids
DES	Motility/Neurologic	Intermittent	Solids **and** liquids (esp. cold)
Systemic sclerosis	Various	Progressive	Solids **and** liquids

Swallow Function

Movement of food through the pharynx and upper esophagus during swallowing

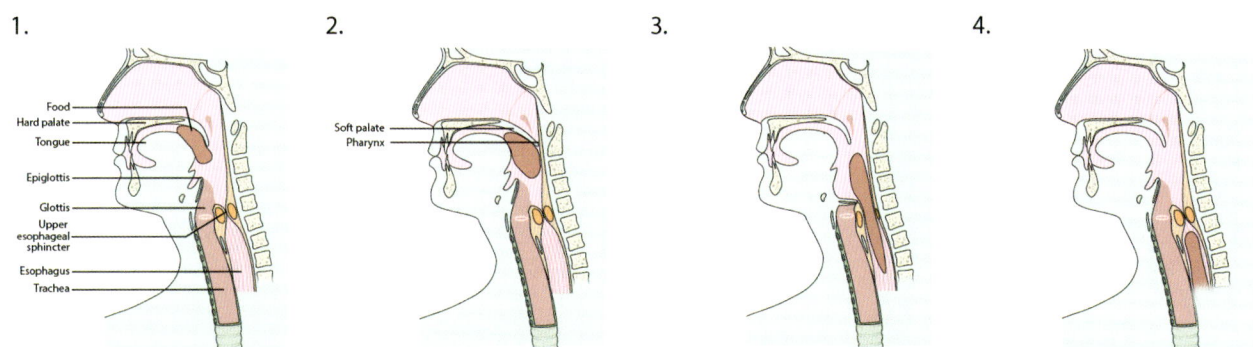

1. Tongue pushes food to the back of the mouth.
2. Soft palate elevates to prevent food from entering the nasal passages.
3. Epiglottis covers the glottis to prevent food from entering the trachea. The upper esophageal sphincter relaxes.
4. Food descends into the esophagus.

Oropharyngeal Dysphagia

- Dysphagia for solids and liquids <u>from the beginning</u>
- **CVA, parkinsonism, ALS, MS**
- Patients may complain of choking, gagging, nasal regurgitation (problems with oropharyngeal transfer), pulmonary aspiration
- PEG/PEJ may be required for nutrition but will not prevent aspiration of oral secretions

Dysphagia — Diagnostic Testing

- <u>EGD</u>: usually the 1st test performed
- <u>Barium swallow</u>
  - May **follow** normal EGD if symptoms persist
  - May **precede** if EGD is risky or more information needed
- <u>Video fluoroscopic swallowing study (VFSS)</u>: video-type x-ray of swallowing various barium consistencies
  - Also called "<u>modified barium swallow</u>": transfer dysphagia
- <u>Esophageal manometry</u>
  - For evaluation of motility disorders (high-resolution manometry [HRM] provides more information than traditional manometry)

ANATOMIC OBSTRUCTION

- Dysphagia initially to solids, **then** liquids
- Can be <u>intermittent</u> or <u>constant/progressive</u>
- Younger patients: Schatzki ring
- Older patients: cancer or peptic stricture

Anatomic — Lower Esophageal Ring (a.k.a. Schatzki Ring)

- Intermittent solid food dysphagia (meat and bread)
- "Steakhouse syndrome"
- Patient may regurgitate impacted bolus for relief
- Symptomatic rings are usually < 13 mm in diameter
- Treatment: dilation followed by PPI (reduces recurrence)

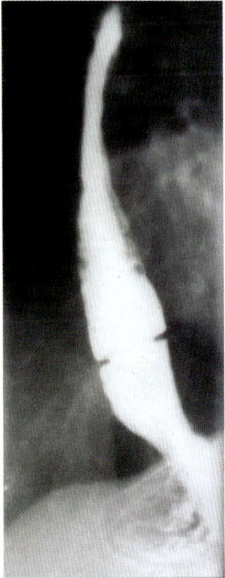

[1]

Anatomic — Esophageal Stricture

- History of slowly progressive, constant dysphagia for solid food
- Long history of **incompletely treated acid reflux** (peptic strictures)
- May also be caused by **prolonged NG tube use** or **lye ingestion** (alkali injury to esophagus)
- Treatment is dilation and PPI therapy (particularly for peptic strictures)

Anatomic — Malignant Obstruction

- Esophageal adenocarcinoma
- Squamous cell carcinoma
- Extrinsic compression
- History of slowly progressive dysphagia to solids, then soft food, then liquid
- **Dysphagia + weight loss = esophageal CA until proven otherwise!**

Anatomic — Plummer-Vinson Syndrome

- Rare disorder, dysphagia due to upper esophageal web
- Generally found in **postmenopausal women**
- Associated with **iron-deficiency anemia (IDA)**; iron deficiency may play a role in web formation
- **Increased risk of squamous cell CA**
- Triad of dysphagia, upper esophageal web, and IDA

Audience Response 1

A 47-year-old presents with persistent and progressive dysphagia over the last 2 years. His wife says he's complained of heartburn more and more over the past several months. Last month he had an episode of regurgitation, and she insisted that he come for evaluation.
A chest x-ray done yesterday at a local urgent care because of mild chest pain shows absence of the gastric air bubble.

Which diagnosis is most likely?

A. Diffuse esophageal spasm
B. Eosinophilic esophagitis
C. Adenocarcinoma of the esophagus
D. Achalasia
E. *Candida* esophagitis

Answer:_____

- Neuronal denervation/ganglion cell degeneration of myenteric plexus
  - Absence of organized peristalsis
  - Incomplete relaxation of LES (loss of inhibitory ganglion that normally produce nitric oxide for smooth muscle relaxation)
  - Sparing of cholinergic neurons that cause contraction (botulinum toxin poisons these excitatory neurons)
- Characteristic features
  - Dysphagia for solids and liquids
  - Regurgitation (delayed)
  - Nocturnal cough, aspiration, chest pain

Achalasia — Diagnosis[2]
- Barium swallow
- EGD: helps rule out tumor
- Esophageal manometry: confirms no peristalsis and nonrelaxing LES
- This barium esophagram is classic …

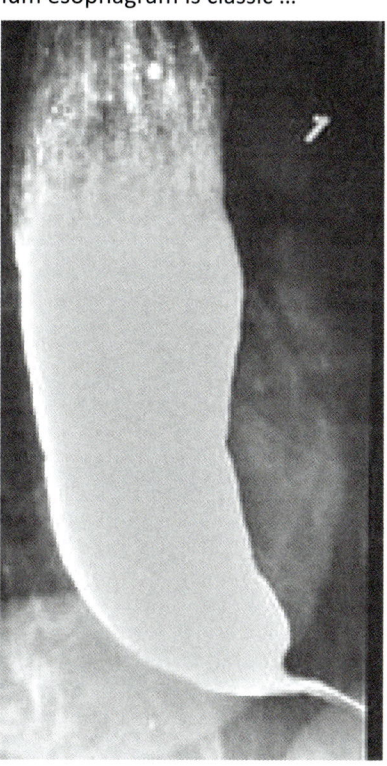

[3]

"Bird-beak" narrowing

Pseudoachalasia
- Tumors can involve neuronal plexuses
- Can be part of a paraneoplastic syndrome
- Gastric and esophageal cancer, lung cancers, others
- Presentation and manometry can appear similar to traditional achalasia
- Need to consider imaging, including CT chest and EUS

Achalasia — Potential Treatments
- Pneumatic dilation using 3- to 4-cm (30- to 40-mm) diameter balloon with 5% risk of perforation
- Surgical/Laparoscopic myotomy
- Peroral endoscopic myotomy (POEM)
- Endoscopic botulinum toxin Type A for high-risk patients
  - May require repeat therapy in 6–12 months
- Treatment decisions depend on patient preference and health and age of patient (i.e., surgery if younger and healthier)

DIFFUSE ESOPHAGEAL SPASM (DES)

Diffuse (Distal) Esophageal Spasm (DES)
- Simultaneous (uncoordinated), non-peristaltic contractions
- Intermittent dysphagia for solids and liquids (especially cold liquids)
- "Atypical" chest pain (atypical for angina)
- Reflux symptoms can mimic DES symptoms, so treat with PPI if you suspect GERD
- Barium swallow can be normal, but may show "corkscrew" pattern
- 1st line: diltiazem or imipramine
- 2nd line: isosorbide or sildenafil
- 3rd line: botulinum toxin injection

Manometry
- Standard manometry
- New high-resolution manometry: general principles
  - Purple/Red = high pressure
  - Blue = low pressure
  - Chicago classification
    - Impaired EGJ relaxation (i.e., achalasia)
    - Normal EGJ relaxation
      - Jackhammer esophagus — hypercontraction
      - Distal esophageal spasm — uncoordinated/simultaneous contraction

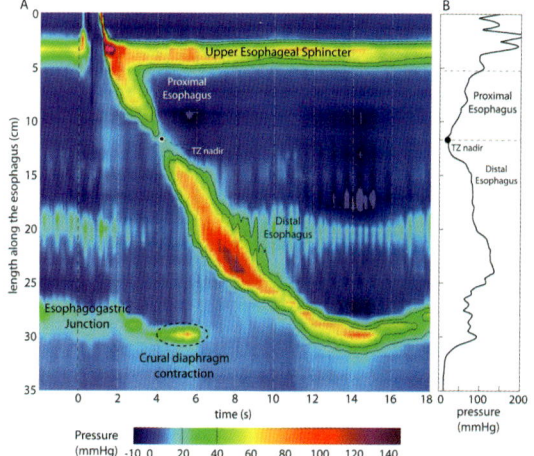

[4]

Normal swallow

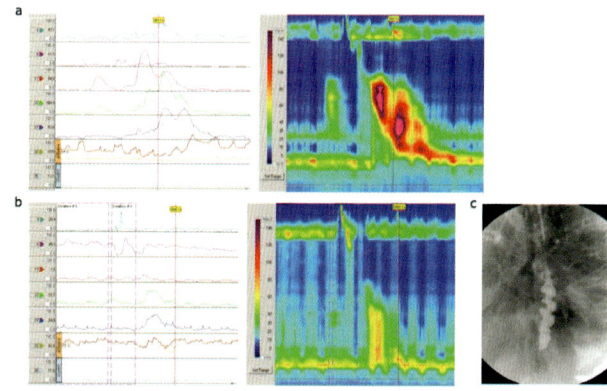

DES: HRM reveals excess, simultaneous (non-peristaltic) contractions with normal LES relaxation (so no achalasia).

SYSTEMIC SCLEROSIS

- When scleroderma involves internal organs, it's called systemic sclerosis (SSc)
- Leads to atrophy of **smooth muscle** in distal 2/3 of esophagus — weakened peristalsis
  - Upper 1/3 esophagus is striated muscle
- LES is "wide open" or "patent"
- Dysphagia may be due to esophagitis, stricture, or dysmotility
- Workup: barium swallow and EGD ± HRM

AR 2

A 26-year-old male presents with intermittent solid food impaction. Regularly, when he eats a bite of meat, he feels like it doesn't go down completely.

For the next 30 minutes, he can't even swallow liquids. Finally, he brings up the piece of meat and is able to swallow afterward.

He denies heartburn or any other GI symptoms. He does have several seasonal allergies for which he takes OTC medications.

Which of the following do you recommend?

A. EGD with biopsies of the esophagus
B. Omeprazole 20 mg q a.m.
C. Prednisone 40 mg PO daily for a week
D. Barium swallow
E. Refer to an allergist.

Answer:_____

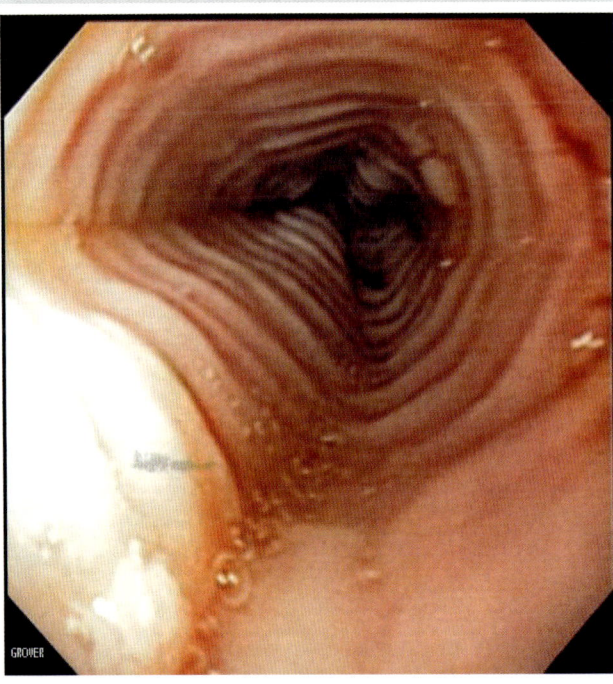

- **EGD shows "feline esophagus" (stacked circular rings), and biopsy reveals infiltrate of eosinophils (> 15 eos/HPF)**
- GERD usually has < 5 eos/HPF

Eosinophilic Esophagitis (EoE)

- Solid food dysphagia/**food impaction**
- Often young males (**20–40 years of age**)
- Often history of allergies (food, environmental), asthma
- Treatments
  - PPI may help those with PPI-REE (clinical and histological EoE but respond to PPI — pathogenesis not completely clear)
  - **Swallowed fluticasone** (bid) or **viscous budesonide** should show response < 1 week
- **Referral to an allergist** — dietary elimination can be considered as initial treatment (ACG)

AR 3

A 17-year-old high school girl, previously healthy, presents to the office with substernal pain when swallowing either solids or liquids. This has been present for 1 day with a sudden onset of the pain. There is no history of heartburn or any other symptoms.

PMH significant for taking OCPs and doxycycline for acne.

PE is normal for exam of oropharynx, neck, and chest.

What is the best recommendation?

A. CT chest
B. EGD
C. Barium swallow x-ray
D. Fluconazole 100 mg a day for 3 days
E. Stop doxycycline and give reassurance.

Answer:_____

Miscellaneous Causes of Esophagitis

- Odynophagia usually due to either **pill-induced** or **infectious** causes
- **Pill induced**
  - **D**oxycycline, **A**SA, **N**SAIDs, **I**ron, **K**Cl, **A**lendronate (bisphosphonates)
- Treatment: Stop the offending medicine and reassure the patient
- EGD may be needed if severe or protracted symptoms or etiology not completely clear based on presentation
- Opportunistic infections (OIs): *Candida*, **HSV**, and **CMV**
- *Candida*: If dysphagia and no improvement with empiric antifungals (oral fluconazole), EGD with biopsy
- Not always 100% correlation between thrush and esophageal candidiasis
- Threshold for EGD lower if no thrush

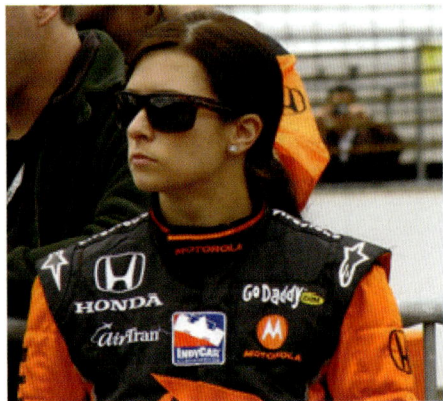

[5]

GASTROESOPHAGEAL REFLUX DISEASE (GERD)

- Transient lower esophageal sphincter relaxations, not preceded by swallow, can lead to GERD (also seen in normal patients)
- LES pressure decreased by progesterone (pregnancy), chocolate, smoking, anticholinergics, fat, EtOH
- Classic Sx: heartburn and regurgitation
- Extraesophageal manifestations
  - Loss of dental enamel
  - Hoarseness/Throat clearing
  - **Chronic cough**, especially nocturnal
  - **Globus sensation** (sensation of fullness)
  - **Noncardiac chest pain** (70% caused by GERD)
  - **Exacerbation of asthma**, especially at night
- Diagnosis
  - Therapeutic trial (PPI) if no alarm signals present
  - **Alarm signals** (need EGD)
    - Dysphagia/Odynophagia
    - Weight loss
    - Anemia
    - Blood in stool or vomitus
    - Iron deficiency anemia
    - Failure to respond to full doses of PPI
  - Prolonged ambulatory pH helpful in atypical cases

AR 4

A 50-year-old female complains of 1 year of daily hoarseness. She has frequent noncardiac chest pain with nocturnal heartburn despite using famotidine. She denies dysphagia and weight loss.

No help with allergist and ENT for the hoarseness.

You recommend:

A. EGD now
B. Esophageal manometry
C. Pantoprazole 40 mg PO bid
D. Famotidine 20 mg bid, plus sucralfate 1 g qid ac

Answer:_____

Treatment of GERD

- Mild-to-moderate GERD
  - Raise head of bed
  - Weight loss
  - Small meals; no fatty meals/EtOH in evening
- Healing rates of esophagitis
  - H_2 blockers 50%
  - **PPIs 80–95%**
- Consider fundoplication in young patients to avoid long-term PPI use
  - **Outcomes best in those who respond to PPIs**
  - Beware!! 60% will still require PPI therapy post-op
- Motility study prior to surgery needed to ensure no impaired peristalsis
- Pre-op ambulatory Ph monitoring needed if no evidence of erosive esophagitis (ACG)
- Metoclopramide (too many side effects) and sucralfate (not very effective) have **little use** in treatment of GERD
- **Long-term use of H_2 blockers is typically ineffective (tachyphylaxis)**
- Patients with atypical symptoms take longer to respond to treatment and may require more aggressive treatment
  - Example: cough/hoarseness from reflux — **treat with PPI bid**

Proton Pump Inhibitors

- Causes mild hypergastrinemia
- Likely increased short-term risk of CAP
- Possible increased bone fracture risk**?** Association only**?** Causality**?**
  - Hypochlorhydria could theoretically decrease calcium absorption
- Hypomagnesemia (muscle spasms, arrhythmias, seizures)
- Increased risk of *C. difficile*
- Maintain patients on lowest effective dose

BARRETT ESOPHAGUS

AR 5

A 55-year-old male patient with a BMI of 40 is seeing you for follow-up of long-standing reflux disease (> 10 years) poorly controlled with a daily H_2 blocker. He is doing well and has no complaints. He undergoes an EGD at your request to rule out Barrett esophagus and is found to have a 2-cm segment of Barrett's with biopsies positive for intestinal metaplasia, but no dysplasia.

He wants to know the follow-up endoscopy schedule.

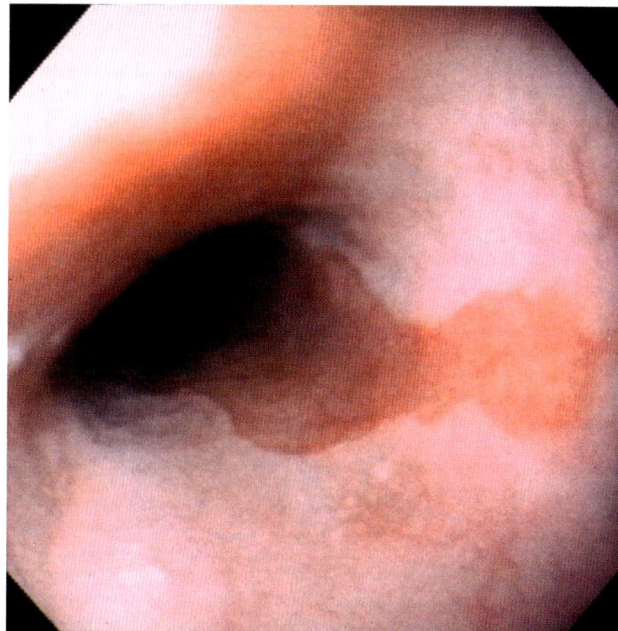

You recommend which of the following?

A. Repeat exam in 3–5 years and switch to PPI daily.
B. Repeat exam yearly; continue H_2 blocker.
C. Treat with radiofrequency ablation and continue H_2 blocker.
D. There is no dysplasia, so there is no need for further endoscopic surveillance.

Answer:_____

Barrett Esophagus (BE)

- Change in cell type from squamous to <u>specialized intestinal columnar epithelium</u> due to chronic GE reflux
  - Biopsies show intestinal metaplasia with goblet cells
- Symptoms of reflux may not be prominent
- Higher risk of having BE in **Caucasian males > 50 years of age**, BMI > 30, longstanding GERD, smoking, known hiatal hernia
- BE associated with 30× risk for esophageal adenocarcinoma (0.1–0.4% per year)
- PPI can decrease dysplasia risk in Barrett's, so treat all patients with Barrett's

Barrett's Surveillance — ACG Guidelines[6]

- <u>No dysplasia</u>: 3–5 years
- <u>Low-grade dysplasia</u>
  - Confirm with 2 pathologists
  - Repeat EGD after intensive acid suppression with 4-quadrant biopsies every 1 cm
  - EMR mucosal irregularities
  - Referral to therapeutic endoscopist to discuss endoscopic eradication therapy

Barrett's Surveillance

- <u>High-grade dysplasia</u>
  - Repeat EGD with 4-quadrant biopsies every 1 cm
  - Confirm with 2 pathologists
  - EMR of any mucosa irregularity (assists with diagnosis — invasive cancer — and treatment)
  - Endoscopic ablation afterwards (i.e., RFA)
  - Caveat: Surgery, as opposed to endoscopic therapy, may be required depending on depth of involvement

ZENKER DIVERTICULUM

AR 6

An 60-year-old patient from the local nursing home is sent to your office after regurgitating undigested food. The "sitter" says the food looked like rice and beans from 2 days ago. In the office you notice the patient's breath is quite foul.

How would you like to proceed?

A. Barium swallow
B. Refer to GI to consider EGD.
C. PPI therapy daily
D. Ignore, since this is only the "1st" episode of dysphagia.

Answer:_____

Zenker Diverticulum[7]

- Outpouching of the hypopharynx (area of muscular weakness)
- Herniation of pharyngeal mucosa posteriorly between the cricopharyngeus muscle and inferior pharyngeal constrictor muscles
- Treatment options include endoscopic therapies vs. surgery with cricopharyngeal myotomy

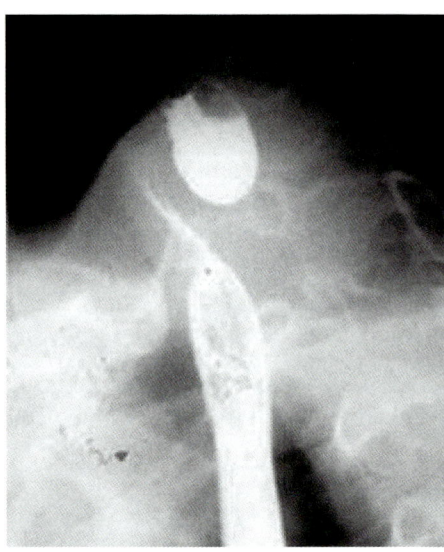

Zenker's

ESOPHAGUS — PEARLS

- **Dysphagia to solids <u>and</u> liquids:** motility disorder (i.e., achalasia), neurologic, cancer/stricture
- **Pseudoachalasia:** <u>cancer</u> mimics achalasia
- **EoE treatments:** PPI, swallowed steroids, elimination diet
- **Pre-op motility study** prior to <u>fundoplication</u>
- **Higher risk of having BE** in Caucasian males > 50 years of age, BMI > 30, longstanding GERD, smoking, known hiatal hernia
- **PPIs** <u>decrease</u> dysplasia risk in Barrett's

STOMACH

The Stomach

- Physiology
- Dyspepsia
- Gastritis
- *H. pylori*
- Peptic Ulcer Disease
- Dumping Syndrome
- Gastroparesis

NORMAL PHYSIOLOGY

- G cells in the antrum release gastrin in response to vagal stimulation, amino acids, and gastric distention
- Gastrin causes parietal cells to secrete HCl into the lumen
- Gastrin also stimulates ECL cells to produce histamine

  Gastrin is the dominant mediator of postprandial gastric acid production.

- Somatostatin and secretin both decrease production of gastrin (and therefore gastric acid)
- In the absence of stomach acid, gastrin levels will increase dramatically
- **PPIs can cause gastrin levels to increase > 500 pg/mL**

DYSPEPSIA

Dyspepsia — A Nonspecific Term
- Can encompass a variety of patient complaints: postprandial fullness, early satiety, epigastric discomfort, heartburn, gnawing pain ...
- Causes include **PUD, gastritis, GERD, gastroparesis, NSAIDs** ...
- New-onset, unexplained dyspepsia in patient > 60 years of age warrants EGD
- In the setting of alarm symptoms ...
  - **Progressive dysphagia**
  - **Unexplained weight loss**
  - **Evidence of GI bleeding**
    ... or failure of therapy, order EGD

ACG and CAG Dyspepsia Guidelines 2017[8]

Algorithm for management of undiagnosed dyspepsia

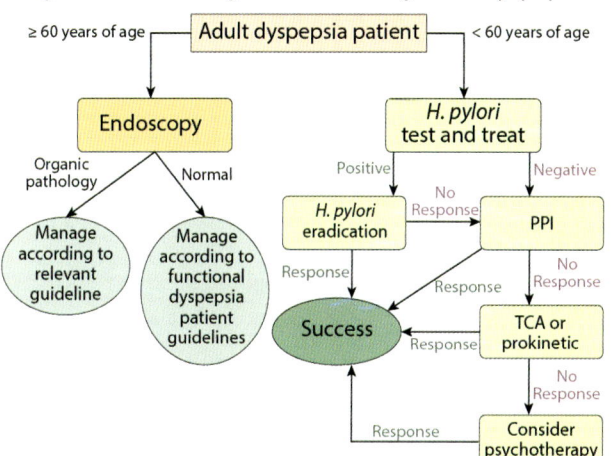

ACG = American College of Gastroenterology
CAG = Canadian Association of Gastroenterology

GASTRITIS
- **Type A (body/fundus)** — **a**utoimmune, **a**trophic, pernicious **a**nemia, **a**chlorhydria
  - Pernicious anemia: antibodies to parietal cells (achlorhydria) and intrinsic factor (B$_{12}$ deficiency)
- **Type B (antrum)** — most common form (80%) and usually due to *H. pylori*
- Achlorhydria = poor absorption of itraconazole, ketoconazole, and thyroxine because they require gastric acid for optimal absorption
- **Fluconazole** does not require gastric acid for proper absorption

Gastritis — Erosive Gastropathy
- Causes include NSAIDs, EtOH, and severe physiologic stress (major surgery, burns)
- Important circumstances to consider gastric acid suppression <u>prophylaxis</u>
  - Prolonged mechanical ventilation
  - Coagulopathy
  - Severe burns
- Most effective <u>treatment</u> for stress-related mucosal bleeding is IV PPI

- Can cause gastritis, PUD, gastric adenocarcinoma, and gastric B-cell (MALT) lymphoma
- 50% of the world's population may be infected
- Test for *H. pylori* when:
  - PUD (history or current)
  - Duodenitis
  - MALT lymphoma
  - Family history of gastric cancer (data unclear)
  - Dyspeptic patients < 60

H. pylori — How to Test?
- Invasive
  - Gastric biopsy — look for organisms on staining
  - Biopsy urease test (*H. pylori* can hydrolyze carbon isotope-labeled urea to CO_2 and ammonia — look for the radiolabeled CO_2)
- Noninvasive
  - Urea breath test
  - Stool antigen
  - Serology (**no longer recommended due to low specificity and low PPV**; < 50%)

PPIs and *H. pylori*
- PPIs can cause false negative for urease biopsy or breath testing, gastric biopsy, and stool antigen
- Hold PPI 2 weeks prior to testing
- Confirmation of eradication should only be done > 4 weeks after completion of antibiotic therapy

H. pylori — Treatment
- Triple-drug therapy (eradication rate of 80%)
- OCLAM (**O**meprazole 20 mg + **Cl**arithromycin 500 mg + **Am**oxicillin 1 g — all bid × 10–14 days) if no risk for macrolide (e.g., clarithromycin, azithromycin) resistance
- If penicillin allergy — metronidazole, clarithromycin, and PPI
- PPI, bismuth, metronidazole, and tetracycline if macrolide resistance concerns
- Salvage (failure of 1st meds) therapy often includes bismuth, metronidazole, tetracycline, and PPI
- Other salvage therapy — levofloxacin (Levaquin), amoxicillin, PPI

AR 7B

Same patient: 35-year-old male with dyspepsia. He was *H. pylori*-positive and received triple therapy. Two months later in office, he feels better. He wants to know if the infection was eradicated.

Which of the following do you recommend?

A. Glucose breath test
B. *H. pylori* antibody (serology)
C. *H. pylori* fecal antigen
D. Upper GI series

Answer:_____

Who Needs Confirmation of Cure (> 4 Weeks Later)?
- Any patient with *H. pylori*-associated ulcer
- Persistent dyspepsia despite "test and treat" strategy
- Those with MALT lymphoma
- Resection of early gastric cancer
- **Do not use serology!**
- ACG guidelines 2017 — "Whenever *H. pylori* infection is identified and treated, testing to prove eradication should be performed using a urea breath test, fecal antigen test, or biopsy-based testing at least 4 weeks after the completion of antibiotic therapy and after PPI therapy has been withheld for 1–2 weeks"

PEPTIC ULCER DISEASE (PUD)

- Causes (1 and 2 most common):
  1) *H. pylori* ~ 50% of PUD
  2) NSAIDs
     - Prevalence in patients on NSAIDs — 25%
     - Not necessarily correlation between ulcers and symptoms
  3) Zollinger-Ellison syndrome/High acid-secreting states (rare)

NSAID-Induced PUD — Risk Factors
- First 3 months of use
- High doses
- Advanced age
- History of ulcer disease/prior UGI bleed
- Concurrent use of corticosteroids or aspirin
- Serious medical illness
- Alcohol is not ulcerogenic, but can cause gastritis
- Corticosteroids alone have small risk of causing ulcers, but when used in combination with NSAIDs, they can significantly increase ulcer development and bleeding risk in hospitalized patients

Treatment of Nonbleeding PUD
- 3 strategies
  1) Treat *H. pylori* if present
  2) Decrease acid secretion
  3) Stop exacerbating processes (smoking, NSAIDs)
- PPIs are 1st line therapy

DUODENAL vs. GASTRIC ULCER

Duodenal and Gastric Ulcers — Treatment
- DUs usually due to *H. pylori* and NSAIDs
- HP+ and uncomplicated DUs — can often just treat the HP
- HP+ and complicated DUs — PPI for 4–8 weeks after HP treatment
- HP+ and GUs — PPI for 8–12 weeks after HP treatment
- NSAID-associated ulcers often treated with PPI for at least 8 weeks
- Repeat EGD is done on some gastric ulcers to rule out underlying cancer
  - **Remember: Cancers can ulcerate**

AR 8

You are called to the ED to evaluate a patient with **severe** epigastric pain. On examination, he displays rebound tenderness. He reports taking high-dose NSAIDs for a back injury for the past 6 weeks. A perforated ulcer is suspected.

What test would you order to evaluate?

A. EGD
B. UGI series
C. CT of abdomen
D. Abdominal x-ray

Answer:_____

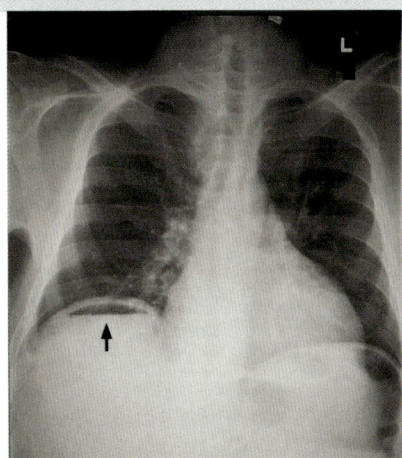

Indications for Surgery in PUD
- UGI bleed (if unable to control endoscopically — surgery needed for 5% of UGI bleeds)
  - Can also utilize interventional radiology
- Gastric outlet obstruction (if refractory to balloon dilation — surgery needed for ~ 25% of cases)
- Perforation
- Recurrent/refractory ulcers (rare)
- ZES (surgery for the underlying gastrinoma)

BLEEDING PEPTIC ULCERS

- **NSAIDs are the <u>leading</u> cause of bleeding ulcers**
  - *H. pylori* also an important cause of bleeding
- Examples when NSAID-related ulcer risk is higher: patients > 65 years of age, concurrent ASA or steroids, prior ulcers
- COX-2 inhibitors have decreased GI side effects (COX-2 is the inducible enzyme involved in inflammatory response; COX-1 produces the protective prostaglandins in the stomach)
- **COX-2 + ASA 81 mg has same risk as regular doses of NSAIDs** (ASA takes away the benefit of COX-2)

Prevention of NSAID-Related Ulcer Complications with Prophylactic PPI[9]

- ACG guidelines risk stratification
- **High risk** (<u>avoid NSAIDs if possible</u>)
  - Prior complicated PUD and/or > 2 general risk factors as below
- **Moderate risk** (<u>PPI needed</u>)
  - 1–2 risk factors as below
  - RFs: Age > 65 years, high dose NSAIDs, prior uncomplicated PUD, concurrent ASA or steroids or anticoagulants
- **Low risk**
  - No risk factors; low-dose NSAID alone (<u>might not need prophylaxis</u>)

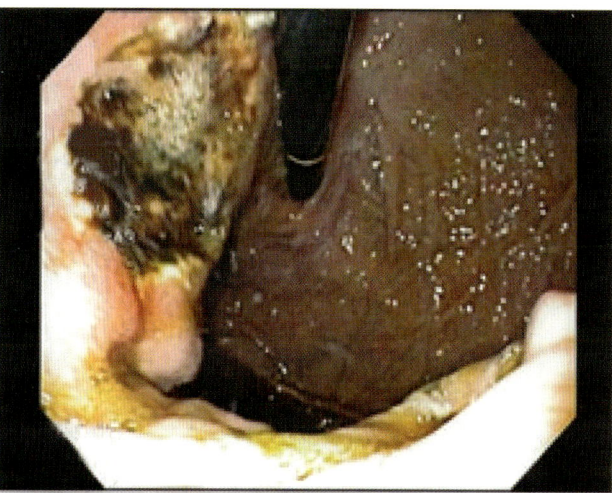

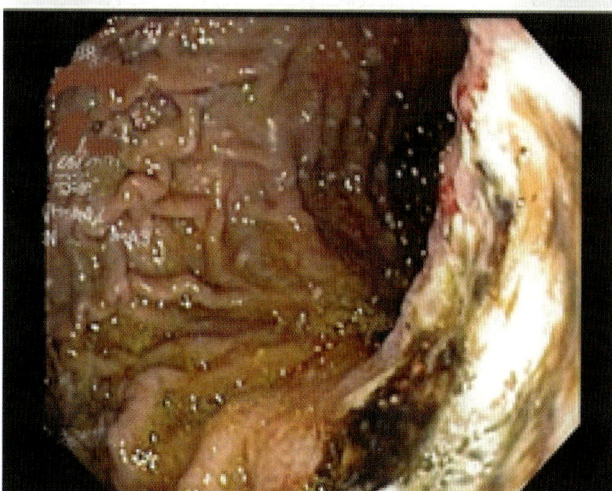

AR 9

62-year-old male with melena for past 3 days; takes daily aspirin for CAD

Hgb 12.0 g/dL; normal BP and HR

PPI drip started

EGD: clean-based gastric ulcer

Which of the following do you recommend?

A. Consider discharge in a.m. if no further bleeding.
B. Keep on IV PPI for 72 hours.
C. Tell patient to never take aspirin again.
D. Refer to interventional radiology because bleeding is likely to restart.

Answer:_____

Workup for Bleeding Peptic Ulcers

- EGD findings that suggest increased risk of rebleed
  - Actively bleeding vessel at time of endoscopy (55%)
  - Nonbleeding visible vessel (43%)
  - Visible clot (22%)
  - Clean-based ulcer (< 10%)
- If there are no other medical comorbidities, **patients with clean-based ulcers can be sent home same day or next day**

Treatment of Bleeding Peptic Ulcers

- Best results are with <u>combination</u> epinephrine injection + cautery or hemoclip
- Most patients with a bleeding ulcer will need prompt IV PPI treatment

Nonulcer Causes of UGI Bleeding
- **Osler-Weber-Rendu** (hereditary hemorrhagic telangiectasia)
  - Telangiectasias on the skin and buccal and nasal mucosa and throughout the GI tract, lungs, and brain
  - Bleeding AVMs may form — commonly in the stomach/duodenum
- **Peutz-Jeghers syndrome**
  - Hamartomatous polyps found between stomach and rectum
  - Dark melanin spots on lips, buccal mucosa, hands, and feet
  - The polyps can cause acute/chronic GI bleeding

Other Issues Involving GI Bleeding
- Video capsule endoscopy of small bowel
  - Useful in workup for small bowel bleeds or occult blood loss with negative EGD and colonoscopy
- Balloon-assisted enteroscopy
  - Allows for evaluation and treatment of small bowel lesions previously out of reach of standard endoscopes

ZOLLINGER-ELLISON SYNDROME (ZES)

ZES and PUD
- Gastrinoma causing diarrhea ± steatorrhea (acid denatures lipase and other pancreatic enzymes), postbulbar duodenal ulcers, esophagitis
- Zollinger-Ellison triangle (90% located between the porta hepatis, mid-duodenum, and head of pancreas)
- 80% are sporadic, **20% are associated with MEN1**
- Fasting serum gastrin > 1,000 pg/mL and low pH (**inappropriately high gastrin**)
- Can normally see moderately increased gastrin in PPI use, atrophic gastritis (high pH can stimulate gastrin release)

ZES
- Workup
  - Secretin stimulation test
  - Marked rise in gastrin with secretin would suggest ZES
  - CT/MRI/EUS and octreotide scan to localize tumor
- Treatment
  - Surgical exploration (**1/2 cured by resection of primary tumor**)
  - High-dose PPI therapy

DUMPING SYNDROME

Dumping Syndrome after Gastric Surgery
- Postprandial symptoms: palpitations, sweating, diarrhea, nausea, lightheadedness
- **Early type** occurs 30 minutes after eating (hyperosmolality of food with fluid shifts)
- **Late type** occurs > 90 minutes after eating and is likely due to hypoglycemia-increased insulin release when food reaches small bowel
- Treatment for both types: Avoid sweets and lactose-containing foods, avoid liquids with meals, and encourage frequent small meals high in protein/complex carbs

GASTROPARESIS
- Delayed gastric emptying — presents as N/V, early satiety, abdominal pain
- Diabetics
  - **Acute hyperglycemia delays gastric emptying**
  - **Hyperglycemia also damages nerves**
- Other causes: systemic sclerosis, viral infection, spinal cord injury, parkinsonism, narcotic pain meds
- Obstruction must be ruled out, and diagnosis confirmed with GES
- Metoclopramide? (FDA warning — beware of permanent **tardive dyskinesia**)

STOMACH AND PUD — PEARLS
- **Dyspepsia** is a nonspecific term: Epigastric pain radiating to back and progressive dysphagia with weight loss are among symptoms that would prompt further testing (e.g., EGD, CT)
- **PPIs** can cause false negatives for urease biopsy or breath testing, gastric biopsy, and stool antigen
- **COX-2 + ASA 81 mg** has same risk as regular-dose NSAIDs (ASA takes away benefit of COX-2)
- GI bleed from **clean-based ulcer** — discharge home!
- **Zollinger-Ellison syndrome:** inappropriately high gastrin level (low pH, but high gastrin!)

SMALL INTESTINE AND COLON

INFLAMMATORY BOWEL DISEASE (IBD)
- Crohn disease (CD) or ulcerative colitis (UC), although a small percentage of people have "indeterminate colitis" with features of both
- See table that follows for comparison of CD and UC

Comparison of CD and UC

Comparison of CD and UC		
	Crohn Disease	**Ulcerative Colitis**
Lesions	Focal, skip, deep	Shallow, continuous
Clinical Course	Indolent	More acute
Prednisone*	Less responsive	Very responsive
Granulomas	Pathognomonic	None
Rectal Involvement	Rectal sparing in 50%	Rectum **always** involved
Perianal Disease	Abscesses, fistulas	None
Small Bowel Involvement	> 50%	Backwash ileitis in < 10%
*For flares; not for long-term maintenance therapy		

- p-ANCA suggests UC
- ASCA suggests CD

AR 10

A 25-year-old male has a 3-year history of abdominal pain and irregular bowel movements. He was diagnosed with Crohn disease 2 years ago and started on mesalamine 4.8 g/day. He seemed to respond at first. He now presents with weight loss and drainage of stool and mucus from around the anus.

PE reveals fullness in the RLQ and a fistula near the anus.

Labs show anemia with Hgb 8.5 g/dL, an albumin of 2.5 g/dL, and a CRP of 50 mg/L.

Colonoscopy reveals ulceration of ileum, ascending colon, and sigmoid colon. The biopsies show chronic and active inflammation.

MRI shows no abscess.

Which of the following do you recommend?

A. Change to sulfasalazine 4 g PO each day.
B. Budesonide 9 g per day
C. Ciprofloxacin 500 mg PO bid for 1 month
D. Infliximab at 5 mg/kg induction and maintenance

Answer:_____

Common Drugs for IBD — 5-ASA
(Mild-to-Moderate UC, Mild Colonic CD)
- Topical antiinflammatory effect
- More effective for UC than CD
- **Mesalamine (5-ASA)*:** Different formulations allow release in distal ileum and colon or given as an enema (proctosigmoiditis) or suppository (proctitis only)
  - Delayed release, colon (Asacol and Lialda [once-daily dosing])
  - Entire GI tract/small bowel disease (Pentasa, Apriso)
- **Sulfasalazine: Split** by bacteria in the colon into 5-ASA + sulfapyridine, therefore not effective for CD of small bowel
  - Sulfapyridine is responsible for reversible infertility in men, leukopenia, and headaches

*While there may be other brand name medications available for the generic medications mentioned here, the speaker notes the brands cited here are among the most commonly encountered. MedStudy does not endorse any brand biases.

Common Drugs for IBD — Steroids (UC or CD)
- **Prednisone, IV steroids**
- **Budesonide:** Enteric-coated; released mainly in ileum/ascending colon
  - Metabolized in liver to inactive products (90% first-pass effect so fewer systemic side effects); still, monitor bone mineral density yearly
  - Ileal release for small bowel Crohn's (Entocort EC)
  - Extended release/MMX technology for mild-to-moderate UC

"Biologics" (UC or CD)
- Monoclonal antibodies to TNF (a.k.a. tumor necrosis factor-α [TNF-α]), others (Ab to integrin)
- Moderate-to-severe Crohn disease, fistulous Crohn's, and refractory UC
- Evaluate for latent TB and HBV and administer all recommended age-appropriate vaccinations before initiation of therapy
- Infliximab (Remicade)* = TNFi, UC/CD
- Adalimumab (Humira, Amjevita)* = TNFi, UC/CD
- Vedolizumab (Entyvio) = Ab to integrin, CD/UC
- Others

*While there may be other brand name medications available for the generic medications mentioned here, the speaker notes the brands cited here are among the most commonly encountered. MedStudy does not endorse any brand biases.

Immunomodulators (6-MP / AZA) and Other Drugs
- May be used with TNFi therapy
- **6-MP/AZA** (UC or CD): steroid-sparing drugs that take 3–4 months to show an effect
  - Monitor CBC and liver tests
  - Monitor TPMT activity and metabolites (6-TG = bone marrow suppression, 6-MMP = hepatotoxic)
- **Methotrexate:** toxic folic acid analogue used to maintain remission in Crohn disease
  - Long-term use — hepatotoxicity
  - Contraindicated in pregnancy

Crohn Disease
- Bimodal onset, 1st peak in **20s–30s**, 2nd smaller peak in **70s–80s**
- Transmural inflammation, hence…
  - Can develop **perianal fistulas**, **strictures**, and **abscesses**
- Endoscopy: deep ulcers, granulomas
- Tetrad to remember
  1) **Rectal sparing**
  2) **Skip lesions**
  3) **Perianal disease**
  4) **Ileocecal involvement**
- SBFT may show "string sign"
- CD bowel involvement
  - Colon only: 30%
  - Small bowel only: 30%
  - "Both": 40%

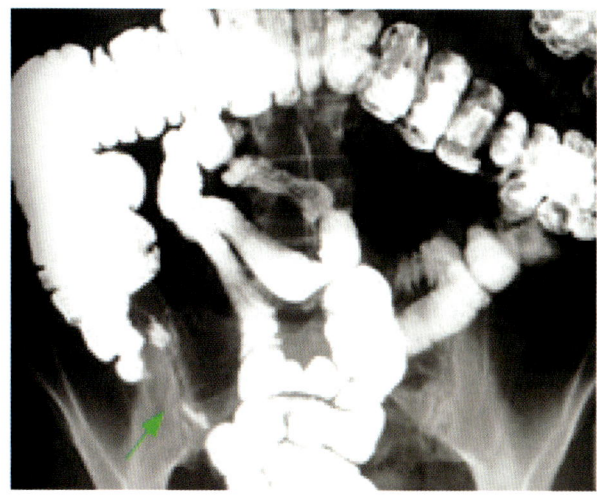

Crohn Disease — Assessment of Disease Activity

- Crohn Disease Activity Index (CDAI) — points associated with the variables below and classified as mild-moderate, moderate-severe, severe-fulminant (**< 150 points = remission**)
  - # of stools per day
  - Need for antidiarrheal medication
  - Abdominal pain
  - General well-being
  - Abdominal mass
  - Anemia
  - Complications (e.g., fistula, arthritis, erythema nodosum)
- Newer focus is on **"deep remission"** — symptom and endoscopic remission (can have significant inflammation with minimal or no symptoms)

Crohn Disease — Complications

- **Fistulas, abscesses** (transmural inflammation)
- **Osteoporosis** is common, vitamin D malabsorption
  - Check vitamin D and BMD
- **B_{12} deficiency/malabsorption** (especially if > 60 cm TI diseased/resected)
- Increased risk of **colon CA** (if involving ≥ 30% of the colon)
  - Initiate screening after 8 years of disease or symptom onset (ACG CD guidelines 3/2018)
- **Toxic megacolon**, CD or UC (colonic dilation and systemic toxicity)

IBD — Extraintestinal Manifestations

These Problems Improve as Disease Activity Improves	These Symptoms Tend Not to Improve with Improvement of Disease Activity (Independent)
RF-negative arthritis (Type 1)	Ankylosing spondylitis (HLA-B27+)
Aphthous ulcers of the mouth	Iritis/scleritis/uveitis (HLA-B27+)
Erythema nodosum	Primary sclerosing cholangitis (HLA-B8+)
Pyoderma gangrenosum (not always parallel to disease activity)	RF-negative arthritis (Type 2)

- Type 1 — acute, pauciarticular (< 6 joints), often knee
- Type 2 — polyarticular, often MCP joints of hands

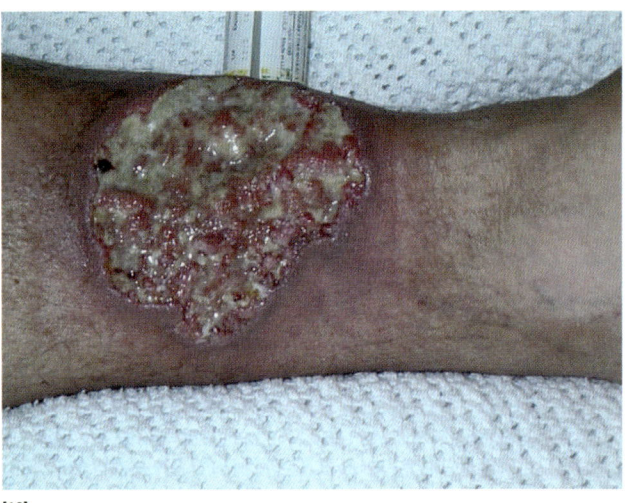

[10]

Pyoderma gangrenosum. Pathergy = deep ulcers develop often at sites of minor trauma, UC > CD.

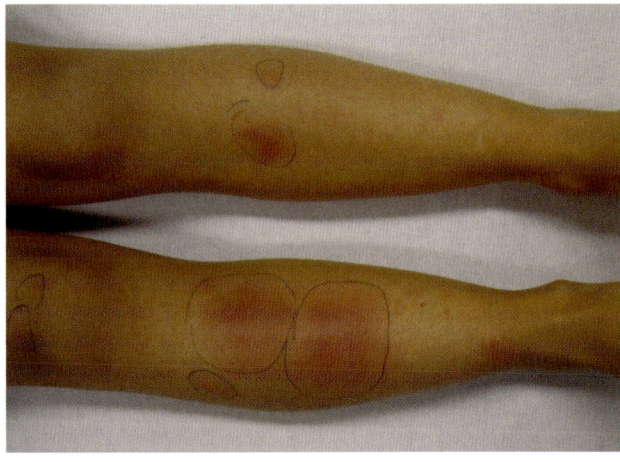

[11]

Erythema nodosum. Erythematous, tender nodules often on shins (UC or CD).

AR 11

A patient with Crohn disease was doing poorly on mesalamine, and a change to a more aggressive therapy (biologic or 6-MP) is planned. She's been on high-dose steroids for 2 months.

Which of the following should be done now?

A. TB interferon-γ release assay
B. Begin to taper off the steroids.
C. Assess for hepatitis B, vaccinate if negative.
D. All of the above

Answer:_____

Crohn Disease / IBD — Treatment

- 5-ASA (rarely used in CD, but can use sulfasalazine in mild-moderate <u>colonic</u> disease)
- Prednisone (avoid long-term use due to side effects)
- Budesonide for mild-to-moderate CD of ileum/cecum
- 6-MP/AZA and biologics: Both steroid sparing
  - Significantly increased risk of lymphoma and skin cancer with 6-MP/AZA
  - Combo therapy 6-MP or AZA and biologic — increased risk of **hepatosplenic T-cell lymphoma**
- Screen patients for HBV and TB before starting biologics or 6-MP/AZA

Crohn Disease — Treatment Scenarios

- Acute small bowel obstruction or "flare": corticosteroids
- Fistula or perianal: 6-MP/AZA or biologic; may add ciprofloxacin/metronidazole
- Steroid-dependent or moderate-to-severe: biologic ± 6-MP/AZA (steroid-sparing agents)
  - Biologic ± 6-MP/AZA for <u>induction</u> of remission in moderate-to-severe
  - 6-MP/AZA alone not good for <u>induction</u> of remission (take too long to work)
  - Biologic ± 6-MP/AZA for <u>maintenance</u> of remission in moderate-to-severe

Surgery and Recurrence in CD

- Need for surgery decreasing (improved medications)
- Most common site for surgery is **ileocolonic**
- Surgery may be needed for obstruction, perforation, abscesses, cancer
- Assess **risk factors for post-op recurrence** to decide need for prophylactic treatment (i.e., 6-MP/AZA, infliximab)
  - RFs for post-op recurrence include <u>penetrating</u> or <u>fistulizing</u> disease, more <u>extensive</u> bowel involvement, <u>prior surgery</u> for CD, <u>smoking</u>, <u>shorter</u> pre-op disease duration, <u>younger</u> patients
- Do colonoscopy 6 months post-op to assess for endoscopic evidence of recurrence to help guide need for medical therapy

AR 12

A 30-year-old female has had ulcerative colitis for about 10 years. 5 years ago, azathioprine was added to her daily mesalamine after she had several flares requiring prednisone. With the current combination, she has been in clinical remission. She presents now with persistent watery diarrhea. There is no blood or tenesmus or abdominal pain. There is no history of recent antibiotic use.

PE: There is mild diffuse abdominal tenderness.

Labs: WBC 13,000/mm³; Hgb 10 g/dL; MCV 103 fL

Which of the following do you recommend as the next step?

A. Empiric prednisone, starting at 40 mg PO daily
B. Colonoscopy
C. Stool for *C. difficile*
D. No treatment because this is likely viral gastroenteritis.
E. Start infliximab for refractory ulcerative colitis.

Answer:_____

Ulcerative Colitis

- Inflammation begins in the rectum and extends proximally (contiguous)
- Confined to colon except for rare cases of "backwash ileitis"
- 70–80% of UC patients are p-ANCA positive
- Main symptoms are abdominal pain and bloody diarrhea
- Infectious causes must be ruled out
  - *C. difficile* (most important to rule out)
  - *Campylobacter* (relapsing course can mimic UC flares)
  - *E. histolytica*
- Consider *C. difficile* infection whenever an IBD (UC or CD) patient presents with a "flare"

Ulcerative Colitis — Assessing Disease Activity

- Mayo Score
  - Stool frequency
  - Rectal bleeding
  - Endoscopic findings (degree of inflammation)
  - Global assessment of well-being by physician (i.e., normal, mild disease, moderate, severe)
- Scores range from 0–12 (12 most severe)

Ulcerative Colitis — Treatment

- <u>Mild</u>/<u>Moderate</u> disease options
  - Rectal 5-ASA (enemas or suppository, treats proctitis)
  - Rectal steroids can be used as 2nd line for proctitis
  - Oral 5-ASA: added to enemas/suppository if topical ineffective (combo of rectal/oral very effective)
  - 5-ASAs can induce and maintain remission
- <u>Moderate</u>/<u>Severe</u> disease options
  - Initial therapy often oral prednisone (outpatient)
  - Initial inpatient therapy (severe disease) can involve prednisone IV, biologic (i.e., infliximab), or IV cyclosporine
    - If "fulminant," patient may need colectomy, particularly if poor response to meds
- Maintenance therapy after remission for severe disease, especially if steroid dependent
  - 6-MP/AZA or biologics (both are steroid sparing)
- Newer biologics
- Vedolizumab (antibody to integrin), may be used if ...
  - Primary failure to TNFi
  - Secondary failure (respond at first, then lose response) to TNFi

Ulcerative Colitis — Surveillance and Surgical Indications

- Polypoid dysplastic mucosa on surveillance colonoscopy, often can be resected endoscopically
  - Surgery sometimes needed
  - IBD specialist needed, particularly in more complex cases
- Flat/Invisible dysplasia harder to manage — refer to IBD specialist, chromoendoscopy, possible surgery
- Guidelines frequently being updated
- Noncancer indications for surgery include:
  - Intractable disease
  - Toxic megacolon/perforation
  - Exsanguinating hemorrhage

Ulcerative Colitis and
Primary Sclerosing Cholangitis (PSC)
- When to suspect: UC patient with jaundice, itching, or cholestatic LFTs
- 5% of UC patients will develop PSC (also seen in CD but less frequently)
- Next step: Abdominal U/S → MRCP
- These patients have a high risk of both <u>colon cancer</u> and <u>cholangiocarcinoma</u>
- Start CRC annual surveillance at time of PSC diagnosis, regardless of disease duration!!

PSC

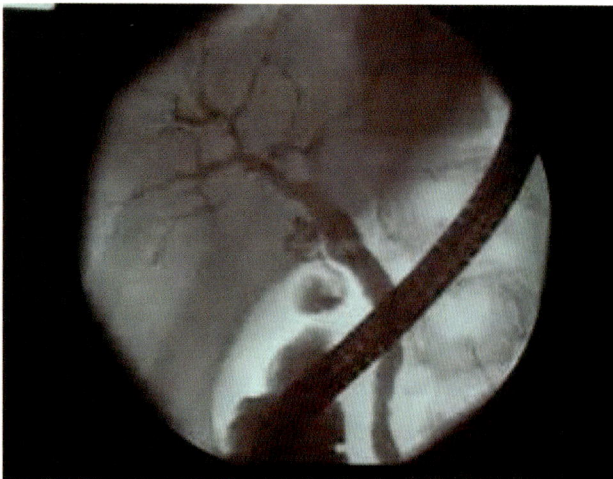

- Be on the lookout for UC patient with elevated alkaline phosphatase (ALP) > 2× normal
- Multifocal strictures involving intrahepatic bile ducts —"string of pearls"

IBD — Pearls
- **UC** — <u>contiguous</u> inflammation starting in rectum
- **CD** — skip lesions, granulomas, <u>transmural</u> inflammation with fistulas and abscesses
- **Biologics and AZA/6-MP** are **steroid sparing**
- Rule out **C. difficile** in any IBD flare
- **Risk of colon cancer** increases with <u>duration</u> of disease and in setting of <u>pancolitis</u>, <u>active inflammation</u>, and <u>PSC</u>
- **Elevated LFTs** and IBD — rule out <u>PSC</u>!
- Start **surveillance** colonoscopy at time of <u>PSC diagnosis</u>!

DIARRHEA
- > 200–250 g/day of stool, where normal is 150–180 g/day
- Normal stool frequency is 3/day to 3/week
- General divisions
  - Acute: ≤ 2 weeks
  - Persistent: 2–4 weeks
  - Chronic: > 4 weeks

Acute Diarrhea
- Frequently has an infectious etiology
1) Take history (e.g., travel, meds, food, sick contacts)
2) Physical exam (signs of dehydration)
3) Stool studies may include culture, O&P, *C. difficile*, and fecal WBCs
4) Colonoscopy/Sigmoidoscopy with biopsies can differentiate infectious from inflammatory disease (IBD)
   - Crypt abscesses seen in both, **crypt distortions are found <u>only</u> in IBD**

Chronic Diarrhea Workup
- Loose stools > 200–250 g/day for **> 1 month**
- Potential contributing mechanisms
  1) Osmotic
  2) Secretory
- Stool osmol gap = 290 − 2[stool Na$^+$ + stool K$^+$]
- For the 290 above, stool osmolality is assumed to be equal to serum osmolality of 290
- Any significant difference/gap is due to <u>unmeasured osmoles</u>

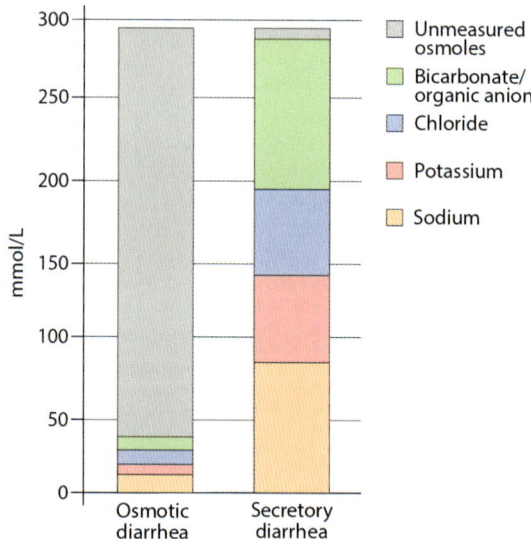

Stool Osmolality = Serum Osmolality
- Extremely low stool osmolality suggests a dilute sample (fluid/urine — factitious)
- Secretory diarrhea — gap often < 50 (Na$^+$ and K$^+$ make up greater % of osmolality compared to osmotic)
- **Osmotic diarrhea** contains <u>unmeasured osmoles and lower Na$^+$/K$^+$</u>, so 2[Na$^+$ + K$^+$] will be <u>much less</u> than 290 mOsm/kg
  - The difference will be > 50 mOsm/kg, often greater than 100
- Many causes of diarrhea have both osmotic and secretory components
- Causes of **secretory diarrhea**
  - Enterotoxin from *E. coli*, cholera, and *S. aureus*
  - Gastrinomas and VIPomas

Osmotic Diarrhea

- A 24-hour fast <u>does</u> greatly improve the diarrhea
- Causes of **osmotic diarrhea**
  - Lactase deficiency (increased lactose in lumen)
  - Mg-containing laxatives/antacids
  - Sugar alcohols (xylitol, sorbitol)
  - Malabsorption (pancreatic insufficiency, celiac disease, bacterial overgrowth)
  - Most laxatives, including castor oil

Causes of Chronic Diarrhea to Consider

- **Diabetes mellitus (DM); multiple factors**
  - Visceral autonomic neuropathy
  - Pancreatic insufficiency (DM can cause pancreatic damage and pancreatic damage can cause DM)
  - Bacterial overgrowth (enterocyte damage and malabsorption)
- **Amyloid**
  - Visceral autonomic neuropathy, gastroparesis (like DM) and postural hypotension
- **Carcinoid syndrome**
  - Release of vasoactive mediators
  - GI tumors
    - This occurs when primary <u>tumor</u> (usually midgut-distal SB and proximal colon) <u>metastasized to liver</u>
    - Can't deactivate vasoactive mediators

Carcinoid Syndrome

- Most neuroendocrine tumors (NETs) are asymptomatic and do not metastasize
- Presentation: paroxysmal flushing; crampy, explosive diarrhea; hypotension; tachycardia
- Diagnosis: 24-hr urine 5-HIAA (> 25 mg/day; normal is < 10 mg/day); CT will show mets in the liver
- MRI and OctreoScan often used as well (many tumors express somatostatin receptors — OctreoScan utilizes a radiolabeled somatostatin analogue called octreotide)

AR 13

A 48-year-old male comes to see you for chronic diarrhea. Symptoms began 2 years ago, and he reports passing 3–4 loose stools daily (his norm was previously 1–2 solid stools/day). After going online he's convinced he must have IBD since his neighbor was diagnosed with ulcerative colitis last month.
The patient denies blood in the stool, and there has been no weight loss.

He does complain of occasional generalized abdominal discomfort. Biopsies from a recent colonoscopy indicate presence of a "lymphocytic infiltrate." The colonoscopy report indicates the mucosa looked normal.

What is the likely diagnosis?

A. Bile acid diarrhea
B. Microscopic colitis
C. Ulcerative colitis
D. *C. difficile* colitis

Answer:_____

Causes of Chronic Diarrhea to Consider

- **Microscopic colitis** (<u>collagenous</u> and <u>lymphocytic</u>)
  - Associated with celiac disease (<u>72-fold</u> increased risk of microscopic colitis in celiac patients)
  - Normal-looking mucosa with chronic, watery diarrhea
  - Biopsy gives Dx: collagenous band in submucosa or lymphocytic infiltrate
  - Treatment
    - If mild, antidiarrheals (loperamide)
    - If symptoms more severe/if diarrhea persists, budesonide

Collagenous Colitis

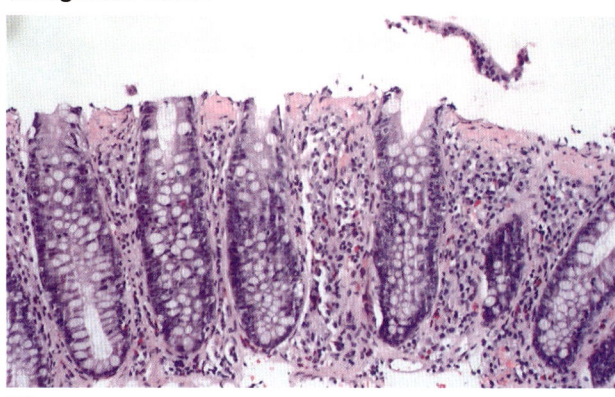

[12]

Causes of Chronic Diarrhea to Consider

- **Lactase deficiency**: volume generally < 200 g/day; common disorder
- **IBS-D**: Patients generally have loose stools with normal daily volume
- **Bile acid diarrhea**
  - Bile acids produced in liver and stored in gallbladder
  - Released to digest fat in SB
  - Normally absorbed back at terminal ileum (TI)
  - Can spill into colon causing increased fluid secretion from colonic mucosa

Diarrhea — Pearls

- **Stool osmol gap** — <u>greater than 50–100</u> = <u>osmotic</u>
- **Stool osmol gap** — <u>less than 50</u> = <u>secretory</u>
- 24-hour fast improves osmotic diarrhea
- Carcinoid **syndrome** occurs if mets to liver
- **Microscopic colitis** — appears normal during colonoscopy, but abnormal under the microscope
- **Celiac** patient with persistent diarrhea — consider concurrent <u>microscopic colitis</u>!

Malabsorption

- Patients can present with "chronic diarrhea" and the following "Big 6":

"PIC ACC"

1) **P**T (INR) — vitamin K
2) **I**ron deficiency
3) **C**alcium deficiency
4) **A**lbumin (low)
5) **C**holesterol (low)
6) **C**arotene (vitamin A) deficiency

- **Decreased mucosal transport** (enterocyte damage or SB resection)

or

Decreased digestion (not enough enzymes; i.e., pancreas)

Malabsorption from Decreased Mucosal Transport

- Small bowel diseases (e.g., celiac disease, Whipple disease, intestinal lymphoma)
- **Celiac disease**
  - 1% of population
  - Autoimmune intestinal disorder with altered response to dietary gluten (**wheat, barley, malt, rye**)
  - Results in small bowel villous atrophy (but many things can cause this!)
  - **Iron deficiency anemia is the most common sign**; also beware of osteoporosis/osteomalacia
  - If you see this …

… Think Celiac Disease!

- **Dermatitis herpetiformis**: itchy vesiculopapular eruptions on the face, trunk, buttocks, sacrum, and extensor surfaces of elbows and knees

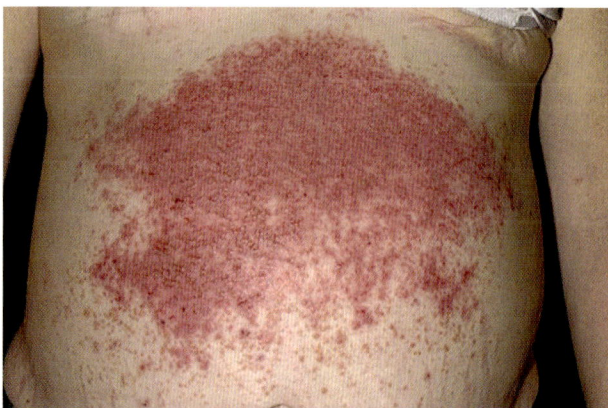

Dermatitis herpetiformis

Celiac Disease Diagnosis

- Dx of celiac disease may include:
  1) IgA tTG (90% sensitivity)
  2) Check serum IgA (increased rates of IgA deficiency in celiac patients — false-neg tTG)
  3) Abnormal duodenal biopsy (do EGD if + serology or patients with high probability regardless of serology)
- Response to a gluten-free diet not necessarily indicative of celiac disease — could be **nonceliac gluten sensitivity** (syndrome of symptomatic response to gluten avoidance but no serologic or histologic evidence of disease)

Other Causes of Malabsorption
Due to Decreased Mucosal Transport

- **Collagenous sprue**: variant of celiac disease; biopsies show flattened mucosa with large masses of subepithelial eosinophilic hyaline material in lamina propria
- **Tropical sprue**: caused by infectious organism (?) and endemic in Caribbean, South Africa, Venezuela, India, and Southeast Asia
  - Treat with tetracycline/doxycycline 3–6 months and/or folic acid replacement
- **Olmesartan-associated enteropathy**: Angiotensin II receptor antagonist causes sprue-like enteropathy

Decreased Mucosal Transport

- **Whipple disease**: rare; tetrad of Sx (i.e., arthralgias, abdominal pain, weight loss, diarrhea/malabsorption)
  - Caused by *T. whipplei* (gram-positive bacillus)
  - Neurologic symptoms (depression, paranoia, dementia)
  - Small bowel Bx: foamy macrophages +PAS staining bacterial remnants
  - Tx: ceftriaxone or PCN IV × 14 days, then TMP/SMX × 1 year
- **Eosinophilic gastroenteritis**: weight loss, low albumin, iron-deficiency anemia; peripheral eosinophilia
  - Elimination diet (type can vary) ± corticosteroids

Decreased Mucosal Transport — Consequences of Small Bowel Resection (e.g., Ischemia, Crohn's)

- Bile acid–induced diarrhea
  - When **< 100 cm** TI resected, overflow causes secretory diarrhea
  - Bile acids are secretagogues in colon
- Steatorrhea
  - When **> 100 cm** TI resected, bile acids are eventually lost and malabsorption/steatorrhea results
- CaOx kidney stones
  - Fatty acid diarrhea due to ileal disease if > 100 cm
  - FA binds calcium in lumen so it can't bind oxalate — oxalate absorbed into blood
- Gallstones
  - Usually **pigment** gallstones
  - Altered balance of bile acids and cholesterol that make up gallstones
- Hypocalcemia (from vitamin D malabsorption)

Decreased Mucosal Transport — Short Bowel Syndrome

- **Short bowel syndrome**: after <u>massive</u> resection of small bowel
- Likely to occur with < 2 feet (60 cm) of remaining small bowel
- Possible lifelong TPN if < 100 cm and IC valve removed
  - ICV removal — leads to reduced transit time and SBBO
- Leaving colon in <u>helps</u> due to its absorptive capacity of H_2O, electrolytes, and short-chain fatty acids
- SBS: low-fat diet, small frequent meals, and vitamin supplementation

Malabsorption Due to Decreased Digestion

- **2 main causes**
  1) **Pancreatic insufficiency** (chronic pancreatitis, pancreatic cancer, cystic fibrosis)
     - Positive response to treatment with pancreatic enzymes
     - Always think of pancreatic CA if new-onset steatorrhea or weight loss (particularly if no clear cause), or older age
  2) **Bile acid deficiency** (also decreased transport): Bile acid needed for fat digestion and enabling nutrient absorption
     - <u>Ileal</u> resection > 100 cm/Ileal disease (Crohn's)
     - <u>Severe liver disease</u> (decreased production of bile acids)
     - <u>ZES</u> (lipase is inactivated and bile acids precipitate)
     - <u>SIBO</u> with subsequent breakdown of bile acids (bacteria can also damage enterocytes and lead to malabsorption)

Malabsorption from Bacterial Overgrowth

- Presenting complaint is usually abdominal distension ± steatorrhea
- Intestinal bacteria make folate but block absorption of B_{12} **(high folate levels, low B_{12})**
- Potential causes
  - Structural abnormalities (after ICV or other small bowel resection)
  - Motility disorders (DM, systemic sclerosis)
  - Achlorhydria
  - Immune disorders

Tests for Malabsorption — Bacterial Overgrowth

- **Dx: lactulose hydrogen breath test** (give PO lactulose, measure hydrogen in breath — bacteria produce hydrogen from lactulose)
- Consider treatment with rifaximin, or amoxicillin/clavulanate, or cephalexin + metronidazole

Tests for Malabsorption — Steatorrhea

- Fecal fat
  - **Gold standard** is 3-day quantitative fecal fat measurement (> 6 g/day is pathologic)
  - **Sudan stain is also used as a spot screening test**
- Any patient who frequently has <u>> 40 g/day of fecal fat</u> likely has <u>pancreatic insufficiency</u> (unless history of <u>massive</u> intestinal resection)

Tests for Malabsorption — Transport / Mucosal Problem vs. Digestion

- <u>D-xylose absorption test</u>: measures absorptive capacity of proximal SB; PO ingestion of D-xylose, measure in urine and blood
  - This allows you to exclude some small bowel diseases, and now pancreatic insufficiency is more likely
  - Low D-xylose absorption may be from small bowel disease; send for EGD to obtain small bowel biopsy
  - **Normal D-xylose = normal small bowel mucosa**

Malabsorption — Pearls

- **Celiac disease** is an example of decreased mucosal transport and is associated with the rash <u>dermatitis herpetiformis</u>
- **Bile acid diarrhea** = < 100 cm TI resected
- **Fatty acid diarrhea** = > 100 cm TI resected
- The 2 main causes of <u>decreased digestion</u> are **pancreatic insufficiency** and **bile acid deficiency**
- **SIBO** can be decreased transport or decreased digestion; test with <u>lactulose breath test</u>
- **SIBO clues** = high folate, low B_{12}

CONSTIPATION

Constipation — Causes

- Majority of cases are idiopathic, but look for **colonic inertia** (slow transit) or **pelvic floor dysfunction**
- Anticholinergic drugs (antipsychotics, antidepressants, 1st generation antihistamines)
- Opioids/Narcotic pain meds
- Iron preparations
- Calcium supplements/Calcium channel blockers
- Endocrine: DM and hypothyroidism
- Pregnancy (altered progesterone and estrogen)
- Injury/Disease of parasympathetics to distal colon/rectum can cause megacolon
  - **Sacral nerve damage**
  - **MS**
  - **Chagas disease** (*Trypanosoma cruzi*)
    - Infection can lead to alterations of the enteric nervous system
  - **Hirschsprung disease** (aganglionic megacolon)
    - Internal anal sphincter denervated so won't relax with rectal distention
    - Colon itself also can be aganglionic
- Pelvic floor dysfunction (PFD)
  - Unable to properly relax muscles during defecation
  - Normally during defecation, relax puborectalis muscle and external anal sphincter and get pelvic floor descent; in dyssynergic defecation, these processes may not occur

AGA Position Statement on Constipation — Take-Home Points
- 3 major categories: normal transit, slow transit, and defecatory disorders (difficulty evacuating rectum)
- In general, assess for <u>defecatory disorder</u> **earlier** on in workup and transit problems later on in workup
- Defecatory disorders include increased resistance to evacuation (high anal pressure or paradoxical contraction of pelvic floor and anal sphincter muscles; i.e., PFD)

Constipation — Diagnosis
- Workup if patient also has weight loss, rectal bleeding, anemia, FH of CRC, recent onset without explanation, or no recent screening
  - Colonoscopy
  - Serum Ca^{2+} and TSH
- Other tests include:
  - **Anorectal manometry (ARM)** to measure sphincter pressures, rectal sensation, and rectal compliance (i.e., PFD)
  - **Defecogram** (barium x-ray during defection)
  - **"Sitz markers"** (patient takes capsule with 24 radio-opaque markers, abdominal x-ray 5 days later; abnormal if multiple markers retained)

Constipation — Defecogram and Sitz Markers
- **Defecogram** can indicate presence of prolapse, rectoceles, or occult intussusception — all may require surgical correction
- **Sitz marker study**
  - Delay in left and/or right colon in slow transit constipation
  - Stagnation/collection of markers in rectum if outlet delay

Constipation — Treatment
- If **idiopathic**, treat by increasing dietary fiber* to 25–30 g/day and avoid dehydration
- **Colonic inertia:** fiber or bulking agents may help
- **Pelvic floor dysfunction:** retraining ± biofeedback
*Warning: Fiber can also cause bloating and abdominal cramping

Next Steps If Fiber and Water Do Not Work …
- Polyethylene glycol (PEG) powder (osmotic laxatives)
- Lubiprostone (Amitiza) or linaclotide (Linzess) = stimulate intestinal fluid secretion
- Hirschsprung disease: surgical treatment
- Opioid/Narcotic-related constipation: μ-opioid antagonists (naloxegol, methylnaltrexone)
- Stimulant laxatives (senna or bisacodyl)
  - Cause colonic muscles to contract
  - Indicated for <u>short-term</u> use

Fecal Incontinence vs. Impaction
- **Incontinence** a major problem for patients ≥ 65 years of age, especially women S/P vaginal delivery
- Workup may include anorectal manometry, defecography, colonoscopy (assess for inflammation, lesions)
- Goal to increase stool bulk, improve anal tone
- Consider biofeedback (can work in certain cases of FI; i.e., if weakness of EAS) and sacral nerve stimulation
- Watery incontinence can occur with **impaction** (large mass of dry, hard stool in rectum)
  - Tx: Remove impaction with mineral oil enema or manually

Constipation — Pearls
- **Medications**, especially opioids, are very <u>common</u> causes (check med list!!)
- Think **defecatory disorders**, such as PFD, <u>early</u> on in differential
- **PFD** = assess with ARM and consider biofeedback

IRRITABLE BOWEL SYNDROME (IBS)
- 15% of the population!
- Abdominal pain/discomfort associated with disturbed defecation
- Psychological dysfunction is common (neuroses, anxiety, or depression)
- Exclude
  - Celiac disease
  - Lactose intolerance
  - Bacterial overgrowth
  - Dietary factors

Rome IV Criteria — IBS
- Recurrent abdominal pain/discomfort on average at least 1 day per week in the last 3 months, associated with 2 or more of the following:
  1) Related to defecation
  2) Change in frequency of stool
  3) Change in stool form
- IBS-C
- IBS-D
- IBS-mixed
- Confirm no alarm symptoms (e.g., rectal bleeding, weight loss, IDA, nocturnal symptoms, FH of CRC, FH of IBD)

IBS Treatment
- Treatment — reassurance/therapeutic physician-patient relationship followed by:
  - Diet (low **FODMAPs** = **f**ermentable **o**ligo-, **d**i-, and **m**onosaccharides **a**nd **p**olyols)
  - Behavioral/Cognitive therapies
  - Antispasmodics (for abdominal pain)
  - Tricyclic antidepressants (abdominal pain, more beneficial in IBS-D)
  - Fiber and osmotic laxatives/PEG (IBS-C)
  - Linaclotide, lubiprostone (IBS-C) = stimulate intestinal secretion
  - Antidiarrheals (IBS-D)
  - Possibly rifaximin (IBS-D, esp. with bloating)
  - Eluxadoline in IBS-D (μ-opioid receptor agonist, Δ-opioid antagonist)

DIVERTICULAR DISEASE AND LOWER GI BLEED

Other Intestinal Diseases — Diverticular Disease
- 4 types of diverticular disease
    1) **Asymptomatic diverticulosis** (most common; 80–85%)
    2) **Painful diverticulosis** (contraction of hypertrophied colonic muscle; 10–15%)
    3) **Diverticular bleeding**
    4) **Diverticulitis**

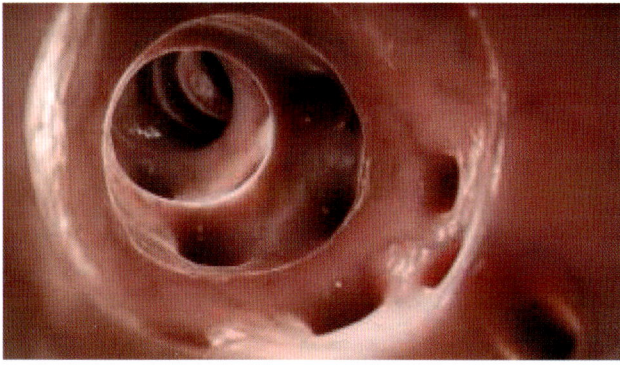

Diverticular Bleeding
- Most common cause of GI bleeding in patients ≥ 65 years of age (angiodysplasia is 2nd most common cause)
- Typically stops spontaneously
- Classic presentation: "painless, maroon stool" (color can vary from red to black)

Diverticulitis
- Caused by inflamed diverticula, due to microperforations
- Occurs in **< 5% of patients** with diverticulosis
- SSx
    - LLQ pain/tenderness
    - Fever
    - High WBC
    - No bleeding
- CT useful in evaluation — **avoid colonoscopy for 4–8 weeks**
- Presentation depends mainly on 2 factors: **severity** and presence of **complications**
- Uncomplicated (localized) vs. complicated (e.g., abscess, phlegmon, fistula — all require specific treatments [i.e., drainage])
- Patients with uncomplicated disease sometimes can be sick with <u>severe</u> disease (i.e., sepsis, high fever) and require inpatient admission
- AGA suggests colonoscopy after resolution in appropriate candidates to exclude CRC if no recent high-quality exam
- **Mild diverticulitis** (Tx): can tolerate PO and no peritoneal signs; <u>metronidazole</u> (gram-negative anaerobic) + <u>ciprofloxacin or TMP/SMX</u> (gram-negative aerobic)

- **Moderate/Severe** (IV indicated) give either:
    - Dual-drug therapy **(best)** — 3rd generation cephalosporin or ciprofloxacin (gram-negative aerobic) <u>plus</u> clindamycin or metronidazole (gram-negative anaerobic)
                or
    - Single-drug therapy — ticarcillin/clavulanate, piperacillin/tazobactam, imipenem/cilastatin, cefotetan (all of these cover both aerobic and anaerobic gram-negatives)

Other Intestinal Diseases — Angiodysplasia (AVM)
- 2nd most common cause of bleeding in patients ≥ 65 years of age
- Most common site is from right colon/cecum
- <u>Angiography</u> may help Dx/Tx (embolization or injection of vasopressin) in severe disease
    - Also used for mesenteric ischemia, any severe upper/lower GI bleeds
- AVMs frequently can be controlled endoscopically

INTESTINAL ISCHEMIA

Other Intestinal Diseases — Intestinal Ischemia — 4 Types
1) Acute mesenteric ischemia
    - 70% mortality
    - Caused by lodging of thromboembolus in a mesenteric artery (i.e., SMA) with acute loss of blood flow
    - **Classic presentation**: <u>lactic acidosis</u> and abdominal pain <u>out of proportion to exam</u>
    - Often history of AFib
    - Dx with CT angiography if patient is stable, or straight to surgery (peritoneal signs/ intraperitoneal air)
    - If not as sick, possible candidate for interventional radiology (endovascular thrombectomy, angioplasty)
2) Ischemic colitis
    - Most common form of bowel ischemia
    - Nonocclusive ischemia, often around splenic flexure ("watershed")
    - Sudden LLQ pain and bloody stools
    - Often no clear cause, but consider low-flow conditions (e.g., hypotension, HF, arrythmias) and hypercoagulable states
    - Most cases resolve quickly without intervention, but ABX should be considered in moderate or severe disease
    - Isolated <u>right-sided</u> ischemic colitis associated with **higher mortality** (? overlap with SMA disease)

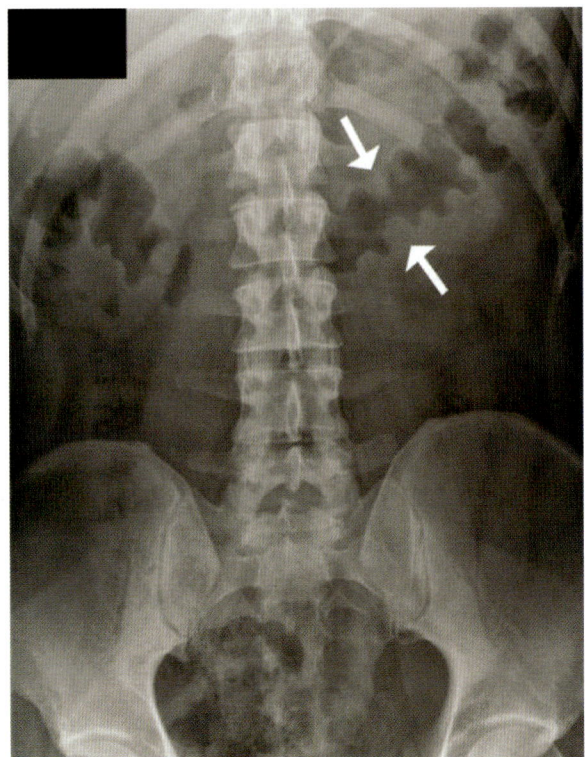

- Ischemic colitis
  - "Thumbprinting" seen on abdominal film/KUB is not specific for type of ischemia, but does represent submucosal edema/hemorrhage
3) Chronic mesenteric ischemia
  - "Intestinal angina" with **classic triad** of abdominal pain after meals, abdominal bruit, weight loss
  - Pain due to episodes of inadequate blood flow brought on by digestion (1–3 hours of dull, gnawing abdominal pain about 30 minutes after eating)
  - Often history of PVD or smoking
  - Dx by MRA or CT angiogram, and **Tx is angioplasty or surgical bypass**
4) Mesenteric venous thrombosis
  - Associated with **hypercoagulable** states
  - Also associated with **pancreatitis** (splenic vein thrombosis), **cirrhosis** (portal vein thrombosis), **SCD**, **PNH** (paroxysmal nocturnal hemoglobinuria), **intraabdominal sepsis**
  - Bleeding from gastroesophageal varices may occur if portal or splenic veins are involved
  - Dx with CT (> 90% sensitivity)
  - Tx acute MVT may include thrombolytics and long-term anticoagulants

ACUTE APPENDICITIS

Surgical Issues — Acute Appendicitis
- Usually diagnosed clinically
- SSx: RLQ pain, anorexia with low grade fever, and mild leukocytosis
- In > 50% of cases the pain starts "periumbilical" and migrates to RLQ
- Dx: abdominal CT or U/S (sonography if CT not available and possibly for children, pregnant women — avoid radiation)

BOWEL OBSTRUCTION

Surgical Issues — Bowel Obstruction
- Small intestine: post-op adhesions, tumor
- Colonic: carcinoma, diverticulitis, volvulus
- **Confirm Dx with flat and upright abdominal film** (SBO = air-fluid levels at different heights; same height suggests paralytic ileus)
- **Tx SBO:** IVF and NG suction for 1–2 days while correcting electrolytes and minimizing narcotics, surgical consultation
- **Tx sigmoid volvulus:** can be acutely decompressed by sigmoidoscopy/colonoscopy, but need surgical correction ultimately

Sigmoid Volvulus — "Coffee Bean" on X-ray

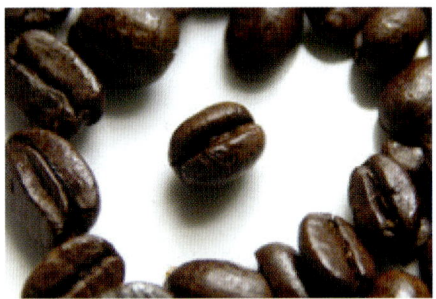

[13]

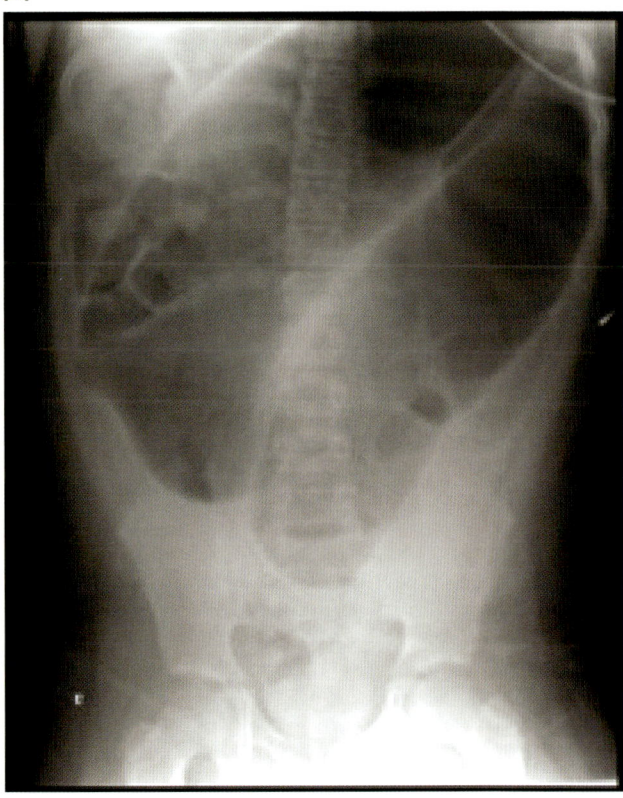

PANCREAS

AR 14

A 35-year-old female presents to the ED with severe epigastric pain for the past 12 hours. The pain radiates to the back and is associated with vomiting. It's a constant pain, and she's never had a pain similar to this in the past.

Past medical history: negative

Social history: She admits to "social" drinking; she is a nonsmoker
Physical exam: moderate-to-severe epigastric pain

T bili 2.1
AST 120
ALT 140
Lipase 800 U/L (normal is up to 160)

Of these listed options, what should be ordered next?

A. ERCP
B. MRCP
C. Surgery consult for cholecystectomy
D. EGD

Answer:_____

ACUTE PANCREATITIS

Pancreas — Acute Pancreatitis (AP) Etiology
- Main causes: **EtOH** abuse and **gallstones**
- **Post-ERCP pancreatitis** occurs in up to 5% of patients getting ERCP (so mainly done for impending cholangitis or +MRCP or high suspicion of stone in bile duct [i.e., T bili > 2.5])
- **Drug induced**
  - Diuretics (furosemide)
  - Estrogens
  - Azathioprine
  - Anti-HIV drugs
  - Oral hypoglycemics

AP — Etiology
- **Hypertriglyceridemia** (> 1,000 mg/dL), **hypercalcemia**, and **trauma**
- **"Idiopathic"** causes may include biliary microlithiasis, hereditary pancreatitis, and cystic fibrosis
- **Occult malignancy**, particularly in older patients (ACG guidelines — always consider pancreatic tumor in patients > 40 years of age with AP)

AP — Diagnosis
- 2 of the following required for diagnosis (ACG, 2013):
  - **Upper abdominal pain radiating to back**
  - **Amylase or lipase 3× ULN**
  - **CT/MRI consistent with acute pancreatitis**
- Lipase (more specific) often stays elevated beyond day 7
- Other causes of high amylase
  - **M**acroamylasemia (benign macromolecules with low urinary excretion)
  - **S**alivary amylase
  - **A**cute cholecystitis
  - **P**erforated ulcer
  - **D**KA
  - **I**ntestinal infarction
  - **E**ctopic pregnancy

AP Severity Classification — 2012 Atlanta Classification
- **Mild** — no organ failure, no local or systemic complications
- **Moderate** — transient organ failure (resolves within 48 hours) and/or local or systemic complications (e.g., CV, resp.) without persistent organ failure (> 48 hours)
- **Severe** — persistent organ failure that may involve 1 or more organs
- 2 main types of pancreatitis are **interstitial** and **necrotizing**
- AGA 2018 — necrotizing pancreatitis is characterized by pancreatic or peripancreatic necrosis and is typically seen in patients with moderately severe or severe AP

Findings Associated with Severe Course — ACG 2013
- Patient characteristics — Age > 55, BMI > 30, altered MS, comorbid disease
- Evidence of systemic inflammatory response syndrome (SIRS)
- Labs abnormalities — BUN > 20, rising BUN, Hct > 44, rising Hct, elevated Cr
- Radiology findings — pleural effusions, pulmonary infiltrates, multiple or extensive extrapancreatic collections
- **SIRS (requires 2 of the following):**
  - Temp < 96.8°F (36.0°C) or > 100.4°F (38.0°C)
  - Tachycardia (HR > 90)
  - Respirations (RR > 20 or pCO_2 < 32 mmHg)
  - WBC abnormal

AP — Clinical Signs

- <u>Cullen sign</u> — faint blue discoloration around umbilicus indicating hemoperitoneum
- <u>Turner (Grey-Turner)</u> — bluish to reddish/purple to greenish/brown discoloration of flanks from retroperitoneal blood

Cullen Sign

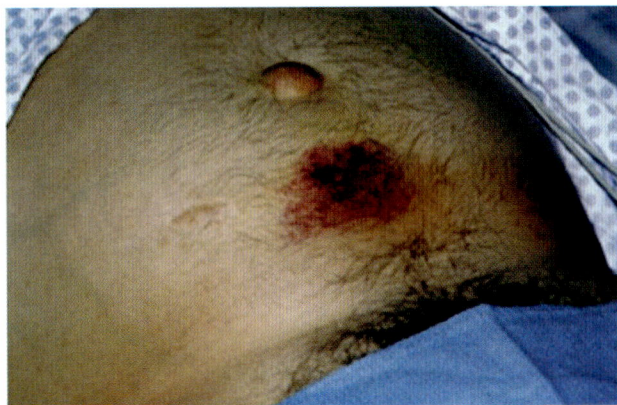

[14]

AP — Scoring Systems

- Scoring systems: Ranson, Glasgow, APACHE II, BISAP
- **BISAP**
  - **B**UN
  - **I**mpaired mental status
  - **S**IRS
  - **A**ge > 60
  - **P**leural effusion
- **Higher points = higher mortality**

AP — Assessment and Management

- Physical exam — assessment for fluid loss, cardio/pulmo involvement
- Labs — including CBC, CMP, amylase and lipase, TG, calcium
- Sonogram to rule out GS
- Routine CT **not always recommended at initial presentation** unless diagnostic uncertainty; additionally, necrosis may not fully manifest until several days after admission
- CT may be required later in admission in moderate-to-severe cases, not doing well clinically (assess for necrosis)
- Early, aggressive IVF replacement (AGA 2018 — no recommendation on NS vs. RL)
  - Overly aggressive can also lead to harm (cardio/resp) so monitor closely, titrate to clinical and biochemical targets
- Monitor BUN with IVF; change in BUN **can predict mortality** (aim for decrease in BUN)
- Early, adequate fluid replacement may be associated with **decreased morbidity and mortality**
- Persistent hemoconcentration can be associated with the development of **necrotizing pancreatitis**

AP — Management

- Try for early **oral** refeeding, particularly if no N/V or evidence of ileus
- If can't tolerate POs or moderate-to-severe AP, consider **enteral** feeding
- Enteral feeding is better than TPN; can maintain intestinal barrier and prevent gut bacterial translocation
- Prophylactic antibiotics **are not recommended** regardless of severity or type of pancreatitis (interstitial vs. necrotizing) — use if concern for infection
- AGA 2018 — if gallstone-related pancreatitis, consider CCY during same admission due to better clinical outcomes

Complications

- **Acute fluid collections**, < 4 weeks
- **Acute necrotic tissue collections**, < 4 weeks
- **Pseudocysts**
  - > 4 weeks, encapsulated wall (generally, no need to drain if no symptoms)
- **Walled-off necrosis**
  - > 4 weeks, encapsulated wall
- Acute necrotic tissue collections and walled-off necrosis can <u>become infected</u> — need to consider this if patient fails to improve, gets worse, or develops signs of sepsis
  - If so:
    - Start on antibiotics
    - Possible CT with FNA with Gram stain and culture to confirm infection
    - May require debridement (ideally, if patient is stable, try to wait > 4 weeks so areas of necrosis become walled off)

CHRONIC PANCREATITIS

Chronic Pancreatitis (CP) — Overview

- Commonly (60–70%) as a result of chronic (> 10 years) EtOH ingestion
- Initial, asymptomatic phase followed by recurrent bouts of abdominal pain
- Steatorrhea and DM may develop late in disease once > 80–90% of **endocrine** (hormones)/**exocrine** (enzymes) function is lost
- Increased risk of pancreatic CA (chronic inflammation is a risk factor for pancreatic cancer)

CP Risk Factors

- EtOH
- Smoking
- Genetics
  - ***CFTR*** gene mutations (cystic fibrosis)
  - Hereditary pancreatitis: ***PRSS1*** (encodes cationic trypsinogen) and ***SPINK1*** genes (encodes a pancreatic secretory trypsin inhibitor)
  - These various mutations are associated with <u>poor control of trypsin activity</u>, which leads to pancreatic damage
- Autoimmune pancreatitis
- Systemic diseases, including SLE

Diagnosis of CP

- Classic diagnostic triad seen in < 20% of cases
  1) Pancreatic calcification
  2) Diabetes
  3) Steatorrhea
- Abdominal x-ray only 30% sensitive but <u>very</u> specific
- CT of abdomen (80–85% sensitivity): pancreatic calcifications or dilated pancreatic duct (PD), and/or pancreatic atrophy
- MRI/MRCP often used instead of CT (hence ERCP rarely used unless need for therapeutic intervention)
- **"Double duct sign" (dilated PD and common bile duct [CBD]):** rule out pancreatic head mass (can also be seen in CP)
- EUS often used in specialized centers — EUS features/criteria include dilated PD, visible side branches, PD stones, and lobularity
- Amylase and lipase <u>not helpful</u> with diagnosis of chronic pancreatitis (fibrosis as opposed to acute inflammation)
- **Fecal elastase** (a pancreatic protease, see low values in CP) can be helpful with sensitivity and specificity > 90%
- **Secretin stimulation test** (collect duodenal fluid after stimulation and assess for bicarb — low bicarb in chronic pancreatitis)

Complications of CP

- With continued abdominal pain
  - Rule out continued EtOH
  - Rule out **pseudocyst**
  - Rule out **cancer**
- Pancreatic CA develops in 4% after > 20 years
- **Gastric varices** can develop from splenic vein thrombosis
- **Endocrine insufficiency** can be seen in up to 50% of patients with CP, including DM (lose insulin)
- Pancreas can produce **less glucagon**, so patients are prone to developing <u>hypoglycemia</u> (no glucagon to increase glucose)

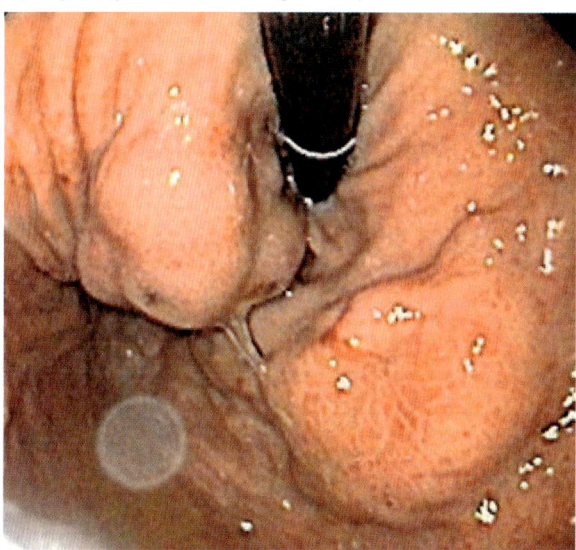

Treatment of CP —

Focus on Pain and Steatorrhea

- **EtOH** and **tobacco cessation**
- Small meals, low fat meals
- Ensure **adequate fat-soluble vitamin** levels
- **Pancreatic enzyme supplementation** for steatorrhea (30,000 international units of pancreatic lipase per meal)
  - May assist with <u>pain</u> (exogenous enzymes can reduce endogenous enzyme secretion and pancreatic pressure)
- **Endoscopic therapy** — removal of PD stones, PD stents, celiac nerve block may be options, but data limited
- **Surgery** — decompress PD (Puestow procedure to decompress dilated PD — pancreaticojejunostomy)

AUTOIMMUNE PANCREATITIS

Autoimmune Pancreatitis (Acute or Chronic Pancreatitis)

- Occurs in < 5% of cases of chronic pancreatitis
- CT will show <u>head mass lesion</u> or <u>diffuse enlargement</u> ("sausage-shaped pancreas") — can look like cancer
- **Type 1** = elevated IgG4, associated with <u>systemic</u> disease including salivary gland disease, bile duct disease (IgG4-associated cholangitis)
- **Type 2** = normal IgG4, younger patients, not systemic
- Histology: dense lymphoplasmacytic infiltrate
- Tx: prednisone 40 mg/day with slow taper (5 mg/week)

Sausage-Shaped Pancreas

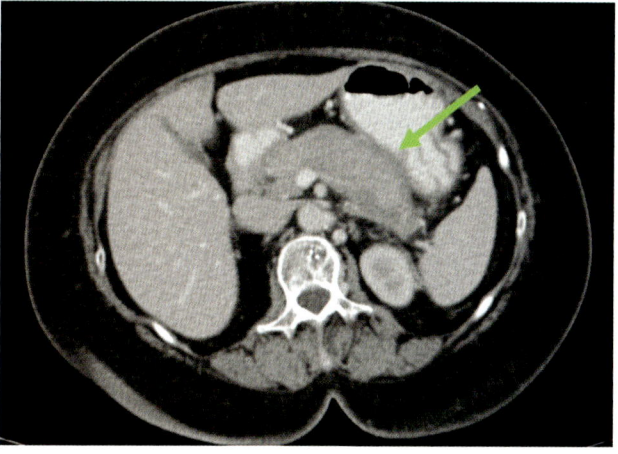

PANCREATIC DISEASE — PEARLS

- **EtOH** and **gallstones** are main risk factors for <u>acute pancreatitis</u>
- **Routine CT** <u>not always</u> recommended at initial presentation unless diagnostic uncertainty
- **Early, adequate fluid replacement** may be associated with <u>decreased</u> morbidity and mortality
- **Routine prophylactic antibiotics** are <u>not</u> recommended
- **Double duct sign:** Rule out pancreatic <u>cancer</u>!!
- **Autoimmune pancreatitis:** Treat with <u>steroids</u>

BILIARY SYSTEM

AR 15

49-year-old male with long-standing ulcerative colitis developed mild RUQ discomfort several weeks ago. He denies diarrhea and has not seen any blood in his stool. He went to a local urgent care last week after his wife complained that he looked "yellow." Labs were drawn, and he's here today to review them with you.

PMH: hypertension, cluster headaches

Past surgical Hx: appendectomy (13 years of age), colonoscopy (6 months ago)

Meds: mesalamine

Labs: T Bili 3.5 mg/dL; AST 42 U/L; ALT 36 U/L; amylase 36 U/L; alkaline phosphatase 375

You are most concerned about ...

A. Gallstones, so you order an abdominal U/S.
B. PUD, so you refer to GI for an EGD.
C. Colon CA, so you refer to GI for a colonoscopy.
D. PSC, so you order an MRCP.

Answer:_____

CHOLELITHIASIS

Biliary System — Gallbladder Stones

- Cholelithiasis is common (20% of women, 8% of men; usually asymptomatic)
- 75% of stones are cholesterol stones (pure or mixed); the rest are bile pigment stones (contain bilirubin)
- Profile for **cholesterol** stones: elevated BMI, rapid weight loss, female, pregnancy
- Profile for **pigment** stones: old age, SCD, or other cause of hemolysis (increased unconjugated bilirubin)

Dx / Tx of Cholelithiasis

- Abdominal U/S is 90% sensitive
- HIDA can confirm cystic duct obstruction if concerned about <u>acute cholecystitis</u>
- **Symptomatic patient**: elective cholecystectomy because 70% have recurrent symptoms if not treated
- **Asymptomatic patient**: Only 20% of these patients ever develop symptoms within 10–20 years, so do nothing in most cases
  - May need to consider prophylactic CCY in certain populations (i.e., if increased risk GB cancer as in <u>porcelain GB</u> or <u>large gallstones</u>)
- **Acalculous cholecystitis** occurs in very ill, ICU patients; CT or U/S will show large, tense, often thickened GB with pericholecystic fluid (no stones, but +HIDA)

Biliary System — Ductal Stones

- CBD stones
  - **Choledocholithiasis**, including post cholecystectomy from retained stone
  - **Mirizzi syndrome:** obstruction of the common hepatic duct due to extrinsic compression from a stone in the cystic duct (not CBD!)
  - CBD stones can lead to **cholangitis**
  - CBD stones are removed by ERCP (± sphincterotomy, stent, balloon sweep)
- Clinical predictors of choledocholithiasis in patients with symptomatic cholelithiasis, ASGE
  - **Very strong:** CBD stone on sonogram, bili > 4.0, or clinical ascending cholangitis
  - **Strong:** dilated CBD > 6 mm, bili 1.8–4.0
  - **Moderate:** > 55 years of age, clinical GS pancreatitis or abnormal liver test other than bili

CHOLANGITIS

- Acute cholangitis suggested by <u>Charcot triad</u>
  1) Biliary colic
  2) Fever
  3) Jaundice
- <u>Reynolds pentad</u> adds
  4) Altered mental status/mental confusion
  5) Bacteremia/septic shock

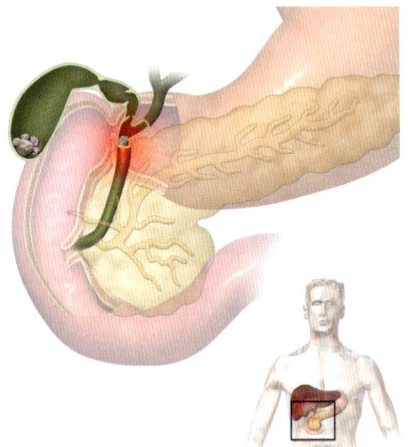

[15]

- Tx: broad spectrum IV ABX with a focus on colonic type bacteria, IVF and **urgent biliary drainage**
  - i.e., piperacillin-tazobactam, ampicillin-sulbactam
- Adjust to blood culture results

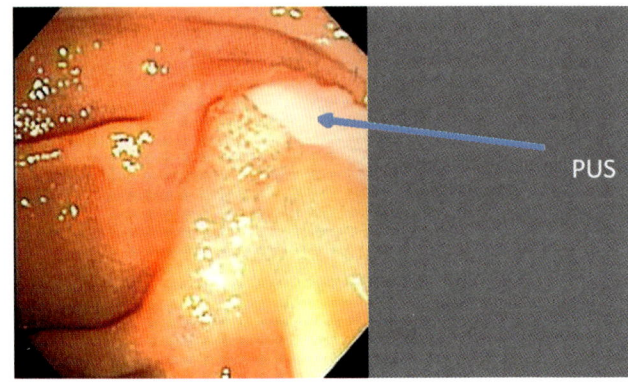

PUS

PRIMARY BILIARY CHOLANGITIS (PBC)

Biliary System — Non–Stone Disease:
Primary Biliary Cholangitis (PBC)
- Formerly primary biliary cirrhosis
- 95% are women, typically middle-aged, considered "autoimmune"
- Toxic bile acids can accumulate in liver
- Bile ducts chronically inflamed — can lead to cirrhosis
- Common presentation: fatigue, **elevated ALP** (> 2–5× ULN), pruritus
- 90% have **+AMA** (> 1:40) but degree of elevation <u>does not</u> correlate with severity of disease
- Can see fat-soluble vitamin deficiencies including A/D/E/K
  - Decreased bone mineral density (need bone density studies in PBC patients)
- Can see high cholesterol levels (difficulty secreting cholesterol into bile)

Dx / Tx of PBC
- Liver biopsy sometimes performed (biopsy if diagnostic uncertainty, staging, prognosis)
  - Can see **florid duct lesions** (inflammation around bile ducts) and granulomas; later on, can see bile duct loss
- **Ursodiol** (synthetic bile acid — reduces toxicity of bile salt pool) slows progression of disease; <u>can decrease mortality</u> and need for liver transplant
- May ultimately require liver transplantation, however

PRIMARY SCLEROSING CHOLANGITIS (PSC)

Biliary System — Non–Stone Disease: PSC
- Occurs more frequently in males (70%), middle-aged
- Cause unknown; inflammation leads to sclerosis/scarring throughout biliary tree
- Negative AMA, often +p-ANCA
- 75% of PSC patients have UC (less common in CD)
  - 5% of UC patients have PSC, and 2% of CD patients have PSC
- IBD patients with persistent increase in ALP should be screened
- Diagnosis: usually start with MRCP, not ERCP (increased risk of cholangitis)

Primary Sclerosing Cholangitis
- Similar to PBC, can see deficiencies in fat-soluble vitamins
- 8–15% develop **cholangiocarcinoma**
  - MRCP/ERCP can show "dominant stricture" but can be difficult to distinguish benign dominant stricture from cholangiocarcinoma
  - Biliary brushing/biopsy can help diagnosis, but not always
- Patients with UC and PSC are at increased risk of CRC compared to UC alone
- Increased risk of GB cancer

Onion Skin Fibrosis

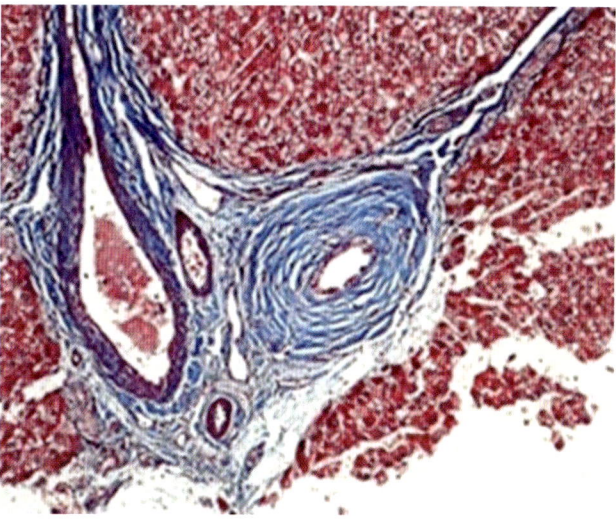

[16]

- In PSC on liver biopsy, see fibrous portal expansion
- True "onion skin lesion" is not always seen
- Liver biopsies infrequently done to diagnose PSC; diagnosis can frequently be made on bile duct imaging

PSC

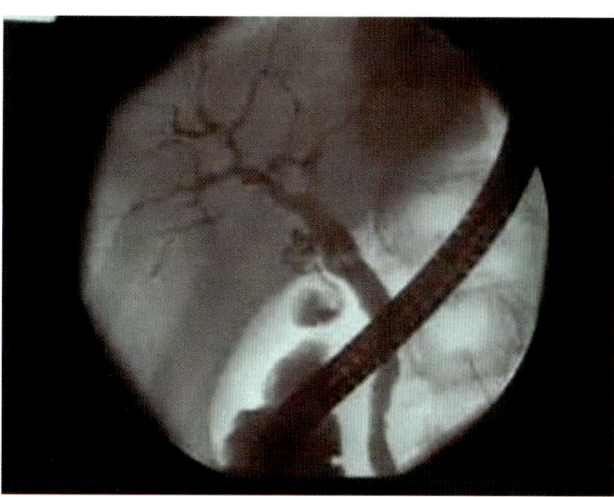

Intra- and/or extrahepatic, "beaded appearance" leads to obstructive jaundice and cirrhosis

Tx of PSC
- The only sure treatment of PSC is **liver transplantation**
- Colectomy can "cure" UC, but will not affect course of PSC
- Remember: Rule out PSC in any patient with jaundice/elevated ALP and history of IBD!

BILIARY DISEASE — PEARLS
- **Pigment** gallstones associated with <u>hemolysis</u>
- **Acalculous cholecystitis:** <u>sick</u> ICU patient
- **Mirizzi** syndrome: stone in <u>cystic duct</u> pushes on biliary tree
- **PBC:** <u>+AMA</u>, fat-soluble vitamin <u>deficiencies</u>, <u>ursodiol</u>
- **PSC:** IBD patients with increased <u>ALP</u>

LIVER

Liver Disease — Overview

	Differential Diagnosis of Chronic Hepatitis
A	Autoimmune hepatitis
B	Hepatitis B
C	Hepatitis C
D_1	Hepatitis D (only with hep B)
D_2	Drugs
D_3	Diseases: • Wilson disease • α_1-Antitrypsin deficiency • Hemochromatosis
F	NAFLD

Liver Disease / Liver Tests — Overview
- With viral hepatitis, the ALT is often higher because toxicity is more liver specific, and ALT is more specific than AST
- AST also present in muscle and other extrahepatic organs
- Transaminase levels > 1,000 U/L may be from liver ischemia, HSV, CMV or DILI (drug-induced liver injury/acetaminophen) as well as acute viral hepatitis
- Causes of elevated ALP: **B**one, **K**idney, **I**ntestine, **P**lacenta
- GGT rises in parallel with ALP from the liver

Bilirubin and Jaundice — Unconjugated Hyperbilirubinemia
- Overproduction of bilirubin (product of heme breakdown) or defects in uptake or conjugation
- **Gilbert's** (benign inherited disorder of bilirubin conjugation; 7% of population)
  - Defect in gene underlying bilirubin glucuronidation
  - Triggers often include fasting, illness (e.g., cold, flu)
- **Crigler-Najjar** syndrome (inherited disorder of bilirubin conjugation, can be severe and present in infancy)
- **Hemolysis** (releases unconjugated bilirubin)

Bilirubin and Jaundice — Conjugated Hyperbilirubinemia
- Associated with **cholestasis** — decrease in bile flow due to impaired secretion of hepatocytes or obstruction of bile ducts
- Acute and chronic liver injury (e.g., viral hepatitis, meds), obstructive jaundice (i.e., bile duct tumor, stone)
- Inherited conjugated — **Dubin-Johnson's** (disorder of bilirubin excretion into bile, with dark pigment accumulation in liver)
- Inherited conjugated — **Rotor syndrome** (same as above but no pigment in liver)
- Unconjugated bili is tightly bound to albumin, and the complex is too large to pass through glomerulus (so won't show up in urine until it eventually becomes conjugated)
- Conjugated bili is less tightly bound and can pass into the urine

Assessment of Severity of Liver Dysfunction
- **Child-Pugh classification** = A, B, or C
  - Calculator based on HE grade, degree of ascites, degree of bilirubin elevation, degree of low albumin, degree of prothrombin time prolongation
- **MELD score** (**M**odel for **E**nd-Stage **L**iver **D**isease)
  - Calculator based on creatinine, bilirubin, and INR
  - Helps accurately predict 3-month survival

HEPATITIS

Viral Hepatitis — Serological Tests

Hepatitis — Serological Tests									
	Anti-HAV IgM	Anti-HAV IgG	HBs Ag	Anti-HBs IgG	Anti-HBc IgG	Anti-HBc IgM	HBeAg	Anti-HDV	HBV DNA
Acute Hepatitis A	+	−	−						−
Previous HAV	−	+	−						−
Acute HBV	−		+ Early	−	−	+	+	−	+
Acute HBV — Window			−	−	−	+	−	−	−
Chronic Active HBV			+	−	+	−	Usually +	−	+
Remote HBV (Immune)			−	+	±	−	−	−	−
Vaccinated (Immune)			−	+	−	−	−	−	−
Acute Hepatitis D (w/ Acute Hep B = Coinfection)			+ Early	−	−	+	+	+	+
Acute Hepatitis D (w/ Chronic Active Hep B = Superinfection)			+	Rarely +	+	−	Usually +	+	+

Core window = HBsAg cleared, but no HBsAb yet;
only +hepatitis B core IgM

Hepatitis A
- RNA virus transmitted by fecal-oral route
- Jaundice begins 3 weeks after exposure,
  with prolonged cholestasis up to 4 months possible
- Majority of infections associated <u>with symptoms</u> but overwhelming majority recover fully
- 1% chance of fulminant hepatitis
- HepA vaccine is given as 2 doses > 6 months apart: Some important groups to consider for vaccine ...
  – All children at 1 year of age
  – Endemic areas
  – Chronic liver disease
  – HIV+, etc.
- Following exposure to HAV — HepA vaccine and/or immunoglobulin can be effective as prophylaxis after exposure to HAV
- CDC is a great resource for your clinical practice

Hepatitis B — Overview
- Key points
  – HBsAg: Means you are producing hepatitis B virus
  – HBsAb: Indicates past exposure to <u>either</u> virus or vaccine; usually indicates immunity
  – HBcAb: The Ab appears early as IgM, then IgG, so **HBcAb IgG is best marker for previous infection**
  – **HBeAg+**: Correlates with <u>**quantity**</u> of intact virus and <u>**infectivity**</u>
  – Maternal-to-fetal transmission more likely if HBeAg+

Acute Hepatitis B
- ALT rises between months 2–3; jaundice month 3
- Window period (around 4th month): **HBcAb IgM must be done to confirm acute HBV** because HBsAg is undetectable, and weeks/months go by before HBsAb becomes detectable
- 70% patients can be asymptomatic with no jaundice
- Some can get serum sickness — like picture with arthralgias and fever
- Fulminant hepatic failure in 0.1–0.5%
- In general, treatment often supportive but can give antiviral therapy in some cases (e.g., severe disease, protracted course)

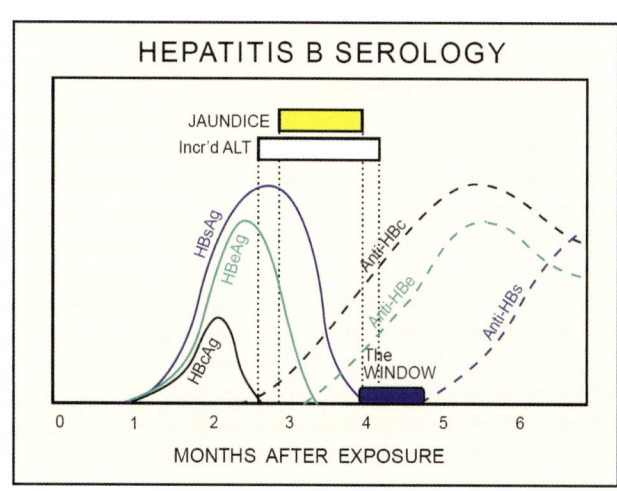

Hepatitis B Vaccination
- Some important groups to consider for **vaccination** ...
  - Universal vaccination in **neonates**, regardless of hepatitis B status of mother
  - **High-risk adults** (e.g., health care workers, dialysis, household contacts) should be vaccinated
- Postvaccination testing to assess titer is done in patients at high risk for continued exposure (i.e., health care workers) or those less likely to mount an immune response (e.g., dialysis, immunosuppressed)
- Can also give immunoglobulin after exposure (i.e., needlestick), ideally within 24 hours, along with vaccine
- Immunoglobulin and vaccine in other potential exposures as well — ocular, mucosal, sexual
- Hep B+ in pregnancy — give immunoglobulin and vaccine to neonate
- Individual with acute HBV — Give HBIG and HepB vaccination to sexual contacts of this individual and infants cared for by this individual
- CDC website is a great resource for your clinical practice

Chronic Hepatitis B
- Occurs when virus remains > 6 months (risk of chronicity 90% for infants, 5% for adults = infants have greater rates of chronicity once exposed compared to adults)
- 2 types of carrier states
  1) Inactive carrier state (asymptomatic with normal liver enzymes)
     - Need med prophylaxis if they become **immunocompromised** (e.g., chemo, IBD Tx)
     - Always check HBsAg and HBsAb prior (even +core alone increases reactivation risk if immunocompromised)
  2) Chronic active hepatitis B (abnormal liver enzymes)
- Check labs including LFTs, platelet count, INR, HBsAg, HBsAb, HBeAg, HBeAb, HBV DNA

Treatment of Chronic HBV
- Complex, depends on multiple variables including HBsAg, eAg status, VL, presence of cirrhosis
- Guidelines can vary by society recommending treatment — "general" recs are below (consult hepatology)
- **If eAg+, treat if DNA > 20,000 and ALT > 2× ULN**
- **If eAg−, DNA > 2000 and ALT > 2× ULN**
- Generally treat most cirrhotic patients
- If lower VL or ALT or uncertainty, may need liver biopsy to help with decision treatments
- Meds include antivirals (i.e., tenofovir and entecavir)
- Sometimes pegylated interferon (younger patients who may want shorter treatment duration; however, increased side effects)

Hepatitis B and Hepatocellular Carcinoma (HCC)
- HCC; 2% conversion per year (lifetime risk for HCC is 20%)
- Screen q 6 months if cirrhosis
- If noncirrhotic, some important groups to screen ...
  - Active hepatitis with abnormal LFTs
  - Elevated VL
  - FH of HCC
  - African American or African descent
  - Asian male > 40, Asian female > 50
  - Others
- Generally screen with sonogram ± AFP (AFP can increase sensitivity but can lead to false positives); AASLD 2018 says "with or without" AFP
- Some centers also may use CT or MRI

Hepatitis C
- 2nd only to NAFLD for number of new cases per year
- Mostly genotype 1 in U.S.
- 1/4 of HIV patients are coinfected with HCV
- 70–80% of acute HCV becomes chronic, so 2–4 months after infected/diagnosed recheck to confirm persistent HCV RNA
- 25% with chronic HCV will get cirrhosis in 25 years
- Recommend screening all **baby boomers** born 1945–1965
- Screen if risk factors (guidelines vary somewhat) (e.g., IVDU, exposure to contaminated blood products, dialysis, HIV, elevated LFTS)

Hepatitis C and HCC
- Chronic HCV with cirrhosis (different from Hep B) — screen every 6 months for HCC, sonogram ± AFP
- 2–8% annual risk of developing HCC in Hep C cirrhotics
- Some suggest HCC screening in advanced fibrosis as well (Stage 3; not yet cirrhosis)

Hepatitis C — Associated Conditions
- **Mixed cryoglobulinemia** strongly associated with chronic HCV
- Presents as small vessel vasculitis with rash consisting of "palpable purpura"
- Hepatitis C also associated with ...
  - **Immune complex glomerulonephritis**
  - **Lymphoma**
  - Porphyria cutanea tarda (photosensitivity leading to skin blistering)

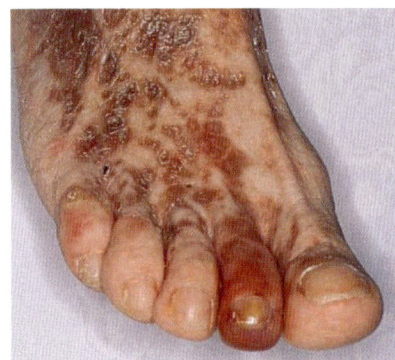

Mixed cryoglobulinemia. Residual brown discoloration after purpura resolves; ischemic toe.

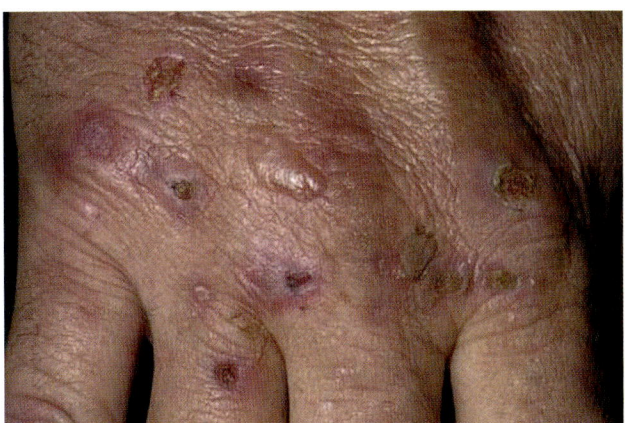

Porphyria cutanea tarda

Treatment of Chronic HCV
- Guidelines are constantly evolving for HCV treatment
- Older drugs (pegylated interferon/ribavirin) much less effective than new antivirals used today
- Newer direct antivirals ± ribavirin have excellent viral clearance **(> 95% cure rate, pan-genotypic options, well tolerated with few side effects, and 12 weeks or less of therapy for most)**
- Newer drugs also effective in those who failed prior pegylated interferon and ribavirin

Hepatitis D
- RNA virus that requires coexistent HBV
- Can occur acutely with HBV (**coinfection**) or as <u>**superinfection**</u> in those with previously established chronic HBV
- Immunity to HBV (HBsAb+) implies immunity to HDV
- Suspect this if sudden decompensation in patient with chronic HBV and <u>Dx with anti-HDV IgM</u>

Hepatitis E
- Transmission can vary (e.g., fecal-contaminated water, zoonotic [contaminated meat and shellfish], blood transfusion)
- Found globally but more common in Asia, Africa, Central America — often due to contamination of water supplies
  - Can also be seen in travelers
- Most patients asymptomatic and clear the virus
- Neurologic symptoms relatively common if symptomatic (e.g., meningitis, neuropathy)
- Hepatitis E in endemic areas carries **high risk for fulminant hepatitis**, particularly **in 3rd trimester of pregnancy (20% maternal fatality rate)**

Viral Hepatitis — Pearls
- **Hep A:** Majority of infections associated with <u>symptoms</u> but overwhelming majority <u>recover fully</u>
- **Hep B:** 70% patients can be <u>asymptomatic</u> with no jaundice
- **Hep B carriers** who need <u>immunosuppressive</u> meds may require <u>prophylaxis</u>
- Multiple <u>noncirrhotic</u> Hep B patients require **HCC screening**
- Screen all <u>baby boomers</u> for **Hep C**
- **Hep D** requires coexistent <u>Hep B</u>
- **Hep E** can be <u>lethal</u> in <u>pregnant females</u>

Autoimmune (Chronic) Hepatitis
- Autoimmune hepatitis (AIH)
  - Female > male, often 40s or 50s
  - Can be asymptomatic or present with ALF
- **Type 1** — classic type, ANA ± anti-smooth muscle Ab
  - +ANA (most sensitive but least specific)
  - +Anti-smooth muscle Ab (SMA) (more specific than ANA)
  - Can check anti-actin Ab, but less widely available (more specific and sensitive than anti-SMA)
- **Type 2** — Anti-LKM (liver/kidney microsome) or anti–LC-1 (liver cytosol antigen)

Autoimmune (Chronic) Hepatitis

Scoring System (6 points = probable AIH; 7 or more points = definite AIH)		
ANA or SMA	> 1:40, 1 point	> 1:80, 2 points
IgG	IgG > ULN, 1 point	IgG > 1.1× ULN, 2 points
Liver Bx	"Compatible," 1 point	"Typical," 2 points
Absence of viral hepatitis		2 points

- Liver biopsy (opinions vary on need) — some groups say biopsy if unclear diagnosis based on clinical picture and labs
- Liver Bx: portal mononuclear cell infiltrate spreads into hepatic lobule (sometimes referred to as interface hepatitis [a.k.a. piecemeal necrosis])
- Generally treat if elevated transaminases, elevated IgG, abnormal histology or symptoms: <u>treatment improves survival</u>
- **Treat with prednisone ± azathioprine**
- No cure; liver transplant indicated for end-stage disease

DRUG-INDUCED LIVER INJURY

Drug-Induced Liver Injury — Overview
- <u>Pure cholestasis</u> vs. <u>mixed cholestasis</u> (mixed = increased bili and ALT = worse prognosis)
- DILI mechanism = **dose dependent/predictable** (i.e., acetaminophen) vs. **idiosyncratic** (most common mechanism in general)
- Key examples
  - **Acute DILI:** In U.S., acetaminophen most common cause (LFTs abnormal < 3 months), followed by ABX
  - **Chronic DILI and possible cirrhosis**; i.e., methotrexate and isoniazid
  - **Pure cholestasis:** anabolic steroids, OCPs
  - **Mixed cholestasis:** amoxicillin/clavulanate

Drug-Induced Liver Injury — Acetaminophen
- **Mechanism of toxicity**
  - Goes through P-450 system to NAPQI (liver toxic)
  - Glutathione reduces NAPQI to nontoxic metabolites
  - EtOH induces P-450, so increased NAPQI (increased risk APAP toxicity)
  - Alcoholics may also have decreased glutathione
- **Management**
  - If suspected, check acetaminophen level, LFTS, INR
  - Activated charcoal if recent ingestion (< 4 hours)
  - Treat with *N*-acetylcysteine (NAC = glutathione precursor)
  - Try to give as early as possible (prior to ALT increase)

Drug-Induced Liver Injury — Alcohol
- AST:ALT ratio of 2:1
- **Discriminant function** (alcoholic hepatitis): **(4.6 × [PT in sec – PT control]) + (bili/17.1)**
- DF = ≥ 32: prednisolone

Drug-Induced Liver Disease — Others
- <u>Methotrexate</u>
  - Can cause indolent, asymptomatic liver disease that progresses to cirrhosis
  - LFTs often normal after initial treatment despite ongoing liver injury, so may need periodic liver biopsy after certain cumulative doses are reached
- **OCPs**
  - Associated with <u>hepatic adenoma</u> (generally benign but can have malignant transformation)
  - <u>Peliosis hepatis</u> (cystic blood-filled cavities)
  - <u>FNH</u> (focal nodular hyperplasia = nonmalignant hepatic tumor)

NONALCOHOLIC FATTY LIVER DISEASE (NAFLD)

Nonalcoholic Fatty Liver Disease — Overview
- NAFLD = hepatic steatosis with no other etiology (i.e., EtOH)
- Other causes of fat in liver — EtOH, meds (amiodarone), Wilson disease
- NAFLD = **Most common liver disorder in Western countries**
- PMH — obesity, DM, high cholesterol
- Nonalcoholic steatohepatitis (NASH) = **fat and inflammation**
- ALT > AST (in contrast to EtOH liver disease); however, LFTS can be normal
- Diagnosis — often <u>radiologic</u> (i.e., sonogram) but sometimes liver biopsy is done (e.g., diagnosis uncertain, fibrosis concern)
- **Vibration-Controlled Transient Elastography:** vibrates liver to see how stiff, measures fibrosis without biopsy
- **APRI** (AST-to-platelet ratio index) can help identify risk of fibrosis (if <u>low platelets</u>, <u>APRI increases</u>)
- Treatment is not standardized: "weight loss" (e.g., diet/exercise, meds, bariatric endoscopy, surgery)
- Confirm vaccinated for HAV and HBV
- HCC screening if cirrhosis

CIRRHOSIS
- Physical exam findings
  - Hepatosplenomegaly
  - Jaundice
  - Caput medusae (engorged superficial veins near umbilicus)
  - Spider angiomas (cutaneous telangiectasia)
  - Ascites
  - Palmar erythema
  - Asterixis

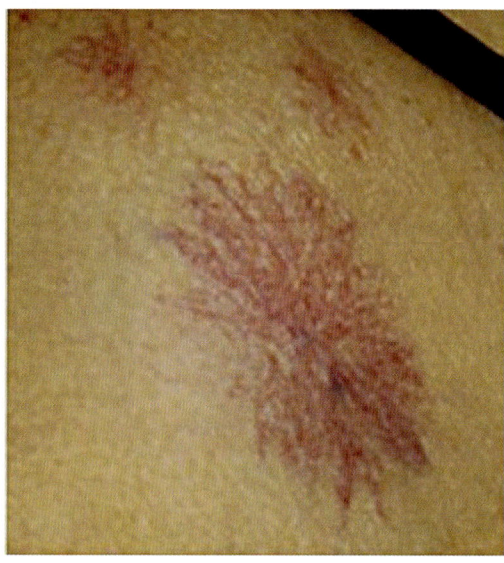

[17]

Cirrhosis Complications — HCC
- 75% have antecedent cirrhosis (so not all!)
- Can be associated with chronic liver disease of any type (e.g., Hep B, Hep C, PBC, hemochromatosis, NAFLD/NASH)
- Generally screen cirrhotic patients with any type of CLD every 6 months
- Generally use sonogram ± AFP (some centers use CT or MRI)
- Also screen some **noncirrhotic Hep B** patients and possibly **Stage 3 Hep C** patients
- Consider new HCC in any cirrhotic who decompensates suddenly with no obvious reason

HCC Treatment
1) Consider resection of localized HCC if Child-Pugh A or B, no portal HTN
2) If Child Class C, consider transplant
3) Transplant possible for **single lesion < 5 cm, or up to 3 lesions < 3 cm** (assuming no extrahepatic disease or vascular invasion — <u>Milan criteria</u>)
4) With advanced disease consider: RFA, transarterial chemoembolization and oral-targeted therapies (sorafenib)

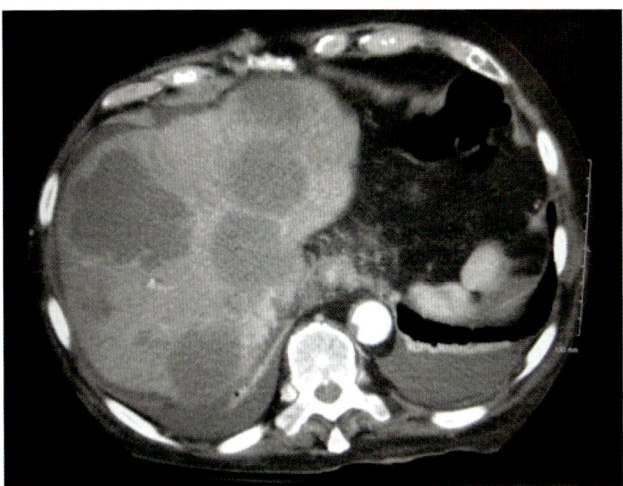

Cirrhosis Complications — Esophageal Variceal Hemorrhage
- 1/3 with varices will bleed, with 30% mortality rate
- Only 50% of bleeding varices stop spontaneously
- Varices **size** important (correlates with risk of bleeding)
- **Hepatic venous pressure gradient (HVPG)** is the difference between the wedged HV pressure and the free hepatic venous pressure
    - = Estimate of pressure gradient between PV and IVC
    - Quantifies degree of portal HTN
- Normal HVPG is < 6 (portal HTN > 6)
    - > 10 mmHg = varices form
    - > 12 mmHg = varices bleed and develop ascites

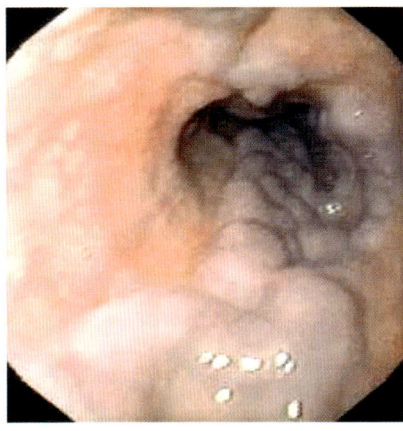

Cirrhosis Complications — Variceal Bleeding
- Primary therapy is **endoscopic banding**
- **Octreotide** is a splanchnic vasoconstrictor (decreases splanchnic blood flow and varices filling) given IV along with endoscopic therapy
- Give all cirrhotics with bleeding prophylactic ABX, which decreases mortality (ceftriaxone, AASLD 2017)
- If can't control bleeding, Blakemore tube and TIPS (transjugular intrahepatic portosystemic shunt — channel between PV and HV)
- Gastric varices harder to treat endoscopically than EV (particularly GV further away from the GEJ in the fundus)

Primary Prophylaxis (to Prevent Bleeding)
- Small EV, Child Class A, no red wale signs = no treatment but need to rescreen periodically
- Small EV, Child Class B or C, or red wale signs = nonselective β-blocker (i.e., nadolol or propranolol)
- Medium or large EV = β-blocker or banding (but banding may be more effective, especially if larger)
- For **secondary prophylaxis** (after acute bleeding is treated) = band to eradication and give β-blockers

Cirrhosis Complications — Hepatic Encephalopathy
- Reversible brain dysfunction in liver failure (ammonia is a neurotoxin that enters PV from GI tract, normally liver clears ammonia)
- Can be due to intrinsic liver issues or vascular (i.e., shunting due to TIPS)
- Serum ammonia levels are far less important than physical exam
- Rule out contributing causes (i.e., **UGIB** [can lead to increased ammonia levels in blood] and **primary peritonitis**)
- Try to avoid restricting dietary protein because many patients already malnourished
- **Lactulose** (goal is 2–3 BMs/day) = decreases ammonia absorption in GI tract
    - Osmotic laxative has "purging" effect and ...
    - Also leads to lower gut pH which inhibits bacterial ammonia (NH_3) production and traps NH_3 as inactive NH_4.
- **Rifaximin** if lactulose not working or not tolerated
- **Neomycin** infrequently used — has nephro-/ototoxicity

Cirrhosis Complications — Hepatorenal Syndrome
- In cirrhosis, get production of vasodilators (i.e., nitric oxide) — leads to activation of renin-angiotensin system with secondary increased renal vascular resistance and decreased renal perfusion
- Must first rule out prerenal azotemia, obstruction, and drugs as etiology of acute renal injury
- Urine Na^+ is very low (often < 10 mEq/day)
- Type 1 = more severe, 50% decrease in creatinine clearance
- Type 2 = less severe
- Management
    - Volume management (IV **albumin** infusion)
    - Potential medications include **midodrine** (α1-agonist vasoconstrictor), **octreotide** (decreases splanchnic flow and increases MAP and SVR), and **terlipressin** (vasopressin analogue, vasoconstrictor)

Cirrhosis Complications — Ascites
- **SAAG (serum-to-ascites albumin gradient) > 1.1** seen with any disease associated with portal HTN (cirrhosis, HF, Budd-Chiari = HV clot, PVT)
- **SAAG < 1.1** = nonportal HTN-related disease — nephrotic syndrome, malignancy, TB (increased lymphocytes), lymphoma (increased triglycerides = chylous ascites)
- **Low total protein** mainly in cirrhosis (fenestrations between capillaries close and protein can't get into ascites), TP < 2.5 g/dL (SAAG > 1.1)
- In general, patients with a TP < 1 g/dL have an increased risk of primary peritonitis (a.k.a. spontaneous bacterial peritonitis; opsonins in high TP ascites can prevent primary peritonitis)

Cirrhosis Complications — Primary Peritonitis
- Fever most common sign; can also see abdominal pain, change in MS
  - Many patients may lack fever and pain
- Peritoneal fluid has > 250 PMN/mL and positive bacterial culture
- You <u>must</u> consider primary peritonitis if there is deterioration in <u>any</u> patient with ascites (and do not forget to consider HCC, too)
- Usual suspects: *E. coli*, then *S. pneumoniae*, then *Klebsiella*
- Treat with broad spectrum ABX, taking into account local resistance patterns
  - IV albumin on day 1 and 3 can <u>decrease mortality</u>
  - <u>Primary prophylaxis</u> (prevent 1st episode) = **TP < 1.5 g/dL** (if concurrent chronic kidney disease [CKD] or liver failure)
  - <u>Primary prophylaxis</u> if **TP < 1.0 g/dL** and in hospital
  - <u>Primary prophylaxis</u> if **bleeding** in setting of portal HTN
  - Give patients with prior bout of primary peritonitis prophylaxis (<u>secondary prophylaxis</u>)
  - Prophylactic antibiotics in general may include daily norfloxacin or trimethoprim/sulfamethoxazole
- Do not confuse with <u>secondary</u> bacterial peritonitis (due to perforated viscus)
- **Ascitic fluid** in <u>secondary</u> bacterial peritonitis
  - Protein > 1 g/dL, frequently > 3 g/dL
  - Glucose < 50 g/dL
  - WBC elevated, often > 5,000
  - Ascites fluid LDH > serum LDH
  - Multiple organisms on Gram stain and culture
- Mortality 100% in patients who do not go to surgery

Treatment of Ascites
- Dietary Na$^+$ (< 2 grams per day)
- Water restriction (if Na$^+$ < 125 mEq/L) and follow daily weight
- **Spironolactone** and **furosemide** (100 mg/40 mg)
  - Avoid NSAIDs (precipitate acute renal injury)
- Presence of peripheral edema can help determine how much fluid can be removed per day — if peripheral edema, can remove more (> 1 liter) because edema fluid can be mobilized to intravascular space
- With large volume paracentesis (≥ 5 L), replace 6–8 g of albumin for each liter of fluid removed
- TIPS can be used in some cases of refractory ascites, which will decompress the portal system

Cirrhosis — Pearls
- **HCC** — Transplant possible for single lesion < 5 cm, or up to 3 lesions < 3 cm (<u>Milan criteria</u>)
- Acute variceal **bleeding** — <u>banding</u> and <u>octreotide</u>
- **Antibiotics** <u>decrease mortality</u> in bleeding cirrhotics
- Ascites: **SAAG > 1.1** means <u>portal HTN</u> associated
- **Primary peritonitis**: > 250 PMNs
- **Primary peritonitis**: IV albumin on day 1 and 3 can <u>decrease mortality</u>

HEREDITARY LIVER DISEASE

Hereditary Liver Disease — Hemochromatosis
- Inherited form of iron overload (common = 10% Caucasians in U.S. heterozygote carriers)
- Distinguish from secondary iron overload (e.g., SCD/thalassemia [multiple transfusions])
- Type 1: Associated with mutations in *HFE* gene (also rarer forms Type 2–4)
- *HFE* is autosomal recessive — increased gut iron absorption
- Iron in liver (cirrhosis, HCC), pancreas (diabetes), skin (bronzing), heart (CM), hypogonadism (infertility), arthritis (2nd and 3rd MCP joints, wrists)
- HCC (usually if cirrhosis) = very high (> 20-fold risk) and **#1 cause of mortality**
- Screen with iron panel (AASLD): **≥ 45% iron sat** and/or **elevated ferritin** (ferritin above ULN)
- Confirm with HFE genotype (*C282Y/C282Y* or compound heterozygote *C282Y/H63D* [less severe phenotype])
- Liver biopsy (not always required) — generally ordered when elevated LFTS or ferritin > 1000 (more to look for fibrosis)
- Tx: phlebotomy in patients with evidence of iron overload (on labs) or organ damage with goal of ferritin level 50–100 ng/mL
- Consider screening family members

Hereditary Liver Disease — Wilson Disease
- Autosomal recessive
- Can't incorporate copper into ceruloplasmin and excrete into bile — copper accumulates in body tissues — especially liver
- Typically presents as liver disease and/or neurologic/psychiatric dysfunction in adolescents (between 10 and 25 years of age), but can be seen in 70s
  1) **Serum ceruloplasmin is <u>low</u>**
  2) Accumulation of copper in liver — inflammation
  3) Serum and **urinary copper** are <u>high</u>
  4) **Kayser-Fleischer rings** are <u>pathognomonic</u> (slit-lamp exam) — seen in > 95% of patients who have neuropsychiatric symptoms

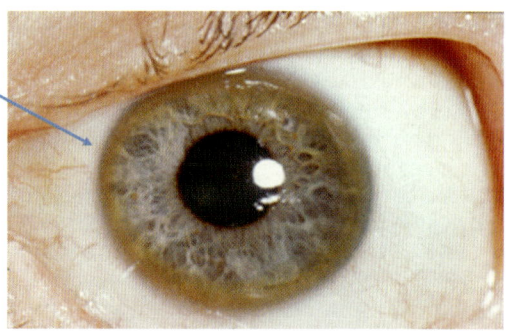

[18]

Kayser-Fleischer ring. Copper deposition at the corneoscleral junction

Hereditary Liver Disease — Wilson Disease

- Children more likely to present with liver disease, older patients neuropsychiatric
- Other findings: increased AST/ALT ratio (hemolysis — copper may damage RBC membrane), low ALP, hypouricemia
- Liver Bx confirms diagnosis with high copper level in the liver, but not always needed (i.e., if KF rings present)
- Tx is a 2-phase process:
  - **Phase 1: Chelation** — binds Cu and excretes into urine with <u>penicillamine</u> (inactivates pyridoxine/vitamin B_6 — so give pyridoxine supplement) or <u>trientine</u> (less neuro SEs)
    - Zinc (3rd option) — prevents copper gut absorption
  - **Phase 2: Maintenance** therapy with 1 of the 3 drugs listed above, along with low-copper diet (avoid nuts, chocolate, shellfish, mushrooms)
- The only treatment for fulminant Wilson disease is transplant
- Consider genetic testing in family members

Hereditary Liver Disease — α_1-Antitrypsin Deficiency

- Autosomal co-dominant transmission (another example of this type of inheritance is blood type)
- AAT is a serine protease (i.e., elastase) <u>inhibitor</u> that folds and is not released from liver (AAT damages liver = chronic liver disease)
- Leads to lung disease (elastase not inhibited so digests elastin in lung)
- Check **serum α_1-antitrypsin level** (<u>low</u>)
- Check genotype (normal allele is "M"; "ZZ" genotype most commonly associated with disease)
- Liver biopsy — PAS+, diastase-resistant globules
- Patient may require liver transplantation

Liver Disease during Pregnancy

- **Hyperemesis gravidarum:** T1; hypovolemia and weight loss
- **Intrahepatic cholestasis of pregnancy:** T2 and early T3; pruritus, elevated ALP, increased serum bile acids
  - Can lead to fetal morbidity and mortality
  - Treat with ursodiol (nontoxic bile acid — dilutes out toxic bile acids); possible early delivery
- **HELLP syndrome** — often part of preeclampsia: HTN + proteinuria
  - Develops at 28–36 weeks with hemolysis, elevated liver enzymes, low platelets
  - Often requires prompt delivery
- **Acute fatty liver of pregnancy:** most frequently T3; rapid development of liver failure and encephalopathy (liver manifestations can be more severe than HELLP)
  - Prompt delivery

Liver Transplant

- Indications — cirrhosis with complications, HCC, ALF, others (i.e., Wilson disease)
- ALF — emergent transplant
- CLD — start evaluation MELD > 10; **candidates once MELD ≥ 15** (risk/benefit ratio generally becomes favorable at MELD 15)
- MELD exception points can be given to transplant at a lower MELD (i.e., HCC)
- Contraindications to transplant include: severe cardiopulmonary disease, metastatic HCC, sepsis

NUTRITION

Nutrition — Overview

- **Water-soluble vitamins:** generally not stored in the body and can sometimes deplete quickly
  - Vitamin C, vitamin B_1 (thiamin), vitamin B_2 (riboflavin), vitamin B_3 (niacin), pantothenic acid, vitamin B_6 (pyridoxine), folic acid, vitamin B_{12} (exception; can be stored in liver), biotin
- Fat-soluble vitamins
  - Vitamin A (retinol), vitamin D, vitamin E (tocopherols), vitamin K
- Others (e.g., **electrolytes** [magnesium, potassium], **trace elements** [iron, selenium, copper, chromium, zinc])

AR 16

A 46-year-old executive had her gallbladder removed 2 days ago after presenting with RUQ pain and fever. You are consulted by the surgery resident after the patient develops ophthalmoplegia and nystagmus.

AR 16A
What likely led to this condition?

A. Side effect of anesthesia during surgery
B. IV dextrose prior to giving thiamine in an alcoholic (closet drinker)
C. Use of tricyclic antidepressants
D. Urinary tract infection

Answer:_____

AR 16B
What is the treatment?

A. Give thiamine 500 mg IM or IV immediately.
B. Give pyridoxine immediately.
C. High-flow oxygen, mannitol, and consult a neurologist.
D. Give thiamine 500 mg slow-drip over 6–8 hours.

Answer:_____

Specific Deficiencies — B Vitamins

- **Vitamin B$_1$ (thiamine):** can occur quickly, weeks to months
  - Wet beriberi — HF
  - Dry beriberi — neuropathies
  - Wernicke encephalopathy (confusion, ataxia, oculomotor dysfunction)
  - Korsakoff syndrome (memory loss, confabulation — make up info they can't remember)
- **Vitamin B$_2$ (riboflavin)** — angular cheilitis, glossitis
- **Vitamin B$_3$ (niacin)** — pellagra (dermatitis, photosensitivity, diarrhea, dementia)
- **Vitamin B$_6$ (pyridoxine)** — cheilitis, nasolabial dermatitis

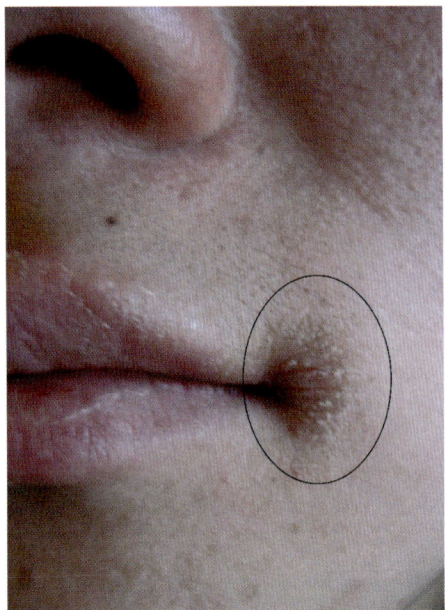

[19]

Angular cheilitis (inflammation corner of mouth)

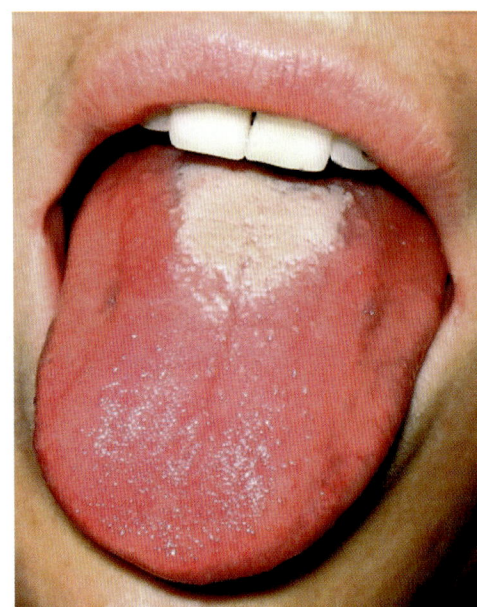

[20]

Glossitis

Niacin (B$_3$) Deficiency

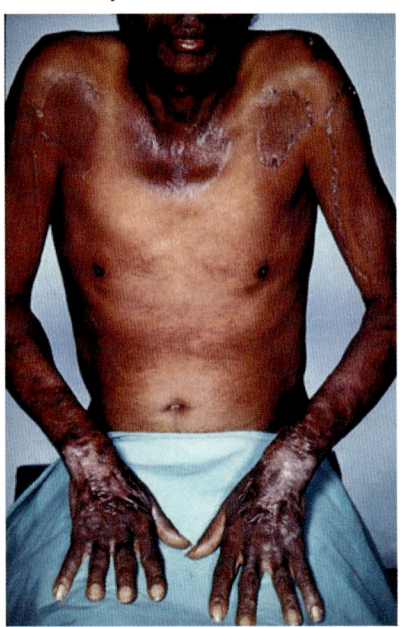

[21]

Pellagra

- The 3 Ds …
  1) Dermatitis
  2) Diarrhea
  3) Dementia

Specific Vitamin Deficiencies — B$_{12}$ (Cobalamin)
- Food-cobalamin complex hydrolyzed by stomach acid
- Binds to R protein in stomach — this complex is then hydrolyzed
- B$_{12}$ binds to IF (secreted by parietal cells) and absorbed in TI
- Causes: **low stomach acid** (pernicious anemia, PPI), **celiac** (absorption), **CP**, **SBBO** (bacteria compete for B$_{12}$), **TI disease**, **diet** (vegans)

B$_{12}$ Deficiency
- See increased homocysteine and methylmalonic acid on labs, macrocytic anemia
- Peripheral neuropathies
- <u>Subacute combined degeneration</u> (**dorsal** [sensory = proprioception/position sense and vibration] and **lateral** [motor] columns of spinal cord)
- Can take months to deplete due to increased body stores

Specific Deficiencies — Folate
- Alcoholics, meds (sulfasalazine and methotrexate interfere with folate metabolism), pregnancy
- Limited body stores — can be depleted in weeks, in contrast to B$_{12}$
- Normal MMA but increased homocysteine
- Macrocytic anemia

Specific Deficiencies — Vitamin C
- Vitamin C deficiency causes **scurvy**
- Issues with collagen and connective tissue
  - Petechiae, ecchymoses, purpura, perifollicular hemorrhage (fragile collagen in vessels)
  - Gingivitis
  - Poor wound healing
  - Hyperkeratotic papules around hair follicles
- **Vitamin C overdose:** Increases incidence of oxalate renal stones, false-negative stool guaiac, and can possibly lead to iron overload (vitamin C helps with iron absorption)

Fat-Soluble Vitamins
- **Vitamin A**
  - <u>Deficiency</u> associated with decreased night vision, rash
  - <u>Chronic toxicity</u> associated with liver disease/cirrhosis (accumulates in liver stellate cells) and bone disease (increased fracture risk)
- **Vitamin D**
  - Fatty fish, synthesized in dermis from sunlight
  - Hydroxylated to 25 vitamin D in liver (blood test), 1-25 vitamin D in kidney
  - Calcium absorption gut and bone metabolism
  - <u>Deficiency</u> — rickets (children) and osteomalacia (adults)
  - <u>Toxicity</u> — results in increased calcium absorption from the bowel, hypercalcemia, and hypercalciuria
- **Vitamin E**
  - Antioxidant; protects cell membranes
  - <u>Deficiency</u> — neuropathy, ataxia, hemolytic anemia
  - <u>Excess vitamin E</u> — associated with increased all-cause mortality (so be careful recommending supplementation)
  - Can cause marked potentiation of oral anticoagulants
- **Vitamin K**
  - Green vegetables
  - Involved in clotting factor activity (2, 7, 9, 10, prothrombin) and bone metabolism
  - <u>Deficiency</u> in **liver disease** (vitamin K clotting factors synthesized in liver), **malabsorption**, **antibiotics** (can kill bacteria that help to synthesize vitamin K)
  - Bleeding, bruising, increased INR
  - Also associated with low bone density

Nutrition — Other
- **Magnesium:** deficiency can be seen with PPI use — tetany and seizures
- **Copper:** deficiency associated with microcytic/hypochromic anemia (can be confused with IDA and if give iron, can make anemia worse — copper competes with iron for absorption)
- **Zinc:** deficiency associated with impaired taste, perioral, perianal, and acral (toes and fingers) dermatitis
- **Selenium:** deficiency associated with cardiomyopathy (Keshan disease in China), skeletal muscle disorders
- **Iron:** deficiency due to bleeding or decreased absorption (celiac, bariatric surgery) — see hypochromic/microcytic anemia

Nutrition Pearls — Rapid-Fire Associations
- **Thiamine:** Beriberi, Wernicke encephalopathy, and Korsakoff syndrome
- **Niacin:** pellagra (the 3 Ds — dermatitis, dementia, diarrhea)
- **Vitamin B$_{12}$:** subacute combined degeneration
- **Vitamin C:** scurvy
- **Vitamin A deficiency:** decreased night vision
- **Magnesium deficiency:** tetany and seizures (i.e., with PPI)

AUDIENCE RESPONSE ANSWERS AND EXPLANATORY INFORMATION

Audience Response 1
D. Achalasia
Clinical presentation and absence of gastric air bubble suggest achalasia (impairment of swallowed air into the stomach). Esophageal cancer would also be in the differential diagnosis; however, adenocarcinoma would have a more rapid onset than 2 years, and the patient would be older.

AR 2
A. EGD with biopsies of the esophagus
Rule out eosinophilic esophagitis, which is common in this age group and also associated with allergies, including seasonal allergies.

AR 3
E. Stop doxycycline and give reassurance.
EGD if severe symptoms, atypical symptoms (hematemesis, prolonged symptoms [i.e., > 7 days]). Doxycycline is commonly associated with pill esophagitis.

AR 4
C. Pantoprazole 40 mg PO bid
- Extraintestinal manifestation of GERD warrants PPI trial to help with both diagnosis and treatment
- EGD guidelines vary — discuss with GI doctor need for EGD (obviously alarm signals but also chronic symptoms, risk factors for Barrett's and cancer including older age, male, smoking, obesity)

AR 5
A. Repeat exam in 3–5 years and switch to PPI daily.
PPIs can better control heartburn and can help decrease dysplasia and cancer risk in Barrett's. Ensure that 4-quadrant surveillance biopsies were in fact done and not just 1 or 2 biopsies to establish the diagnosis of Barrett's.

AR 6
A. Barium swallow
- Clinical presentation suggestive of Zenker's; will see barium collect in diverticula
- EGD can be potentially dangerous due to risk of perforation
- EGD would be indicated if concern for other diagnosis, alarm symptoms, or concern for cancer

AR 7A
D. *H. pylori* testing and treatment if positive
This patient is young, with no alarm symptoms.

AR 7B

C. *H. pylori* fecal antigen

Serum antibody can remain + after successful treatment. EGD with biopsies for HP can also be done in some cases but is not needed in this particular patient.

AR 8

D. Abdominal x-ray

Upright chest and abdominal films are a reasonable first test to do quickly. If no free air on AXR or concern for other diagnosis, may require alternative imaging including CT scan.

AR 9

A. Consider discharge in a.m. if no further bleeding.

Clean-based ulcers have low risk of rebleeding and do not require endoscopic therapy.

AR 10

D. Infliximab at 5 mg/kg induction and maintenance
- CDAI estimated (but not enough data points from case to calculate 100% accurately) to be at least 300 (moderate-severe)
- Active inflammation on colonoscopy
- Indication for biologic treatment
- The other therapies can be used in Crohn's in some cases but would be less effective in this clinical scenario
- With regard to antibiotics specifically, there is little role for these agents in UC as opposed to CD

AR 11

D. All of the above
- Need to assess for TB and HBV prior to treatment with immunosuppressing medications
- 6-MP and biologics are steroid-sparing agents; hence steroids should be tapered off when on these medications
- Try to vaccinate for HBV prior to starting immunosuppressives given risk of nonresponse when immunosuppressed

AR 12

C. Stool for *C. difficile*

It is critical to rule out *C. difficile* in IBD patients. *C. difficile* is a common complication of IBD and can lead to poor outcomes in IBD patients, including increasing the risk for needing a colectomy.

AR 13

B. Microscopic colitis

Normal-looking mucosa is typical of microscopic colitis. Can see 2 subtypes:
1) Lymphocytic colitis (increased intraepithelial lymphocytes)
2) Collagenous colitis (thickened subepithelial collagen band)

AR 14

B. MRCP

MRCP is the best choice of the listed options. Reasonable to proceed with MRCP given elevated liver tests which can suggest gallstone pancreatitis.
- If evidence of cholangitis, ERCP might be required
- EGD would not be helpful
- Cholecystectomy would not be indicated until more objective information is obtained

AR 15

D. PSC, so you order an MRCP.
- MRCP would be the best option to assess for PSC (less invasive than ERCP), particularly given history of IBD
- Because gallstone disease is so common, a sonogram may also be reasonable as a first step to assess for gallstone disease, including choledocholithiasis
- Viral hepatitis would also be in the differential

AR 16A

B. IV dextrose prior to giving thiamine in an alcoholic (closet drinker)

Ophthalmoplegia and nystagmus would be typical of thiamine deficiency.

AR 16B

A. Give thiamine 500 mg IM or IV immediately.
- Immediate (not "slow drip") parenteral therapy is needed and can be followed afterwards by PO therapy
- Intravenous dextrose may precipitate cardiovascular collapse and lactic acidosis in thiamine-deficient patients (due to complex interplay of pyruvate, glucose, and the TCA cycle — see reference below)

ebmconsult.com/articles/thiamine-administration-before-iv-glucose-alcoholics

[1]   James W. Smith, MD

[2]   *American Journal of Gastroenterology*. 2013.

[3] Farrokhi F and Vaezi M. Idiopathic (primary) achalasia. *Orphanet Journal of Rare Diseases*. 2007, 2:38.

[4]   Ghosh S. University of Cincinnati.

[5]   Manningmbd https://creativecommons.org/licenses/by-sa/3.0/legalcode

[6]   Sharma P, Shaheen NJ, et al. Clinical Practice Update: Endoscopic treatment of Barrett's esophagus with dysplasia and/or early cancer. Gastroenterology. 2019 Nov 12. pii: S0016-5085(19)41537-0. doi: 10.1053/j.gastro.2019.09.051

[7]   Dionigi G, et al. *World Journal of Surgical Oncology*. 2006; 4:17 [doi:10.1186/1477-7819-4-17]

[8]   gi.org/guideline/management-of-dyspepsia-2/

[9]   Lanza FL, et al. *The American Journal of Gastroenterology.* volume 104, pages 728–738 (2009)

[10]   James Heilman, MD

[11]   James Heilman, MD

[12]   Ed Uthman, MD [CC BY-SA 2.0 (https://creativecommons.org/licenses/by-sa/2.0)], via Wikimedia Commons

[13]   Robert Knapp [CC BY-SA 3.0 (https://creativecommons.org/licenses/by-sa/3.0)], from Wikimedia Commons)

[14]   Herbert L. Fred, MD and Hendrik A. van Dijk [CC BY 2.0 (https://creativecommons.org/licenses/by/2.0)], via Wikimedia Commons

[15]   Bruce Blaus

[16]   E M Said, MD

[17]   Herbert L. Fred, MD and Hendrik A. van Dijk

[18]   Herbert L. Fred, MD, Hendrik A. van Dijk [CC BY 3.0 (https://creativecommons.org/licenses/by/3.0)], via Wikimedia Commons

[19]   James Heilman, MD https://creativecommons.org/licenses/by-sa/3.0/legalcode

[20]   Martin Kronawitter https://creativecommons.org/licenses/by-sa/2.5/legalcode

[21]   Herbert L. Fred, MD, Hendrik A. van Dijk [CC BY-SA 3.0 (https://creativecommons.org/licenses/by-sa/3.0)], via Wikimedia Commons

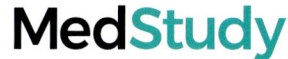

INTERNAL MEDICINE REVIEW

General Internal Medicine

Presented by

Leonard A. Mankin, MD

GENERAL INTERNAL MEDICINE

TABLE OF CONTENTS

General Internal Medicine Outline
- Drug Interactions and Important Side Effects
- Geriatrics
- Urology and Sexual Health
- Ethics
- Perioperative Care
- Preventive Medicine
- Overdose and Poisoning
- Eyes, Ears, Nose, Throat
- Pregnancy and Women's Health

DRUG INTERACTIONS AND IMPORTANT SIDE EFFECTS

Drug-Drug Interactions
- Account for ~3% of hospitalizations in U.S.
- A few drugs account for majority of problems
- ABIM wants you to recognize drug-drug interactions and important adverse effects of commonly used drugs

Warfarin
- Mechanisms for ↑ INR
  - Altered intestinal flora (↓ intestinal vitamin K synthesis)
    - TMP/SMX
    - Metronidazole
    - Macrolides
    - Fluoroquinolones
  - Decreased breakdown by liver (cytochrome P450)
    - Statins, gemfibrozil
    - Amiodarone
    - Azole antifungals
    - SSRIs
- Mechanisms for ↓ INR
  - Dietary vitamin K (leafy green vegetables)
  - Rifampin (induces catabolism of warfarin)

Warfarin and Analgesics
- NSAIDs increase risk of bleeding in patients on warfarin, without raising the INR
- Acetaminophen, used regularly, increases INR
  - > 9,100 mg/week (325 mg q 6 hours) has led to 10× risk of having INR > 6.0[1]
  - Small RCTs suggest ↑ INR (~ 1.0) if using > 2 g/day for > 3 days[2]
- No interaction with opioids and warfarin

Direct Oral Anticoagulants (DOACs)
- Advantages
  - Significantly fewer drug-drug interactions than warfarin
  - No drug-food interactions
  - No need to measure INR
- Concerns
  - Drugs that ↑ bleeding risk while on DOACs:
    - Azole antifungals (ketoconazole, fluconazole)
    - Amiodarone

Other Common Drug-Drug Interactions
- PDE-5 inhibitors + nitrates
  - Phosphodiesterase-5 (PDE-5) inhibitors (sildenafil, tadalafil, vardenafil) potentiate the hypotensive effects of nitrates
- Lithium + hydrochlorothiazide
  - Combination increases retention of lithium by the kidneys, causing lithium toxicity
- Clonidine + β-blockers
  - If clonidine is withdrawn, unopposed α-receptor stimulation can cause fatal rebound hypertension
- Gabapentin/Pregabalin + opioids or benzos
  - May cause respiratory suppression, esp. in older patients, COPD

Hyperkalemia — Drug Induced
- ↓ Aldosterone production
  - ACEIs/ARBs
  - NSAIDs
- Aldosterone resistance
  - K^+-sparing diuretics (spironolactone/eplerenone)
  - TMP/SMX

Trimethoprim / Sulfamethoxazole
- Hyperkalemia has been reported in older patients and those with HIV
- Mechanism: Acts like amiloride, blocking the sensitive Na^+ channels in the distal collecting tubule, reducing renal K^+ excretion
- Use TMP/SMX with caution in patients with baseline elevated K^+ or who are taking ACEs/ARBs/spironolactone

Amiodarone and the Thyroid
- Hypothyroidism (5% overt, 25% subclinical)
  - Increased iodine load suppresses thyroxine production
- Hyperthyroidism (3–5%)
  - Direct toxic effects on thyroid gland, leading to thyroiditis
  - Iodine uptake in autonomous functioning nodule or Graves'
- Important to monitor TSH every few months while on amiodarone

The Patient with Increased Thyroxine Requirements
- Assess compliance
- Malabsorption
  - Celiac disease
  - Chelating agents
    - Iron, sucralfate, PPI, aluminum, calcium, and magnesium
- Increased T_4 catabolism
  - Phenytoin, CBZ, rifampin, cholestyramine
- Iodine overload
  - Amiodarone

Side Effects of Statins
- Myalgias: 5–18%
- Rhabdomyolysis (rare): 0.1%
- Abnormal LFTs: 0.5–3% (usually reversible)
- Liver failure: 0.0001%

Major Interactions with Statins

- Certain drugs ↓ metabolism and increase risk of myopathy
  - Amiodarone
  - Clarithromycin
  - Azole antifungals (keto, fluc, itra)
  - Grapefruit juice (≥ 8 oz/day)
  - Fibrates (gemfibrozil >> fenofibrate)
  - Calcium blockers (amlodipine or diltiazem) have a specific interaction with simvastatin
- In general, must lower dose of statin or change to a statin that is metabolized by different enzyme system (e.g., pravastatin or rosuvastatin)

QT Interval Prolongation

- People on ≥ 2 QT-prolonging agents are at highest risk for torsades de pointes, especially in the setting of low magnesium or low potassium
- Common agents
  - Antiarrhythmics (e.g., amiodarone, dronedarone, sotalol)
  - Antipsychotics (e.g., quetiapine, ziprasidone)
  - Antimicrobials (quinolones, macrolides, antiretrovirals)
  - Antidepressants (TCAs, fluoxetine, citalopram, escitalopram)
  - Methadone
  - Triptans

Serotonin Syndrome

- Triad of symptoms
  1) Mental status changes (agitation, delirium, disorientation)
  2) Autonomic hyperactivity (diaphoresis, hyperthermia, tachycardia, HTN, diarrhea)
  3) Neuromuscular abnormalities (hyperreflexia, clonus, rigidity)
- May be due to overdose of a single drug (e.g., SSRI), but more often associated with drug-drug interactions of ≥ 2 serotonergic drugs; common drugs include:
  - SSRIs
  - SNRIs
  - TCAs
  - Trazodone
  - Tramadol
  - Triptans
  - Cocaine
  - Methamphetamine
  - Fentanyl

Most Important Drug Causes of Hyponatremia

- Hydrochlorothiazide
- SSRIs
- Carbamazepine
- TMP/SMX

Drugs That Increase Serum Uric Acid

- Diuretics, especially thiazides
- Niacin
- Cyclosporine

Audience Response 1

A 66-year-old houseless man is diagnosed with TB. He is started on a 4-drug regimen (isoniazid, rifampin, pyrazinamide, and ethambutol).

PMH: atrial fibrillation, hyperlipidemia, hypothyroidism, depression

Meds: warfarin, metoprolol, atorvastatin, levothyroxine, and citalopram

Which of the following adjustments would be most appropriate for his medication regimen?

A. Increase warfarin and increase levothyroxine.
B. Increase warfarin and decrease levothyroxine.
C. Decrease warfarin and increase levothyroxine.
D. Decrease warfarin and decrease levothyroxine.

Answer:_____

AR 2

You get called with a panic lab value (INR 5.8) for a 52-year-old woman with PMH of HTN, DM, and AFib. When you review her records, her INR has been stable between 2.0 and 3.0 for the last 8 months. She is finishing a 7-day course of an antibiotic prescribed by an ED physician for "bronchitis"; she does not recall the name.

Meds: warfarin 5 mg daily, metformin 1,000 mg bid, HCTZ 25 mg daily

Which antibiotic was she likely prescribed?

A. Linezolid
B. Azithromycin
C. Cefixime
D. Cephalexin
E. TMP/SMX

Answer:_____

AR 3

You are seeing a 38-year-old woman in clinic with a prosthetic mitral valve. Her main complaint is severe bruising with minimal trauma, if any. INR 6 weeks ago was 2.9; today's INR is 6.9.

Which of the following, when taken on a daily basis, could explain her increased INR?

A. Acetaminophen
B. Calcium carbonate
C. OCP
D. Famotidine
E. Docusate sodium

Answer:_____

AR 4

A 60-year-old man comes in complaining of aching in his shoulders and thighs.

He is currently taking benazepril, amlodipine, warfarin, omeprazole, simvastatin, and loratadine.

Which of these drugs is most likely contributing to his symptoms?

A. Loratadine
B. Amlodipine
C. Omeprazole
D. Warfarin
E. Benazepril

Answer:_____

AR 5

A 73-year-old man with bipolar disorder, CAD, HTN, and systolic HF presents for syncope. He has the following rhythm strip:

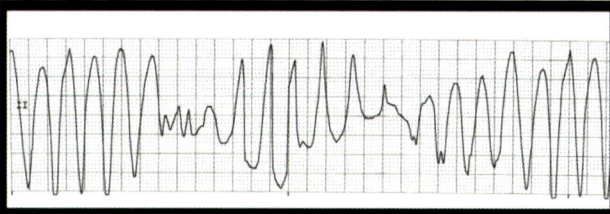

Which of the following medications most likely contributed to his arrhythmia?

A. Metoprolol and clonidine
B. Lithium and HCTZ
C. Amlodipine and simvastatin
D. Quetiapine and methadone
E. Sildenafil and isosorbide

Answer:_____

AR 6

A 63-year-old woman with bipolar disorder, HTN, CKD, and hyperlipidemia has blood pressures consistently > 160/90.

Her most recent labs showed a potassium of 5.3 and creatinine of 1.9.

Meds: atorvastatin, lithium, metoprolol

Which of the following medications would be reasonable to add for her hypertension?

A. Clonidine
B. Lisinopril
C. Spironolactone
D. Amlodipine
E. HCTZ

Answer:_____

GERIATRICS

- Osteoporosis
- Falls
- Insomnia
- Dementia and Delirium
- Urology and Sexual Dysfunction

Rule #1
for Geriatrics Exam Questions
If you can stop a medication, do it!!!!

Rule #2
for Geriatrics Exam Questions
If you can't stop a med, then order physical therapy.

NSAIDs in Older Patients
- 2017 systematic review
  - 8.7% of hospitalizations in older patients were due to adverse drug reactions, with NSAIDs being the most common etiology
- Older patients at highest risk of GI bleeding, renal impairment, and heart failure from NSAIDs

OSTEOPOROSIS

Osteoporosis — Prevention
- Calcium and vitamin D in premenopausal women are controversial
  - USPSTF recommends against unless patient lives in institutional setting
  - NOF recommends supplementation
- 2014 Cochrane review
  - Ca^{2+} + vit D reduced hip fracture risk: 1 fewer hip fracture per 1,000 older adults per year (9 if high risk)
- Vitamin D alone may have a role in preventing falls

Risk Factors for Osteoporosis
- Age > 65
- History of a fragility fracture — personal, or in a 1st degree relative
- Weight < 127 lb or BMI < 21
- Current smoker
- Alcohol intake of > 2 drinks daily
- Menopause before 40 years of age
- Currently or previously treated with > 3 months of steroid therapy at a dosage of ≥ 5 mg/day of prednisone
- Malabsorption

Who Should Get a DXA Scan?
- Women ≥ 65 years of age
- Postmenopausal women < 65 years of age with additional risk factors
- NOF also recommends screening in:
  - Men > 70 years of age (or > 50 years of age with risk factors)
  - Men and postmenopausal women > 50 who have had a fracture
- USPSTF has no recommendation for or against screening men who have not had a fracture

Medications and Osteoporosis
- Glucocorticoids
- Antiseizure medications (phenobarbital, phenytoin, carbamazepine)
- Drugs associated with hypogonadism (depot medroxyprogesterone, GnRHs, aromatase inhibitors, methotrexate, chronic opioids)
- Thyroid overreplacement
- Cyclosporine
- Lithium
- PPIs

Diseases to Screen for Osteoporosis
- Gastrointestinal diseases
  - Inflammatory bowel disease, celiac disease, gastric bypass, or gastrectomy
- Endocrine diseases
  - Primary hyperparathyroidism, Cushing syndrome, hypogonadism, hyperthyroidism
- Chronic kidney disease/failure
- Prolonged bed rest or wheelchair bound
- Rheumatoid arthritis, SLE
- Anorexia nervosa

WHO Diagnostic Categories — BMD-Based Definition of Osteoporosis / Osteopenia
- A T-score represents the number of standard deviations the bone mineral density (BMD) measurement is above or below the young-normal mean bone mineral density

Condition	T-Score (SD)
Normal	≥ −1.0
Osteopenia	Between −1.0 and −2.5
Osteoporosis	≤ −2.5
Severe osteoporosis	≤ −2.5 with fracture(s)

Osteoporosis — Therapy
- Calcium, vitamin D, weight-bearing exercise, and fall risk assessment should be part of all prevention and treatment plans
- Target 1,000–1,200 mg calcium, 800–1,000 units vitamin D per day **including dietary intake**
- USPSTF recommends against low-dose supplements (< 1,000 mg/< 400 units)

Who Should Receive Drug Therapy for Osteoporosis?
- Postmenopausal women and men > 50 years of age with these findings:
  - Any hip or vertebral compression fracture
  - T-score < −2.5 SD
  - T-score between −1.0 and −2.5 **and** 10-year probability of hip fracture ≥ 3% **or** 10-year probability of any major osteoporosis-related fracture ≥ 20% based on FRAX

Osteoporosis — Therapy
- Bisphosphonates
  - Alendronate, ibandronate, risedronate, zoledronate (IV)
- Calcitonin: 2nd line therapy only; helpful for acute pain of osteoporotic fractures (injectable form)
- Teriparatide (SQ PTH): useful for those who are at high risk and cannot tolerate bisphosphonates
- Denosumab: injectable anti-RANKL therapy; effective, but $$$
- Raloxifene
- Estrogens (HRT): Should no longer be used solely for prevention or treatment of osteoporosis

Osteoporosis Therapy — Duration
- Controversial topic!
- Ongoing bisphosphonate therapy comes with risk of complications, namely osteonecrosis of the jaw and transverse long bone fractures
- Bisphosphonate therapy should be continued for at least 5 years
- At 5-year mark, reassess fracture risk
  - Low risk (stable BMD, no prior fractures), then can stop medication and monitor
  - High risk (BMD < −3.5, prior fractures), continue medication

AR 7
A 56-year-old postmenopausal woman presents with concern for osteoporosis because her 50-year-old sister-in-law just fractured her hip. The patient has never been on HRT. She is an obese, nonsmoking woman without any underlying medical problems. She has no perimenopausal symptoms.

She has no family history of osteoporosis.

What would you recommend for her?

A. DXA scan
B. Estrogen/Progestin HRT
C. Alendronate
D. Encourage weight-bearing exercise.
E. Raloxifene

Answer:_____

AR 8
A 65-year-old woman has a screening DXA scan. She has no family history of osteoporosis. She drinks alcohol occasionally and does not smoke. PMH negative except for DVT while on oral contraceptives.

Meds: calcium 1,000 mg/vit D 800 IU daily

DXA scan: T −2.7 at hip, −1.8 at the vertebra

What would you recommend?

A. Teriparatide
B. Alendronate
C. Raloxifene
D. Calcitonin
E. Estrogen/progestin HRT

Answer:_____

AR 9

A 72-year-old woman with history of osteoporosis presents to follow up on her DXA scan results. She has taken alendronate 70 mg weekly for the past 6 years.

She had a DXA scan 6 years ago with a T-score of −1.8 at the hip and −1.6 at the spine with a FRAX 10-year risk of hip fracture of 3.5%. Her current DXA scan shows a T-score of −1.9 at the hip and −1.7 at the spine.

What would you recommend?

A. Continue alendronate.
B. Switch to raloxifene.
C. Switch to teriparatide.
D. Switch to denosumab.
E. Stop alendronate.

Answer:_____

AR 10

A 63-year-old woman with a family history of osteoporosis presents with a vertebral fracture. She has a workup that reveals no complicating causes other than osteoporosis. Other history includes Type 2 DM, prior DVT, and severe reflux esophagitis with stricture in the past. Her exam is unremarkable except for spinal tenderness over T7.

What would you recommend?

A. Teriparatide
B. Alendronate
C. Estrogen
D. Zoledronate
E. Kyphoplasty

Answer:_____

FALLS

- Increasing age increases fall risk
  (25% at 70 years of age, 50% at 80 years of age)
- Risks for falls
  - Prior falls
  - Poor vision
  - Unsteady gait
  - Lower-extremity weakness
  - Medications
  - Cognitive impairment
  - Musculoskeletal and cardiovascular disease

Medications and Fall Risk

- Benzodiazepines
- Antihypertensives
- Antidepressants (especially tricyclics)
- Antipsychotics
- Opioids
- Sleep medications

INSOMNIA

- A very common and vexing issue in older adults
- Look for conditions that could be responsible (pain, nocturia, restless legs, dyspnea, OSA, anxiety)
- SSRIs/SNRIs may cause insomnia in up to 20% of patients
- Stimulants, corticosteroids, diuretics should be administered early in the day
- Counsel on avoidance of caffeine, alcohol, and nicotine

Insomnia — Treatment

- **CBT for insomnia (CBT-I) is 1st line therapy** — safer than medication with superior outcomes, but limited availability
- Ideally, medications should be used only to supplement CBT-I
- Benzodiazepines and non-BZD "Z drugs" effective, but associated with falls, amnesia, somnambulism, dementia, and habituation
- Low-dose trazodone or gabapentin are reasonable alternatives to habit-forming drugs (off-label)
- Anticholinergics (antihistamines, tricyclics, neuroleptics), including OTC sleep aids, have many adverse effects
- Ramelteon (melatonin agonist) seems safe and may be helpful; melatonin untested but might be worth a try
- α-Blockers useful for PTSD with nightmares

RESTLESS LEG SYNDROME

- Leg discomfort ± paresthesias at rest that:
  - Is worse at night
  - Causes a strong urge to move the legs
  - Is relieved by movement
- Occurs more frequently with advancing age; 20% in those > 80 years of age

Restless Leg Syndrome — Treatment

- **Check for Fe deficiency in all patients — Tx with iron only if deficiency present**
- Gabapentin or pregabalin are now considered first line therapy
- Dopaminergic agonists (pramipexole, ropinirole) may be considered, but have the following downsides:
  - Augmentation — increased symptom severity with ongoing use (earlier onset, higher intensity, spread to other areas of the body)
  - Compulsive behaviors — pathologic gambling, eating, shopping, and hypersexuality

DEMENTIA AND DELIRIUM

Dementia

- Chronic, progressive cognitive deterioration
- Differential diagnosis
  - Alzheimer's (80%)
  - Multiinfarct
  - Lewy body (sleep disturbances, hallucinations, parkinsonian features)
  - Parkinson's
  - Depression (pseudodementia)

Alzheimer's Treatment

- Mild/Moderate disease: Cholinesterase inhibitors (donepezil, rivastigmine) are 1st line and may slow the progression of decline
- Cholinesterase inhibitors most helpful for quieting behavioral disturbances in patients with dementia
- NMDA receptor antagonists (memantine) may offer small benefit in moderate-to-severe dementia
- Severe disease: Minimize medications and focus on nonpharmacologic Tx
- Neuroleptics increase mortality

Delirium
- Acute, transient alteration in consciousness
- Somnolence more common than agitation
- Differential diagnosis
  - Systemic illness (especially infection)
  - **Medications**
  - Surgery
  - Uncontrolled pain
  - Restraints
  - Bladder catheters
  - Sundowning

Managing Delirium
- Prevent, prevent, prevent!
- Search for underlying cause
- Stop all nonessential medications, especially psychoactive ones
- Reorient patient frequently
- Avoid restraints
- Avoid neuroleptics if possible
- No BZD

AR 11
A 76-year-old woman is brought in for evaluation of several recent falls. She lives in a nearby nursing home. She spends much of her day in bed, getting up for lunch and dinner. She has Type 2 diabetes, hypertension, coronary disease, and reflux.

Meds: omeprazole, nortriptyline, hydrochlorothiazide, calcium/vit D

In addition to exercise training, which would you recommend?

A. 24-hour Holter monitor
B. Event-recorder monitor
C. Stop nortriptyline.
D. Begin alendronate.
E. Order soft restraint while in bed.

Answer:_____

AR 12
A 72-year-old woman reports discomfort in both her lower extremities. The discomfort is present when she is seated, occurring in both calves. It improves when she is walking. She describes it as a deep ache, sometimes with an itching or pulling feeling. She has increased symptoms at nighttime when she is in bed. She has a history of DM and HTN.

Meds: hydrochlorothiazide, lisinopril, metformin

Exam: unremarkable

AR 12A
Which is the most appropriate test?

A. Ankle brachial indices
B. Serum potassium level
C. Iron studies
D. CPK
E. CT scan

Answer:_____

AR 12B
The patient's labs return normal: ferritin 80 ng/mL, creatinine 0.9 mg/dL.

Which is the most appropriate pharmacologic therapy?

A. Gabapentin
B. Pramipexole
C. Felodipine
D. Oxycodone
E. Topiramate

Answer:_____

AR 13
You are called to evaluate a 74-year-old man with Parkinson disease. He has been hospitalized twice in the last year for urosepsis. Because of incontinence, he has required a chronic indwelling urinary catheter. He is currently afebrile and has no abdominal pain. He has had no mental status changes or recent falls.

Labs (from 48 hours ago):

WBC 8,000/mm³; Hct 42%; Na⁺ 137 mEq/L; K⁺ 3.6 mEq/L; BUN 20 mg/dL; Cr 1.2 mg/dL;
Urine culture > 100,000 colonies of *Enterococcus*

Which therapy do you recommend?

A. No therapy at this time
B. Ceftriaxone
C. Ampicillin
D. Vancomycin
E. Imipenem

Answer:_____

UROLOGY AND SEXUAL HEALTH

URINARY INCONTINENCE
- Normal micturition requires appropriate cerebral cortex and brainstem function, sacral nerve function (S2–S4), and bladder muscle function (detrusor and sphincter muscles)

Types of Urinary Incontinence
- Incontinence due to reversible causes
- Functional incontinence
- Lower urinary tract causes
  - Urge incontinence (detrusor overactivity)
  - Stress incontinence (sphincter dysfunction)
  - Incomplete bladder emptying: "overflow" incontinence (detrusor underactivity)
  - Mixed incontinence
- Incontinence due to reversible conditions (and treatment)
  - UTI — antibiotics
  - Atrophic vaginitis/urethritis — topical estrogen
  - Pregnancy/Vaginal delivery/Episiotomy — self-limited usually
  - Postprostatectomy — self-limited usually
  - Stool impaction — disimpaction, stool softeners
  - Drugs

Drug Causes of Urinary Incontinence
- Diuretics: polyuria, frequency, urgency
- Caffeine: aggravates or precipitates incontinence
- Anticholinergics (including tricyclics): impaired bladder emptying and/or retention*
- Sedatives: sedation, muscle relaxation
- Opioids: impaired bladder emptying and/or retention

*Anticholinergics can sometimes be used as treatment for urge incontinence

Types of Urinary Incontinence
- **Urge incontinence**
  - "Overactive" detrusor muscle produces urge to void even at low volumes
  - Sx: not being able to reach restroom in time, small-volume voiding
- **Stress incontinence**
  - Bladder functions normally but sphincter weak
  - Incontinence with cough, sneezing, jumping, laughing, standing
- **Mixed incontinence**
  - Features of both urge and stress
- **Overflow incontinence**
  - Overactive bladder ± outlet obstruction (e.g., due to BPH)
  - Underactive bladder (diabetes, MS, Parkinson's, spinal cord injury)

Urinary Incontinence — Therapy
- Bladder training: urge, stress, and mixed
- Kegel exercises: urge, stress, and mixed
- Drugs for urge and mixed
  - Anticholinergics (e.g., oxybutynin, tolterodine)
  - β-Agonists (mirabegron)
- Surgery: last resource for stress
- Drugs for stress: none!!
- Overflow
  - Treat underlying cause
  - Intermittent catheterization (neurogenic bladder)

SEXUAL DYSFUNCTION

Erectile Dysfunction (ED) — Etiology
- Vascular (most common!): diabetes, cardiovascular disease
- Neurogenic: diabetes, peripheral neuropathy
- Hypogonadism (low testosterone): low libido along with ED
- Medications: antihypertensives, SSRIs
- Psychogenic: acute onset; may be partner specific, depression related; responds well to PDE-5 drugs

ED — Therapy
- PDE-5 inhibitors: all contraindicated with nitrates!
  - May cause visual changes, especially color vision
  - Tadalafil now approved for BPH
- Vacuum device: safe but inconvenient
- Intraurethral alprostadil (MUSE): safe but uncomfortable
- Penile injections: alprostadil, papaverine, phentolamine
- Penile implants: Use only after other therapies have failed

Other Sexual Dysfunction
- Dyspareunia: usually due to postmenopausal atrophic vaginitis — treat with lubricant or vaginal estrogen
- Decreased libido: Look for hypogonadism or meds, especially SSRIs
- Delayed orgasm: occurs in up to 30% of patients on SSRIs

Benign Prostatic Hyperplasia (BPH)
- Prevalence: 60% at 60 years of age, 80% by age 80 years of age
- Presents with nocturia, hesitancy, weak stream, dribbling
- Clinical diagnosis
- BPH symptoms alone should not prompt PSA testing
- Behavioral therapy first (decrease fluids, caffeine, EtOH)
- α-Blockade (terazosin, tamsulosin) — watch for orthostasis
- 5-α reductase inhibitor (finasteride) — takes up to 6 months to have effect
- If medications not effective, consult a urologist for procedural approach

AR 14
A 79-year-old woman reports problems with urinary incontinence on a daily basis. She has to void many times during the day and leaks urine frequently before she can get to the restroom. She has not had hematuria or dysuria.

Meds: omeprazole, sertraline, and enalapril

U/A is normal.

Which is the most likely cause of the incontinence?

A. Detrusor hypoactivity
B. Sphincter hypoactivity
C. Detrusor hyperactivity
D. Side effect of sertraline
E. Side effect of enalapril

Answer:_____

AR 15
A 76-year-old woman is evaluated for urinary incontinence. She reports a 6-year history of incontinence occurring when she laughs, coughs, or sneezes. Recently, she has had incontinence with standing.

U/A is normal.

BUN 14 mg/dL, Cr 1.1 mg/dL, Glu 111 mg/dL

Which would you recommend?

A. Oxybutynin 2.5 mg PO bid
B. Doxazosin 2 mg PO bid
C. Kegel exercises
D. Imipramine 25 mg PO q hs
E. Mirabegron 25 mg PO daily

Answer:_____

GENERAL INTERNAL MEDICINE

© 2022 MedStudy Internal Medicine Review – General Internal Medicine   219

AR 16

A 76-year-old man presents for evaluation of urinary frequency and decreased urinary stream. The symptoms have been present for the past 3 years but have worsened in the last 6 months. He is now getting up 4 times per night to urinate. On exam, his prostate is 3+ enlarged without nodularity.

What do you recommend for short-term relief?

A. Tamsulosin
B. Finasteride
C. TURP
D. Prostate ultrasound and biopsy
E. PSA testing

Answer:_____

AR 17

A 74-year-old diabetic man reports increasing problems with sexual functioning. He reports normal sexual desire but inability to sustain an erection sufficient for intercourse. It has been slowly worsening for the past 3 years.

Testicular and prostate exams are normal.

Meds: metformin, insulin, atorvastatin, famotidine, and ginkgo biloba

What is the most likely cause of his erectile dysfunction?

A. Atorvastatin
B. Famotidine
C. Ginkgo biloba
D. Low testosterone
E. Vascular disease

Answer:_____

AR 18

A 67-year-old man presents for treatment of erectile dysfunction. He has had problems sustaining erections for the past year. He has a normal libido. Testicular and prostate exams are normal.

Meds: simvastatin, omeprazole, isosorbide mononitrate, lisinopril, aspirin

What would you recommend for therapy?

A. Intraurethral alprostadil
B. Sildenafil
C. Testosterone patch
D. Testosterone injections
E. Referral for penile implant

Answer:_____

Sedentary Lifestyle

- Excessive sitting has been linked to increases in all-cause mortality, CV mortality, cancer, and diabetes

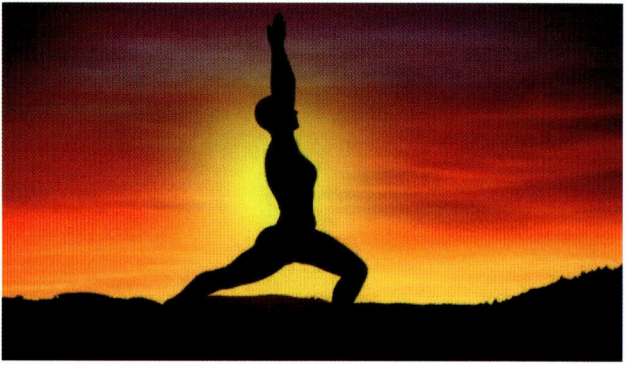

ETHICS

PRINCIPLES OF PHYSICIAN-PATIENT INTERACTION

- **Respect** for patient autonomy: helping patients make free, noncoerced choices
- **Beneficence**: to act in the best interests and welfare of the patient
- **Nonmaleficence**: the duty to do no harm to the patient
- **Justice**: equitable care for all patients

An Approach to Ethical Dilemmas

- Clarify ethical issues
    - What weighs on either side of the decision?
    - What ethical principles are at stake?
    - What cultural issues are relevant?
- Consider ethics consult (slow)
- Court decision: last resort (really, really slow)

Respect for Patient Autonomy

- Religious differences
    - Cannot force adults to receive care if contrary to religious preferences
- Pregnancy
    - Pregnant women usually cannot be forced to have care for themselves <u>or</u> the fetus
- Paternalism
    - Practice of overriding or ignoring patient's preferences in order to enhance welfare: ethically improper
    - Patients should be active participants in decision-making process; "informed consent"

DECISION-MAKING CAPACITY AND COMPETENCY

Decision-Making Capacity
- Decision-making capacity refers to the act of comprehending, evaluating, and choosing among realistic options: it is **decision specific**
- **Different from competency — determined by the courts**
- If patient can't make decisions due to incapacitating illness, someone can decide on their behalf: "surrogate" or "proxy"
- Surrogate decision-maker governed by state law: spouse > parents > children > siblings
- Durable power of attorney (DPOA) for health care **supersedes** family
- Surrogate should be representing what the patient would want/decide

ADVANCE DIRECTIVE
- A tool for patients to direct health care should they lose decision-making capacity
- **Living will or POLST** (**p**hysician **o**rder for **l**ife-**s**ustaining **t**reatment): more focused, allows persons to express their preferences regarding specific treatments (e.g., mechanical ventilation, hemodialysis, nutrition)
- **DPOA**: legal surrogate decision maker in case patient loses medical decision-making capacity
- **DPOA** supersedes living will; important that they are aware of its content

CONFIDENTIALITY AND PUBLIC WELFARE

Confidentiality
- Doctor-patient confidentiality not absolute, particularly if:
  - Patient confides plan to harm self or others
  - Patient conveys plans to harm named individual, these plans must be reported; level of specificity varies by state
  - Patient requests to withhold medical info from person at risk (HIV, TB, STI exposures); must make sure person at risk is notified (usually by contacting public health)

Physician-Patient Sexual Relationships
- Any intimate relationship between patient and physician is inappropriate
- A physician needs to terminate the professional relationship with a patient and wait a period of time before pursuing a personal relationship with a former patient
- Avoid sexual contact with patient surrogates as well (parents, children, power of attorney)

PHYSICIAN ERROR

Disclosure of Medical Errors[3]
- A medical error should be disclosed if a physician suspects or knows that it has an actual or potential impact on the patient's health, well-being, or medical decision making
- Disclosure is not conditioned by the likelihood that the error will be otherwise recognized
- Errors do not necessarily imply negligent or unethical behavior, but failure to disclose them may
- Health care professionals are ethically obligated to be forthcoming about health care injuries and errors
- Virtually all patients want physicians to acknowledge even minor errors
- Action to prevent future errors is important

AR 19
A 29-year-old woman presents with hematemesis. Her Hct is 20%. She receives IVF and is T&S for transfusion.

A repeat Hct 2 hours later is 14%. When a blood transfusion is recommended, the patient refuses because of religious convictions. Her husband, who is in the room with her, supports her stance. She has another episode of hematemesis during the discussion.

What would you do?

A. Obtain a court-appointed representative.
B. Get a hospital ethics consult.
C. Give blood because this is a life-threatening emergency.
D. Give blood because of the principle of beneficence.
E. Expedite endoscopy and consider non–blood volume expanders if hypotensive.

Answer:_____

AR 20
A 21-year-old college student is brought to the ED by her roommate for symptoms of headache and fever with stiff neck over the past 6 hours. On exam, she is somnolent but arousable, with a temp of 102.2°F (39.0°C), BP 100/52 mmHg, HR 112 bpm. Nuchal rigidity is present.

WBC is 24,000/mm^3

She consents to a lumbar puncture. You obtain CSF and send it to the lab. The nurse arrives with an IV bag with antibiotics, and the patient starts to scream, "I won't allow it!" When asked why not, she screams, "You are trying to poison me with pesticides!"

You carefully explain the high risk of death from untreated meningitis. The patient continues to scream, "Everyone here is trying to kill me!"

What should you do?

A. Treat with IV fluids only because antibiotics carry a risk and should not be given without patient consent.
B. Treat with antibiotics because the patient has questionable decisional capacity.
C. Obtain a court order urgently for treatment.
D. Obtain consent from the patient's roommate and give antibiotics.

Answer:_____

AR 21

A 44-year-old woman presents to clinic upset because she was found to be HIV positive at a recent health fair screening. Her husband, also your patient, doesn't know about her HIV status, and she refuses to tell him because she is afraid that disclosure would destroy their marriage. HIV is a reportable illness in your state.

In addition to encouraging disclosure, which should you do?

A. Honor her request for confidentiality.
B. Tell the husband immediately and recommend HIV testing.
C. Recommend the husband be HIV tested at next visit as routine screening.
D. Test the husband for HIV without his knowledge.
E. Report her illness to the health department.

Answer:_____

AR 22

An 86-year-old woman who lives in a nursing home is admitted with severe aspiration pneumonia. She is unconscious with a fever of 104.0°F (40.0°C); ABG 7.22/52/66. She has been started on IV antibiotics and fluids.

Her nephew is the durable power of attorney for health care. The patient has never completed a living will or advance directives.

The nephew meets with you, stating that his aunt has become demented over the past few years. The nephew would like IV fluids and antibiotics discontinued, with comfort care only.

You understand the patient's son is also present.

Which of the following statements about the nephew is true?

A. Because the patient has not left specific advance directives, the nephew's instructions to discontinue IVF and antibiotics should not be carried out.
B. The patient has a son, who is next of kin, and therefore the nephew cannot make medical decisions for her.
C. The nephew's request to discontinue IVF and antibiotics is within his capacity to act as the patient's durable power of attorney.
D. The nephew's instructions can be carried out only if it is determined that he had discussed this specific situation with his aunt and is carrying out substituted judgment.

Answer:_____

AR 23

A 56-year-old man with Type 2 diabetes is hospitalized for treatment of cellulitis. He is given 100 units of NPH insulin instead of the 10 units that he usually takes. This is discovered 15 minutes after he receives the dose. He is placed on a D10 drip.

What should the physician tell the patient?

A. He is at risk for low blood sugar, so he will be receiving a drip with glucose in it.
B. A dosage error was made, and he received 10× the insulin dose he was supposed to receive. He is receiving glucose to help prevent low blood sugar.
C. He may have too much insulin right now, so he is being put on a glucose drip to avoid low blood sugar.
D. You are concerned that he could develop low blood sugar today, so you will be monitoring him closely and will have him on a glucose drip to prevent low blood sugar.
E. You will discuss this if he asks about it.

Answer:_____

PERIOPERATIVE CARE

PREOPERATIVE CARDIAC RISK ASSESSMENT

Pre-Op Cardiac Risk Assessment — Basic Algorithm
- Does patient need emergency surgery? Yes → proceed to surgery
- For nonemergent surgery:
  - Estimate risk of **MACE** (RCRI):

MACE = **m**ajor **a**dverse **c**ardiovascular **e**vent (MI, CVA or CV death); RCRI = Revised Cardiac Risk Index

Revised Cardiac Risk Index (RCRI)
- 5 independent predictors of MACE:
  1) History of ischemic heart disease
     - History of MI
     - +Exercise test
     - Current chest pain
     - Use of nitrates
     - ECG with pathologic Q waves
  2) History of heart failure
  3) History of stroke
  4) DM requiring insulin
  5) CKD; pre-op creatinine > 2 mg/dL

Pre-Op Cardiac Risk Assessment — Basic Algorithm
- Does patient need emergency surgery? Yes → proceed to surgery
- For nonemergent surgery:
  - Estimate risk of **MACE** (RCRI):
    - **MACE** risk low (< 1%) → proceed to surgery
    - **MACE** risk high (> 1%) → what is the functional capacity?

- Functional capacity:
  - ≥ 4 METs → proceed to surgery
  - < 4 METs → stress testing and possible revascularization or consider nonsurgical approach

METs = metabolic equivalents

Pre-Op Cardiac Risk Assessment — Key Points
- Active heart disease should be addressed before elective surgery
- Chronic heart disease — most patients with good exercise capacity do not need a workup
- Low-risk surgeries (cataract, vasectomy, minor biopsies) rarely need workup

Preoperative β-Blockers
- β-Blockers should be continued if patients have been taking them chronically for a good reason (arrhythmia, ischemia)
- Do not abruptly withdraw β-blockers in the perioperative period
- Starting β-blockers in patients with high cardiac risk before an elective procedure is controversial

Labs to Check
- Routine preoperative labs in healthy adults are not advised
- Selective testing for specific circumstances
  - Hemoglobin/Hematocrit
    - If > 65 years of age undergoing major vascular surgery
    - All surgeries that would/could result in major blood loss
  - Creatinine
    - If > 50 years of age undergoing major surgery
- CBC: Not recommended unless cheaper than hematocrit alone
- Electrolytes: Not recommended unless history suggests reason to check
- Glucose, liver function tests, PT/PTT, U/A: Not recommended unless clinical signs/symptoms

ECG
- **No** for low-risk surgery
- **Yes** for patients with CAD, arrhythmias, PAD, cerebrovascular disease, or other significant structural heart disease
- Age alone not a factor

CXR / PFTs
- CXR
  - Suspected cardiac or pulmonary disease
  - Not indicated in patients with unremarkable history and physical exam
- PFTs
  - Unexplained dyspnea
  - Before lung volume reduction surgery in COPD

Stents and DAPT
- Elective noncardiac surgery
  - DAPT can be stopped:
    - After 2 weeks of balloon angioplasty
    - ≥ 30 days of bare-metal stent implantation
    - DES
      - 3–6 months, "may be considered"
      - > 6 months OK

PERIOPERATIVE MEDICINE — MANAGEMENT
- Antiplatelet
  - ASA — continue for minor surgery or recent (6 months) MI, PCI, stroke; for major surgery, stop 7–10 days before
  - Clopidogrel — stop 5–7 days before surgery
  - NSAIDs and COX-2 — stop 1–3 days before surgery
- Anticoagulant
  - Minor surgery — continue
  - Major surgery
    - 4–6 hours for IV heparin (can reverse with protamine)
    - 24 hours for LMWH
    - 24–72 hours for DOACs
    - 5 days for warfarin

Heparin Bridging
- Replacement of warfarin with heparin to minimize time that patient is anticoagulated
- Appropriate for patients with a very high risk of thromboembolic event such as:
  - Embolic stroke, cardiac stent or VTE within past 3 months
  - Mechanical mitral valve
  - Mechanical aortic valve + other stroke risks
  - AFib only if extremely high risk (CHADS-VASC$_2$ of 5–6)

Perioperative Medicine — Management
- Cardiovascular: Continue β-blockers, calcium channel blockers, nitrates, statins; diuretics often held to help with volume management; ACEIs and ARBs controversial
- Estrogen: Discontinue hormone replacement several weeks before surgery (if continued, increase level of DVT prophylaxis)
- Diabetes agents
  - Oral hypoglycemics — stop 24–72 hours before surgery depending upon half-life of drug and risk of hypoglycemia
  - No short-acting insulin the morning of surgery
  - Reduce intermediate-acting insulin by 25–50%
  - Basal insulin — continue same dose or reduce to 2/3
- Psychiatric meds
  - MAOI — stop 10–14 days before surgery
  - SSRIs — consider withholding 2–3 weeks before neurosurgery
  - Antipsychotics — continue
  - Tricyclic antidepressants and lithium — continue
- Neurologic medications
  - Antiseizure medications — continue
  - Antiparkinsonian — continue
  - Alzheimer drugs — discontinue

AR 24

A 78-year-old man with a history of hypertension and DM falls and fractures his hip. He will require hip surgery. Prior to this fracture, he could mow the lawn without any difficulty.

Exam

Vitals: BP 150/90 mmHg, HR 90 bpm

Chest: clear

Cardiac: Nl S_1S_2, no murmur

Ext: no edema

ECG: NSR, LVH

Labs: Hgb 11 g/dL, Hct 33%, Glu 148 mg/dL

What would you recommend?

A. Nuclear medicine stress test
B. Echocardiogram
C. Transfuse 2 units of blood.
D. Okay for immediate surgery.

Answer:_____

PREVENTIVE MEDICINE

SCREENING TESTS

Important Screening Exams to Know

- **Blood pressure**: annually for adults ≥ 40 years of age (or increased risk), every 3–5 years between 18 and 39 years of age if BP < 130/85 mmHg

Important Screening Exams to Know[4]

- **Diabetes**
  - All adults starting at 45 years of age
  - Screen earlier if BMI > 25* and ≥ 1 risk factor
    - HTN
    - 1° relative with DM
    - Vascular disease
    - Gestational DM
    - PCOS
    - Physical inactivity
    - HDL < 35 and/or TG < 250
    - High-risk ethnicity**
  - Screen with fasting glucose, 2-hour OGTT, or HbA1c
  - If screening is normal, repeat screening q 3 years

*BMI > 23 in Asian Americans
**African American, Latino, Native American, Asian American, Pacific Islander

- **Cholesterol**: Measure lipids every 5 years, adults 40–75 years of age
- **Statin for primary prevention of CVD**: adults 40–75 years of age with no history of CVD, 1 or more CVD risk factors, and calculated 10-year ASCVD event risk ≥ 7.5% (ACC-AHA) or ≥ 10% (ACP)

CANCER SCREENINGS

Important Cancer Screening

- **For all screening, do not screen if life expectancy < 10 years**
- **Breast cancer**: biennial mammography for women 50–74 years of age
  - 40–49 years of age, individualize; lower disease reduction and higher false-positive rate in this age group
- **Prostate cancer**: USPSTF recommends against PSA screening; ACP says shared decision-making between 50 and 69 years of age
- **Colorectal cancer**: USPSTF recommends screening with colonoscopy (q 10 years), FIT (annually) or DNA testing (q 3 years) for:
  - 50–75 years of age (Grade A)
  - 45–50 years of age (Grade B)
  - Selectively for 75–85 years of age (Grade C)

Cervical Cancer Screening — Caveats

- Primary HPV testing is equally sensitive but more specific than PAP or PAP/HPV for prevention of cervical dysplasia (fewer false positives)
- New American Cancer Society guidelines recommend starting later (age 25) than USPSTF guidelines and remove emphasis on cytology
- Stop screening if cervix removed for benign disease
- Pelvic exam with bimanual exam no longer recommended

Cervical Cancer Screening — USPSTF vs. ACS[5]

Years of Age	2018 USPSTF	2020 ACS
21–24	PAP q 3 years	No screening
25–29	PAP q 3 years	HPV q 5 years*
30–64	HPV q 5 years or HPV/PAP q 5 years or PAP q 3 years	HPV q 5 years*
≥ 65	Stop screening if 3 consecutive normal PAPs or negative HPV tests × 2	Stop screening if 3 consecutive normal PAPs or negative HPV tests × 2

HPV/PAP q 5 years or PAP q 3 years still an option if primary HPV testing not available

CT Screening for Lung Cancer

- NLST shows 20% reduction in lung cancer mortality in smokers screened with LDCT; NNS to prevent one lung cancer death at 3 years: 320
- High false-positive rate
- USPSTF B: annual screening between 55 and 80 years of age with ≥ 30 PY smoking Hx and current smoker or quit within past 15 years

Screening Guidelines for AAA

- USPSTF and ACC/AHA recommend one-time screening (ultrasound) for AAA in <u>men</u> 65–75 years of age who have ever smoked
- Evidence insufficient for screening in women

VACCINATIONS

Adult Immunization Schedule

Age	Schedule
Young adults	Completion of childhood immunizations (MMR, Tdap or Td, polio, HepA and HepB vaccines)
11–45 years of age (males too!)	HPV vaccine
Every year	Influenza
Every 10 years	Tdap once, then Td booster
> 50 years of age	Recombinant zoster vaccine (2-dose series spaced 2–6 months apart)

Pneumococcal Vaccine[6]
- Two types of pneumococcal vaccines:
  1) PCV13
     - Optional! No longer routinely recommended
     - ≥ 65 years of age, CDC suggests "shared decision-making" for those who reside in care facilities or who are burdened with chronic disease (heart, lung, liver, DM, alcoholism, or active tobacco use)
     - If using PCV, administer > 1 year before PPSV23
  2) PPSV23
     - ≥ 65 years of age — give once
     - < 65 years of age, may give single dose early if chronic disease (same as above), and then repeat at age 65
       - If given early between 60 and 64 years of age, wait 5 years before 2nd dose

Pneumococcal Vaccine — Special Considerations
- ≥ 19 years of age with severe immunocompromising conditions: PCV13 + PPSV23 8 weeks apart, 2nd PPSV23 given 5 years later
- ≥ 19 years of age with CSF leak or cochlear implant: PCV13 + PPSV23 8 weeks apart

Immunization Don'ts
- Pregnancy: Do not give attenuated live vaccines (MMR, oral polio, yellow fever, typhoid, varicella, nasal influenza, VZV live attenuated)
- HIV: Avoid MMR and VZV live attenuated in individuals with very severe immunosuppression (CD4 counts < 200/mm^3)

Vaccinations for Patients at Risk

Group	Vaccines
Asplenia	Hib, pneumococcal (PCV13 and PPV23), meningococcal
Chronic liver disease	Hepatitis A and B
Health care worker	Hepatitis B, influenza, MMR, Tdap
IVDU	Hepatitis A and B, Tdap
Lung disease	Pneumococcal, influenza

AR 25
A woman makes an appointment for a physical exam when she turns 65. She has not seen a physician for 12 years, and that visit was for a skin rash. She has not had a regular doctor because she lacked insurance.

In addition to mammography, appropriate preventive care should include:

A. Pap smear
B. CBC
C. CBC and FIT
D. Pap smear and FIT
E. Pap smear, CBC, and FIT

Answer:_____

AR 26
Which patient meets guideline criteria for AAA screening?

A. 50-year-old man who presents with chest pain
B. 55-year-old woman who presents with a stroke
C. 60-year-old woman with a 100-pack-year history of smoking
D. 75-year-old woman with 100-pack-year history of smoking
E. 66-year-old man with 60-pack-year history of smoking, quit 10 years ago

Answer:_____

AR 27
In November, a 34-year-old woman (G1P0) comes to see you at 24 weeks of gestation. She reports no history of chickenpox. She received all regular immunizations growing up, with her last immunizations received prior to college 16 years ago.

Which immunizations would you recommend?

A. No immunizations
B. Varicella, Tdap
C. Varicella, influenza
D. Varicella, Tdap, influenza
E. Tdap, influenza

Answer:_____

AR 28
A 61-year-old healthy man comes in for a first visit. He has not seen a doctor since 50 years of age.

In addition to seasonal flu, which immunizations would you recommend for him?

A. PPSV23
B. Tdap, PPSV23
C. Tdap, varicella zoster
D. Varicella zoster, PCV13
E. Tdap, varicella zoster, PPSV23
F. No vaccines are indicated at this time.

Answer:_____

AR 29

A 19-year-old woman is evaluated in the ED for severe headache and altered consciousness. She has a lumbar puncture and is found to have meningococcal meningitis. Her mental status deteriorates, and she requires intubation for airway protection.

Who should receive meningococcal prophylaxis?

A. The 3rd year medical student who did the ED workup
B. The resident who did the lumbar puncture
C. The anesthesiologist who intubated the patient
D. All of them

Answer:_____

AR 30

An influenza epidemic strikes a nursing home at which you are the medical director. The patients received the influenza vaccine yesterday, but cases began appearing 5 days ago. You now have 11 confirmed cases of influenza A.

What do you recommend?

A. Treat patients with oseltamivir as soon as any symptom of influenza occurs.
B. Isolate all patients without symptoms to a separate wing of the nursing home.
C. Begin all nursing home residents on a 14-day course of rimantadine.
D. Begin all nursing home residents on a 14-day course of oseltamivir.
E. Give all residents pneumococcal vaccine.

Answer:_____

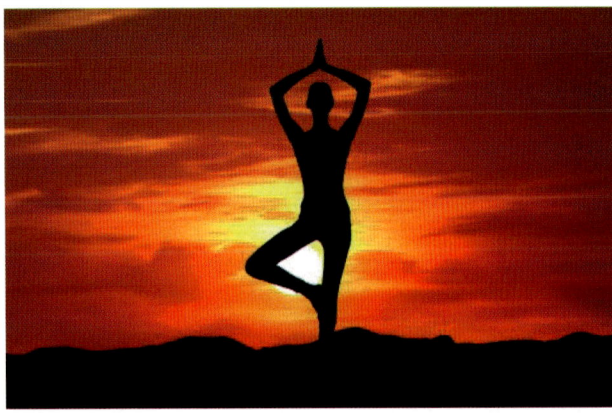

OVERDOSE AND POISONING

General Principles
- Protect airway
- D50, naloxone, thiamine
- BMP, ABG with carboxyhemoglobin, urine, and serum toxicology screen
- Calculate anion and osmol gaps
- Measure serum acetaminophen and salicylate levels
- Gastric decontamination (charcoal/lavage)

Charcoal Not Effective for the Following
- Caustics
- Cyanide
- Electrolytes
- Alcohols (e.g., ethanol, ethylene glycol, methanol)
- Hydrocarbons
- Heavy metals (e.g., iron, lithium, lead, mercury)

Anion Gap Acidosis
- Methanol
- Uremia
- Ketones
- Paraldehyde
- Isoniazid, iron
- Lactate (e.g., metformin, HIV meds)
- Ethanol and ethylene glycol
- Salicylates

Important Toxins to Review
- Anticholinergics
- Tricyclic antidepressants
- Acetaminophen
- Nitrites
- Lithium

Anticholinergic Overdose
- **Red** as a beet: cutaneous vasodilation
- **Dry** as a bone: anhidrosis
- **Hot** as a hare: hyperthermia
- **Blind** as a bat: mydriasis
- **Mad** as a hatter: hallucinations
- **Full** as a flask: urinary retention
- **Antidote**: physostigmine

TCA Overdose
- Common cause of hospitalization and death from prescription drugs on exams
- Effects: cardiovascular toxicity, CNS effects, anticholinergic effects
- Block absorption: charcoal, lavage, charcoal (if within 2 hours)
- **Antidote: sodium bicarbonate (not physostigmine or procainamide)**
- Benzos if seizures (not phenytoin)
- Drug levels do not rule out significant toxicity

The Stages of Poisoning with Acetaminophen
- Stage 1: (0–24 hours)
  - Asymptomatic or flu-like (nausea, vomiting, malaise)
- Stage 2: (24–48 hours)
  - Asymptomatic
  - Liver enzymes may start to rise
- Stage 3: (49–96 hours)
  - Peak symptoms
  - Peak liver abnormalities
  - Death may occur from coagulopathy or liver failure
- Stage 4
  - Recovery

Acetaminophen Overdose
- > 7.5 g ingestion in healthy adult can cause liver damage
- Toxic dose less if patient has underlying liver disease or chronic alcohol use

Acetaminophen Nomogram

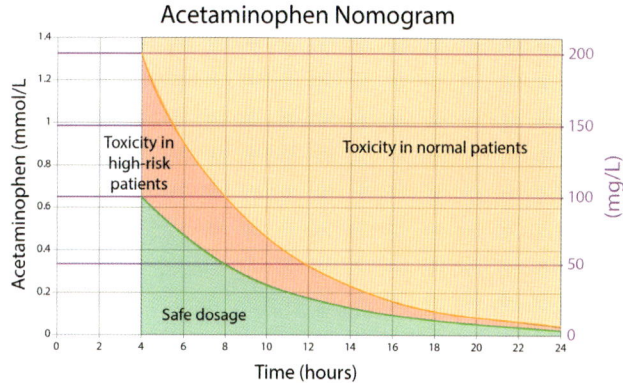

Management of Acetaminophen Overdose[7]
- Gastric emptying if within 1–2 hours of ingestion
- Activated charcoal if within 2–4 hours of ingestion
- *N*-acetylcysteine (17 doses) should be administered, PO or IV, at 4 hours after ingestions for anyone who falls in the toxic range on the nomogram

Clinical Features of Nitrite Abuse
- Tachypnea
- Tachycardia
- Headache
- Hypotension
- Cyanosis unresponsive to oxygen (methemoglobinemia)

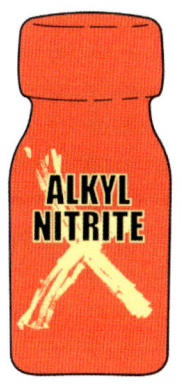
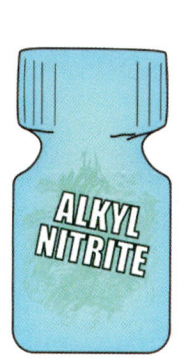
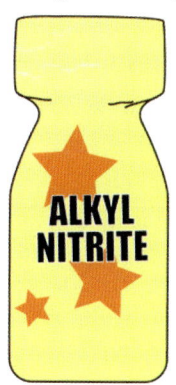

Features of MDMA (Ecstasy) Intoxication
- Common features
  - Euphoria
  - Increased sexual arousal
  - Bruxism
  - Tachycardia
- Serious side effects
  - Severe hypertension
  - Hyperthermia
  - Hyponatremia
- Distinguishing features
  - Bruxism and hyponatremia

Methamphetamine Abuse
- Important clinical features
  - Hypertension/Tachycardia
  - Diaphoresis
  - Severe agitation or psychosis
  - "Meth mouth" with chronic use (less saliva/bruxism leads to dental cracking, decay, and severe caries)
  - Skin excoriations
  - Delusions of parasitosis

Meth Mouth

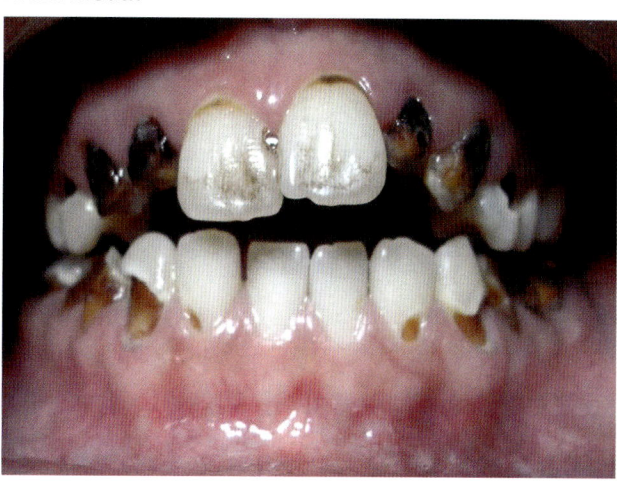

Poisoning and Overdose Antidotes

Toxin	Antidote
Acetaminophen	*N*-acetylcysteine
Narcotics	Naloxone
Benzodiazepines	Flumazenil*
Nitrites	Methylene blue
Iron	Deferoxamine
Methanol, glycols	Fomepizole
Organophosphates	Atropine/Pralidoxime (2-PAM)
Cyanide	Nitrites, sodium thiosulfate

*Flumazenil not recommended for someone who is a chronic user of benzodiazepines because it can induce seizure

AR 31
The agent of choice for treatment of the arrhythmia associated with a tricyclic antidepressant overdose is which of the following?

A. Sodium bicarbonate
B. Procainamide
C. Amiodarone
D. Naloxone
E. Physostigmine

Answer:_____

AR 32

A 20-year-old woman presents to the ED tearful and agitated. She reports taking a bottle of extra-strength acetaminophen 2 hours ago in a suicide attempt. Her physical exam is normal.

Labs: Hgb 13 g/dL, Hct 39%, WBC 9,000/mm³; acetaminophen level 280 mg/mL (toxic) at 4 hours

What is the most appropriate management?

A. Gastric lavage and deferoxamine
B. Activated charcoal alone
C. Activated charcoal and *N*-acetylcysteine
D. *N*-acetylcysteine alone
E. Deferoxamine alone

Answer:_____

AR 33

A 29-year-old man is brought to the ED by friends. The patient was at a party with his friends when he became confused and then unresponsive.

On exam: BP 60/30 mmHg, HR 140 bpm, T 97.0°F (36.1°C), O₂ saturation 88%, extremities with marked cyanosis; Mouth: cyanosis of lips

Labs:

Hgb 14 g/dL, Hct 42%, WBC 1,000/mm³

ABG: pH 7.32, pO₂ 86 mmHg, pCO₂ 44 mmHg

Na⁺ 136 mEq/L, K⁺ 4.0 mEq/L, Cl⁻ 105 mEq/L, HCO₃⁻ 20 mEq/L

The patient is placed on 100% O₂ by mask without improvement in his cyanosis.

What therapy should he receive?

A. Amyl nitrite
B. Methylene blue
C. Bicarbonate drip
D. Naloxone
E. IV alcohol

Answer:_____

AR 34

A 45-year-old male patient of yours calls you on a Sunday afternoon. He has been having nausea, vomiting, and diarrhea today. He also has had a headache and mild dyspnea. These symptoms actually improved when he was shoveling snow earlier in the day but have now returned. He reports his wife is sick in bed with the same "flu-like" syndrome.

What do you recommend?

A. See you in clinic tomorrow if the symptoms persist.
B. You will make a house call today.
C. Have the patient call 911 for emergent evaluation/transport to ED.
D. Prescribe oseltamivir for both the patient and his wife.

Answer:_____

EYES, EARS, NOSE, THROAT

AR 35

An obese, 36-year-old woman presents for evaluation of headaches. She has had increasing problems with headaches over the past 6 months. She has had no visual symptoms. She has occasional nausea but no focal neurologic symptoms. The headaches keep her home from work.

Exam: BP 120/70 mmHg, HR 80 bpm

Skin: without lesions

Fundi: as shown

Neurologic exam: normal

Meds: CaCO₃, OCP, fluoxetine

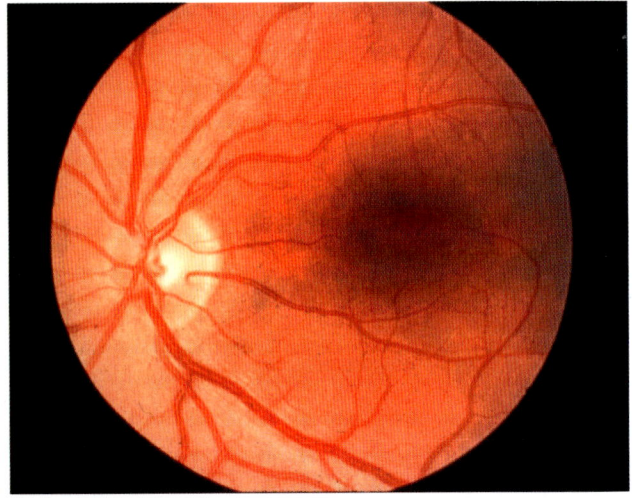

What is the most likely diagnosis?

A. Glioblastoma
B. Idiopathic intracranial hypertension (formerly known as pseudotumor cerebri)
C. Tuberous sclerosis
D. Prader-Willi syndrome
E. Headache from oral contraceptives

Answer:_____

Headaches in Reproductive-Age Women
- Incidence of OCP-associated HA: 600/100,000
- Incidence of idiopathic intracranial hypertension (IIH): 3.3/100,000

Idiopathic Intracranial Hypertension (IIH)
- 90% of patients are female, and obese
- Headaches (94%) — diffuse, worse in a.m.
- Visual disturbances (blurring, scotomas)
- Pulsatile tinnitus
- Papilledema
- 6th nerve palsy (diplopia)
- Diagnosis: CSF normal and OP > 250 mmH₂O
- Treatment: acetazolamide

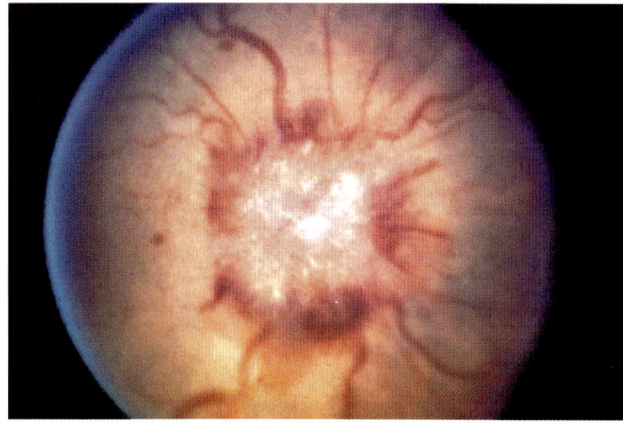

Ophthalmologic Emergencies (Emergent Consultation)
- Alkali burn — profuse water irrigation
- Central retinal artery occlusion — sudden, painless unilateral blindness, cherry-red spot
  - Ocular massage, Trendelenburg position, breathe into paper sack
- Angle-closure glaucoma ("closed-angle")
- Penetrating injury
- Endophthalmitis — bacterial or fungal
- Retinal detachment — photopsias, shade/curtain coming down, black dots showers
- Orbital cellulitis: EOM exam, diplopia, pain with eye movement

Pharyngitis

Etiology	Clinical Features
Group A strep	Tonsillar exudates, no cough, tender adenopathy, fever
Mononucleosis	Tonsillar exudates, palatal petechiae, splenomegaly
Chlamydia pneumoniae	Hoarseness
Mycoplasma	Erythema multiforme Bullous myringitis
Viral pharyngitis	Rhinorrhea, URI symptoms
Acute HIV	Rash, lymphadenopathy, oral ulcers, risk factors

Chronic Cough — Differential Diagnosis
- Upper airway cough syndrome (formerly known as postnasal drip)
- Reflux disease (GERD)
- Asthma
- Nonasthmatic eosinophilic bronchitis
- Medications (inhalers, ACEIs)
- Malignancy

Acute Sinusitis — Diagnosis
- Clinical
- Etiology: viral (90%), bacterial, fungal
- Save sinus CT for patients with recurrent or refractory disease

Guidelines for Antibiotic Use for Sinusitis
- Persistent symptoms > 10 days
- Onset with severe symptoms: T > 102.0°F (38.9°C) and purulent nasal discharge or facial pain for > 3–4 days
- Worsening symptoms: "double sickening," new onset of fever, headache, or increase in nasal discharge 5–6 days after initial URI

Acute Sinusitis — Therapy
- Decongestants/Saline irrigation
- 1st line — amoxicillin or amoxicillin/clavulanate
- Penicillin allergic: doxycycline or 3rd generation cephalosporin
- Reserve respiratory quinolones (levofloxacin, moxifloxacin) due to higher risk of toxicity
- 5- to 7-day duration of therapy
- TMP/SMX or macrolides no longer recommended due to high rates of resistance

Hearing Loss
- Conductive (bone conduction > air conduction): otitis media, TM perforation, eustachian tube blockage, otosclerosis, cerumen
- Sensorineural (air conduction > bone conduction): presbycusis, drugs, meningitis, Ménière disease, acoustic neuroma, environmental
- **Sudden** sensorineural hearing loss must be seen by ENT ASAP! + MRI, start prednisone 40–80 mg

AR 36
A 63-year-old woman with diabetes presents with right ear pain and right facial nerve palsy. She has had a fever for the past 24 hours and the draining ear shown.

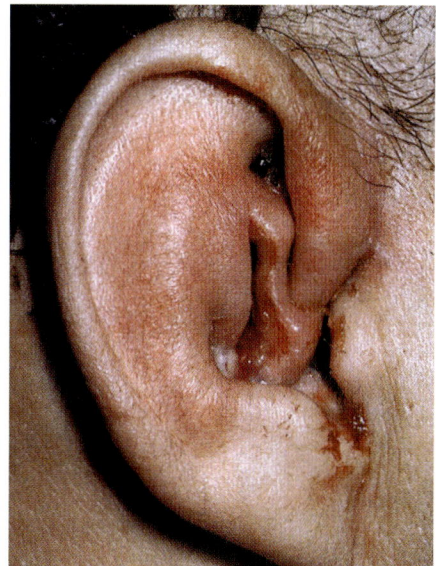

Which is the most appropriate treatment?

A. Amoxicillin PO
B. Vancomycin and clindamycin
C. Ciprofloxacin otic
D. Piperacillin-tazobactam and ciprofloxacin IV
E. Isoniazid/Rifampin

Answer:_____

AR 37

A 33-year-old woman presents with sore throat, rhinorrhea, maxillary sinus pressure, and green nasal discharge present for 3 days.

Exam: T 99.2°F (37.3°C); HR 90 bpm; BP 110/70 mmHg

Nose: swollen turbinates

Neck: no adenopathy

Chest: clear

What would you recommend?

A. Decongestants/Nasal irrigation
B. A + azithromycin
C. A + TMP/SMX
D. A + amoxicillin/clavulanate
E. A + metronidazole

Answer:_____

AR 38

A 67-year-old woman comes in with 1 hour of unilateral right eye pain. The pain started while watching a movie at the theater. PMH notable for hypertension, osteoporosis, and migraines.

Meds: alendronate, hydrochlorothiazide

Exam: Left eye is normal. Right eye has mild conjunctival injection; cornea is slightly hazy; pupil is 6 mm and poorly reactive to light. She reports halos around the light during exam.

In addition to calling an ophthalmologist, what treatment would you recommend?

A. Sumatriptan SQ
B. Ketorolac IV
C. Timolol eyedrops
D. Acyclovir IV
E. Gabapentin PO

Answer:_____

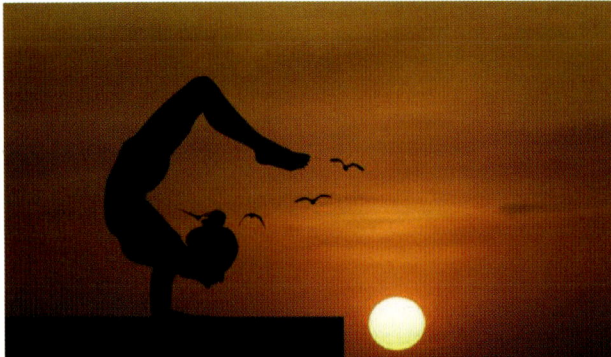

PREGNANCY AND WOMEN'S HEALTH

AR 39

A 29-year-old G1P0 female with Type 1 DM presents at 22 weeks of gestation with increasing pedal edema. Her BP is 170/110 mmHg. U/A reveals 3+ proteinuria. She has no headaches or neurologic symptoms.

Which treatment would you recommend?

A. Hydrochlorothiazide
B. Lisinopril
C. Labetalol
D. Nitroprusside drip
E. Spironolactone

Answer:_____

Hypertension and Pregnancy
- Treat usually only if SBP ≥ 160 mmHg and/or DBP ≥ 100 mmHg, regardless if they have preeclampsia or not
- Treatment goals: SBP 140–150 mmHg; DBP 90–100 mmHg
- Preferred meds
  - Labetalol
  - Methyldopa
  - Long-acting nifedipine
  - Hydralazine
  - Other CCB
- **Stop** ACEI/ARB and diuretics

Preeclampsia / Eclampsia — Clinical Features
- SBP ≥ 140 mmHg or DBP ≥ 90 mmHg after 20 weeks of gestation
- Edema
- Proteinuria
- Headache, visual disturbances
- Hyperreflexia
- **GTC seizures**

Preeclampsia / Eclampsia — Lab Abnormalities
- Proteinuria (protein:creatinine ≥ 0.3)
- Increased Cr (≥ 1.1 mg/dL)
- Increased uric acid
- Increased transaminases
- Decreased platelets (< 100,000)

SLE and Pregnancy
- Normal fertility, but miscarriage rate 1.5–3× increased
- Anti-Ro(SSA) or anti-La (SSB) antibodies in the mother are associated with neonatal lupus and congenital heart block
- If SLE active (especially with renal involvement) or if APLA+ or anti-dsDNA+, increased risk of SLE flares and fetal problems
- Treat with steroids or hydroxychloroquine
- Avoid methotrexate

Hyperthyroidism in Pregnancy

- Mild hyperthyroidism is normal, does not require treatment
  - Goal of treatment is to prevent fetal hypothyroidism and to control maternal symptoms
- If symptomatic, β-blocker 1st line
- If needed, PTU for early pregnancy, and methimazole after 1st trimester
- No radioactive iodine
- If hypothyroid, increase levothyroxine dose by 30–50%

Hypothyroidism in Pregnancy

- Need for thyroid hormone increases 30–50% during pregnancy
- Thyroid replacement is crucial to prevent neurocognitive deficits
  - Treat all women with TSH > 4.0
  - Increase dose of levothyroxine and monitor TSH frequently

AR 40

A 36-year-old woman (G3P2) comes to see you regarding her blood sugars. She was diagnosed with gestational diabetes during her first pregnancy and subsequently was diagnosed with diabetes.

What goal(s) would you recommend for glycemic control?

A. Postmeal sugars < 240
B. Premeal sugars < 180
C. Premeal sugars < 150
D. Premeal sugars < 120
E. Premeal sugars < 90 and HbA1c < 6%

Answer:_____

Diabetes and Pregnancy[8]

- Screen for gestational DM with 75-g OGTT at 24–28 weeks of gestation in women who do not have known DM
- Women with DM
  - Tight control before conception (1–2 months before stopping birth control) and throughout pregnancy
  - Goal = HbA1c < 6% if can be done without hypoglycemia

Hypercoagulability in Pregnancy

- 5-fold increased risk
- **No** CT pulmonary angiogram
- LMWH
- Warfarin **only** for mechanical heart valve

Drugs to Avoid Absolutely During Pregnancy

- Isotretinoin
- ACE inhibitors, ARBs, and spironolactone
- Benzodiazepines
- Quinolones and tetracyclines
- Nitroprusside
- Warfarin
- Fluconazole (even for yeast infection!)[9]

Asymptomatic Bacteriuria of Pregnancy

- Screening done at 12–16 weeks of gestation
- 1/3 go on to develop pyelonephritis if not treated
- Associated with preterm birth, low birth weight, and increased perinatal mortality
- Appropriate length of treatment controversial

Hot Flashes

- Therapy — extremely high placebo effect (20–50%!)
- Low-dose estrogen is most effective therapy
  - Use in combo with progestin in women with an intact uterus
- Do not use estrogen in women at higher risk (breast cancer, VTE or CV disease)
- SSRIs (paroxetine, citalopram), SNRIs (venlafaxine), and gabapentin are alternatives for women unable to take estrogens
- Paroxetine prevents activation of tamoxifen, so should not be used together

AR 41

A 25-year-old woman G1P0 presents at 10 weeks of gestation for evaluation. She is asymptomatic.

Labs: Hgb 12 g/dL, Hct 36%;
Urine culture: 100,000 colonies *E. coli*

What would you recommend?

A. Amoxicillin
B. Ciprofloxacin
C. TMP/SMX
D. No treatment

Answer:_____

AUDIENCE RESPONSE ANSWERS

Audience Response 1
A. Increase warfarin and increase levothyroxine.

AR 2
E. TMP/SMX

AR 3
A. Acetaminophen

AR 4
B. Amlodipine

AR 5
D. Quetiapine and methadone

AR 6
D. Amlodipine

AR 7
D. Encourage weight-bearing exercise.

AR 8
B. Alendronate

AR 9
E. Stop alendronate.

AR 10
D. Zoledronate

AR 11
C. Stop nortriptyline.

AR 12A
C. Iron studies

AR 12B
A. Gabapentin

AR 13
A. No therapy at this time

AR 14
C. Detrusor hyperactivity

AR 15
C. Kegel exercises

AR 16
A. Tamsulosin

AR 17
E. Vascular disease

AR 18
A. Intraurethral alprostadil

AR 19
E. Expedite endoscopy and consider non–blood volume expanders if hypotensive.

AR 20
B. Treat with antibiotics because the patient has questionable decisional capacity.

AR 21
E. Report her illness to the health department.

AR 22
C. The nephew's request to discontinue IVF and antibiotics is within his capacity to act as the patient's durable power of attorney.

AR 23
B. A dosage error was made, and he received 10× the insulin dose he was supposed to receive. He is receiving glucose to help prevent low blood sugar.

AR 24
D. Okay for immediate surgery.

AR 25
D. HPV and FIT

AR 26
E. 66-year-old man with 60-pack-year history of smoking, quit 10 years ago

AR 27
E. Tdap, influenza

AR 28
C. Tdap, varicella zoster

AR 29
C. The anesthesiologist who intubated the patient

AR 30
D. Begin all nursing home residents on a 14-day course of oseltamivir.

AR 31
A. Sodium bicarbonate

AR 32
C. Activated charcoal and *N*-acetylcysteine

AR 33
B. Methylene blue

AR 34
C. Have the patient call 911 for emergent evaluation/ transport to ED.

AR 35
E. Headache from oral contraceptives

AR 36
D. Piperacillin-tazobactam and ciprofloxacin IV

AR 37
A. Decongestants/Nasal irrigation

AR 38
C. Timolol eyedrops

AR 39
C. Labetalol

AR 40
E. Premeal sugars < 90 and HbA1c < 6%

AR 41
A. Amoxicillin

ENDNOTES

[1] *JAMA*. 1998;279(9):657–662.

[2] *Blood*. 2011;118(24):6269.

[3] Disclosing a Medical Error. *PIER ACP*. 2013.

[4] Diabetes Care 2020;43;S1-S212

[5] CA Cancer J Clin 2020;70:321-346

[6] (MMWR 68[46]:1069).

[7] *Ann Emerg Med* 2007;50:292-313

[8] Diabetes Care 2020;43:S183-S192

[9] *JAMA* 2016, 315:58-67.

MedStudy

INTERNAL MEDICINE REVIEW

Hematology

Presented by

Rishi Sawhney, MD

HEMATOLOGY

TABLE OF CONTENTS

Why Some Topic Names Are Not Printed in This Section

At MedStudy, we do all we can to optimize your self-testing and learning.

In this section, the speaker has chosen to introduce topics with an Audience Response question to help you learn.
In the syllabus, we've intentionally "hidden" some topic names that would give away the answers—so you can self-test more effectively. Where we've done this, instead of the topic name, you'll see an empty teal band or some extra space, but you can still find the topic on the page using the Table of Contents.

Presentation Outline
- **Red Cell Disorders**
  - Anemias
  - Hemochromatosis
- **Disorders of Hemostasis**
  - Bleeding Disorders
  - Thrombotic Disorders
- **Bone Marrow Disorders and Hematologic Malignancies**
  - Aplastic Anemia
  - Myeloproliferative Neoplasms
  - Lymphomas and Leukemias
  - Plasma Cell Disorders

RED CELL DISORDERS

ANEMIA
Determine Type and Look for Cause

Approach to Anemias
- **Kinetic** approach — look at **reticulocyte** count
  - Decreased production/maturation — low retic
    - Nutrient deficiency, marrow injury
  - Increased destruction — high retic
    - Hemolysis, microangiopathy
  - Sequestration — high retic
  - Blood loss — high retic
- **Morphologic** approach — look at **MCV**
  - Microcytic (MCV < 80)
    - Iron def, thalassemia
  - Macrocytic (MCV > 100)
    - B_{12}/Folate def, alcohol abuse, liver disease
  - Normocytic (MCV 80–100)

Iron Deficiency Anemia (IDA)
- Most common cause of anemia
- Presentation
  - Fatigue and weakness
  - ± Occult blood loss
  - Insufficient dietary intake
  - Malabsorption
  - Pregnancy
  - Pica: dirt (geophagia), ice (pagophagia)
  - Restless leg syndrome

IDA — Diagnosis
- Microcytosis and hypochromia
- Elevated RDW
- Decreased reticulocyte count
- Elevated platelet count

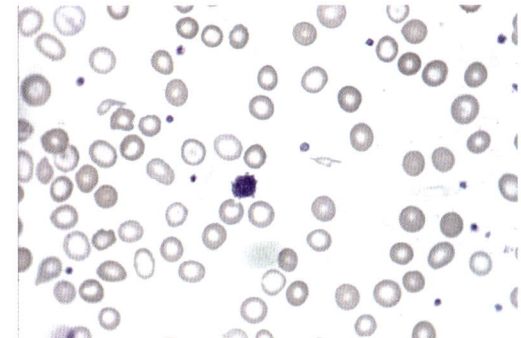

IDA

Ferritin	↓
Iron	↓
TIBC	↑
% Saturation (Fe/TIBC)	< 20%
Transferrin receptor	↑

- Serum ferritin: best test to assess iron stores
  - < 40 ng/mL = IDA
  - Less sensitivity in inflammatory states
- Must pursue etiology of Fe deficiency
  - Young females: GYN blood loss
  - Older adults: GI blood loss
  - ↓ Absorption: sprue, gastric bypass, gastritis, *H. pylori*
- Treatment: Replace iron!
  - PO or IV replacement

Audience Response 1
An 18-year-old female presents complaining of fatigue. She has normal menses.

Exam:

Pallor

Hgb 10 g/dL, MCV 70 fL, Platelets 450,000 cells/mcL

Fe is low, TIBC is increased, ferritin is low, % sat 10.

Rx: iron supplements

On follow-up 2 months later, patient has fatigue, abdominal fullness, and nausea; bowel movements are "dark" and voluminous. She reports adherence to the oral iron.

Repeat CBC shows a microcytic anemia that is unimproved.

Which of the following is the most appropriate next step in management?

A. Coombs test
B. HIV ELISA
C. IgA tTGA
D. Emphasize a need for strict adherence to the iron supplements.
E. Measurement of haptoglobin

Answer:_____

Anemia of Inflammation → AI (ACD)
- Infection, inflammation, malignancy, trauma, heart failure, diabetes, elderly
  - Decreased RBC production and impaired iron utilization despite normal or increased iron stores
    - Mediated by IL-6 and hepcidin
- Normochromic, normocytic RBCs or hypochromic, microcytic
- Decreased reticulocyte count

HEMATOLOGY

Anemia of Inflammation

Ferritin	↑
Iron	↓
TIBC	↓
% Saturation (Fe/TIBC)	Normal – ↓
Transferrin Receptor	Normal

- Measurement of CRP, ESR, fibrinogen helpful to interpret ferritin measurement
- Bone marrow exam for difficult cases: ↑ storage iron
- Treat underlying conditions, transfusions, erythropoietin

Compare and Contrast!

	IDA	AI
Ferritin	↓	↑
Fe	↓	↓
TIBC	↑	↓
% Saturation	↓	↓
Soluble Transferrin Receptor	↑	Normal

Anemia and CKD

- Due to decreased erythropoietin (EPO) production
- Responsive to recombinant EPO-stimulating agents (ESAs)
- **Screen for iron deficiency**
  - Transferrin saturation < 20% and ferritin < 100 ng/mL
  - Correct before starting ESA therapy
    - Target saturation ≥ 20% and ferritin > 100 ng/mL
  - Oral replacement okay, but watch for poor absorption → IV
  - Several options available for IV replacement
- ESAs: **Start only if Hgb < 10 g/dL**
  - **Target: Hgb 10–12 g/dL**
  - Contraindicated in uncontrolled HTN

Megaloblastic Anemias — B$_{12}$ and Folate Deficiencies

B$_{12}$ Deficiency

- Deficiency common
- Anemia not so common
- Causes
  - Pernicious anemia
  - Malabsorption
  - Malnutrition
- Associations
  - Hashimoto's or other autoimmune diseases
  - "White forelock"
  - *H. pylori*
  - Bacterial overgrowth
  - Long-term use of H$_2$ blockers or PPIs
  - Metformin
  - Alcoholism
  - Gastric bypass
  - Pancreatic exocrine failure
  - Sjögren's
  - Ileal disease
  - Vegetarianism
- Presentation
  - Signs/Symptoms of underlying cause, plus …
    - GI
      - Atrophic glossitis
      - Diarrhea
    - Neurologic
      - Paresthesias
      - Numbness
      - Dementia/Personality changes
  - Not all patients have the hematologic changes!

Folate Deficiency

- Causes
  - Malnutrition: <u>alcohol</u>, anorexia
  - Increased requirement
    - Pregnancy
    - Hereditary hemolytic anemias
  - Drugs: trimethoprim, pyrimethamine, methotrexate, phenytoin
- No neurologic manifestations

B$_{12}$ / Folate Deficiency — Clues

- **MCV > 100 fL + hypersegmented polys** = pathognomonic
- Mild hemolysis
  - Slightly ↑ indirect bilirubin
  - ↑ LDH
  - ↓ Haptoglobin
- Decreased reticulocyte count
  - Hemolysis is intramedullary
- ± Leukopenia and thrombocytopenia

Megaloblastic Anemias

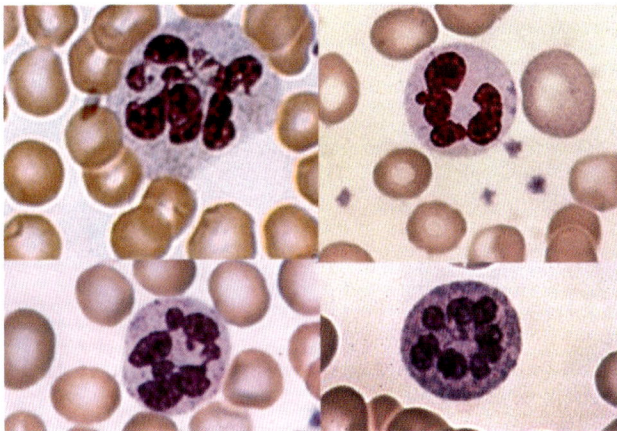

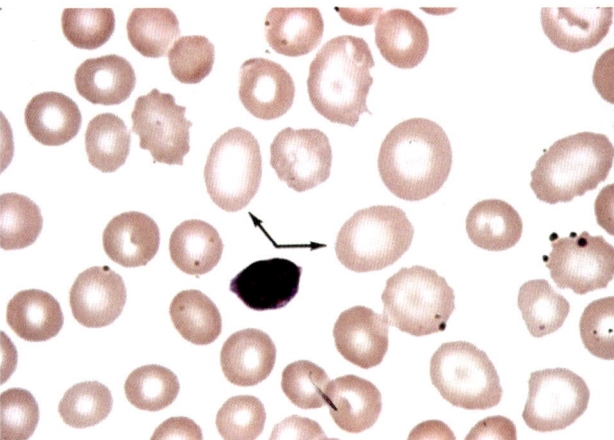

MCV > 100 fL

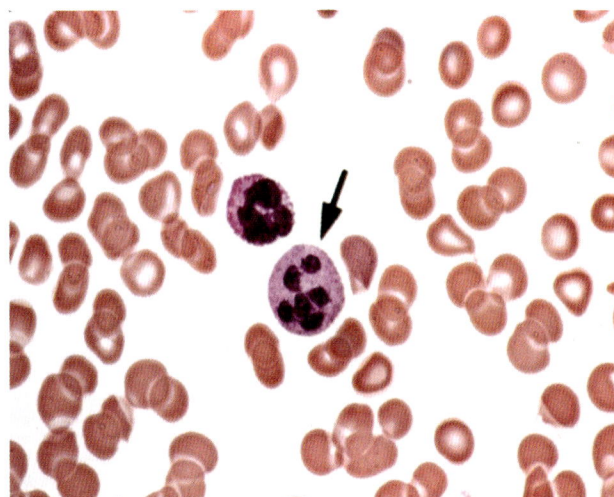

Various views of hypersegmented neutrophils

Definition: 5% with 5 lobes or any 6 lobes

B₁₂ Deficiency

- Diagnose: serum B₁₂ level
    - B₁₂ < 200 = B₁₂ deficiency
    - B₁₂ 200–400 = possible B₁₂ deficiency
        - Check methylmalonic acid (MMA) and homocysteine (HC)
        - MMA ↑, HC ↑ = B₁₂ deficiency
- Diagnosis of pernicious anemia (PA)
    - Intrinsic factor (IF) antibodies
    - Antiparietal cell antibodies
    - Check for elevated serum gastrin and pepsinogen in suspected PA with negative IF antibodies

Megaloblastic Anemias

	B₁₂	Folate
B₁₂	↓	Nl
Folate	Nl	↓
MMA	↑	Nl
HC	↑	↑
Intrinsic Factor Ab	+	N/A

- Treatment
    - B₁₂ injections or high-dose oral therapy
        - Watch for hypokalemia
    - Oral folate replacement
    - Do not treat B₁₂ deficiency with folate alone → anemia will improve but neuro symptoms worsen!

Hemolytic Anemia

Recognizing Hemolysis
- Pallor
- Jaundice
- Gallstones
- Splenomegaly
- Abnormal heart valves
- Symptoms of TTP or DIC
- Symptoms of malaria
- Lab clues
    - ↑ Reticulocyte count
    - ↑ Indirect bilirubin
    - ↑ LDH
    - ↓ Haptoglobin
    - + Coombs if AIHA
- Smear clues
    - Spherocytes
    - Schistocytes
    - Spur cells
    - Bite cells
    - RBC inclusions

Hemolytic Anemia — Keeping It Simple
- Intrinsic: **Problem is within the red cell itself; usually hereditary**
  - Molecular defect inside RBC
    - G6PD, hemoglobinopathies
  - RBC membrane problem
    - Hereditary spherocytosis/elliptocytosis
- Extrinsic: **Problem is in environment outside red cell; usually acquired**
  - Autoimmune hemolysis
  - Microangiopathy
    - DIC, TTP, mechanical heart valves

Hemoglobinopathies
- Sickle cell disease
- α-Thalassemia
- β-Thalassemia
- Likely questions
  - Complications of sickle cell anemia
  - Recognition of the spleen in Hgb SC disease
  - Recognize α-thalassemia misdiagnosed as chronic iron deficiency anemia

Sickle Cell Disease
- Hemoglobin AS
  - Sickle cell trait
  - One affected gene
  - No clinical significance
  - Unable to fully concentrate urine
- Hemoglobin SS
  - Substitution of valine for glutamic acid on the β-globin gene
  - Sickle cell disease with varied expression
- **Clinical presentation**
  - Aplastic crisis from parvovirus B19
  - Functional asplenia
  - Microinfarcts of organs such as brain — CVA
  - Priapism and retinal detachment
  - Pain crisis
  - Acute chest syndrome
  - Nonhealing leg ulcer
  - Avascular necrosis of the hip
- **Management**
  - Acute vasoocclusive crisis
    - Empiric antibiotics
    - Oxygen
    - IV fluids
    - Pain management
  - Supportive
    - Iron chelation
    - Folic acid
  - Disease modifying
    - Hydroxyurea
    - Voxelotor
    - Crizanlizumab

Hemoglobin SC Disease
- 50:50 Hgb S:C
- Severity is between SS and SA disease
- **Milder anemia**
- **Splenomegaly**
- Many do not lose their spleens in childhood!
- At risk for splenic sequestration
  - Vasoocclusive crisis in the spleen
  - Acute anemia
  - Reticulocytosis
  - Shock
  - Can occur at any age!
  - Transfusion and splenectomy

Thalassemias
- Inherited gene defects
- Abnormal Hgb production → hemolysis and ineffective erythropoiesis

	α-Thalassemia Minor	β-Thalassemia Minor
Mechanism	Decreased α-chain production	Decreased β-chain production
Presentation	Mild anemia, with very low MCV Target cells on smear; no iron deficiency	Mild anemia, with very low MCV Target cells on smear; no iron deficiency
Diagnosis	Normal Hb electrophoresis	Elevated HbA$_2$ on Hb electrophoresis
Misc.	Can be misdiagnosed as iron deficiency; and inappropriately treated with iron → secondary hemochromatosis	Can be misdiagnosed as iron deficiency; and inappropriately treated with iron → secondary hemochromatosis

Hemoglobinopathies

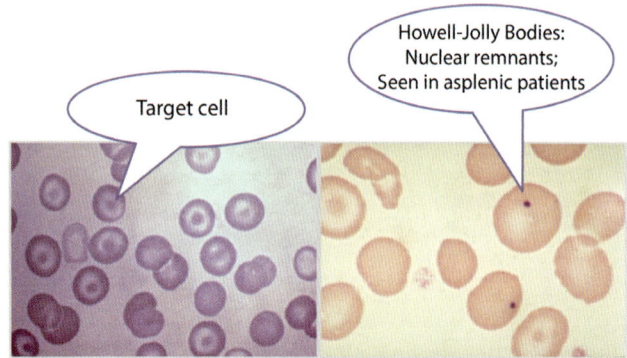

Target cell

Howell-Jolly Bodies: Nuclear remnants; Seen in asplenic patients

AR 2

A 17-year-old female:

RUQ pain × 2 weeks

Gallbladder U/S = cholelithiasis

WBC 10,500 cells/mcL (normal differential)

Hgb 10.2 g/dL, MCV 94 fL

Platelets 400,000 cells/mcL

Reticulocyte count 5.7%

Normal chemistries

AST 24 U/L, ALT 35 U/L, Alk phos 110 U/L

Total bilirubin 4.5 mg/dL, direct bilirubin 0.5 mg/dL, indirect bilirubin 4.0 mg/dL

Which of the following is the most likely associated laboratory finding?

A. Spherocytes on smear
B. Hypercholesterolemia
C. Hypertriglyceridemia
D. Teardrops on smear
E. Smudge cells on smear

Answer:_____

Hereditary Spherocytosis (HS)
- Autosomal dominant, northern European
- RBC membrane disorder
- Chronic hemolysis
- Cholelithiasis, splenomegaly
- Smear — spherocytes
- Dx: EMA binding test; osmotic fragility test
- Management
  - Transfusions
  - EPO, iron
  - Splenectomy

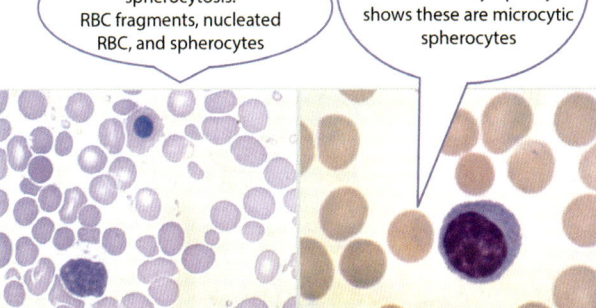

Evidence of hemolysis in spherocytosis: RBC fragments, nucleated RBC, and spherocytes

Hereditary spherocytosis: Lack of central pallor; Normal-sized lymphocyte shows these are microcytic spherocytes

G6PD Deficiency
- X-linked
- Hemolysis with oxidative stress
  - Drugs (antimalarials, sulfa, dapsone)
  - Fava beans
  - DKA
- Smear — bite cells; Heinz bodies
- Dx: G6PD assay
  - Wait 2–3 months after acute episode to avoid false negatives
- Management
  - Avoidance of triggers
  - Transfusion

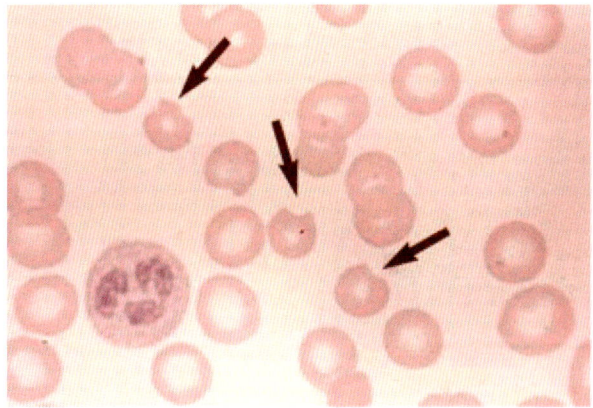

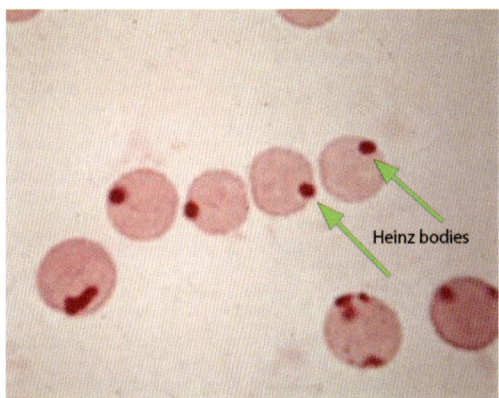

Heinz bodies

Paroxysmal Nocturnal Hemoglobinuria (PNH)
- Acquired stem cell disorder with defective *PIGA* gene
- Loss of membrane-bound protein rendering cells sensitive to **complement-mediated lysis**
- Clinical presentation
  - Intravascular hemolysis
  - Arterial/Venous thrombosis
  - Risk of aplastic anemia/leukemia
- Diagnose by flow cytometry for CD55, CD59
- Treatment
  - Hematopoietic stem cell transplant (HSCT)
  - Steroids for hemolysis
  - Eculizumab

AR 3

A 67-year-old female:

Rapidly growing neck swelling, progressive fatigue

Weight loss of 15 lb in 2 months

Exam = multiple rubbery lymph nodes and palpable spleen

WBC 9,500 cells/mcL (70% segs, 15% eos, 10% lymphs, 5% monos)

Hgb 9.5 g/dL (MCV 90 fL)

Platelets 350,000 cells/mcL

Reticulocyte count 4.5%

LDH 884 U/L

Total bilirubin 3.7 mg/dL, indirect bilirubin 3.2 mg/dL

AST 15 U/L, ALT 25 U/L

BUN 10 mg/dL, creatinine 0.6 mg/dL

Which of the following is the most likely cause of the patient's anemia?

A. Iron deficiency
B. B_{12} deficiency
C. Inflammation
D. Autoimmune hemolytic anemia
E. Acute leukemia

Answer:_____

- Look for an associated condition
  - Warm (IgG): lymphoma, CLL, SLE, viruses, PCN
  - Cold (IgM): lymphoma, CLL, EBV mono, *Mycoplasma* (acral cyanosis)
- Reticulocytosis, high LDH; labs indicate hemolysis
- **Diagnose with Coombs test**
- Treatment
  - Warm Ab: steroids, splenectomy, rituximab
  - Cold Ab: Treat underlying cause, keep warm!

Autoimmune Hemolytic Anemias (AIHAs)

	Warm Ab	**Cold** Ab
Temperature at Which RBCs Agglutinate	Body temp	Room temp
Ab Type	IgG	IgM
Causes	Viral, connective tissue disease, malignancy (CLL)	Infection (*Mycoplasma*, EBV), malignancy (lymphoma)
Diagnosis	DAT positive IgG or C3	DAT positive C3, but negative for IgG
Treatment	Steroids 1st line; rituximab, splenectomy	Keep warm; rituximab

HEMOCHROMATOSIS

Hereditary Hemochromatosis
- Autosomal recessive
  - Caucasians: 5 in 1,000 homozygous
  - *C282Y* (and/or *H63D*) mutation(s) of *HFE* gene
    - Modulates iron absorption via HFE protein
    - Affects hepcidin production
  - Clinical manifestations later in ♀ (menstruation)
- Distinguish from secondary iron overload
- Iron accumulation leads to organ damage
  - Diabetes
  - Arthropathy of iron overload and CPPD
  - Cirrhosis and hepatocellular carcinoma
  - Impotence
  - Skin hyperpigmentation
  - Dilated cardiomyopathy ± conduction defects
  - Susceptibility: *Vibrio*, *Yersinia*, and *Listeria*
- Screen family members of index case
  - Iron saturation, ferritin, *HFE* gene mutation
- Diagnosis
  - Fe/TIBC (≥ 45%), ferritin (> 200 ng/mL ♀ and > 300 ng/mL ♂)
  - Genetic testing for ***C282Y* and *H63D*** mutations
  - Liver biopsy in selected cases
- Treatment is phlebotomy
  - Slows progression and prevents new organ damage
- Guidance: Avoid excessive alcohol intake, vitamin C supplements, and uncooked seafood

HEMOSTASIS

BLEEDING

General Approach to Bleeding Disorders
- Primary hemostasis
  - 90% involve platelet problems
  - Superficial hemorrhage and mucocutaneous bleeding
- Secondary hemostasis
  - Usually clotting factor problems
  - Deep tissue bleeding; i.e., hematomas, hemarthroses
- Useful tests to start workup
  - PT
  - Platelet count
  - PTT
  - Platelet function tests

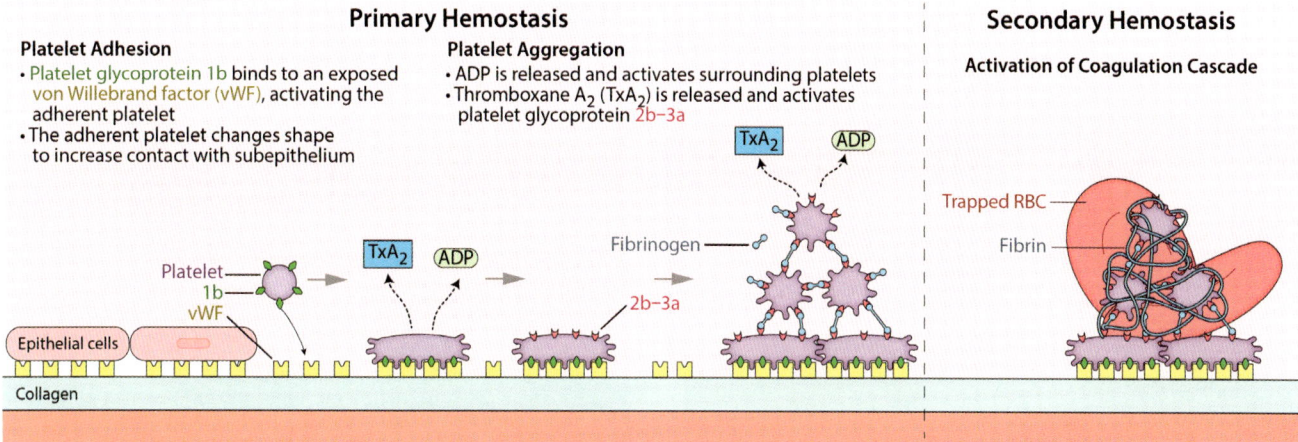

Primary Hemostasis

Platelet Adhesion
- Platelet glycoprotein 1b binds to an exposed von Willebrand factor (vWF), activating the adherent platelet
- The adherent platelet changes shape to increase contact with subepithelium

Platelet Aggregation
- ADP is released and activates surrounding platelets
- Thromboxane A_2 (TxA_2) is released and activates platelet glycoprotein 2b–3a

Secondary Hemostasis

Activation of Coagulation Cascade

Thrombocytopenia

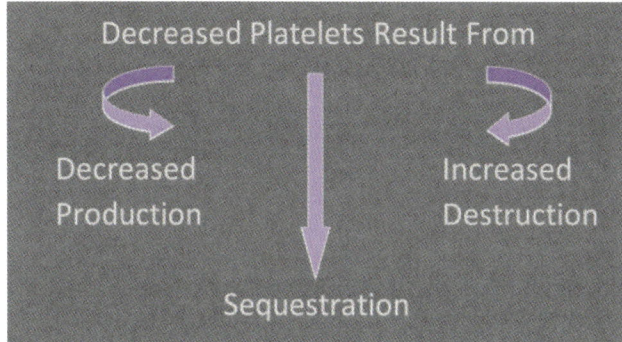

Decreased Platelets Result From

Decreased Production

Sequestration

Increased Destruction

Thrombocytopenia — ↓ Production
- Primary marrow failure
  - Aplastic anemia, B_{12}, and folate deficiencies
- Marrow replacement
  - Acute leukemia, infiltration
- Viral suppression/damage
  - HCV, EBV, HIV
- Drug suppression
  - EtOH, trimethoprim/sulfamethoxazole, MMR

Thrombocytopenia — Sequestration
- Hypersplenism
- Generally mild and trilineage suppression
- Evidence of liver disease

Thrombocytopenia — ↑ Destruction
- ITP
- TTP
- DIC
- HIT: heparin-induced thrombocytopenia
  - HIT Type I: mild
  - HIT Type II: autoimmune, severe

ITP
- Adults = chronic disease
- Etiologies
  - Idiopathic
  - Drugs
  - Disease states, such as lymphoma, CLL, collagen vascular diseases
  - Viral illnesses, such as HCV, HIV
- Easy bruising, petechiae, purpura, mucosal bleeding
- Significant bleeding rare
- Antibody-mediated — IgG
  - Do not order the antiplatelet antibody test
  - No diagnostic test; R/O HIV, HCV, SLE, and drugs
- Treatment
  - Platelets > 30,000 cells per mcL: Observe
  - Platelets < 30,000 cells per mcL: Tx
    - Steroids or
    - IVIG or
    - Splenectomy — remember to vaccinate Capsule
    - Rituximab
    - Thrombopoietic agonists

Thrombotic Microangiopathies
- TTP
- Atypical HUS
- Diarrhea-associated HUS
- HELPP syndrome

TTP
- TTP pentad
  1) Fever
  2) **Anemia* (microangiopathic, hemolytic)**
  3) Renal dysfunction
  4) **Thrombocytopenia***
  5) CNS
- Peripheral smear
  - Schistocytes
  - Thrombocytopenia
  - Normal WBC series
- **Normal PT/PTT**
- Abnormal hemolysis labs

*Dyad required for diagnosis.

Schistocytes

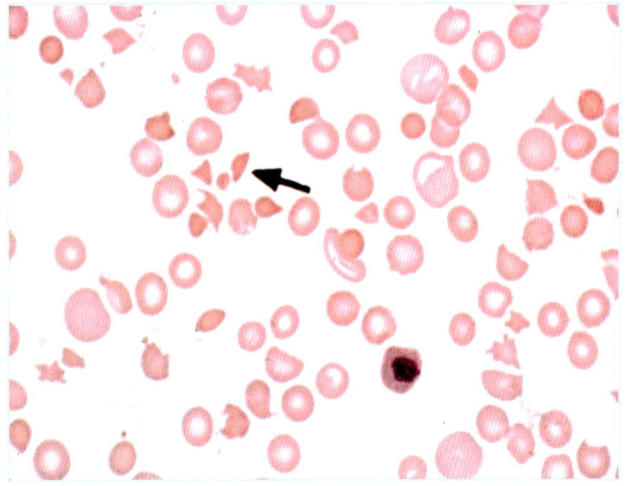

platelet clumping

ADAMTS13 — Central Role in Pathogenesis
- Normal: Endothelial cells make large vWF multimers that are broken down by the *ADAMTS13* gene product
- *ADAMTS13* deficiency causes accumulation of these large multimers
- The multimers stick to the platelets and cause clumping; in some cases of TTP, the clumping is severe → systemwide intravascular hemolysis

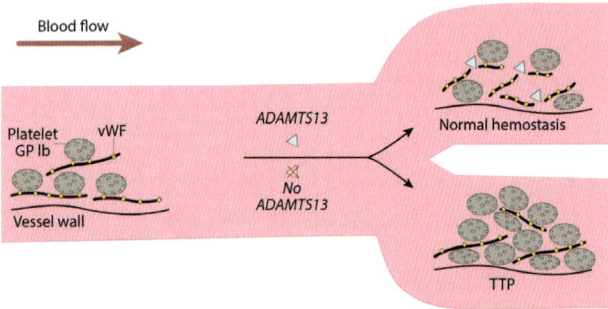

TTP — Etiologies
- Inherited: *ADAMTS13* gene defect
- Acquired: Anti-*ADAMTS13* antibody
  - Idiopathic
  - Drugs
    - Quinine, cyclosporine, ticlopidine, clopidogrel, OCPs
  - Autoimmune disease
    - SLE
    - Antiphospholipid antibodies
  - Infections
    - HIV, pneumococcus
  - Pregnancy/Postpartum
  - Shiga toxin
  - Stem cell transplants
  - Disseminated malignancy

TTP — Treatment
- Medical emergency
  - Plasma exchange is treatment of choice
    - **Except in TTP related to chemotherapy or after HSCT**
  - ± Steroids
  - Rituximab
  - Platelet transfusions are contraindicated

Thrombotic Microangiopathies
- Atypical HUS
  - Similar to TTP, but more renal involvement, and less neuro involvement
  - Caused by complement dysregulation
  - Treat with eculizumab (mAb inhibits terminal complement cascade)
- Diarrhea-associated HUS
  - Similar to TTP; prodrome of bloody diarrhea
  - Caused by *E. coli* 0157:H7 or *Shigella*
  - Treatment is supportive
- HELPP syndrome
  - In pregnancy; eclampsia or preeclampsia
  - Treatment is delivery of fetus

DIC
- Activation of clotting cascade secondary to an underlying illness
  - OB catastrophes
  - Malignancy, trauma, sepsis
- Laboratories
  - Schistocytes, ↓ PLT
  - Reticulocytosis
  - **Abnormal PT/PTT**
  - Low fibrinogen

PT	↑
PTT	↑
PLT CT	↓
Fibrinogen	↓
Fibrin Degradation Products	↑
D-dimer	↑
Protamine	+

DIC — Treatment
- Treatment of the underlying disorder
- Support with appropriate products
  - Cryoprecipitate
  - FFP
  - Platelets
  - PRBCs
- Heparin therapy in malignancies with chronic form

Thrombocytopenias — Simplifying the "Alphabet Soup"

	ITP	TTP	DIC
Pathogenesis	Anti-PLT Ab	Endothelial defect	Thrombin excess
Clinical	Not sick	Ill appearing	Ill appearing
Red Cells	Normal	Schistocytes	Schistocytes
PT	Normal	Normal	Increased
PTT	Normal	Normal	Increased
Fibrinogen	Normal	Normal	Decreased
D-dimer	Normal	Normal	Increased
Management	Steroids, IVIG, splenectomy, TPA-agonists	Plasma exchange; supportive	Supportive

AR 4

A dialysis patient on heparin develops thrombocytopenia (PLT count drops from 220K to 60K), associated with pain and swelling of right calf and leg. Venous duplex U/S of RLE confirms DVT.

What are you going to do?

A. Stop heparin and prescribe bivalirudin.
B. Change the heparin to LMWH.
X C. Stop heparin and prescribe argatroban.
D. Recommend plasma exchange transfusion.
E. Stop heparin and start aspirin for prophylaxis.

Answer: ___C.___

HIT Type II

- Autoimmune
  - Ab vs. heparin-PLT complex
  - 5–8 days after exposure
  - Anamnestic response → 1–2 days
- Less risk with LMWH
- Arterial + venous clots
- PLT < 50% of initial
  - Can be in normal range!
  - Stop heparin
- **Initial Dx is clinical!**
- 4 Ts
  1) **T**hrombocytopenia present?
  2) **T**iming of thrombocytopenia
  3) **T**hrombosis?
  4) **T**hrombocytopenia — other causes?
- Remain hypercoagulable for weeks after improvement

HIT Type II — Diagnosis

- <u>Recognize syndrome</u>
- Assays have slow turnaround time
  - ELISA "HIT antibody panel"
  - Serotonin release assay-gold standard
  - Platelet aggregation assay
  - Clinical presentation consistent and (+) ELISA = probably HIT
- Watch for other causes of ↓ platelets

HIT Type II — Treatment

- **Stop any heparins**; do not switch
- At risk for clot as long as antibodies are present, so …
  - Start alternative anticoagulation: argatroban, fondaparinux, bivalirudin, or direct oral anticoagulant, in all settings — clots or no clots
    - Use argatroban with caution in <u>liver dysfunction</u>
  - Initiate warfarin only after platelet count > 100,000 cells per mcL and anticoagulation with alternate agent is established
  - **No platelet transfusions**

von Willebrand Disease (vWD)

- Most common inherited bleeding disorder
  - 3 types + acquired form
  - Autosomal dominant
  - Type O blood = lower levels vWF
  - Bruising, skin and mucous membrane bleeding
    - Epistaxis
    - Uterine bleeds/menorrhagia
    - Dental bleeding
    - Bleeds with NSAIDs
    - PTT prolonged (decreased Factor 8)
    - Bleeding time/PFA-100: May be normal in mild-to-moderate disease

vWD — Evaluation

- Screening tests
  - vWF:Ag
  - vWF activity tests
    - vWF:RCoF and vWF:CB
  - Factor 8 activity
- Confirmatory tests
  - Ristocetin-induced platelet aggregation (RIPA)
  - vWF multimer distribution on gel electrophoresis

vWD — Diagnosis and Treatment

- Interpretation of vWD labs = Complex; Recognize vWD or, more often, what is <u>not</u> vWD, and know the tests to order
- Treatment is very specialized
  - **Desmopressin (DDAVP),** except Type 2B!
    - Release of vWF and Factor 8 from endothelial cells
  - Cryoprecipitate
  - Factor 8 concentrates, with vW factor

Coagulation Cascade

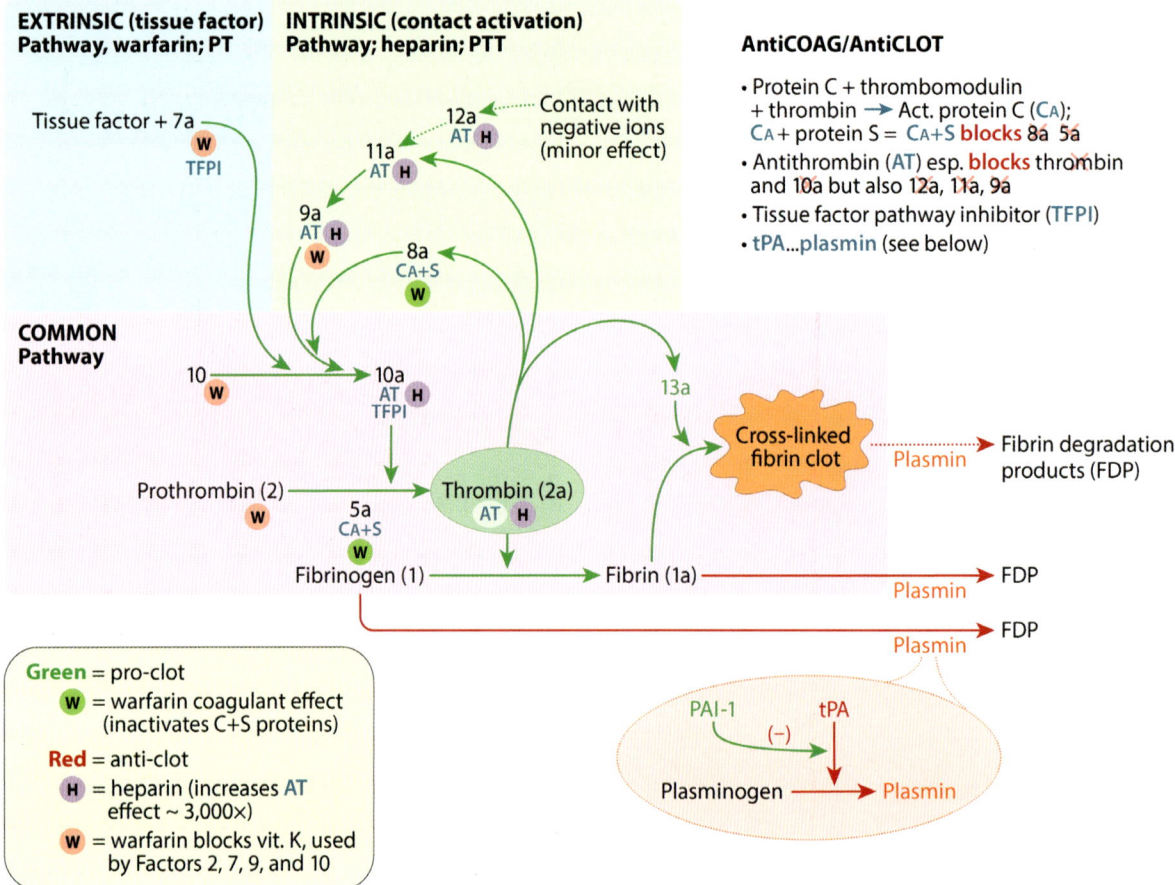

EXTRINSIC (tissue factor)
Pathway, warfarin; PT

INTRINSIC (contact activation)
Pathway; heparin; PTT

Tissue factor + 7a
W
TFPI

12a
AT
←···· Contact with
negative ions
(minor effect)

11a
AT H

9a
AT H
W

8a
CA+S
W

AntiCOAG/AntiCLOT

- Protein C + thrombomodulin
  + thrombin → Act. protein C (CA);
  CA + protein S = CA+S **blocks** 8a 5a
- Antithrombin (AT) esp. **blocks** thrombin
  and 10a but also 12a, 11a, 9a
- Tissue factor pathway inhibitor (TFPI)
- tPA...plasmin (see below)

COMMON
Pathway

10 → 10a
W   AT H
     TFPI

13a

Cross-linked
fibrin clot
→ Fibrin degradation
products (FDP)
Plasmin

Prothrombin (2)
W
5a
CA+S
W

Thrombin (2a)
AT H

Fibrinogen (1) → Fibrin (1a) → FDP
Plasmin

→ FDP
Plasmin

Green = pro-clot
W = warfarin coagulant effect
(inactivates C+S proteins)

Red = anti-clot
H = heparin (increases AT
effect ~ 3,000×)
W = warfarin blocks vit. K, used
by Factors 2, 7, 9, and 10

PAI-1   tPA
(−)
Plasminogen → Plasmin

Evaluation of Prolonged PT / PTT
- Is it a "factor deficiency" problem
  or a "factor inhibitor" problem?
  - 1:1 mix of patient's plasma
    with "normal" plasma
    - Factor deficiency: correction of PTT
    - Inhibitor: no correction of PTT
    - Delayed incubation may reveal an inhibitor
    - Antiphospholipid antibodies
      will not correct
      - Clots! Not bleeds!
  - Factor 8 inhibitor: life-threatening bleeds
    - Hemophiliacs, solid tumors, CLL,
      postpartum, autoimmune disease (RA and SLE),
      > 55 years of age

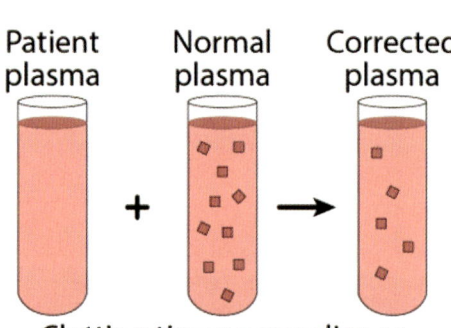

Patient plasma + Normal plasma → Corrected plasma

Clotting times normalize or
decrease to near-normal =
factor deficiency

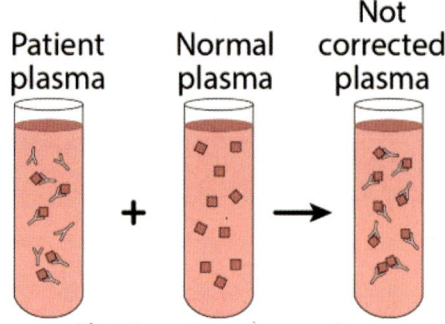

Patient plasma + Normal plasma → Not corrected plasma

Clotting times remain
prolonged = inhibitor

Bleeding Disorder Evaluation: PT, PTT, Bleeding Time, and Platelet Aggregation	
Lab Results	**Etiology**
Elevated PT **and** PTT	Factor deficiency from common pathway Multiple factor deficiency Warfarin affects Factors 2, 7, 9, and 10, so it can affect both PT and PTT, but PT is more sensitive to warfarin
Elevated PT, nl PTT	Factor 7 deficiency
Elevated PTT, nl PT: immediate and sustained (2 hours) correction of PTT by addition of normal plasma	Factor 8, 9, 11, or 12 deficiency

Elevated PTT, nl PT: PTT **not** corrected (or no sustained correction at 2 hours) by addition of normal plasma	Inhibitor syndrome (circulating anticoagulant):
	If clotting:
	    Antiphospholipid synd (esp. lupus anticoagulant)
	    PTT not normalized immediately
	If bleeding:
	    Factor 8 inhibitor
	    PTT initially normalized but not normalized at 2 hours

Elevated PTT, nl PT — but **no** clinical bleeding disorder	Factor 12 deficiency
Normal PT and PTT — but post-op bleeding	Factor 13 deficiency

Normal PT/PTT, but elevated bleeding time:
  Elevated bleeding time with nl plt aggregation
  Elevated bleeding time with nl plt aggregation and decreased plt count
 	
  Elevated bleeding time with abnl plt aggregation
	Platelet problem
	vWD (has decreased plt adhesion but nl aggregation)
	Bernard-Soulier (giant plt) synd (absent GP1b) has similar presentation as vWD except lab also shows decreased plt count
	Glanzmann thrombasthenia (absent GP2b/3a)

Bleeding Disorders — Pearls

- Superficial bleeding (mucosal, ecchymosis), with normal PT/PTT — think **platelet** problem
  - Quantitative — thrombocytopenias
  - Qualitative — von Willebrand's, other platelet function disorders
- Deeper soft tissue bleeding (hematomas, hemarthrosis) with prolonged PT and/or PTT — think **clotting factor** problem
  - Prolonged PT only — think about warfarin, liver disease, vitamin K deficiency
  - Prolonged PTT only — think about Factor 8, 9, 11, 12 problem
    - Check mixing study

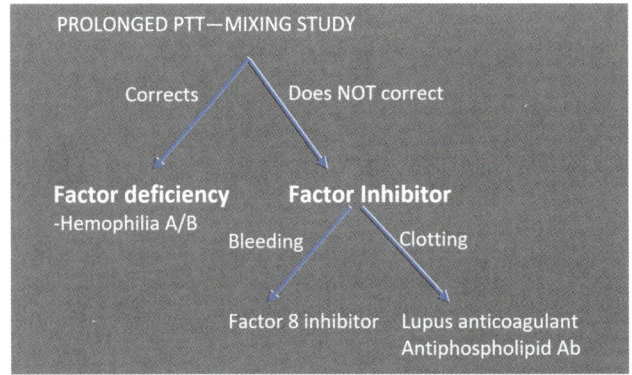

- Isolated prolonged PTT, but with **no** clinical bleeding — Factor 12 deficiency
- Normal PT/PTT, but with postsurgical bleeding — Factor 13 deficiency

Hemophilia A

- Low levels of Factor 8: prolonged PTT
- Corrects with 1:1 mix, unless inhibitor present
- Usually diagnosed shortly after birth if severe
- X-linked recessive
- With mild or moderate disease; may not bleed until older with trauma
- Treatment is very complicated and specialized!
- Bottom line: Give factor if at risk for a bleed

Vitamin K Deficiency

- Vitamin K dependent on:
  - Absorption of diet
  - Synthesis in gut
  - Recycling in liver
- ↓ K → levels of Factors 2, 7, 9, 10, and proteins C and S → prolonged PT
- Treat with vitamin K
  - If bleeding, use FFP
- Causes
  - Liver disease
  - Warfarin
  - Malnutrition/Absorption (TPN!)
  - Antibiotics
    - Cefotetan, cefoperazone, cefamandole, cefazolin = NMTT side chain
    - Broad spectrum = Reduces synthesizing organisms in intestine

HEMATOLOGY

AR 5

Which of the following disorders may present with a normal PT and normal aPTT but evidence of bleeding with a prolonged bleeding time?

A. Factor 8 deficiency
B. Factor 5 deficiency
C. Factor 7 deficiency
D. von Willebrand disease
~~E.~~ Factor 12 deficiency

Answer: _E._

AR 6

A 36-year-old postpartum woman returns within 48 hours of birth complaining of abdominal pain and epistaxis. She had a normal pregnancy and delivery. Exam is benign except for fresh blood in the posterior oropharynx. Labs at discharge were normal.

WBC 15,000 cells/mcL (75% segs, 10% bands, 15% lymphs)

Hgb 8 g/dL, Hct 24%, platelets 4,000 cells/mcL

PT 12 sec, PTT 32 sec, fibrinogen 350 mg/dL

LDH 12,000 U/L

BUN 25 mg/dL, creatinine 3.5 mg/dL

Reticulocyte count 5%

Total bilirubin 5.0 mg/dL, indirect bilirubin 4.5 mg/dL

AST 30 U/L, ALT 35 U/L

Which of the following is the most appropriate next step in management?

A. Platelet transfusion
B. Heparin infusion
C. Platelet transfusion and FFP infusion
D. Bone marrow biopsy
E. Therapeutic plasma exchange

Answer: _____

THROMBOTIC DISORDERS

Thrombophilia
- Inherited
  - Factor 5 Leiden mutation
  - Prothrombin gene mutation
  - Protein C and S deficiency*
  - Antithrombin deficiency*
- Acquired
  - Surgery
  - Central venous catheters
  - Malignancy
  - Nephrotic syndrome
  - Pregnancy
  - Smoking
  - OCPs
  - Heparin
  - Tamoxifen
  - Myeloproliferative disorders
  - Antiphospholipid antibodies
  - Travel (2–4× risk)

*Levels reduced during acute clot. Heparin and warfarin also reduce levels. Test 2 weeks after completing 3–6 months of anticoagulation.

Think about testing for thrombophilia when:
  - VTE at young age (< 50)
  - Recurrent VTE
  - Strong family history of VTE
  - Atypical site of VTE (cerebral, mesenteric)
- Screening panel should include:
  - Factor 5 Leiden mutation
  - Prothrombin gene mutation
  - Protein C and S, AT3
  - Lupus anticoagulant/Cardiolipin Ab/ β_2-glycoprotein I Ab

Primary Antiphospholipid Syndrome
- Need: 1 clinical feature + 1 antibody
  - Clinical features
    - Paradoxical venous/arterial thromboses
    - Pregnancy "morbidity"
      - Recurrent spontaneous embryonic or fetal loss or
      - Prematurity due to (pre)eclampsia/placental insufficiency
  - Antiphospholipid antibodies
    - Lupus anticoagulants
    - Anticardiolipin
    - β_2-Glycoprotein-1
- Other manifestations
  - Livedo reticularis
  - Thrombocytopenia (50,000–140,000/mL)
  - Cardiac valvular thickening/vegetations, heart murmurs
  - Nephropathy
  - Prolonged PT or PTT; no correction with 1:1 mix

AR 7

A pregnant patient, at 28 weeks of gestation, presents with an uncomplicated DVT of her left lower extremity.

What are you going to prescribe for treatment?

A. "Pregnant?" — refer to OB!
B. Unfractionated heparin
~~C.~~ LMWH
D. Rivaroxaban
E. Warfarin

Answer: _C._

Anticoagulants
- Vitamin K antagonists (VKA): DVT/PE, stroke, atrial fibrillation (AFib)
  - Warfarin
- Heparins: DVT/PE, AMI ± PCI
  - UFH, IV or SQ
  - LMWH, SQ (enoxaparin, tinzaparin, dalteparin)
- Factor 10a inhibitors: DVT/PE
  - Fondaparinux (Arixtra), SQ
  - Rivaroxaban (Xarelto): DVT, AFib
  - Apixaban (Eliquis): CVA, AFib
- Direct thrombin (II) inhibitors
  - Argatroban: HIT, PCI
  - Bivalirudin (Angiomax): AMI ± PCI
  - Dabigatran (Pradaxa): nonvalvular AFib, DVT/PE

Anticoagulant Drugs

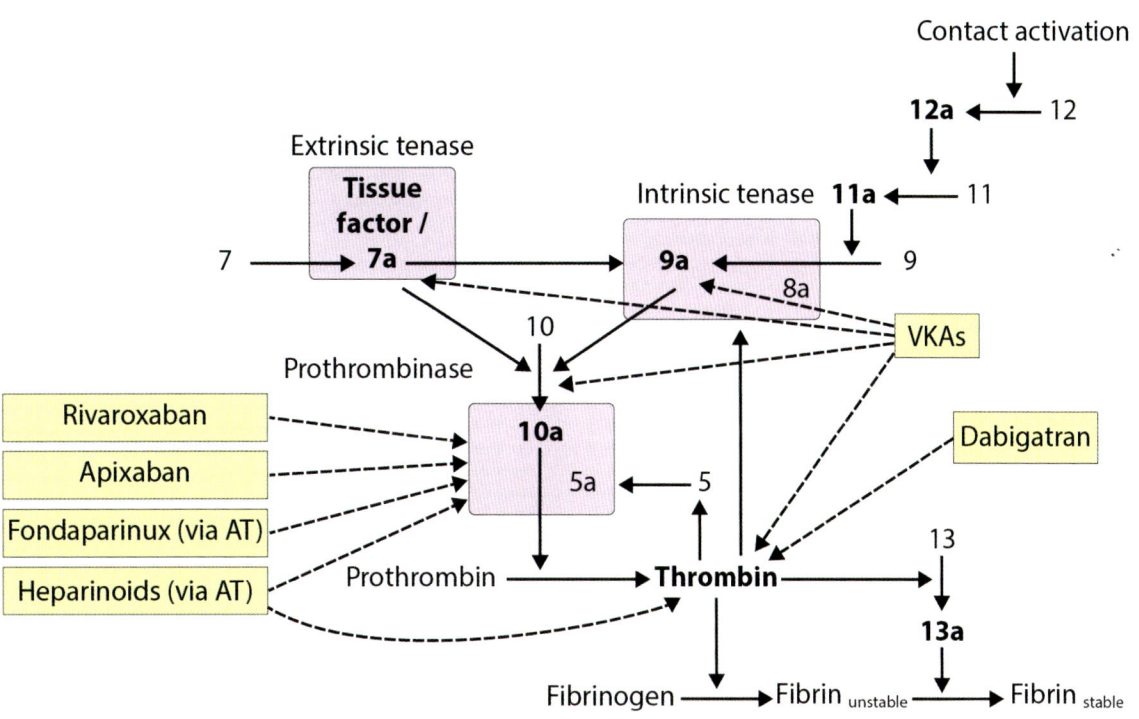

Direct Oral Anticoagulants

	Factor 10a Inhibitors	Thrombin Inhibitors
Drugs	Rivaroxaban Apixaban Edoxaban	Dabigatran
Mechanism of Action	Direct Factor 10a inhibitor	Direct Factor 2a (thrombin) inhibitor
Relevant Indications	VTE treatment and prophylaxis Atrial fibrillation	VTE treatment and prophylaxis Atrial fibrillation
Reversal Agents	Andexanet alfa	Idarucizumab

Venous Thrombosis — Management Pearls
- Initial therapy: LMWH or direct oral anticoagulant (DOAC) for most stable patients
- When is IV UFH preferred? Massive PE, unstable, or renal dysfunction
  - When is thrombolytic therapy considered? Massive PE or iliofemoral thrombus
- Preferred agents in HIT? Argatroban, bivalirudin, fondaparinux
- Preferred agent in malignancy and pregnancy? LMWH
- Renal disease: Avoid LMWH and fondaparinux
- Duration of therapy?
  - Provoked with transient risk factor: 3 months
  - Unprovoked: at least 3 months; consider indefinite
  - Recurrent thrombosis: indefinite

- Indications for IVC filter?
  - Contraindication to anticoagulation
  - Failure of anticoagulation
  - Severe cardiopulmonary compromise
  - Prophylaxis in high-risk surgery

Transfusion Medicine
- Blood products
  - RBC
  - Platelet
    - Target > 10,000 cells/mcL in nonbleeding patients
    - Target > 50,000 cells/mcL for most invasive procedures
    - Do not use in ITP (does not work)
    - Do not use in TTP/HIT (thrombosis!)
  - WBC rarely used!
  - FFP, cryoprecipitate

HEMATOLOGY

Transfusion Reactions

	Signs / Symptoms	Management	Other Info
Acute Hemolytic Transfusion Reaction	Fever, chills, N/V, shock, dark urine	**Stop** transfusion; IVF, supportive care	Due to ABO incompatibility — clerical issue
Delayed Hemolytic Transfusion Reaction	Often clinically silent; drop in Hgb 1–2 weeks after transfusion	Supportive, antipyretics	Rh/Kidd (minor) RBC antigen incompatibility
Febrile Transfusion Reaction	Fever ± chills	Supportive, antipyretics	Most common reaction, self-limited, due to cytokines
Allergic Reaction	Urticaria or hives	Supportive care, antihistamines	IgA-deficient recipients

78-Year-Old Male with Anemia — Acute Dyspnea 3 Hours after Red Cell Transfusion; What Should We Think About?

	TRALI (Transfusion-Related Acute Lung Injury)	TACO (Transfusion-Associated Acute Circulatory Overload)
Mechanism	Immune/Antibody mediated	Fluid overload
Clinical Presentation	"ARDS-like," noncardiogenic pulmonary edema 1–6 hours after transfusion BNP normal	"HF-like," cardiogenic pulmonary edema 1–6 hours after transfusion BNP elevated
Management	Supportive; **stop** transfusion Mechanical ventilation Donor avoidance	Diuretics Transfuse slowly

DISORDERS OF THE BONE MARROW

APLASTIC ANEMIA

- Presentation = **pancytopenia**
- Occurs secondary to a stem cell disorder
- Majority = idiopathic
- Other etiologies
  - Drugs
    - Gold, sulfa, chloramphenicol, carbamazepine, valproic acid, phenytoin, insecticides
  - Viral infection: hepatitis viruses, HIV, parvo B19 (red cells only)
- Presentation is a result of cytopenias
  - Infections
  - Anemia
  - Bleeding
- Diminished cell lines on peripheral smear
- Bone marrow exam is hypocellular; no infiltration of malignant cells or fibrosis
- Prognosis
  - Depends on marrow cellularity, age, and severity of cytopenias
  - Increased risk of future acute leukemia
- Management
  - Immunosuppression
    - Older patients
    - Younger patients with no marrow donor
  - HSCT
    - Younger patients with a donor

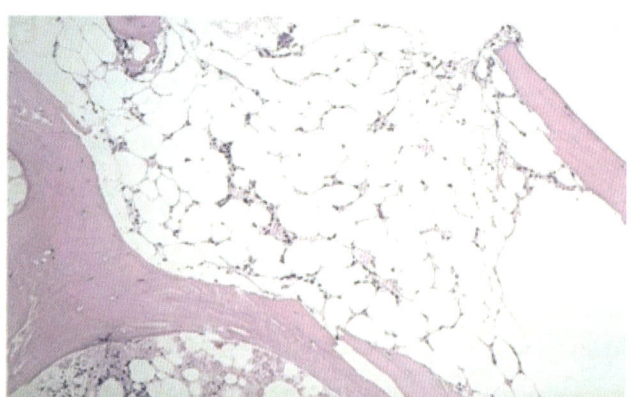

Aplastic anemia

AR 8

A 73-year-old man with history of DM, HTN, presents to the ED with fatigue, headache, and nosebleeds × 1 week. On exam, he is afebrile. Conjunctiva pale. Petechiae noted in oropharynx. Medial deviation of the left eye. Exam is otherwise unremarkable.

Baseline blood work includes: WBC 1.9; Hgb 6.8; Platelet 12

Review of peripheral smear shows blasts without Auer rods. Bone marrow exam shows hypercellular marrow with 68% blasts. Blasts are positive for TdT, CD19, CD20; negative for myeloperoxidase.

CT scan of chest/abd/pelvis shows mild diffuse lymphadenopathy and splenomegaly.

Which is the most likely diagnosis?

A. Large granular lymphocyte leukemia
B. Acute myeloid leukemia (a.k.a. acute myelogenous leukemia)
C. Chronic lymphocytic leukemia
D. Chronic myeloid leukemia (a.k.a. chronic myelogenous leukemia)
E. Acute lymphocytic leukemia

Answer:_____

Heme Malignancies

- Recognize and differentiate:
  - Acute leukemias
  - Myelodysplastic syndrome (MDS)
  - Myeloproliferative disorders
  - Lymphoproliferative disorders (i.e., NHL)
  - Chronic leukemia
  - Hodgkin lymphoma
  - Plasma cell disorders

Acute Leukemias — AML and ALL

- Maturation arrest with accumulation of blasts
- Anemia
- Thrombocytopenia
- Present with symptoms related to cytopenias
  - Infections, fatigue, bleeding
- Workup includes:
  - Bone marrow aspirate and biopsy
  - Special stains and flow to identify type of leukemia
  - Cytogenetic studies on marrow
- Treatment is complex
- May involve induction, consolidation, maintenance, and CNS-directed therapy

Blasts

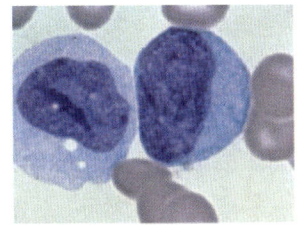
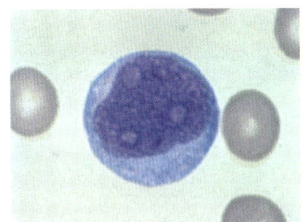
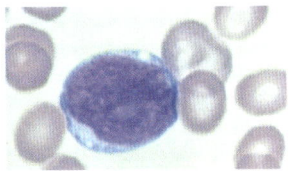
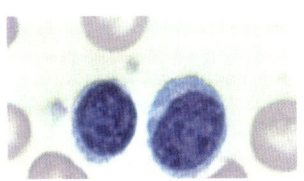

Myeloblast vs. lymphoblast.
UL: young monocyte and a myeloblast
UR: myeloblast
LL: lymphoblast
LR: Normal lymphocytes are smaller.

(Often you cannot differentiate myelo- from lympho- by peripheral smear. Just know that on the exam, it's not acute leukemia if there are no blasts!)

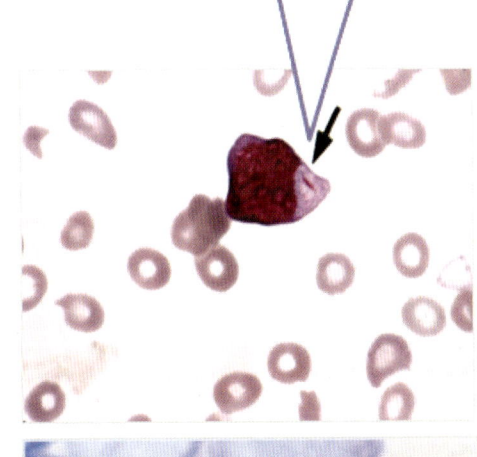

Auer rod in AML: Cell with a splinter

1 leukemia identifiable on peripheral smear!

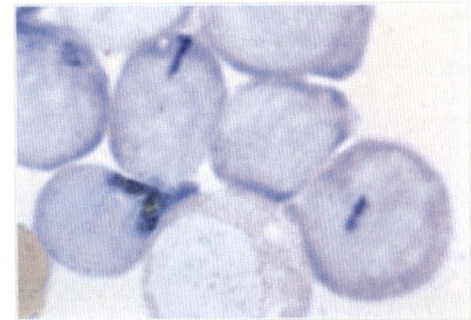

HEMATOLOGY

AML

	Associations	Presents	Specifics	Tx	Misc.
AML	Benzene after MPD Secondary AML always more severe	Cytopenia-related symptoms BM Bx > 20% blasts Hyperviscosity syndrome (CNS, pulmonary)	Auer rods Preceding MDS or complex cytogenetics = worse prognosis Favorable prognosis: t(8;21) t(15;17) inv(16)	Induction CXT ± HSCT APML = ATRA drug (All-**trans** retinoic acid) Blasts > 100,000 require urgent leukophoresis 30–40% cure in adults	APML: t(15;17) (q22;q12) *PML-RARα*: DIC = emergency with high mortality from hemorrhage! Cytopenias ↑ UA ↑ PO₄ ↓ Calcium

PML / RARα
- AML (M3): t(15;17)(q22;q12); *PML/RARα*
  - Retinoic acid receptor α gene is translocated and becomes immune to differentiation effects of retinoic acid → clonal proliferation of myeloid progenitor cells
  - Increased risk of DIC
  - Favorable prognosis
  - All-**trans** retinoic acid (ATRA) induces differentiation in these leukemic cells
    - **"Differentiation syndrome" may complicate therapy**
      - **Volume overload, respiratory distress, hypotension**
      - **Treat with high-dose steroids**

ALL

	Presents	Specifics	Tx	Misc.

ALL	Extramedullary
	Lymphadenopathy (LAD)
	Spleen
	CNS
	Testicles
	Retina
	Ant. mediastinal mass (T-cell subtypes)
		Young do better
		Poor prognosis:
		t(9;22) *BCR-ABL*
		Blasts > 30,000
			CXT
			  Induction
			  Consolidation
			  Maintenance
			  CNS prophylaxis
			30–40% cure in adults
			HSCT for high risk or refractory
				Cytopenias
				Tumor lysis syndrome
				↑ UA
				↑ PO₄
				↓ Calcium

BCR-ABL = Philadelphia chromosome

MYELODYSPLASTIC SYNDROME (MDS)

- Ineffective blood cell production
  - Cytopenias and dysplastic maturation
  - Symptoms include weakness, infection, bleeding
- Bone marrow — hypercellular
- Variable progression to acute leukemia
- Prognosis — IPSS score
  - % of bone marrow blasts
  - # of cytopenias
  - Cytogenetics
- Management
  - Supportive care
    - Transfusions
    - Growth factors
    - Iron chelation
  - Disease modifying
    - Hypomethylating agents
    - Allogeneic stem cell transplant
- 5q deletion syndrome
  - Favorable prognosis
  - Refractory anemia and thrombocytosis
  - Treat with lenalidomide

AR 9

A 32-year-old female develops a large, spontaneous hematoma under her tongue and in her thigh. She is otherwise healthy.

Exam: splenomegaly

CBC:

WBC 110,300 cells/mcL (46% segs, 6% bands, 12% lymphs, 10% myelocytes, 8% metamyelocytes, 5% blasts, 7% eosinophils, 6% basophils)

Hgb 10 g/dL

Hct 30%

MCV 85 fL

PLT 898,000 cells/mcL

PT 12 sec; PTT 30 sec

Which of the following is the most appropriate next step in management?

A. Review the peripheral smear and assess for t(9;22).
B. CT scan of the abdomen
C. FNA of the spleen
D. Assess for the *JAK* mutation.
E. vWF:Ag, vWF:RCoF, and Factor 8 activity

Answer:_____

MYELOPROLIFERATIVE DISORDERS (MPDs)

- Origin = multipotent progenitor cell
- Consequence = overproduction of blood elements without dysplasia

Myeloproliferative Neoplasms

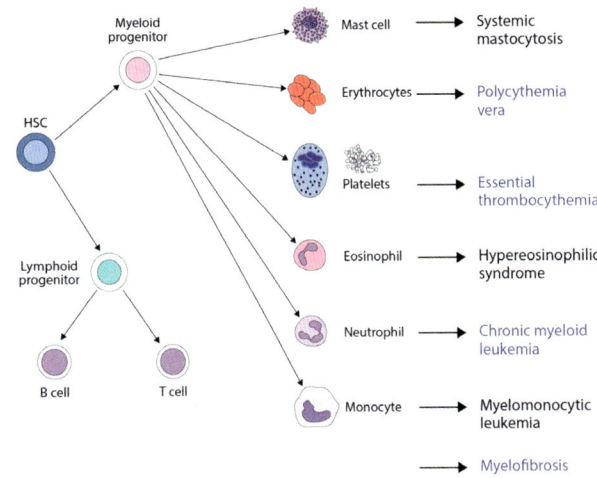

- Elderly
- Classified by the cell line most affected
- Risk of progression to acute leukemia
- Marrow = hypercellular
- Splenomegaly is common
- *JAK2* mutations

JAK2 Mutation

- JAK family of protein kinases
  - Mutations can cause genes to be stuck in the "on" position → Transcription of kinases that result in uncontrolled cell growth
    - Polycythemia vera — nearly 100% *JAK2* positive
    - Essential thrombocythemia — 50% *JAK2* positive
  - JAK-targeted drugs for treatment of cancer and myeloproliferative disorders approved/ under development

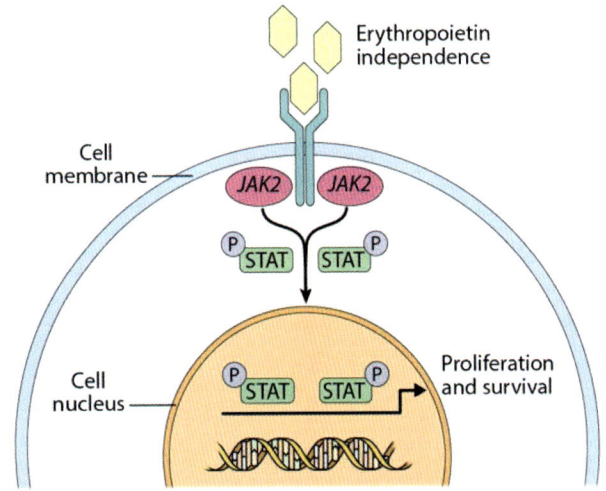

What does *JAK2* normally do? It is a switch that tells blood cells to grow.

HEMATOLOGY

Myeloproliferative — CML

- Clonal expansion of transformed stem cell
  - t(9;22) = *BCR-ABL* (Philadelphia chromosome) →
    BCR-ABL fusion proteins:
    - ABL protein = constitutive (always "on") tyrosine
      kinase → inhibits apoptosis
    - → Imatinib blocks activity of this tyrosine
      kinase → revolutionized treatment of chronic
      phase CML
- Clinical presentation
  - Constitutional symptoms
  - Early satiety and hepatosplenomegaly
  - CBC: ↑ WBC with immature granulocytic cells
    ± anemia, thrombocytosis
    - Thrombocytosis
    - Phases of disease
    - Chronic → accelerated → blast

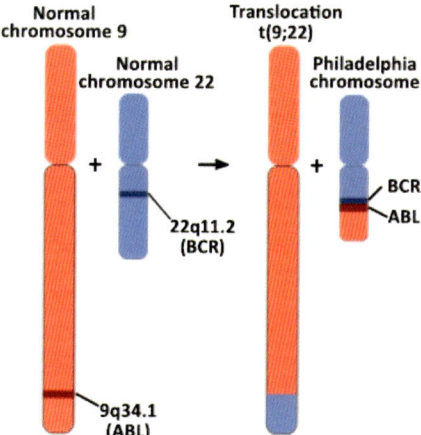

[1]

CML — Chronic Phase

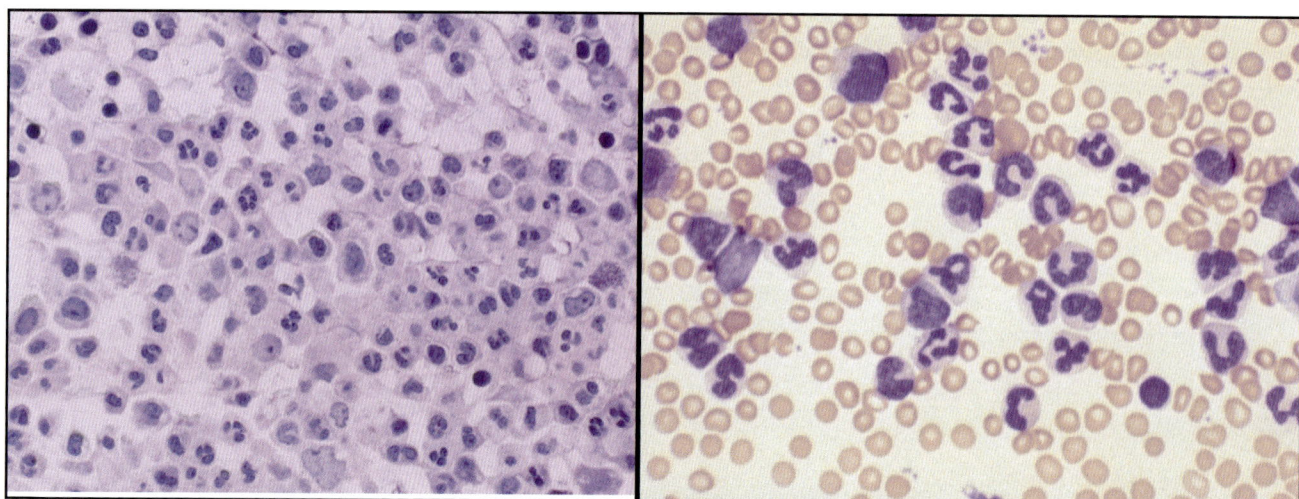

Bone marrow; low power. *Myeloid elements are clearly more abundant than the normal 3:1 myeloid:erythroid (M:E) ratio.*

Peripheral smear *with the pyramid of maturation of granulocytes: promyelocytes, myelocytes, metamyelocytes, bands, and segmented neutrophils*

Myeloproliferative — CML

	Assoc.	Presents	Specifics	Tx	Misc.
CML	XRT	Chronic phase (HSM, leukocytosis) → Accelerated → Blast crisis <u>ALL 1/3</u> <u>AML 2/3</u>	Eosinophils Basophils ↓ LAP score <u>95%: t(9;22)</u> *BCR-ABL*	**TKI 1st line (chronic)** Imatinib Dasatinib Nilotinib Chemo HSCT	Imatinib: Edema HF Hepatotoxicity Cytopenias Hemorrhage

Myeloproliferative — Polycythemia Vera (PCV)

	Presents	Specifics	Tx	Misc.
PCV	Elderly Hyperviscosity: headache, dizzy Splenomegaly Aquagenic pruritus Erythromelalgia Gout, PUD	↑ RBC mass Normal P_aO_2 <u>Low erythropoietin</u> ↑ LAP score 97% (+) *JAK2* Leukocytosis Thrombocytosis	Phlebotomy Hct < 45% ASA reduces MI, CVA If high risk (> 60 years of age or prior thrombosis), use hydroxyurea	Mortality from thrombosis and conversion to AML

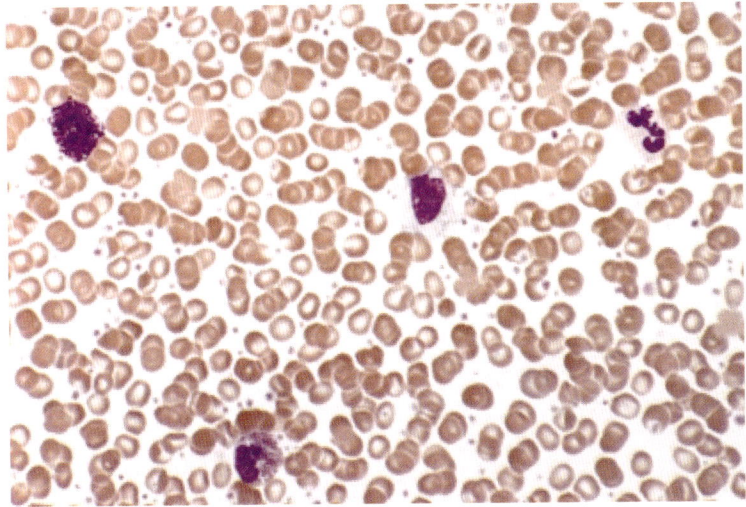

Essential Thrombocythemia

	Presents	Specifics	Tx	Complications
ET	Vasomotor symptoms Erythromelalgia	Thrombocytosis R/O reactive causes JAK2 positive (50%) R/O secondary causes	If high-risk (> 60 years of age or Hx VTE): Use hydroxyurea Target PLT < 400K	Thrombosis (arterial and venous) Hemorrhage progress to myelofibrosis or acute leukemia

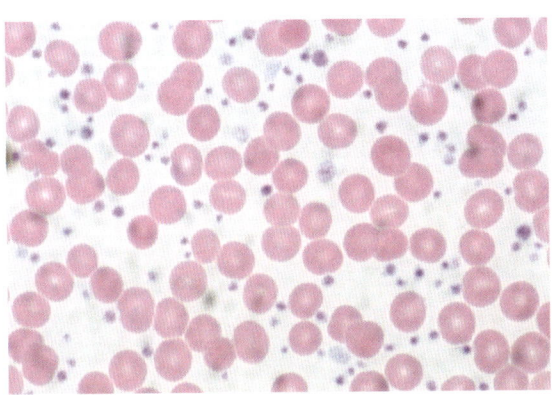

HEMATOLOGY

LYMPHOMAS AND LEUKEMIAS

NON-HODGKIN LYMPHOMA

Non-Hodgkin Lymphoma (NHL) Presentations
- Clinical features
  - Peripheral lymphadenopathy 60%
  - Constitutional symptoms 40%
  - Hepatosplenomegaly
- Variable presentations
  - Cord compression
  - Meningitis
  - CNS mass
  - Monoclonal protein
  - Autoimmune cytopenias

NHL — Subtypes

Types of NHL	
Indolent Lymphomas	**Aggressive Lymphomas**
Elderly Asymptomatic Incurable Delayed Tx	**Variable age Symptomatic Curable Immediate Tx**
Follicular lymphoma	Diffuse large B-cell
Marginal zone (MALT, nodal, splenic)	Burkitt lymphoma
CLL/SLL	Mantle cell
Hairy cell leukemia	B-lymphoblastic
Waldenström macroglobulinemia	Precursor T-lymphoblastic
Mycosis fungoides	Diffuse large T-cell

NHL Evaluation and Treatment
- Excisional biopsy — not FNA
- Imaging studies: CT, PET/CT
- Bone marrow biopsy
- Serum uric acid, LDH
- Prognosis and Tx depend on form/stage
  - Indolent
  - Aggressive
- Complications: CHD, impaired fertility, thyroid disease, and secondary malignancies

NHL Associations
- Viruses
  - HIV, HTLV, EBV, HCV, ? HBV
- Connective tissue diseases
- Autoimmune disorders
- Mixed cryoglobulinemia
- GI lymphoma: Crohn's, celiac disease, *H. pylori* gastritis, GI nodular lymphoid hyperplasia

Aggressive Lymphomas — Symptomatic, Immediate Treatment, Curable (Most)

Subtype	Key Features
Diffuse large B-cell lymphoma (DLBCL)	Most common aggressive lymphoma Early stage — R-CHOP ×3 plus IFRT Advanced stage — R-CHOP ×6 Cure rate 50–60%
Mantle cell lymphoma	Incurable, but aggressive Extranodal involvement — GI tract, spleen, blood t(11;14) → cycle D1 overexpression Chemoimmunotherapy, ibrutinib, lenalidomide
Burkitt lymphoma	Most aggressive Endemic EBV infection (Africa) Sporadic (U.S./Europe) HIV/AIDS Histology — "starry sky" t(8:14) translocation → *C-MYC* oncogene CNS involvement Tumor lysis syndrome

Indolent Lymphomas — Elderly, Asymptomatic, Incurable, Delayed Treatment

Subtype	Key Features
Follicular	Most common indolent lymphoma; t(14/18) leads to BCL-2 overexpression Treat when symptomatic; rituximab ± chemo Risk of transformation to DLBCL (10%)
Marginal zone	3 subtypes (MALT, nodal, and splenic) Chronic antigenic stimulation Gastric MALT — *H. pylori*
Hairy cell	Pancytopenia, splenomegaly, dry tap Lymphadenopathy unusual Flow — CD11c and CD103, *BRAF* mutation Smear — cytoplasmic "hairy" projections on lymphs Treat with purine analogs (cladribine)
Waldenström's	Lymphoplasmacytic IgM monoclonal protein Hyperviscosity syndrome Treat with rituximab ± chemo
CLL/SLL	Discussed later in separate slides

AR 10

A 79-year-old male is noted on a routine physical with an abnormal CBC. He admits to mild fatigue. On exam he has mildly enlarged cervical and axillary lymph nodes, and mild splenomegaly. Lab review: WBC: 68,000, with ALC: 61,000. Hgb: 11.0 g/dL; platelet: 82,000; peripheral blood smear is as shown.

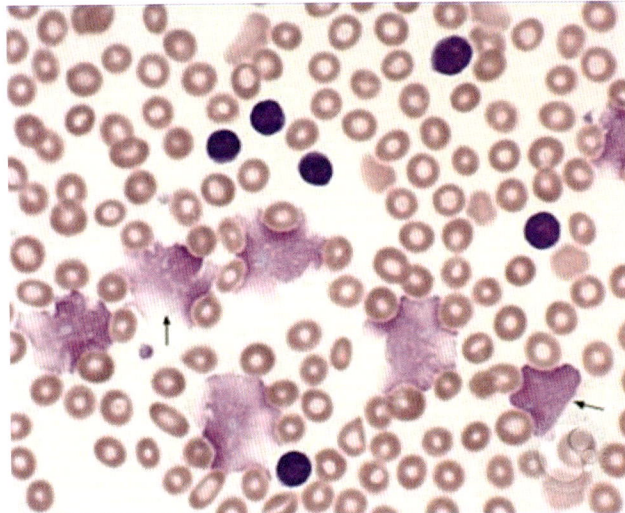

Which of the following is the most likely diagnosis?

A. CML
B. CLL
C. AML
D. ALL
E. HUH?

Answer:_____

CLL / SLL

- Malignant cell is **mature**
- Many times maintains other cell counts
- Presents asymptomatically — discovered on "routine" blood work
- Workup may include review of smear, flow cytometry, marrow, cytogenetics
- "CLL" is a **spectrum** of diseases often referred to as "CLL/SLL"
  - Localized disease = small lymphocytic lymphoma (indolent NHL)
    - Lymphadenopathy without cytopenias and ALC < 5,000 cells/mcL
  - Disseminated = B-cell CLL
    - Peripheral lymphocytosis with ALC > 5,000 cells/mcL
  - <u>Commonly associated with second malignancy</u>
    - Lung cancer, head and neck cancer
- Clinical features
  - Elderly, lymphadenopathy, splenomegaly
  - ± Constitutional symptoms
  - CBC: ↑ WBC, lymphocytosis

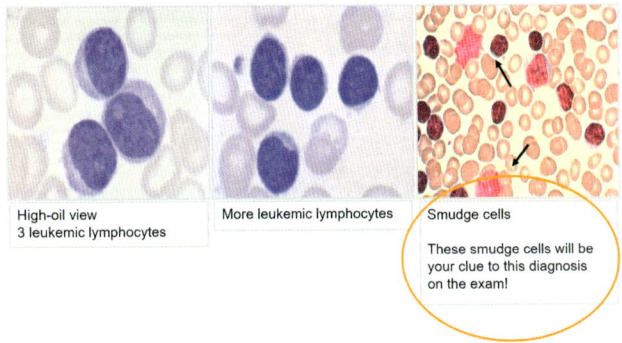

High-oil view
3 leukemic lymphocytes

More leukemic lymphocytes

Smudge cells

These smudge cells will be your clue to this diagnosis on the exam!

B cell that has classic flow pattern: CD5+ with CD19, 20, 23+

Chronic Leukemia — B-CLL

	Assoc.	Presents	Specifics	Tx	Misc.

B-CLL	Most common leukemia
	SLL
		Older
		Chronic
		Asymptomatic
		↑ WBCs
		LAD
		Splenomegaly
		Cytopenias
			Smudge cells
			Prognosis:
			  Rai stage
			  Cytogenetics
				Observation
				Treat rapid disease
				or symptoms
				Drugs
				  Ibrutinib
				  Acalabrutinib
				  Venetoclax
				  Bendamustine
				  Rituximab
				  Fludarabine-based
					Lung CA
					Head & neck CA
					Autoimmune
					  Low platelets
					  AIHA
					↓ Igs — infection risk
					Richter transformation
					to aggressive NHL in 10%

High WBC Count — Pearls

- Mostly mature lymphocytes, not sick appearing? Smudge cells? Think CLL
- Increase in all myeloid precursors (metas, myelos, promyelos, bands?) Philadelphia chromosome? Think CML
- Increase blast forms? Sick patient with severe cytopenias? Think acute leukemia

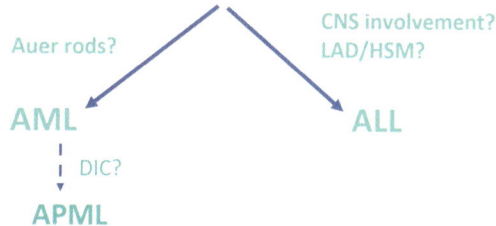

Auer rods?

CNS involvement?
LAD/HSM?

AML   ALL

DIC?

APML

Indolent NHL — Hairy Cell

	Presents	Specifics	Tx
Hairy Cell	Older males <u>Splenomegaly</u> Constitutional Sx Cytopenias <u>LAD unusual</u>! "<u>Dry tap</u>"	Cells seen in peripheral blood with Romanowsky stain Dx: marrow cells and fibrosis; often "dry tap"	Observation Treat rapid disease or symptoms Cladribine > 80% remission rate

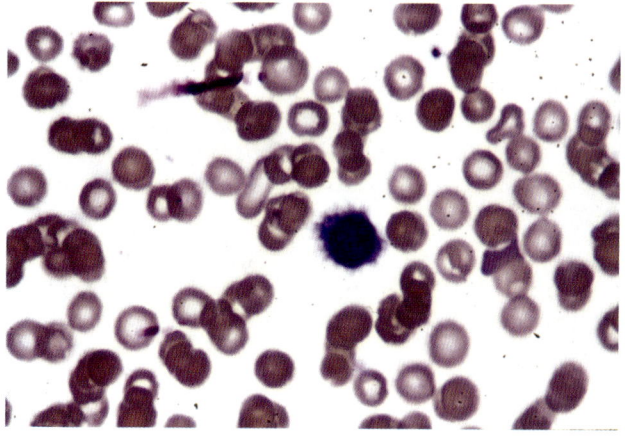

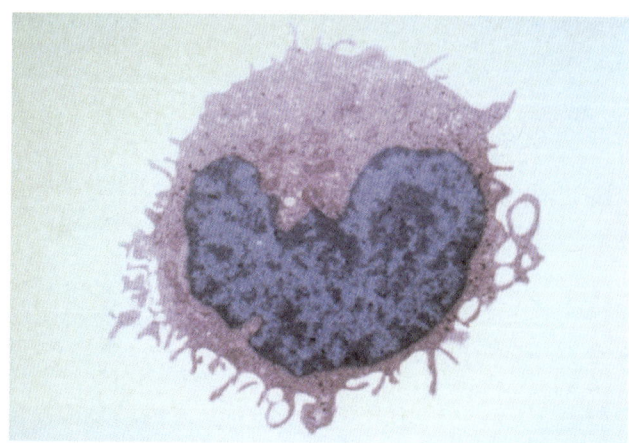

Pancytopenia — Pearls
- Older patient, with hypercellular bone marrow, macrocytic anemia? **Think MDS**
- Younger patient with hypocellular bone marrow? **Think aplastic anemia**
- Associated splenomegaly with "dry tap" on bone marrow aspirate? **Think hairy cell leukemia**

HODGKIN LYMPHOMA (HL)

Hodgkin Lymphoma Presentations
- Bimodal
  - 20–30 years of age
  - > 50 years of age
- Clinical features
  - Asymptomatic cervical node 70%
  - Mediastinal mass on CXR with pain, cough, or dyspnea
  - Constitutional symptoms
  - Splenomegaly 30%
  - Hepatomegaly 5%
  - Generalized pruritus!
  - Alcohol-associated node and bone pain
  - Nephrotic syndrome
  - Eosinophilia
  - AIHA ± ITP

Hodgkin's — Evaluation and Treatment
- Excisional biopsy — not FNA
- Dx: Reed-Sternberg cell
- Treatment based on stage
  - Chemo — ABVD or A-AVD
  - Radiation
- Prognosis — highly curable
  - Even Stage 4 = survival rate of > 60%
- Complications
  - <u>Hypothyroidism</u>
  - Infertility
  - Cardiovascular
    - Premature CAD
  - Secondary malignancy, including:
    - AML
    - Solid tumors, such as breast and lung

Hodgkin Lymphoma — Reed-Sternberg Cell

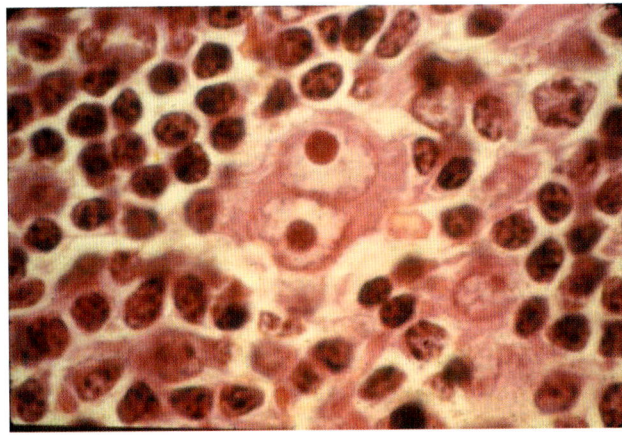

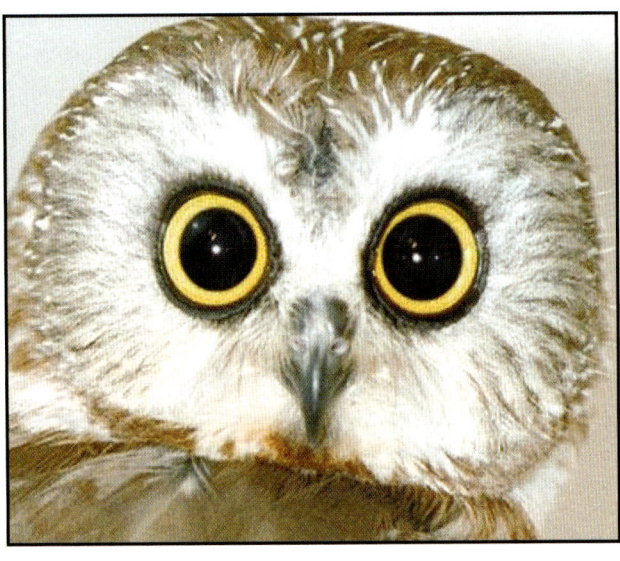

AR 11
A 54-year-old man

PMH: prostate cancer

Fatigue and exertional pain in his back for 2 months

Exam shows normal straight-leg raises, normal hip flexors, and down-going toes.

WBC 8,700 cells/mcL (normal differential)

Hgb 10.5 g/dL

Hct 31%

Platelets 309,000 cells/mcL

Na$^+$ 136 mEq/L

K$^+$ 3.5 mEq/L

Cl$^-$ 114 mEq/L

HCO$_3^-$ 19 mEq/L

BUN 10 mg/dL, creatinine 1.7 mg/dL

Total Protein 8.5 g/dL, Alb 2.9 g/dL

Ca^{2+} 10.4 mg/dL

UA: 2+ glucose, 2+ protein, no blood

Chest radiograph: normal

Which of the following is most likely to diagnose the cause of this patient's back pain?

A. Bone scan
B. Measurement of PSA
C. Serum and urine protein electrophoresis
D. Radiographs of the L-spine
E. MRI of the L-spine

Answer:_____

PLASMA CELL DISORDERS

Multiple Myeloma
- B-cell neoplasm
  - Clonal expansion of plasma cells
  - Produce monoclonal paraprotein (intact Ig or light chain)
- Clinical presentation
  - Lytic bone lesions
  - Hypercalcemia
  - Anemia
  - Acute kidney injury
  - Frequent infections
  - Other clues: rouleaux on smear; increased protein gap
- Dx: SPEP/UPEP, FLC assay, bone marrow biopsy, CT/PET

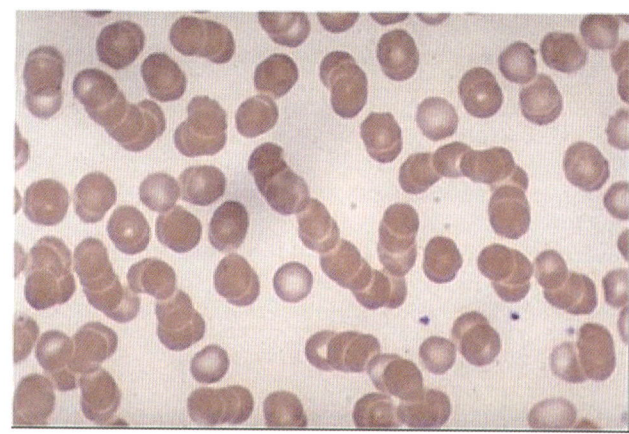

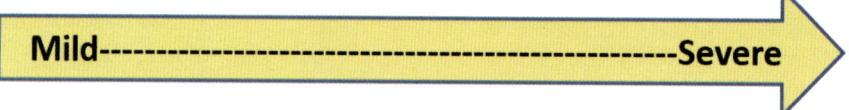

Mild--Severe

	MGUS	Smoldering Myeloma	Multiple Myeloma (Active)
Disease burden	Serum M spike < 3 g/dL Marrow plasma cells < 10%	Serum M spike > 3 g/dL **or** marrow plasma cells > 10%	Marrow plasma cells > 10% or biopsy-proven plasmacytoma
Organ damage (lytic bone lesions, anemia, hypercalcemia, chronic kidney disease)	No	No	**Yes**
Management	Annual labs/H&P	Close surveillance: labs/H&P q3 months	-Imids, bortezomib, daratumumab, HSCT
Risk of transformation to symptomatic myeloma	1% per year	10–20% per year	....

Monoclonal Gammopathies

	Waldenström's	Myeloma
> 10% BM infiltration	Clonal lymphoplasmacytic cells	Clonal plasma cells
M spike	IgM	IgG, A, light chains, D, none
Presentation	60-year-old Caucasian; infiltration of hematopoietic tissues and/or hyperviscosity; "oozing" blood, no bone pain, sausage-link veins on funduscopic exam	Osteolytic lesions (bone pain), anemia, chronic kidney disease, and RTA Type 2, hypercalcemia, recurrent bacterial infections
Evaluation: rouleaux; ↑ T. protein and globulin fraction; SPEP → M spike (✓viscosity when M spike > 4 g/dL); BM biopsy ? MM: Add UPEP and skeletal survey		

Again, Myeloma
- > 10% marrow plasma cells
- > 3 g/dL M spike
- End-organ damage
  - Hypercalcemia, acute kidney injury, anemia, lytic bone disease
  - Frequent infections due to hypogammaglobulinemia
- Workup
  - SPEP, UPEP, serum light chains, skeletal survey, bone marrow biopsy, β_2-microglobulin
- Management
  - Systemic therapies (-imids, bortezomib)
  - Stem cell transplant in younger patients

AUDIENCE RESPONSE ANSWERS

Audience Response 1
C. IgA tTGA

AR 2
A. Spherocytes on smear

AR 3
D. Autoimmune hemolytic anemia

AR 4
C. Stop heparin and prescribe argatroban.

AR 5
D. von Willebrand disease

AR 6
E. Therapeutic plasma exchange

AR 7
C. LMWH

AR 8
E. Acute lymphocytic leukemia

AR 9
A. Review the peripheral smear and assess for t(9;22).

AR 10
B. CLL

AR 11
C. Serum and urine protein electrophoresis

ENDNOTES

[1]   Aryn89 [CC BY-SA 4.0 (https://creativecommons.org/licenses/by-sa/4.0)]

HEMATOLOGY

MedStudy

INTERNAL MEDICINE REVIEW

Infectious Disease

Presented by

Fred Arthur Zar, MD

TABLE OF CONTENTS

Why Some Topic Names Are Not Printed in This Section

At MedStudy, we do all we can to optimize your self-testing and learning.

In this section, the speaker has chosen to introduce topics with an Audience Response question to help you learn. In the syllabus, we've intentionally "hidden" some topic names that would give away the answers—so you can self-test more effectively. Where we've done this, instead of the topic name, you'll see an empty teal band or some extra space, but you can still find the topic on the page using the Table of Contents.

Infectious Disease Outline

- Cellulitis 1
- DM Foot Osteomyelitis
- *Clostridioides* (formerly *Clostridium*) *difficile* Infection
- HIV — CNS Infection
- Febrile Neutropenia
- Tick-Borne Disease 1
- Fungal Disease
- Meningitis
- Cellulitis 2
- Pharyngitis 1
- Botulism
- Sexually Transmitted Infections
- Vaginal Diseases
- Bacterial Diarrhea
- Animal Bites
- Tick-Borne Disease 2
- Cellulitis 3
- Rhinocerebral Infections
- HIV — GI Infections
- Herpes Virus Infection
- Pharyngitis 2
- Parvovirus Infection
- Hemorrhagic Fevers
- Influenza
- HIV Infection
- HIV — Pulmonary Infection
- Infective Endocarditis (IE)
- Community-Acquired Pneumonia
- Urinary Tract Infections
- COVID-19

Case 1 — History and Physical

Hx: A 19-year-old woman comes to the ED with severe left bicep pain of 1-day duration. She is recovering from chickenpox and recalls a very itchy lesion in that area that she has been scratching for 2 days.

PE: T 101.8°F (38.8°C), BP 70/40 mmHg, HR 110 beats/minute, RR 20 breaths/minute

Many healing varicella lesions; L bicep tender, warm 6 × 8-cm swelling with woody induration

Case 1 — Labs, Imaging, Initial Tx

Hgb 11.0 g/dL; WBC 21.0×10^3/mm³: 12% bands; Pl 75,000 cells/mm³

Creatinine 2.0 mg/dL; AST 95 U/L; ALT 100 U/L

MRI: edema of soft tissues above the L bicep muscle belly with early fascial necrosis

She receives a dose of vancomycin and piperacillin-tazobactam and goes for surgical debridement; Gram stain of surgical fluid reveals gram (+) cocci chains.

Audience Response 1
Which of the following would you do now?

A. Continue vancomycin alone.
B. Continue piperacillin-tazobactam alone.
C. Continue vancomycin and piperacillin-tazobactam.
D. Switch to penicillin.
E. Switch to penicillin and clindamycin.

Answer: **E.**

Rapidly progressive Cellulitis

- Group A *Streptococcus* (strep)
  - Lymphatic disease
    - Vein donor leg
    - Mastectomy
- *Pasteurella multocida*
  - Animal bites (e.g., dogs, cats)
- *Clostridium perfringens*
  - Contaminated trauma
- *Vibrio vulnificus*
  - Salt water and cirrhosis
- Necrotizing fasciitis

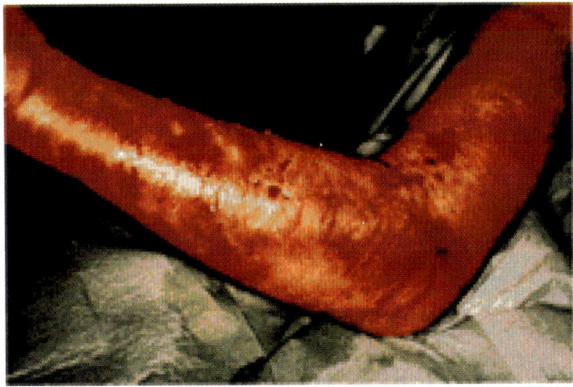

Group A Streptococcus necrotizing fasciitis

The Anatomy of Soft Tissue Infections — "Cellulitis"

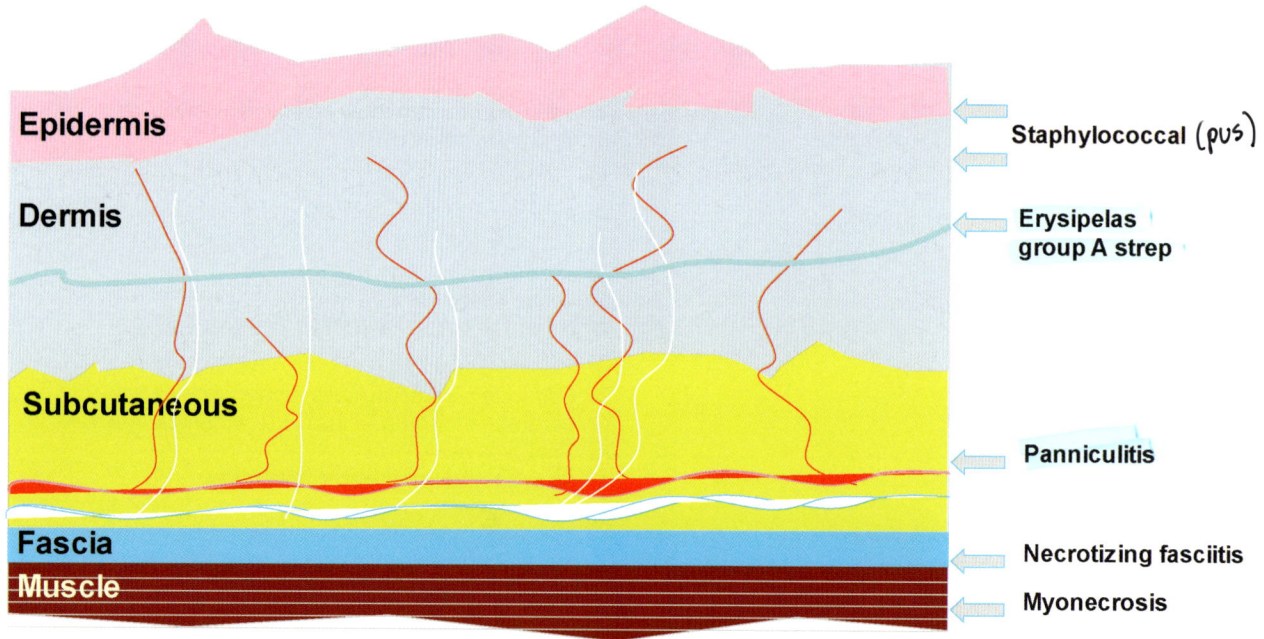

- Epidermis
- Dermis
- Subcutaneous
- Fascia
- Muscle

→ Staphylococcal (pus)

→ Erysipelas group A strep

→ Panniculitis

→ Necrotizing fasciitis

→ Myonecrosis

Necrotizing Fasciitis — Suggestive Findings
- Skin necrosis and blebs
- Disproportionate pain
- Late anesthesia
- Disproportionate systemic toxicity
- Crepitus or gas on x-ray
- Probe passing easily through fascia

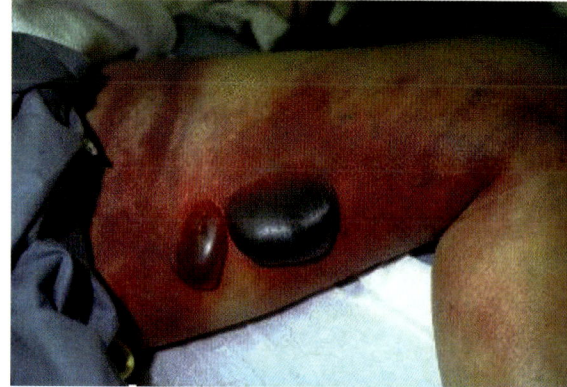

Skin necrosis with blebs

Necrotizing Fasciitis — Microbiology
- Type I (mixed aerobic/anaerobic)
  - At least 1 anaerobe
    - Usually *Bacteroides* or peptostreptococci
  - At least 1 aerobe (not group A strep)
    - Usually enteric GNB
- Type II (group A strep)
  - Group A strep ± *S. aureus*
- Type III (Clostridial)
  - *Clostridium perfringens*
- Other monomicrobial
  - *S. aureus, S. agalactiae, V. vulnificus*
- Treatment
  - Surgery and antibiotics

Toxic Shock Syndrome
- Presenting triad
  - Fever, shock (or orthostatic hypotension), rash (late desquamation)
- Involvement of > 3 organ systems
  - GI (NVD), muscle (myalgia or CPK), AKI, transaminase/bilirubin, thrombocytopenia, altered consciousness
- Sources
  - Strep: soft tissue infection (BC usually positive)
  - Staph: surgical wounds, foreign bodies, pneumonia
- Treatment
  - Site control + organism-specific antibiotics + clindamycin

Case 1 — Key Points
- Recognize rapidly progressive cellulitis and the organisms that cause it
- Recognize necrotizing fasciitis and the approach to treatment
- Recognize toxic shock syndrome and know its treatment

Case 2 — History and Physical
Hx: A 68-year-old man with Type 2 diabetes presents with a draining foot ulcer at the base of his right big toe. The ulcer has been present for 1 week. He denies fever. He takes his metformin regularly.

PE: T 100.2°F (37.9°C); BP, HR, and RR normal

Right-foot circumferential distal redness and a purulent 4- × 5-cm ulcer that probes to bone

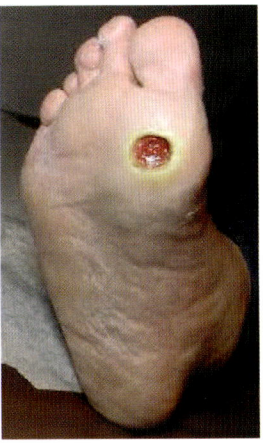

Ulcer over head of 1st metatarsal

Case 2 — Labs and Imaging

CBC: Hgb 12.5 g/dL; WBC 9.7 × 10^3/mm³; Pl 245,000 cells/mm³

Plain radiograph: ulceration of the plantar aspect of the head of the right 1st metatarsal with mild soft-tissue swelling; no gas in tissue; bony structures appear normal without evidence of osteomyelitis

AR 2
Which of the following would you do now?

A. Perform radionuclide bone scan.
B. Conduct MRI of right foot.
C. Start vancomycin and piperacillin-tazobactam.
D. Culture the drainage prior to antibiotics.
E. Obtain a bone biopsy for culture prior to antibiotics.

Answer:_____

Concordance of Bone and Swab Cultures in DM Foot Osteomyelitis[1]
- **The Study**
  - 76 patients with 81 episodes
  - All had bone biopsy for culture
- **The Results**

Organism	Concordance of Both Cultures
S. aureus	**21/49 (42.8%)**
GNB	12/42 (28.5%)
Streptococci	8/31 (25.8%)
Total	43/191 (22.5%)

Sonneville E. *Clin Infect Dis*. 2006

Metaanalysis of Dx Tests for DM Osteomyelitis — 9 Studies; 1,054 Patients[2]

Diagnostic Test	Sens (95% CI)	Spec (95% CI)
Probe-to-bone	0.60 (0.46–0.73)	**0.91 (0.86–0.94)**
MRI	**0.90 (0.82–0.95)**	0.79 (0.62–0.91)
Leukocyte scan	0.74 (0.67–0.80)	0.68 (0.57–0.78)
Radiography	**0.54 (0.44–0.63)**	0.68 (0.53–0.80)
Bone scan	0.81 (0.73–0.87)	**0.28 (0.17–0.42)**

Case 2 — Key Points
- Know the operating characteristics of various tests for diabetic foot osteomyelitis
- Recognize the nonspecific nature of drainage cultures
- Recognize the need for bone cultures for definitive treatment of diabetic foot osteomyelitis

Case 3 — History and Physical

Hx: A 53-year-old woman presents to the ED with a 2-day history of watery diarrhea 10–12 times a day. Three weeks ago, she had a UTI treated with a 7-day course of levofloxacin. She is able to take fluids and her hydrochlorothiazide for blood pressure control.

PE: T 101.5°F (38.6°C), BP 126/80 mmHg, HR 100 beats/minute, RR 16 breaths/minute

Abdomen has minimal bowel sounds and diffuse tenderness.

Case 3 — Labs and Imaging

CBC: Hgb 13.5 g/dL; WBC 19.7 × 10^3/mm³; Pl 245,000 cells/mm³

Creatinine 1.8 mg/dL (baseline 1.0 mg/dL)

Abdominal CT: no free air; slight diffuse thickening of the colonic wall; no evidence of bowel obstruction

AR 3
After obtaining a test for *Clostridioides* (formerly *Clostridium*) *difficile*, what would you do next?

A. Await result prior to treatment.
B. Start metronidazole PO.
C. Start vancomycin PO.
D. Start fidaxomicin PO.
E. Fecal microbiota therapy via colonoscopy

Answer:_____

Response to CDI Treatment When Stratified by Disease Severity[3]

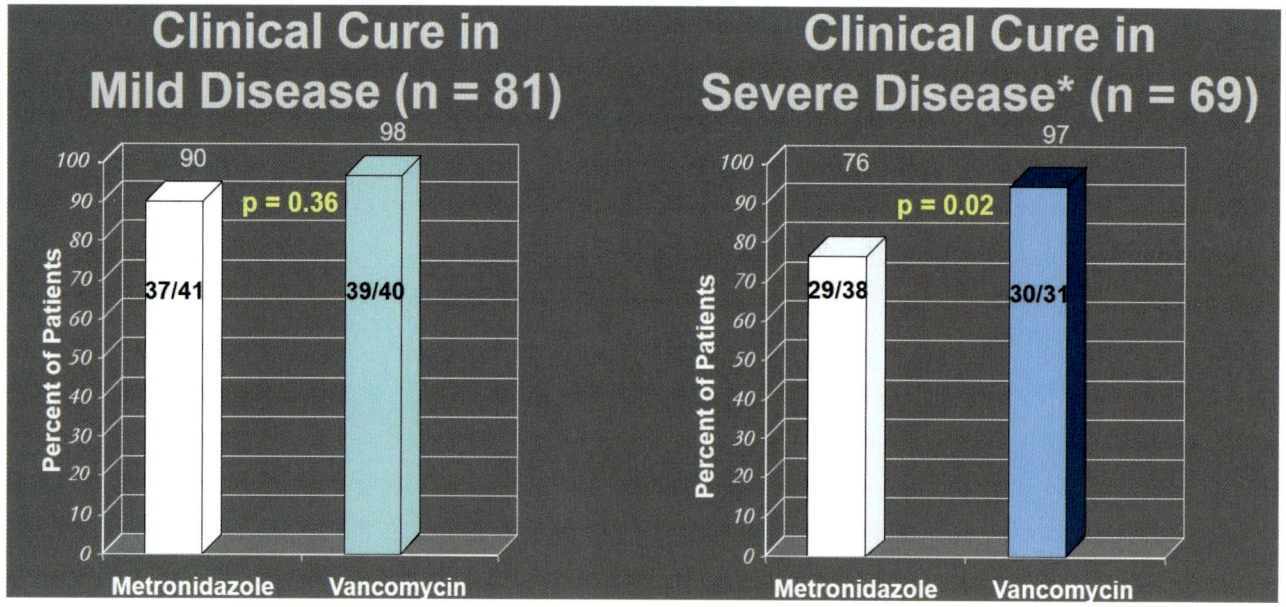

Severe disease defined as intensive care unit admission; pseudomembranous colitis on endoscopy or at least 2 of the following: 1) > 60 years of age; 2) Temperature > 101.0°F (38.3° C); 3) Albumin level < 2.5 mg/dL; 4) White blood cell count (WBC) > 15,000 cells/mm³

Studies Comparing Fidaxomicin to Vancomycin

Study Author	Initial Response		Global Cure	
	Fidaxomicin	Vancomycin	Fidaxomicin	Vancomycin
Louie[4]	253/287 (88%)	265/309 (86%)	214/287 (75%)	198/309 (64%)
Cornely[5]	198/216 (92%)	213/235 (91%)		
Mikamo[6]	87/104 (84%)	95/108 (88%)	70/97 (72%)	71/106 (67%)
Guery[7]	142/177 (80%)	147/179 (82%)	116/177 (66%)	92/179 (51%)
Total	**670/784 (85%)**	**720/831 (87%)**	**400/561 (71%)**	**361/594 (61%)**

Treatment of 1st Episode CDI[8]
- Nonfulminant
  - **Fidaxomicin** PO 200 mg bid × 10 days (preferred)
  - Vancomycin PO 125 mg qid × 10 days (alternative)
  - (Metronidazole PO 500 mg tid × 10 days if above not available/affordable)
- Fulminant*
  - **Vancomycin** PO/NGT or rectal 500 mg qid **and**
  - **Metronidazole** IV 500 mg q 8 h

*Fulminant = hypotension, shock, ileus, megacolon

Treatment of Recurrent CDI[9]
- First recurrence
  - Fidaxomicin PO 200 mg bid × 10 days
- Second or subsequent recurrences
  - Vancomycin taper and pulse*, **or**
  - Vancomycin PO 125 mg qid × 10 days, then rifaximin 400 mg tid × 20 days, **or**
  - Fidaxomicin PO 200 mg bid × 10 days, **or**
  - Fecal microbiota transplantation

*Vancomycin taper and pulse = vancomycin 125 mg qid PO × 2 weeks, then bid × 1 week, then daily × 1 week, then q 2–3 d × 2–8 weeks

Bezlotoxumab Prevention of Recurrent CDI[10]

- **The Study**
  - 2 RDPCT bezlotoxumab ± actoxumab vs. placebo
    - Actoxumab discontinued during interim analysis
  - Standard PO treatment of CDI given
    - Vancomycin or metronidazole
- **The Results**

	Placebo	**Bezlotoxumab**	
Recur at 12 weeks	109/395 (28)	67/386 (17)	**P < 0.001**

Indications For Bezlotoxumab[11]

- In addition to standard treatment if:
  - Recurrent infection within 6 months
  - Initial infection if:
    - Age ≥ 65
    - Immunocompromised
    - Severe CDI on presentation
      - Creatinine increase > 50% or WBC > 15,000

Case 3 — Key Points

- Recognize the typical clinical setting in which *C. difficile* infection occurs
- Know how to treat initial *C. difficile* infection based on severity
- Know how to treat and prevent recurrent *C. difficile* infection

Case 4 — History and Physical

Hx: A 29-year-old man is hospitalized with worsening neurologic symptoms over 8 weeks, which include confusion, dysarthria, left hemiparesis, and poor vision. He was diagnosed with HIV infection 8 years ago and has been noncompliant with therapy. Last CD4 count 2 years ago was 82.

PE: VS are normal; 18/30 on Mini-Mental State Exam; VA 20/200 OU, funduscopy normal; left hemiparesis and hemianopia

Case 4 — Labs and Imaging

CBC: Hgb 9.2 g/dL; WBC 1.5 × 10³/mm³: 12% lymphs; Pl 130,000 cells/mm³

MRI:

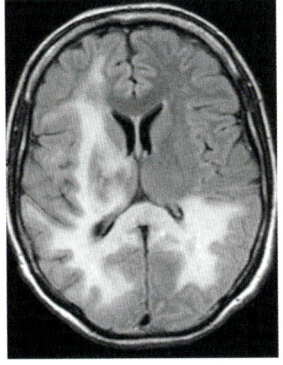

AR 4
Which of the following is most likely?

A. Progressive multifocal leukoencephalopathy
B. Primary CNS lymphoma
C. Toxoplasmosis
D. Cytomegalovirus encephalitis
E. Herpes simplex encephalitis

Answer: **A**

- Virology and pathogenesis
  - JC polyomavirus, > 85% adults infected
  - Dormant in kidney and lymphoid tissue
  - Immunosuppression → lytic infection of oligodendroglia → demyelination
- Clinical manifestations
  - Subacute motor and visual changes
- Diagnosis
  - **Images:** multifocal demyelination, not fitting a vascular territory, no mass effect or enhancement
  - **CSF:** JC virus PCR (+) (70–90% sens)
- Treatment
  - Antiretroviral therapy
  - Decrease immunosuppression

Case 4 — Key Points

- Recognize the clinical presentation of progressive multifocal leukoencephalopathy (PML)
- Know how to diagnose PML

Case 5 — History and Physical

Hx: A 50-year-old man with acute myelogenous leukemia develops fever and chills after completing his 3ʳᵈ round of induction chemotherapy 5 days ago. MRSA screen on admission was negative.

PE: T 104.0°F (40.0°C), BP 136/82 mmHg, HR 128 beats/minute, RR 24 breaths/minute

PICC line in left arm without redness, tenderness, or drainage; rest of exam normal

Case 5 — Labs and Imaging

CBC: Hgb 9.6 mg/dL; WBC 1.2 × 10³/mm³: 20% neutrophils, 5% bands Pl 115,000 cells/mm³

CXR is normal.

Blood and urine cultures are sent.

AR 5A
What is the next step?

A. Await cultures to direct antibiotic therapy.
B. Start cefepime.
C. Start cefepime and vancomycin.
D. Start cefepime and piperacillin-tazobactam.
E. Start cefepime and gentamicin.

Answer: **B.**

Febrile Neutropenia[12]

- Definitions
  - **Fever:** T > 101.0°F (38.3°C) × 1, or 100.4°F (38.0°C) > 1 hour
  - **Neutropenia:** ANC at or expected to be < 500 cells/μL
- Empiric treatment (IDSA 2010)
  - IV monotherapy ~pseudomonal coverage~
    - Piperacillin-tazobactam, imipenem/meropenem, cefepime
  - **Add IV vancomycin only if:**
    - Severe sepsis ✓
    - Blood culture with gram (+) cocci ✓
    - Pneumonia
    - Suspected line sepsis
    - MRSA colonization
    - Soft tissue infection
    - Mucositis
  - Oral outpatient treatment (IDSA 2018)
    - Selected patients based on low risk of complications
      - MASCC and CISNE scores

Case 5 — Initial Course

Antibiotics are started, and his fever resolves over the next 48 hours. Blood and urine cultures are negative. Six days later, fever recurs along with shortness of breath.

Case 5 — Repeat Testing

CBC: Hgb 8.9 g/dL; WBC 1.4 × 10³/mm³: 25% neutrophils, no bands
Pl 100,000 cells/mm³

Chest x-ray and CT are obtained.

Case 5 — Imaging

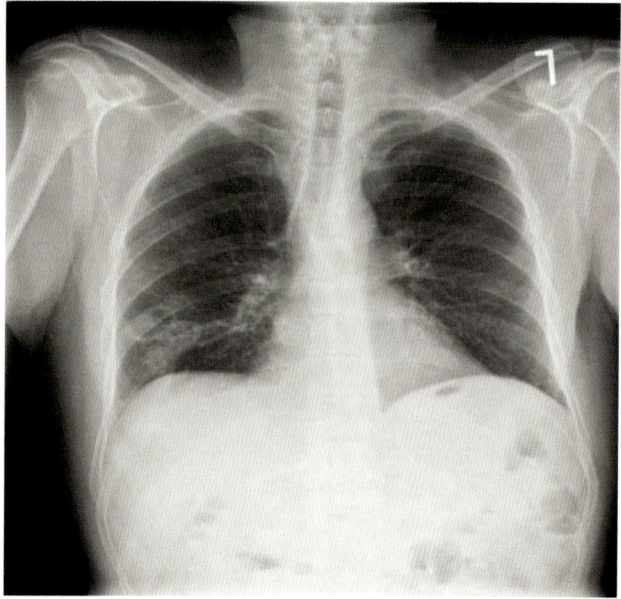

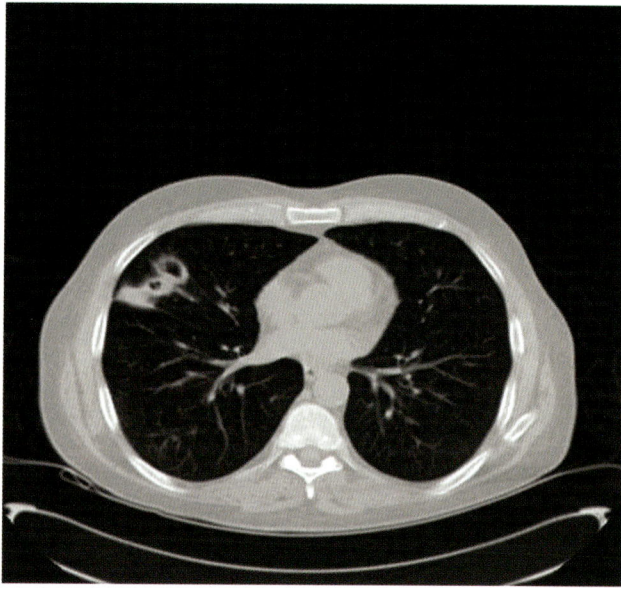

Case 5 — Bronchoalveolar Lavage

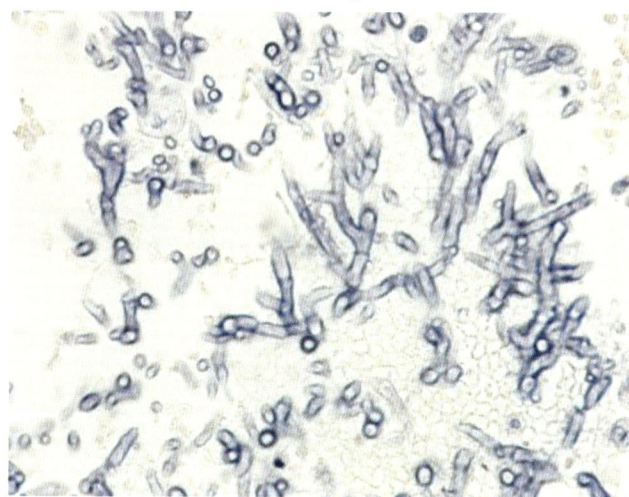

Hyphae with acute angle branching

AR 5B
What would you do now?

A. Start IV fluconazole.
B. Start IV voriconazole.
C. Start IV lipid amphotericin B.
D. Start IV lipid amphotericin B and 5-fluorocytosine.

Answer: **B.** _____

Case 5 — Key Points

- Recognize febrile neutropenia
- Know which immediate antibacterial therapy is indicated
- Know the indications for empiric vancomycin
- Know how to recognize, diagnose, and treat invasive aspergillosis as a complication of prolonged neutropenia

Case 6 — History and Physical

Hx: A 58-year-old man presents to you in August with a 2-day history of fevers with myalgias and a mild headache. He is a Chicago native and returned 6 days ago from a 2-week vacation in Cape Cod, MA. He has rheumatoid arthritis (RA) controlled by etanercept.

PE: T 101.8°F (38.8°C), BP 138/88 mmHg, PR 100 beats/minute, RR 20 breaths/minute

Jaundice;

Heart and lungs are normal;

Mild hepatosplenomegaly;

Chronic changes of RA, no acute inflammation

Case 6 — Labs and Imaging

CBC: Hgb 9.4 g/dL; WBC 9.2 × 10³/mm³:
78% P, 2% bands, 11% L
Pl 85,000 cells/mm³

Haptoglobin < 20 mg/dL, LDH 4× nl, reticulocyte count increased;

AST and ALT 3× nl, total bilirubin 3.8 mg/dL, direct bilirubin 0.8 mg/dL

CXR normal

AR 6A

What diagnostic test would you want next?

A. *Borrelia burgdorferi* serology
B. *Babesia microti* serology
C. *Anaplasma phagocytophilum* serology
D. *Ehrlichia chaffeensis* serology
E. Peripheral smear of blood

Answer:_____

Case 6 — Peripheral Smear

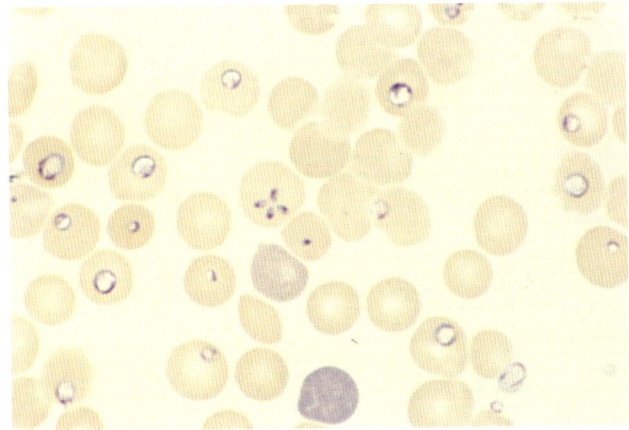

AR 6B

Which antibiotics, if any, do you want to give?

A. Doxycycline
B. Amoxicillin/Clavulanate
C. Chloroquine
D. Azithromycin and atovaquone
E. None

Answer: **D.**_____

Geography of Babesiosis

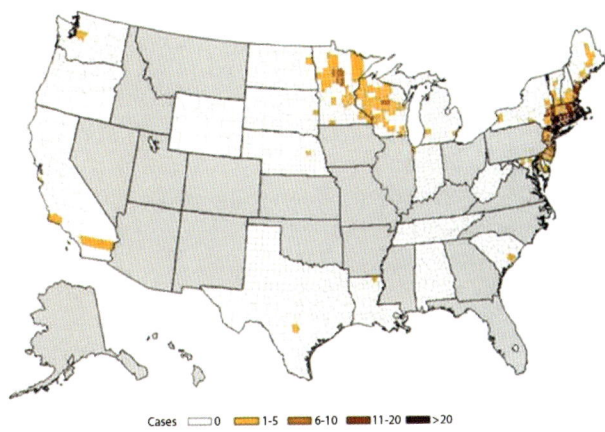

Cases ▭ 0 ▭ 1-5 ▬ 6-10 ▬ 11-20 ▬ >20

[13]

Number of reported cases of babesiosis by county of residence* — 27 states,† 2013

*N = 1,750; county of residence was unknown for 12 of the 1,762 patients. Cases are mapped to the patients' county of residence, which was not necessarily where they became infected.

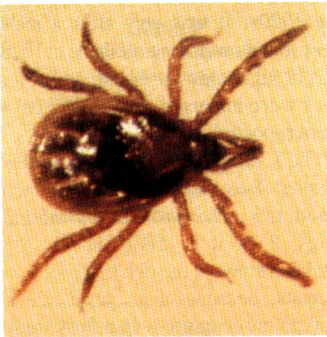

Ixodes scapularis

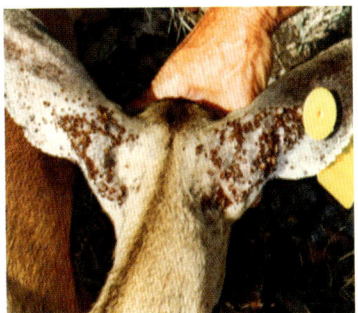

White-tailed deer

Babesiosis
- Microbiology
  - *Babesia microti* (*B. duncani*, *B. divergens*)
  - Transmitted by *Ixodes scapularis*
- Clinical manifestations
  - 1- to 4-week incubation period
  - **Asymptomatic** (~ 40%)
  - **Mild disease** (< 4% parasitemia): fever, malaise, hemolysis, thrombocytopenia, transaminase elevations, jaundice
  - **Severe disease** (≥ 4% parasitemia): asplenic, immunocompromised, ARDS, DIC, AKI, altered mental status
- Treatment
  - Azithromycin (IV if severe) and atovaquone
  - Transfusion may be needed if severe

Case 6 — Continued

He improves over the next 3 days but then fevers—now with chills—recur, and he has a severe headache.

PE: T 104.0°F (40.0°C), BP 140/80 mmHg,
HR 130 beats/minute, RR 20 breaths/minute

Jaundice is gone;

Hepatosplenomegaly unchanged;

Joint exam unchanged

Case 6 — Repeat Labs

CBC: Hgb 10.4 g/dL; WBC 3.2 × 10³/mm³:
40% P, 20% bands, 25% L
Pl 100,000 cells/mm³

Haptoglobin normal;

Transaminases and bilirubin normal

AR 6C

Which diagnostic test would you want next?

A. *Borrelia burgdorferi* serology
B. *Babesia microti* serology
C. *Anaplasma phagocytophilum* serology
D. *Ehrlichia chaffeensis* serology
E. Peripheral smear of blood

Answer: **E.**

Case 6 — Repeat Peripheral Smear

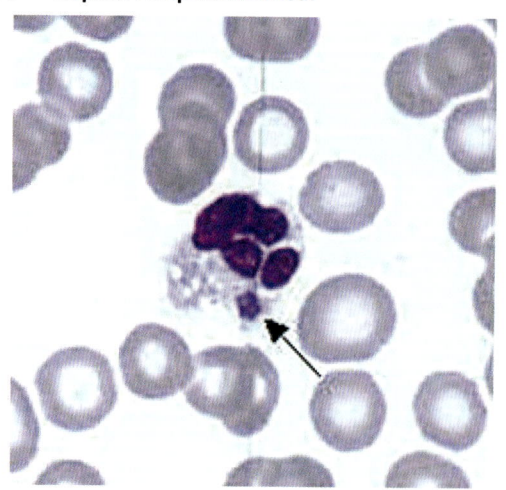

AR 6D

Which antibiotics, if any, do you want to give?

A. Doxycycline
B. Amoxicillin/Clavulanate
C. Chloroquine
D. Azithromycin and atovaquone
E. None

Answer: **A.**

Geography of Ehrlichiosis and Anaplasmosis[14]

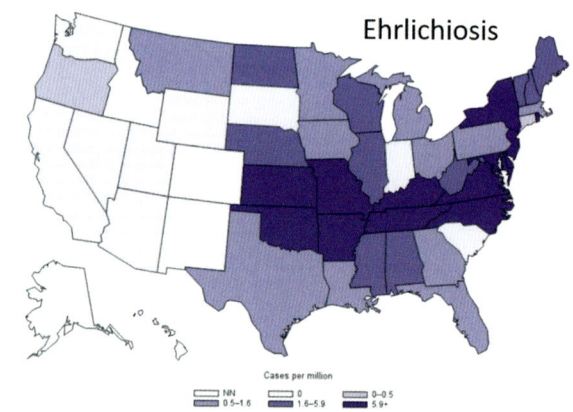

Amblyomma americanum

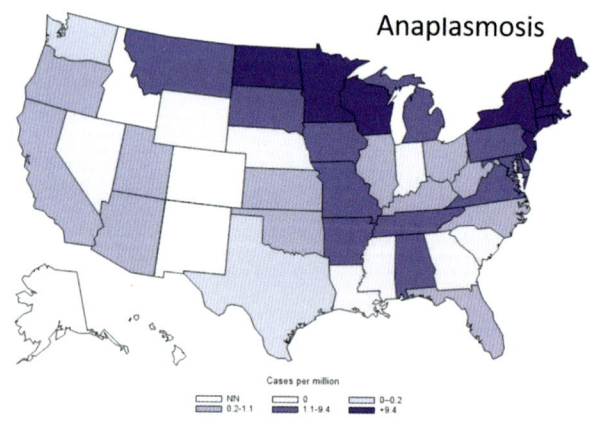

Ixodes scapularis

Tick-borne Intracellular Organisms

	Babesiosis	**Anaplasmosis**	**Ehrlichiosis**
Tick	*Ixodes scapularis*	*Ixodes scapularis*	*Amblyomma americanum*
Organism	*Babesia microti*	*Anaplasma phagocytophilum*	*Ehrlichia ewingii* and *chaffeensis*
Incubation	1–6 weeks	1–2 weeks	1–2 weeks
Presentation	Fever, hemolysis	Flu-like with severe headache	Flu-like with severe headache
Rash	None	< 5%	~ 35%
CBC	Hemolytic anemia	Neutropenia	Lymphopenia ± pancytopenia
Diagnosis	Blood smear (PCR)	Blood smear PMN morulae (PCR)	Blood smear Mono morulae (PCR)
Treatment	Atovaquone + azithromycin	Doxycycline	Doxycycline

Case 6 — Key Points
- Diagnose and treat babesiosis in an immunocompromised host
- Recognize dual infection with tick-borne illnesses
- Diagnose and treat anaplasmosis and ehrlichiosis

Case 7 — History and Physical

Hx: A 31-year-old man presents with a 4-day history of low-grade fever and nonproductive cough. He lives in Chicago. He returned from a golf trip to Phoenix, AZ, 7 days ago. He is otherwise healthy and continues to work as a bank teller.

PE: T 100.0°F (37.8°C); other VS normal

Lungs are clear.

Case 7 — Labs and Imaging

Hgb 14.6 g/dL

WBC 7.2 × 10³/mm³: 54% P, 30% L, no bands; 15% eosinophils

CXR: normal

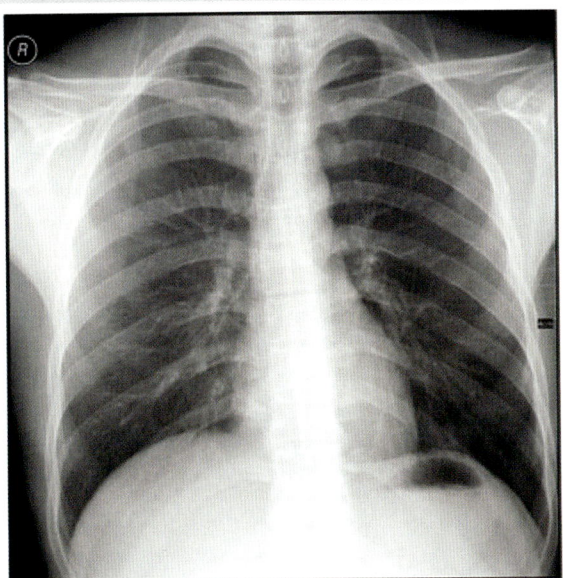

AR 7A
What causative organism do you suspect?

A. *Blastomyces dermatitidis*
B. *Histoplasma capsulatum*
C. *Coccidioides immitis*
D. *Cryptococcus neoformans*
E. *Aspergillus fumigatus*

Answer: _C._

AR 7B
What antifungal, if any, would you give?

A. Fluconazole
B. Itraconazole
C. Liposomal amphotericin B
D. None

Answer: _D._

Coccidioidomycosis
- Epidemiology and pathogenesis
  - Southwestern U.S.
  - **Inhalation of arthroconidia (1)**
  - Worse in persons of color
  - Endospores → dissemination
- Microbiology
  - *Coccidioides immitis* and *posadasii*

Areas Endemic for Coccidioidomycosis

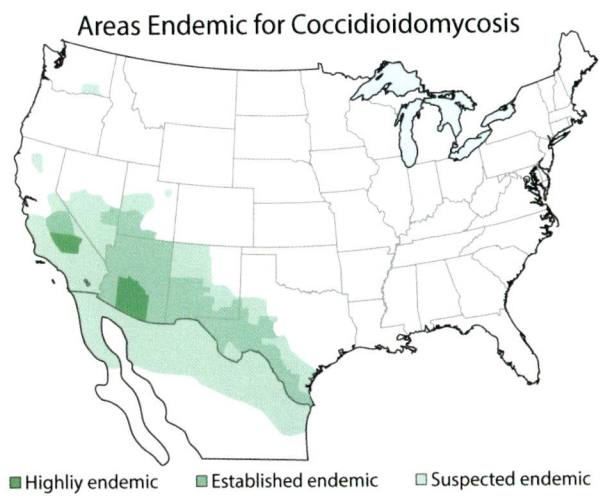

■ Highliy endemic   ■ Established endemic   □ Suspected endemic

[15]

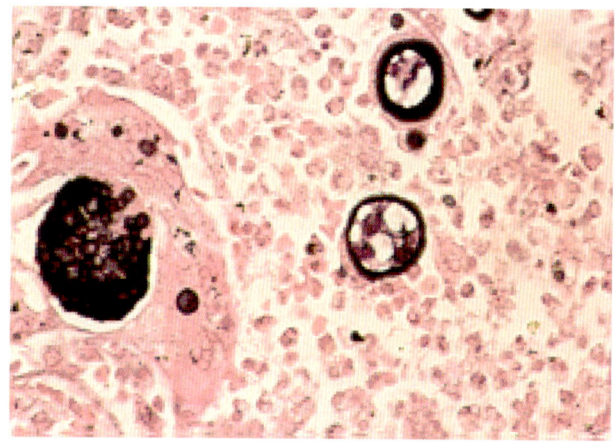

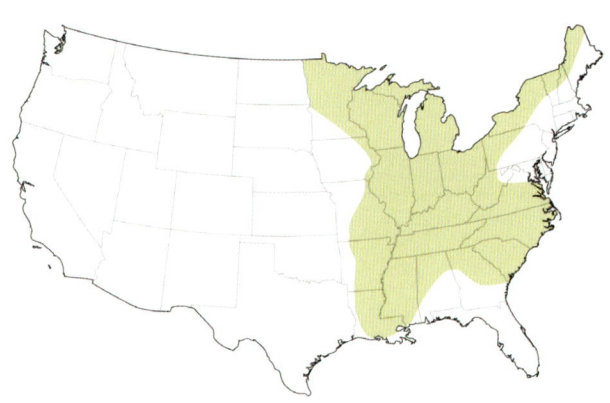

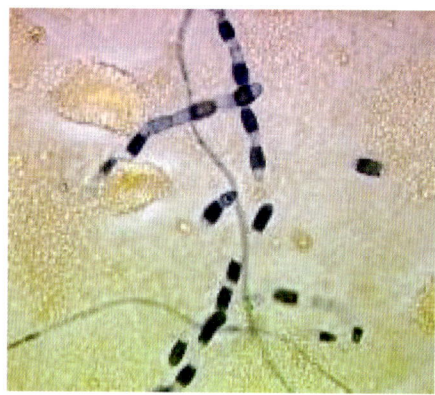

- Clinical manifestations
  - Usually asymptomatic
  - **Valley fever** (fever, cough, flu-like, rash [erythema nodosum], arthritis)
  - Acute/Chronic pneumonia ± cavitation
  - Skin, bone, joints, CNS
  - **Eosinophilia**
- **Treatment**[16]
  - **Nondebilitating/Mild: no antifungal**
  - **Debilitating yet not severe: fluconazole, itraconazole**
  - **Severe/Disseminated: amphotericin B**

IDSA 2016

Blastomycosis
- Epidemiology and pathogenesis
  - **Ohio and Mississippi rivers**
  - Enters through lungs
- Microbiology
  - *Blastomyces dermatitidis*
- Clinical manifestations
  - **Acute or chronic unresolving pneumonia**
  - **Fungating skin lesions**
  - Osteomyelitis
  - Brain abscess

Gilchrist's 1ˢᵗ Case

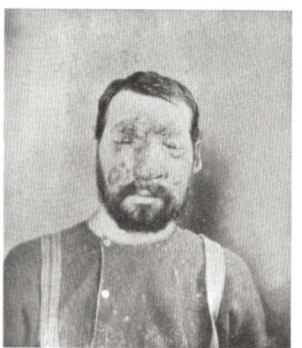

[17]

Blastomycosis
- Diagnosis
  - Tissue/Fluids: broad-based bud
  - Culture
  - **Urinary antigen**
- Treatment[18]
  - **Treat all**
    - Mild to moderate
      - **Itraconazole** × 6–12 months
    - Severe
      - **Amphotericin** B × 1–2 weeks or improvement, then itraconazole for total of 6–12 months

IDSA 2012

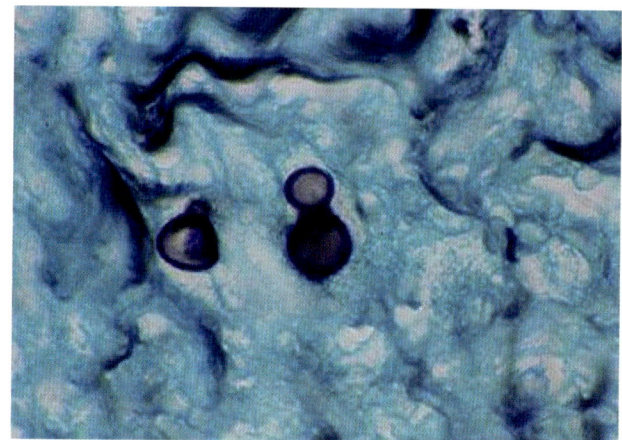

Silver stain

Histoplasmosis

- Epidemiology
  - **Ohio and Mississippi rivers, yet broader distribution**
- Microbiology
  - *Histoplasma capsulatum*
- Clinical manifestations
  - Usually none
  - **Acute/Chronic pneumonia ± cavitation**
  - **Mediastinitis**
  - Dissemination

Areas Endemic for Histoplasmosis

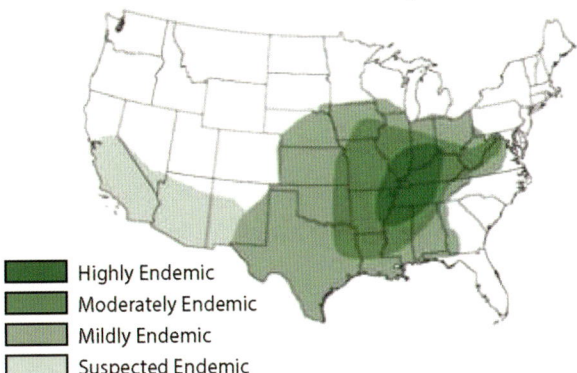

- ■ Highly Endemic
- ■ Moderately Endemic
- ■ Mildly Endemic
- □ Suspected Endemic

- Diagnosis
  - Microscopic appearance
  - Culture
  - Serology
  - **Urinary Ag**
- Treatment[19]
  - Pneumonia
    - Mild: none
    - Moderate: **itraconazole** × 12 weeks
    - Chronic: **itraconazole** × 12 months
  - Severe pneumonia or disseminated:
    - **Amphotericin** B × 1–2 weeks →
      itraconazole to total 12 weeks
  - CNS: amphotericin B × 4–6 weeks,
    then itraconazole × 12 months

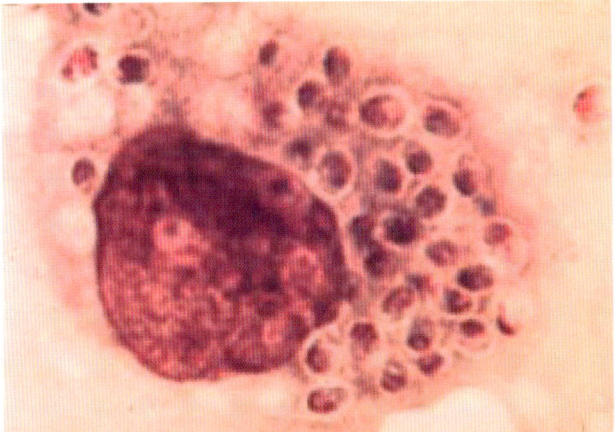

Antifungal Drugs of Choice — 2022

- **Amphotericin B**
  - Severe infection with endemic fungi, crypto, sporo, *Mucor*
- **Azoles**
  - Fluconazole: nonsevere *C. albicans*, *Coccidioides*, *Cryptococcus*
  - Itraconazole: nonsevere endemic fungi, sporotrichosis
  - Posaconazole: invasive aspergillosis, prophylaxis in high-risk patients (SCT, prolonged febrile neutropenia)
  - Voriconazole: invasive aspergillosis
  - Isavuconazole: invasive aspergillosis, mucormycosis
- **Echinocandins** (caspofungin, micafungin, anidulafungin)
  - Prolonged febrile neutropenia
  - Severe candidiasis
- **5-fluorocytosine**
  - Combo Rx of CNS crypto

Antifungal Therapy — 2022

	Cand Non-severe	Cand Severe	Crypt Non-severe	Crypt Severe	Endem Non-severe	Endem Severe	Spor Non-severe	Asp Severe	*Mucor* Severe
Azole									
Fluc	+		+		Cocci				
Itra					+		+		
Vori								+	
Isav								+	+
Posa								+	
Echin		+							
Amph				+		+	(+)		+

For CNS crypto, add 5-FC to amphotericin.
For prolonged febrile neutropenia, add an echinocandin.
For prophylaxis in stem-cell transplant or anticipated prolonged febrile neutropenia, use posaconazole.
Drug levels should be checked when using itraconazole, voriconazole, or posaconazole for invasive fungi or prophylaxis.

Case 7 — Key Points
- Recognize the typical epidemiology and presentations of endemic fungi
- Know the methods of diagnosing these infections
- Understand the treatment of these infections based on severity and underlying host
- Know the antifungal drugs of choice

Case 8 — History and Physical

Hx: An 18-year-old college freshman comes with her 2 roommates to campus health because of fever and a headache for 2 days. She is otherwise healthy.

PE: T 103.2°F (39.6°C), BP 96/66 mmHg, HR 128 beats/minute, RR 20 breaths/minute

Alert and oriented × 3; no papilledema;

Stiff neck; no rash;

Neuro exam normal

AR 8A

Blood cultures are sent. In addition to a lumbar puncture and antibiotics, what would you order next?

A. CT head
B. MRI head
C. Dexamethasone
D. Procalcitonin level

Answer:_____

Dexamethasone for Adult Bacterial Meningitis[20]
- **The Study**
  - PRDBPCT, Netherlands: ≥ 17, *S. pneumoniae* 36%, *N. meningitidis* 32%, other 10%, culture (−) 22%
  - Amoxicillin 2 g q 4 hours IV × 7–10 days, changed PRN, dexamethasone 10 mg 15–20 minutes prior, then q 6 hours × 4 days
  - Glasgow Outcome Scale = 5 (no/mild disability) vs. < 5 (no return to work/school or worse)

- **The Results**

	Dexamethasone (N = 157)	Placebo (N = 144)	P
GOS < 5: all	15%	25%	0.03
S. pneumoniae	26%	52%	0.006
Non–*S. pneumoniae*	8%	11%	NS
Death: all	7%	15%	0.04
S. pneumoniae	14%	34%	0.02
Non–*S. pneumoniae*	3%	4%	NS
Focal deficits: all	13%	20%	0.13
Hearing loss: all	9%	12%	0.54
Hyperglycemia	32%	26%	0.24

Empiric Treatment of Bacterial Meningitis

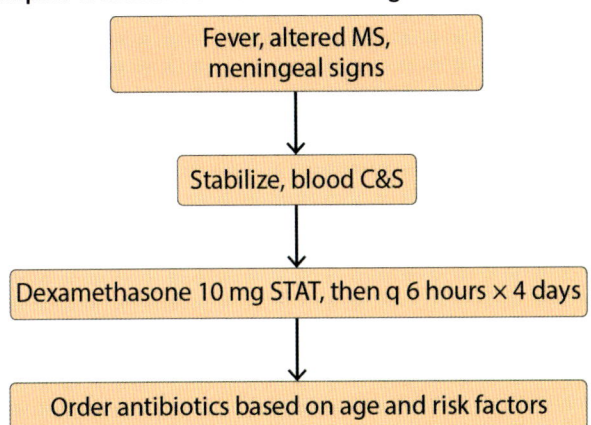

AR 8B

What antibiotics would you give?

A. Ceftriaxone
B. Vancomycin and ceftriaxone
C. Vancomycin, ceftriaxone, and ampicillin
D. Vancomycin and ceftazidime

Answer: ___B___

Empiric Treatment of Bacterial Meningitis

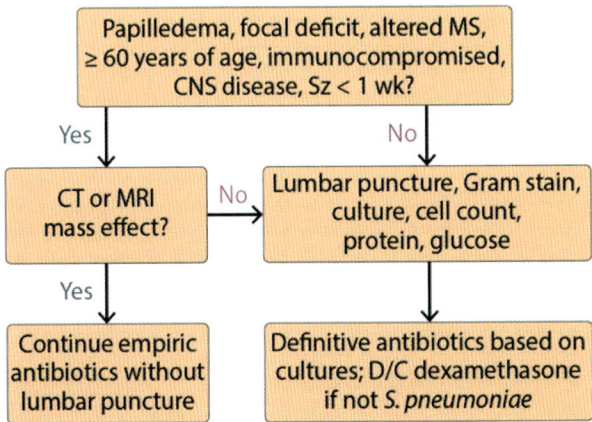

Bacterial Meningitis, United States (1,670 cases)[21]

Years of Age	*S. pneumoniae*	*N. meningitidis*	*L. monocytogenes*
18–34	50%	36%	2%
35–49	75%	8%	2%
50–64	78%	5%	6%
≥ 65	70%	5%	10%

Empiric Therapy of Bacterial Meningitis[22]

Patient	Likely Organisms	Antibiotics
18–50 years of age	*S. pneumoniae, N. meningitidis*	Ceftriaxone + vancomycin
> 50 years of age	Above + *Listeria*	Above + ampicillin
Immunocompromised	*Listeria* + GNB	Vancomycin + ampicillin + cefepime
Neurosurgery	Staph + GNB	Vancomycin + cefepime or meropenem

Case 8 — CSF Findings

Cloudy

WBC 1,300 cells/mm³: 94% P

RBC 2 cells/mm³

Protein 145 g/dL

Glucose 44 mg/dL (serum 120 mg/dL)

Gram stain

Case 8 — CSF Gram Stain

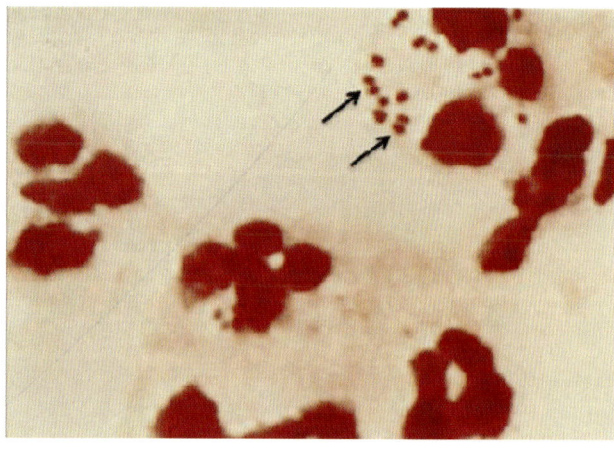

Gram-negative cocci in pairs

Diplococci.

AR 8C
Which of the following is the best therapy pending susceptibilities?

A. Ceftriaxone alone
B. Ceftriaxone and dexamethasone
C. Vancomycin and ceftriaxone
D. Vancomycin, ceftriaxone, and dexamethasone

Answer:_____

AR 8D
Who should receive prophylaxis for exposure to her?

A. Her roommates
B. Her roommates and all health care workers
C. Her roommates, health care workers, and patients in her ward
D. No one

Answer:_____

Chemoprophylaxis for Meningococcal Meningitis
- **Close contact definition**
  - > 8 hours within 3 feet, or
  - Direct contact with secretions
- **Timing of significant exposure**
  - 1 week prior to 1 day after presentation
- **Drugs that are effective**
  - Ciprofloxacin 500 mg PO × 1
  - Rifampin 600 mg PO bid × 2 days
  - Ceftriaxone 250 mg IM × 1

Meningococcal Vaccines[23]
- Vaccine types and age recommendations
  - Quadrivalent (A, C, Y, W135)
    - 11–18 years of age
  - Monovalent (B)
    - 16–23 years of age (shared decision making)
  - Give both to all adults if:
    - Travel to endemic areas
    - Local outbreaks
    - Complement deficiency
    - Asplenia

Case 8 — Key Points
- Recognize the importance of empiric dexamethasone in the treatment of bacterial meningitis
- Know when to do brain images prior to lumbar puncture in suspected bacterial meningitis
- Know the age-based empiric therapies for bacterial meningitis
- Know the definitive therapies for bacterial meningitis
- Know who should receive prophylaxis after exposure to meningococcal meningitis
- Know the current meningococcal vaccine indications for adults

Case 9 — History and Physical

Hx: A 58-year-old man with Type 2 diabetes comes to your office with tender swollen areas on the back of his neck that have been enlarging for the last 5 days. He denies fever.

He is allergic to trimethoprim/sulfamethoxazole.

PE: T 99.5°F (37.5°C), BP 138/88 mmHg,
HR 88 beats/minute, RR 14 breaths/minute

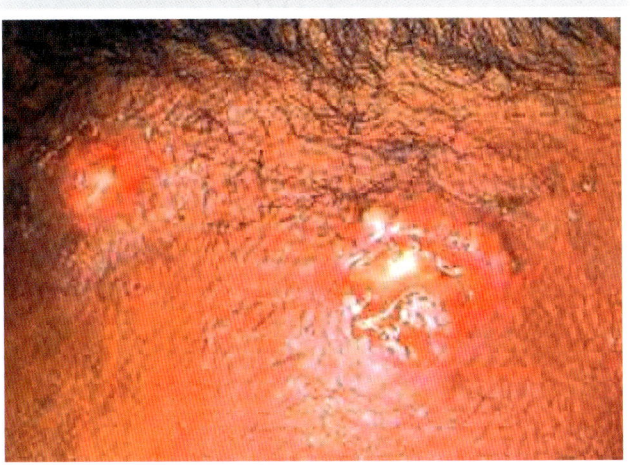

Case 9 — Labs

Blood glucose = 108 mg/dL

Gram stain of pus:

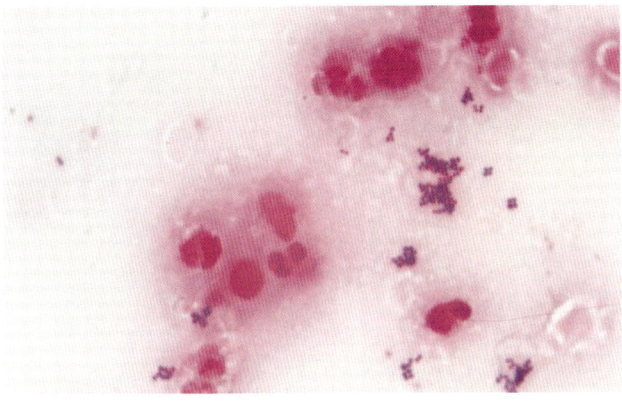

Gram-positive cocci in clusters

AR 9

After draining the lesions in your office, what would you prescribe next?

A. Cephalexin PO
B. Amoxicillin/Clavulanate PO
C. Doxycycline PO
D. Vancomycin IV
E. Daptomycin IV

Answer:____C._____

The Anatomy of Soft Tissue Infections — "Cellulitis"

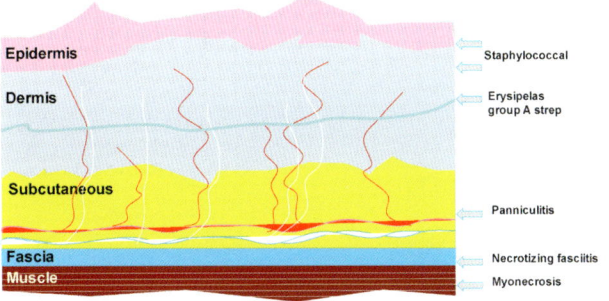

Staphylococcal Infections

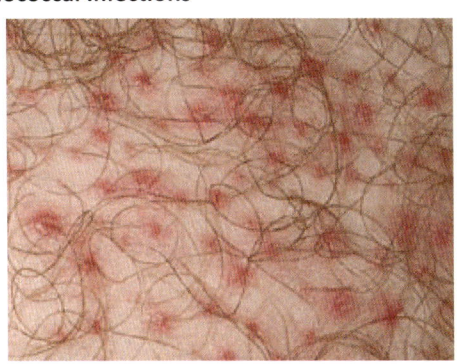

Folliculitis

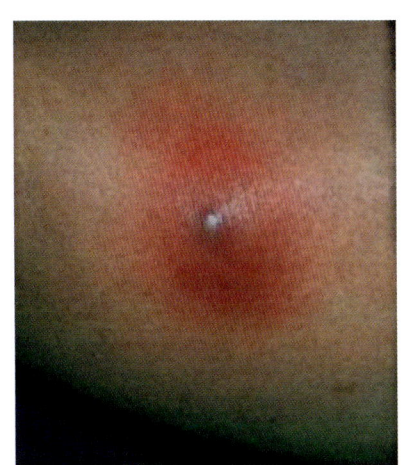

Furuncle (boil)

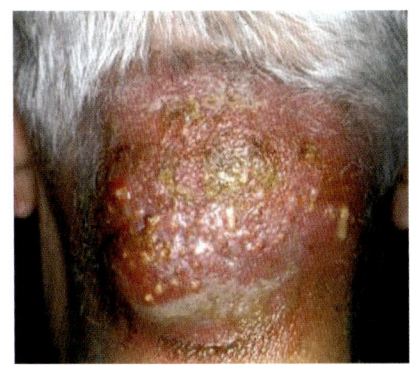

Carbuncle

Streptococcal Lymphangitis (Erysipelas)
- Face
- Arm, post breast surgery
- Post liposuction
- Leg, post saphenous vein harvest

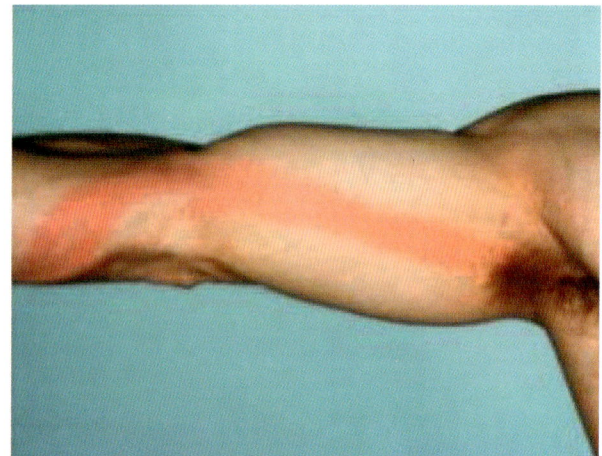

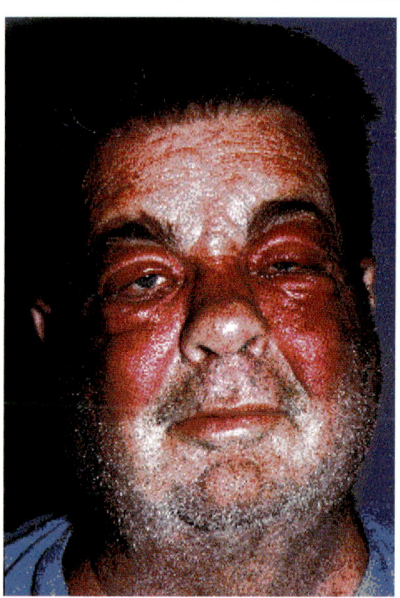

Classification of Skin and Soft Tissue Infections[24]

Severity	Purulent (Staph)	Nonpurulent (Strep)
Mild	No systemic signs	No systemic signs
Moderate	Systemic signs	Systemic signs
Severe	Sepsis or failed Rx, immunocompromised	Sepsis or failed Rx, immunocompromised, bullae/slough, trauma

Treatment of Purulent Cellulitis[25]

- Mild disease
  - **Incision and drainage** only
- Moderate disease
  - **Incision and drainage**
  - Culture
  - Empiric Rx
    - TMP/SMX or doxycycline
  - Definitive Rx
    - MRSA: PO TMP/SMX
    - MSSA: PO dicloxacillin or cephalexin
- Severe disease
  - **Incision and drainage**
  - Culture
  - Empiric Rx
    - Vancomycin, daptomycin, linezolid, telavancin, or ceftaroline
    - Clindamycin if resistance < 15%
  - Definitive Rx
    - MRSA: IV empiric
    - MSSA: IV nafcillin, cefazolin, clindamycin

IDSA 2014

TMP / SMX vs. Placebo for Skin Abscess[26]

- **The Study**
  - Uncomplicated abscess, I+D'd in ED
  - TMP/SMX vs. placebo for 7 days
  - Outcome assessed at 7–14 days
- **The Results** (those who took ≥ 75% of doses)

	TMP / SMX (N = 524)	Placebo (N = 533)	P
Cure	92.9%	85.7%	< 0.001
Repeat I+D	3.4%	8.6%	< 0.05
Infection in HHC	1.7%	4.1%	< 0.05

Treatment of Nonpurulent Cellulitis[27]

- Mild disease
  - PO: PCN, 1° cephalosporin, dicloxacillin, clindamycin
- Moderate disease
  - IV: PCN, cefazolin, ceftriaxone, clindamycin
- Severe disease
  - **Surgery** for debridement and C&S
  - Vancomycin + piperacillin-tazobactam

Case 9 — Key Points

- Recognize a staphylococcal carbuncle by presentation and Gram stain
- Differentiate staphylococcal and streptococcal cellulitis by purulence
- Know the treatments of cellulitis differ based on purulence and severity
- Utilize inexpensive oral drugs to treat uncomplicated *S. aureus* skin infections regardless of methicillin sensitivity

Case 10 — History and Physical

Hx: A 32-year-old man comes to an urgent care center with a 2-day history of a sore throat. He denies cough, runny nose, or hoarseness. No one is sick at home. He works as a real estate agent.

PE: T 99.9°F (37.7°C)

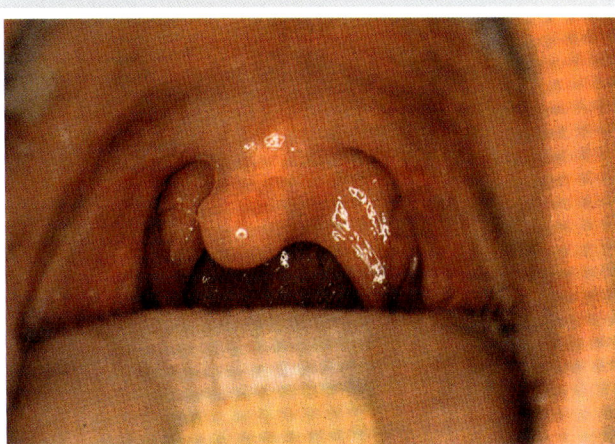

AR 10A
What would you do now?

A. Swab for rapid antigen testing for group A strep prior to treatment.
B. Swab for culture prior to treatment.
C. Swab for rapid antigen and start penicillin.
D. Swab for culture and start penicillin.
E. No testing; no penicillin.

Answer: __A.__

AR 10B
A rapid antigen test is performed and is negative. Now what would you do?

A. Swab for culture prior to treatment.
B. Swab for culture and start penicillin.
C. No further testing; treat with penicillin.
D. No further testing; prescribe no antibiotics.

Answer:_____

Approach to Strep Pharyngitis

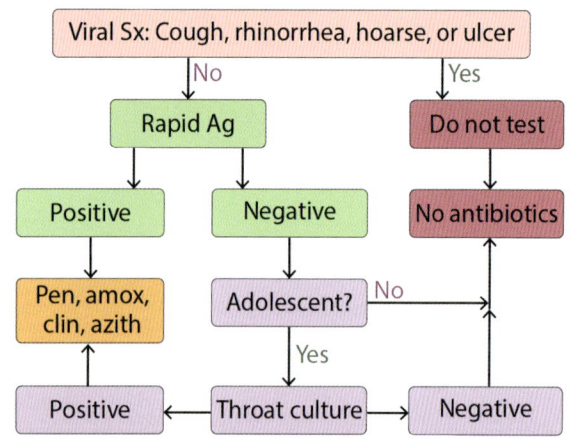

IDSA 2012

Case 10 — Key Points
- Know which adults should be tested for group A strep pharyngitis
- Know the operating characteristics of rapid Ag testing for GABHS
- Know when to treat pharyngitis and with what antibiotics

Case 11 — History and Physical

Hx: A 62-year-old man comes to a Montana ED in February complaining of 2 days of abdominal pain and vomiting and 1 day of blurred vision and trouble talking. His wife is with him and has similar symptoms. They live on a farm and have been eating stored food from their basement, riding out the recent heavy snow fall.

PE: VS are normal, no orthostasis; alert but has dysarthria; pupils and mouth exam.

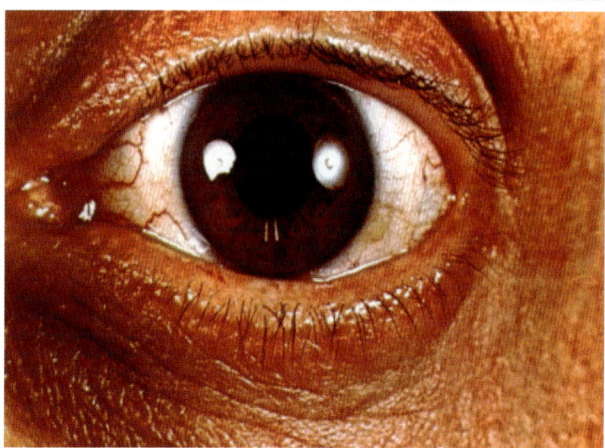

Mydriasis

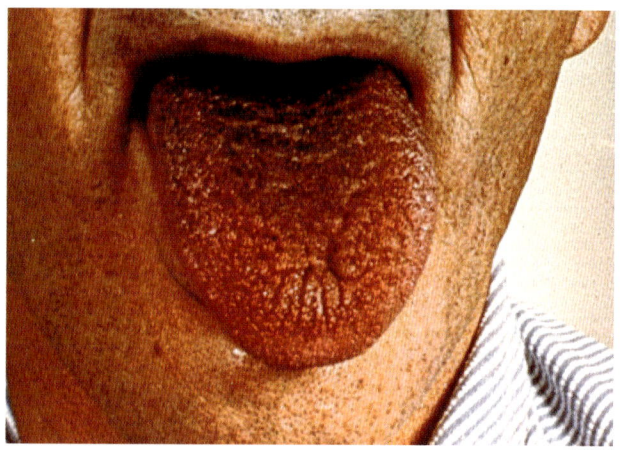

Corrugated tongue

AR 11
What should he be treated with?

A. Plasmapheresis
B. Intravenous immunoglobulin
C. A series of vaccines
D. High doses of an antibiotic
E. An equine antitoxin

Answer:_____

Clostridium botulinum — Botulism
- Toxin acquisition
  - **Foodborne: direct ingestion of preformed toxin**
  - Wound: spores → germinate → toxin production
  - Infantile and unknown: ingestion of spores
- Toxin action
  - Prevents docking of ACh vesicles to presynaptic membrane in peripheral nerves
  - No sympathetic or CNS involvement
- Clinical features
  - Permanent prevention of ACh release
    - Descending motor paralysis
    - Parasympathetic cranial nerve paralysis
      - Dilated pupils, dry tongue, dysarthria, dysphagia, respiratory arrest
    - No fever
- Treatment
  - **Equine antitoxin**
  - Penicillin if wound source
  - Supportive

Case 11 — Key Points
- Recognize the epidemiologic setting of foodborne botulism
- Recognize the clinical manifestations of botulism
- Know the treatment of foodborne botulism

Case 12 — History and Physical

Hx: A 19-year-old man comes to your office complaining of severe burning with urination for 2 days. He noted pus from his urethra today. He had vaginal intercourse without protection with a new female partner 4 days ago. She has no symptoms and denies any prior STIs.

PE: Exam is normal except for easily expressible pus from the urethra.

Case 12 — Labs

Nucleic acid amplification testing (NAAT) is not available in your office. A Gram stain of the urethral pus is performed and is also sent for culture.

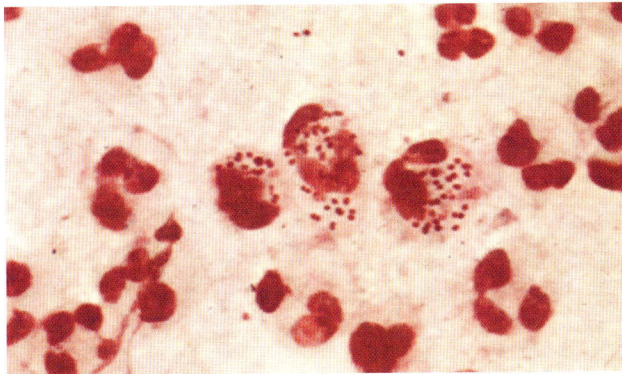

Gram-negative coccobacilli

AR 12

What should be done next?

A. Send him to ED for NAAT prior to treatment.
B. Start ceftriaxone 500 mg IM × 1.
C. Start ceftriaxone 500 mg IM plus azithromycin 1,000 mg PO × 1.
D. Start ceftriaxone 500 mg IM plus doxycycline 100 mg bid x 7 days.

Answer:_____

Neisseria gonorrhoeae in Men[28]
- Purulent, painful urethritis (rarely asymptomatic)
- **Incubation period 3–7 days**
- Complications
  - Epididymitis, prostatitis
- **Diagnosis**
  - **Gram stain or discharge: useful and diagnostic**
    - **Sens = 90–95%; spec = 95–100%**
  - **NAAT of urine**
  - **Culture if above not (+)**
- **Treatment**
  - **Ceftriaxone 500 mg IM × 1**
  - **Doxycycline 100 mg PO bid × 7d <u>if</u> chlamydia not ruled out**
  - **Partner notification and treatment**
  - **Retest 3 months after treatment**

Neisseria gonorrhoeae in Women
- <u>Primary site</u> = **endocervix (80% asymptomatic)**
  - Secondary spread to vagina, urethra, rectum
- Complications
  - Pelvic inflammatory disease
    - TOA, sterility, periurethral abscess
    - Rx: foxy/doxy vs. clinda/gent
  - Disseminated infection
    - Oligoarthritis and cutaneous pustules

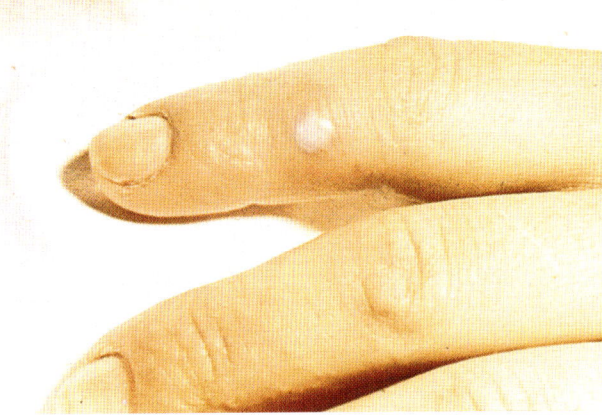

Neisseria gonorrhoeae in Women[29]
- Diagnosis
  - **Gram stain of endocervix: <u>not</u> useful**
    - **Sens = 50–70%; spec = 80%**
  - **NAAT of urine/vaginal swabs or culture required (80–90% sensitive)**
- Treatment
  - **Uncomplicated**
    - **Ceftriaxone 500 mg IM × 1**
    - **Doxycycline 100 mg PO bid if chlamydia cannot be ruled out**
    - **Partner notification and treatment**
    - **Test for cure at 3 months**

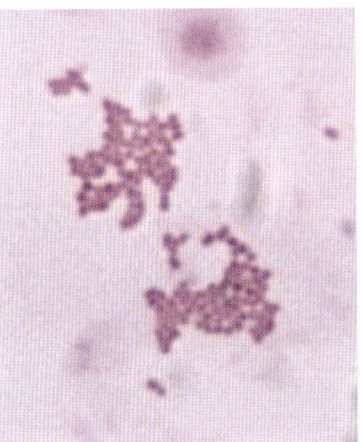

Veillonella spp.

Chlamydia trachomatis[30]

- Epidemiology
  - The most common bacterial STI
  - Majority of women are asymptomatic → continuous reservoir
- Clinical manifestations (7- to 14-day incubation)
  - Women: cervicitis > acute urethral syndrome, > PID, > perihepatitis
  - Men: urethritis > epididymitis
- Diagnosis
  - **NAAT of urine in men, vagina in women**
  - **Ag detection requires urethral or cervical swab, less sensitive**
- Treatment if uncomplicated (test for cure in 3 months)
  - Azithromycin 1,000 mg PO × 1
  - Partner notification and treatment

Case 12 — Key Points

- Know the differing presentations of chlamydia and gonococcal urethritis
- Know the yields of diagnostic tests for chlamydia and gonococcal urethritis
- Know the treatment of uncomplicated infection from each organism
- Understand the need to treat for chlamydia in patients with gonorrhea
- Know the recommended risk groups and frequency of screening for these diseases

Case 13 — History, Physical, and Labs

Hx: A 33-year-old woman returns for follow-up after treatment of a syphilitic chancre on her labia 15 months ago. Her RPR at that time was (+) at a titer of 1:64, and her FTA-ABS was also (+). She was treated with 2.4 MU of benzathine penicillin IM × 1. She has had 3 male sexual partners since then. She has no other medical problems.

PE: Exam is normal.

Lab: RPR (+) at a titer of 1:32

AR 13

What should be done next?

A. Re-treat with benzathine penicillin 2.4 MU IM × 1.
B. Re-treat with benzathine penicillin 2.4 MU IM q week × 3.
C. Perform a lumbar puncture prior to treatment.
D. Have her return in 6 months for repeat RPR.

Answer:_____

Seroreversion of RPR in Treated Syphilis

- Time to seroreversion
  - Primary = 1 year
  - Secondary = 2 years
  - Late latent = 5 years
- Failure to serorevert
  - Reinfection
  - Biological false (+)
  - **Inadequate therapy**
    - **Neurosyphilis does not respond to benzathine penicillin**

Syphilis — CSF Exam in Syphilis[31]

- Indications
  - Neurologic or ophthalmologic signs/Sx
  - Signs of active tertiary syphilis
    - Aortitis
    - Gummas
  - **Treatment failure**
- **Diagnostic of neurosyphilis (any of):**
  - VDRL (+)
  - Protein > 45 mg/dL
  - Lymphocytes > 5 cells/μL

Case 13 — Key Points

- Understand the time frame in which nontreponemal testing for syphilis should serorevert after appropriate Rx
- Know the reasons for failure to serorevert
- Understand the indications for performing a lumbar puncture in patients with syphilis
- Understand how to diagnose neurosyphilis
- Know the recommendations for screening of syphilis

Populations at Increased Risk for STIs

- STI in last 24 months
- New partner in last 3 months
- Multiple partners in last 12 months
- Partner with multiple partners
- Partners found via internet
- Contact with sex workers
- Intravenous drug use
- Recent jail or detention facility
- Exchanging sex for drugs or money
- Men who have sex with men (MSM)

STI Screening of Women[32]

STI	< 25 yo	≥ 25 yo	Pregnant	HIV (+)
GC/Chlamydia	Annual	At risk	< 25 or at risk 1st + 3rd trimester	Annual
Syphilis	At risk	At risk	< 25 or at risk 1st + 3rd trimester	Annual
Trichomonas	At risk	At risk	If HIV (+)	Annual
HBV	At risk	At risk	Once	Once
HCV	At risk	At risk	At risk	Once
HIV	Once	Once	Once	

STI Screening of Men[33]

STI	MSW HIV (-)	MSW HIV (+)	MSM HIV (-)	MSM HIV (+)
GC/Chlamydia	At risk	Annual	Annual	Annual
Syphilis	At risk	Annual	Annual	Annual
HAV			Once	Once
HBV	At risk	Once	Once	Once
HCV	At risk	Once	Once	Annual
HIV	Once		Annual	

Case 14 — History and Physical

Hx: A 24-year-old woman presents with a 3-day history of unpleasant-smelling, continuous vaginal discharge. She is sexually active with 1 partner for 3 years and is currently 10 weeks pregnant.

PE: external genitalia normal; opaque copious vaginal discharge present with an amine odor; underlying vaginal walls and cervix appear normal.

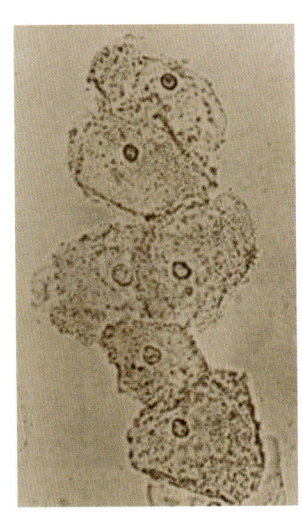

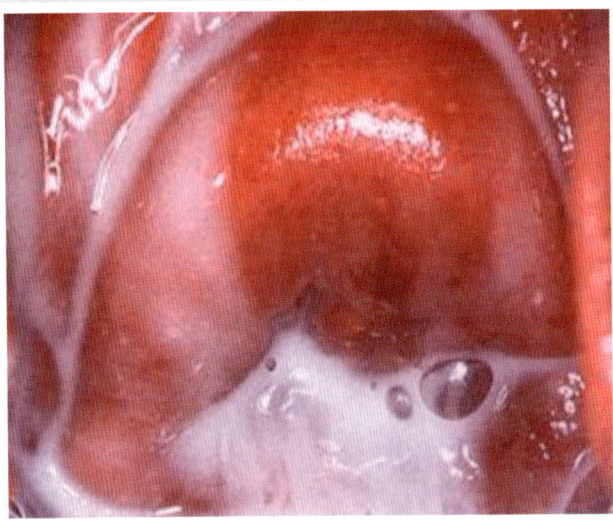

AR 14
What would you do next?

A. Start metronidazole 500 mg bid × 7 days.
B. Start metronidazole 2 g × 1.
C. Start clindamycin 300 mg bid × 7 days.
D. No treatment; have her return in her 2nd trimester and treat if still symptomatic.

Answer: _A._

Case 14 — Labs
A sample of the discharge has a pH of 6.5; addition of KOH produces a fishy odor and reveals no fungal elements on microscopy; a saline prep reveals:

Vaginosis and Vaginitis

- **Bacterial vaginosis**
  - *Lactobacillus* replaced by anaerobes
    - *Mobiluncus*, *Gardnerella*
  - Clinical: amine odor, no irritation
- **Vulvovaginal candidiasis**
  - *C. albicans*
  - Clinical: pruritus, white plaques on red base
  - If recurrent: Rule out DM and HIV
- **Trichomoniasis**
  - *Trichomonas vaginalis*
  - Clinical: profuse discharge, ± foul

Vaginosis and Vaginitis Diagnostic Tests

	Vaginal pH	Wet Prep	KOH Prep
Bacterial Vaginosis	> 5.0	Clue cells	Amine odor
Candida	< 5.0	Fungal elements	Fungal elements
Trichomonas*	> 5.0	Trichomonads	Not diagnostic

*PCR testing, if available, is gold standard

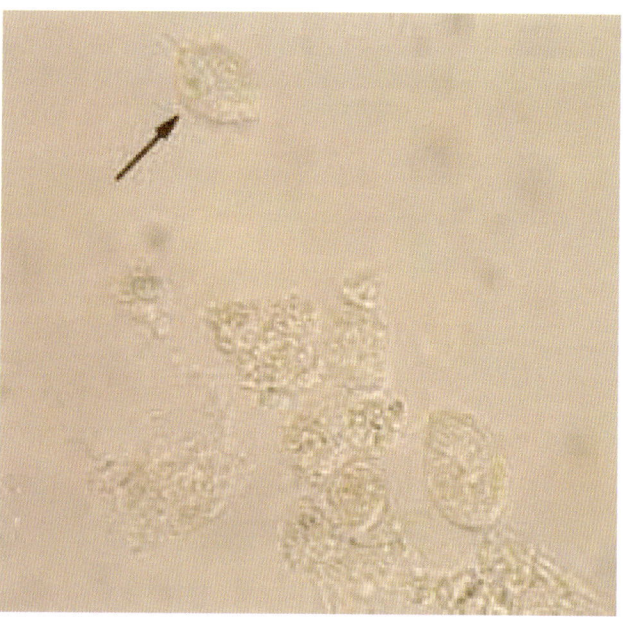

Trichomonas

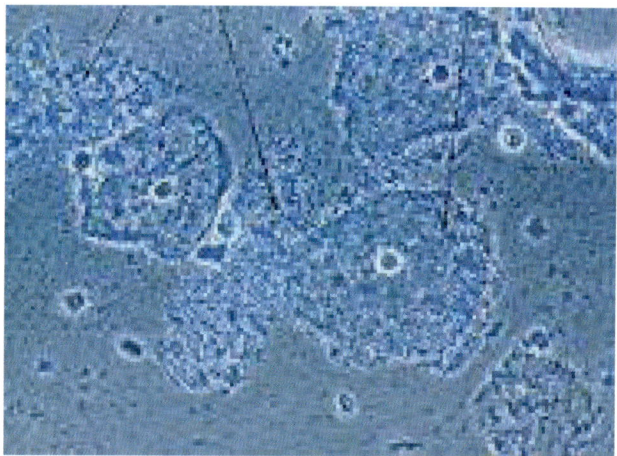

Clue cells

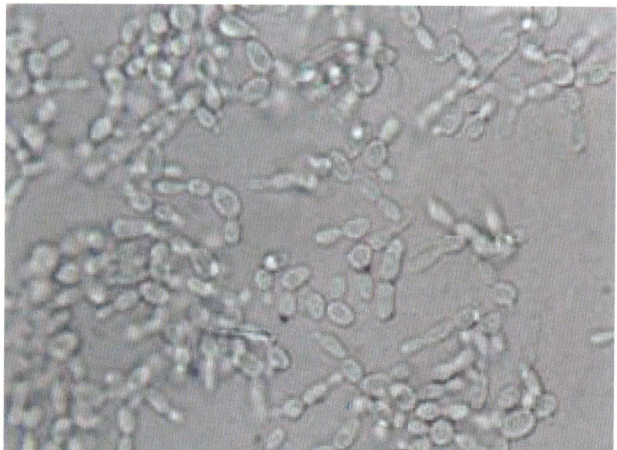

Candida

Vaginosis and Vaginitis Treatment[34]

	1st Line	Other Choices	Pregnancy
Bacterial Vaginosis	Metronidazole 500 mg PO bid × 7 days or 5 g gel × 5 days	Clindamycin cream 5 g × 7 days	Same
Candida	Fluconazole 150 mg PO × 1	Topical clotrimazole or miconazole	Topical clotrimazole or miconazole
*Trichomonas**	Metronidazole PO 500 mg bid × 7 days	Tinidazole	Same

*Retest in 3 months

Fluconazole During Pregnancy[35]
- **The Study (*JAMA* 2016)**
  - Denmark database 1997–2013
  - 1,405,663 pregnancies
    - 3,315 exposed during weeks 7–22
  - 1:4 exposed:not exposed
- **The Results**

	Exposed	Not Exposed	P
Spontaneous Abortion	147/3,315 (4.4%)	563/13,246 (4.2%)	< 0.05
Stillbirth	21/5,382 (0.4%)	77/21,506 (0.4%)	NS

  - Effect seen even if only topical use

Case 14 — Key Points
- Differentiate and diagnose the 3 common causes of vaginal discharge
- Know the treatment of infectious etiologies of vaginal discharge
- Know whether 1st trimester pregnancy affects these treatments

Case 15A — History, Physical, and Labs
Hx: A 38-year-old woman presents with a 2-day history of abdominal cramps and diarrhea 4–5 times per day. She is not vomiting. She was at an office retreat at a resort 2 days prior to becoming ill. Eight of 21 other attendees are similarly ill. The Public Health Department requested stool specimens on all those who were ill, and she is here to follow up on the results.

PE: T 99.4°F (37.4°C), BP 118/80 mmHg, HR 90 beats/minute, RR 14 breaths/minute.

No orthostasis; abdominal exam normal.

Lab: stool culture growing *Shigella sonnei*

AR 15A
In addition to oral hydration, what would you do next?

A. Amoxicillin × 5 days
B. Trimethoprim/Sulfamethoxazole × 5 days
C. Levofloxacin × 3 days
D. No antibiotic therapy

Answer:_____

The Infectious Inoculum of *Shigella*[36]
- The Study
  - Male inmate "volunteers" at Maryland House of Correction given various inocula and observed
- The Results

Inoculum	Disease / Total (%)
< 10^2	27/68 (40)
10^2–10^3	28/84 (33)
10^3–10^4	100/174 (57)
≥ 10^5	38/59 (64)

Shigella — Quinolone Resistance (CDC 2017)
- Plasmid-mediated quinolone resistance (*PMQR*) genes
- Unknown prevalence
- Creates ciprofloxacin MICs of ≥ 0.12 µg/mL
  - Usually MIC is ≤ 0.015 µg/mL
- CLSI guidelines say MIC of ≤ 1.0 µg/mL is **sensitive**
  - Should change to 0.12 is intermediate, > 1.0 is resistant
- *Salmonella* with MIC ≥ 0.12 µg/mL associated with:
  - Prolonged duration of illness and treatment failure
- Common resistance to other agents
  - Macrolides
  - Trimethoprim/Sulfamethoxazole (TMP/SMX)
  - Ampicillin and amoxicillin/clavulanate

Shigella — Approach to Rx
- Culture and sensitivity of suspected cases
- **Do not** routinely treat
  - Usually self-limited (5- to 7-day course)
  - Treatment increases resistance
  - If resistant, treatment increases duration and shedding
- Indications to treat
  - Immunocompromised
  - Severe (hospitalized, invasive, complications)
  - Outbreaks as advised by health department
- Drugs of choice
  - Avoid quinolones if ciprofloxacin MIC ≥ 0.12 μg/mL
- Follow-up cultures if symptoms persist

Case 15B — History, Physical, and Labs
Hx: A 38-year-old woman presents with a 2-day history of abdominal cramps and diarrhea 4–5 times per day. She is not vomiting. She was at an office retreat at a resort 2 days prior to becoming ill. Eight of 21 other attendees are similarly ill. The Public Health Department requested stool specimens on all those who were ill, and she is here to follow up on the results.

PE: T 99.4°F (37.4°C), BP 118/80 mmHg, HR 90 beats/minute, RR 14 breaths/minute

No orthostasis; abdominal exam normal

Lab: stool culture growing *Salmonella enterica*

AR 15B
In addition to oral hydration, what would you do next?

A. Amoxicillin × 5 days
B. Trimethoprim/Sulfamethoxazole × 5 days
C. Levofloxacin × 3 days
D. No antibiotic therapy

Answer:_____

Metaanalysis of Rx of Nontyphoidal *Salmonella* Enteritis[37]
- **The Study**
  - 12 trials of antibiotics vs. placebo, with 778 pts
- **The Results**

	Effect of Antibiotics	P Value
Duration of Illness	−0.07 days	0.76
Duration of Diarrhea	−0.03 days	0.91
Duration of Fever	−0.45 days	0.09
Cure	81% vs. 75%	0.07
C&S (+) > 42 Days	**11% vs. 3%**	**0.01**

Case 15C — History, Physical, and Labs
Hx: A 38-year-old woman presents with a 2-day history of abdominal cramps and diarrhea 4–5 times per day. She is not vomiting. She was at an office retreat at a resort 2 days prior to becoming ill. Eight of 21 other attendees are similarly ill. The Public Health Department requested stool specimens on all those who were ill, and she is here to follow up on the results.

PE: T 99.4°F (37.4°C), BP 118/80 mmHg
HR 90 beats/minute, RR 14 breaths/minute

No orthostasis; abdominal exam normal

Lab: stool culture growing *E. coli* O157:H7

AR 15C
In addition to oral hydration, what would you do next?

A. Amoxicillin × 5 days
B. Trimethoprim/Sulfamethoxazole × 5 days
C. Levofloxacin × 3 days
D. No antibiotic therapy

Answer:_____

Risk Factors for HUS after *E. coli* O157:H7 Infection[38]
- **The Study**
  - Prospective enrollment of 259 children
- **Multivariable Analysis**

Risk Factor	Odds Ratio	P Value
WBC increase*	1.10	0.008
Vomiting	3.05	0.02
Antibiotic Rx	**3.62**	**0.02**
*Each 1.0 above 1.5		

Bacterial Diarrhea Rx Summary

Bacterial	Who to Treat	What to Use
Shigella	Immunocompromised, hospital, outbreak	Not a quinolone
Salmonella	**Comorbid Dx**	**Quinolone**
Campylobacter	< 72 hours or comorbid Dx	Azithromycin, quinolone
E. Coli O157	No one	N/A

Cases 15A, 15B, and 15C — Key Points
- Recognize the presentation of bacterial diarrhea
- Know when bacterial pathogens warrant therapy and what agents to use

Case 16 — History and Physical

Hx: A 28-year-old man comes to the ED 1 hour after a dog bite. It occurred when he tried to break up a fight between his and a neighbor's dog. He has had regular tetanus immunizations; the last one was 4 years ago.

PE: VS are stable.

Hand photo

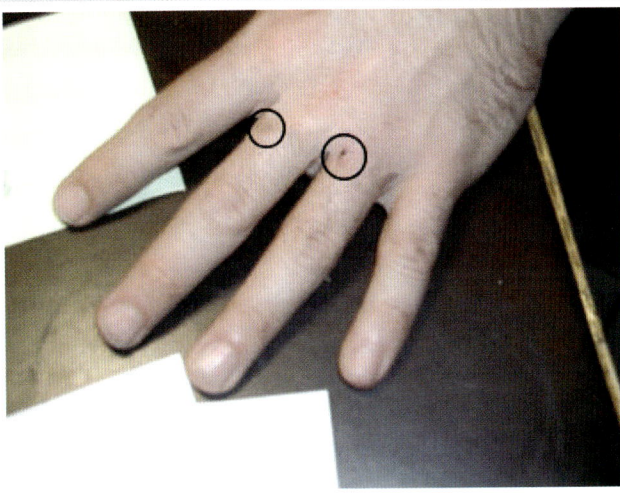

AR 16A
Which tetanus treatment/prophylaxis is needed?

A. Tetanus toxoid alone
B. Tetanus immunoglobulin
C. Tetanus toxoid and tetanus immunoglobulin
D. No tetanus prevention is needed.

Answer:_____

Tetanus — Wound Management

Past Toxoid Doses	Clean and Minor Wound	Tetanus-Prone Wound*
Unknown or < 3	Toxoid	Toxoid + TIG
≥ 3	Toxoid if ≥ 10 years	Toxoid if ≥ 5 years

*Crush, dirt/feces, puncture, missiles
- Give Tdap 1 time in adulthood
- Give Tdap during **each** pregnancy (weeks 27–36)

AR 16B
Which oral antibiotics, if any, should be given?

A. Doxycycline
B. Clindamycin
C. Amoxicillin
D. Amoxicillin/Clavulanate
E. None

Answer:_____

AR 16C
What should be done with respect to rabies?

A. Give rabies vaccine.
B. Give HRIG.
C. Give rabies vaccine and HRIG.
D. Observe dog for 10 days.
E. No prophylaxis needed.

Answer:_____

Animal Bites
- Risk of Infection
  - Humans > cats > dogs
- Approach
  - Debride
  - Image if needed
  - Tetanus prophylaxis
  - Rabies prophylaxis
  - Amoxicillin/Clavulanate indications
    - All human bites
    - Immunocompromised, hand, near joint or bone, severe, crush, edema

Animal Bites — Rabies Prophylaxis
- Animal-specific approach
  - Bat, raccoon, fox, skunk
    - Begin prophylaxis
  - Dog, cat, ferret
    - **Observe × 10 days**
  - Small rodents
    - No prophylaxis needed
- Prophylaxis
  - Human rabies immunoglobulin
    - Infiltrate wound then rest IM
  - Human diploid cell vaccine
    - 1 mL on days 0, 3, 7, and 14

Case 16 — Key Points
- Know the approach to tetanus prophylaxis in the setting of an animal bite
- Know the indications for antibiotics after an animal bite and the antibiotic of choice
- Know the approach to rabies prophylaxis in the setting of an animal bite

Case 17 — History and Physical

Hx: A 35-year-old Wisconsin man presents in August with low-grade fever, myalgias, and rash on his back for 1 week. He is otherwise healthy.

PE: T 100.4°F (38.0°C); other VS normal

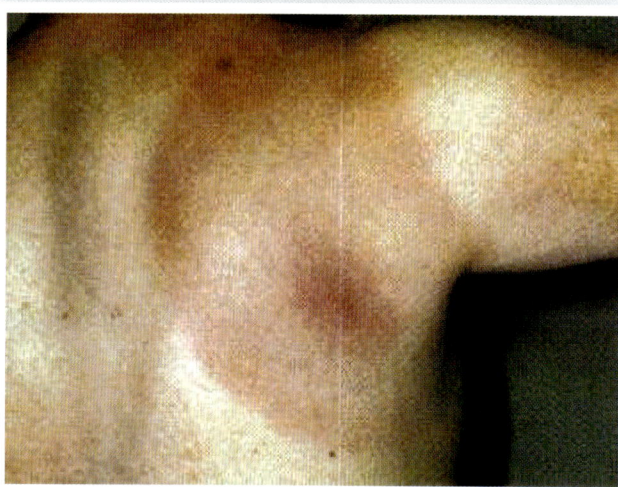

AR 17
What would you do next?

A. Test for Lyme IgM antibody and treat if (+).
B. Test for Lyme IgM antibody but begin treatment for Lyme disease.
C. Treat for Lyme disease without performing serology.
D. Do not test or treat for Lyme disease.

Answer:_____

Lyme Disease Cases U.S.

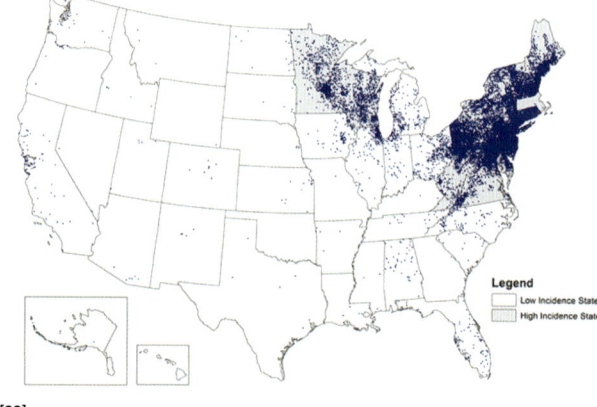

Legend
- Low Incidence State
- High Incidence State

[39]

CDC 2019

Lyme Disease Diagnosis: CDC[40] and IDSA[41]

- Case definition
  - **Erythema migrans (> 5 cm), or**
  - **One late manifestation and lab confirmation of infection**
- Acceptable late manifestations
  - Musculoskeletal: intermittent joint swelling, ± chronic pauciarticular
  - Nervous: lymphocytic meningitis, cranial neuritis, radiculoneuropathy, encephalomyelitis
  - Cardiac: acute 2nd/3rd AVB, resolves in weeks, ± myocarditis
- Lab confirmation of infection
  - **IgM ± IgG Ab by ELISA confirmed with Western blot**
  - PCR and culture not routinely recommended

CDC 2019 and IDSA 2020

Lyme Disease — Treatment[42]

- Antibiotics
  - PO: doxycycline, amoxicillin, cefuroxime
  - IV: ceftriaxone

Manifestation	Route and Duration
EM, cranial neuropathy	PO × 10 (doxy) or 14 (others) days
1° AVB	PO × 14–21 days
Meningitis or radiculopathy	PO or IV × 14–21 days
Carditis	PO or IV × 14–21 days
Arthritis	PO × 28 days
Recurrent/ Refractory arthritis	PO × 28 days (just one course)

Case 17 — Key Points

- Recognize the primary stage of Lyme disease, specifically, erythema migrans
- Know that the presence of erythema migrans is diagnostic of Lyme disease
- Know that serology is not indicated, and may be misleading, in patients with erythema migrans
- Select the appropriate treatment for Lyme disease based on the clinical manifestations

Case 18A — History and Physical

Hx: A 34-year-old man comes to your office with the lesions shown. They started as a solitary bump on the back of the hand and have progressed over the last 2 weeks. They are slightly painful and occasionally drain clear, odorless fluid. He is the owner of the Greenleaf Flower Shoppe in town.

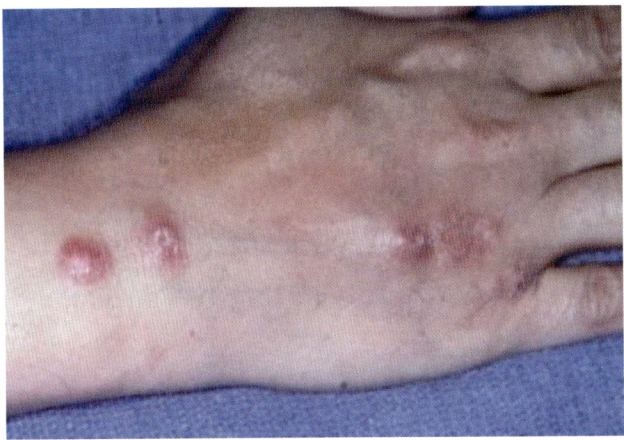

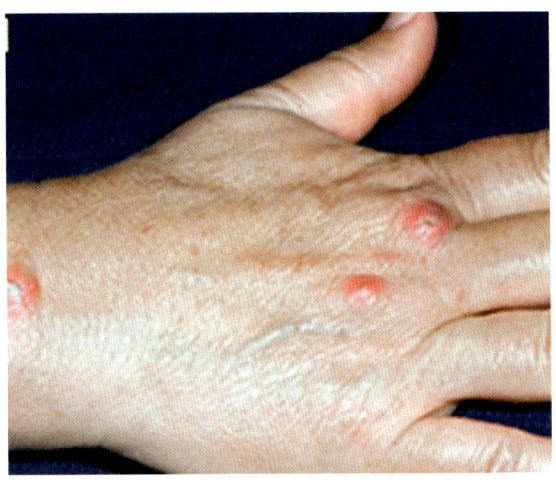

AR 18A

Sending the drainage and/or biopsy for which of the following would be most likely to be diagnostic?

A. Viral culture
B. Bacterial culture
C. Mycobacterial culture
D. Fungal culture

Answer:_____

Sporotrichosis
- Epidemiology and microbiology
  - Inoculation of *Sporotrichum schenckii* in soil
- Clinical manifestations
  - Nodules/ulcers along lymphatic drainage
- Diagnosis
  - Gram stain and culture
- Treatment
  - Itraconazole through 2–4 weeks after resolution

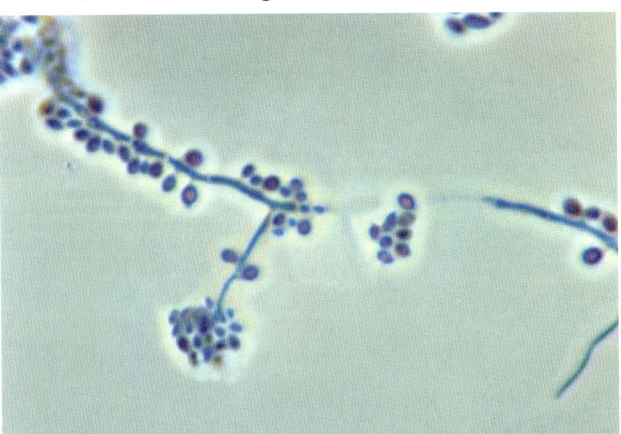

Case 18B — History and Physical

Hx: A 34-year-old man comes to your office with the lesions shown. They started as a solitary bump on the back of the hand and have progressed over the last 2 weeks. They are slightly painful and occasionally drain clear, odorless fluid. He is the owner of the Aquarius Fancy Fish store in town.

AR 18B

Sending the drainage for which of the following would be most likely to be diagnostic?

A. Viral culture
B. Bacterial culture
C. Mycobacterial culture
D. Fungal culture

Answer:_____

Mycobacterium marinum
- Epidemiology
  - Freshwater and saltwater-free living
- Clinical manifestations
  - Indolent nodules without systemic symptoms
- Diagnosis
  - Culture of biopsy or drainage
  - PCR of skin biopsy available
- Treatment
  - Mild: clarithromycin, doxycycline, or TMP/SMX
  - Severe: clarithromycin + ethambutol or rifampin
  - Treat for 1–2 months after resolution of lesions

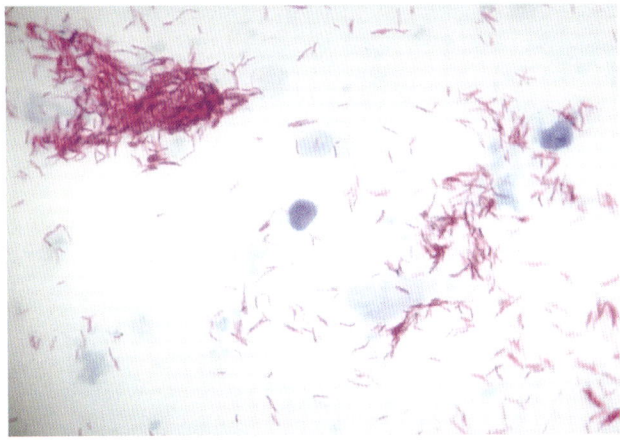

Cases 18A and 18B — Key Points
- Recognize 2 common inoculation soft tissue infections of the hand
- Know the epidemiologic settings in which they occur
- Know what cultures should be taken in each setting
- Know which antibiotics should be administered to treat them

Case 19 — History and Physical

Hx: A 20-year-old woman is brought in by neighbors after being found confused in her home. She wears a medical alert bracelet that says "diabetes" on it.

PE: T 98.6°F (37.0°C), BP 100/68 mmHg,
HR 112 beats/minute, RR 30 breaths/minute

Orthostatic and oriented only to name;

Right-eye proptosis with periorbital swelling and limited EOM on that side;

Dusky area superior lateral nose as shown; mucous membranes dry

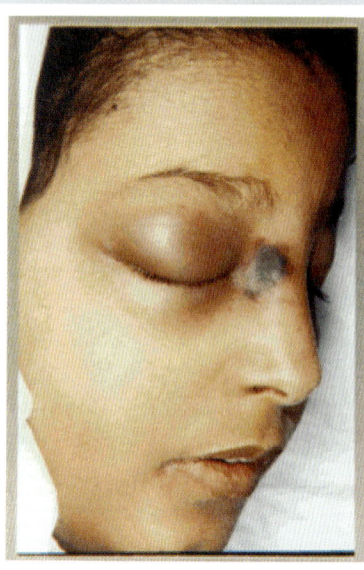

Case 19 — Labs and Initial Care

Labs:

Serum glucose 313, serum ketones (+)

Na^+ 132 mg/dL, K^+ 3.3 mEq/L, Cl^- 95 mEq/L, HCO_3^- 13 mEq/L, AG 24

Phos 2.0 mg/dL, Creat 2.1 mg/dL

WBC 22.3 × 10^3/mm^3 with 11% bands

Initial care:

Receives IVF, insulin bolus and constant infusion, K^+ and phos with resolution of her DKA and improvement in her mental state; CT scan of orbits and sinuses performed

Case 19 — CT Orbits and Sinuses

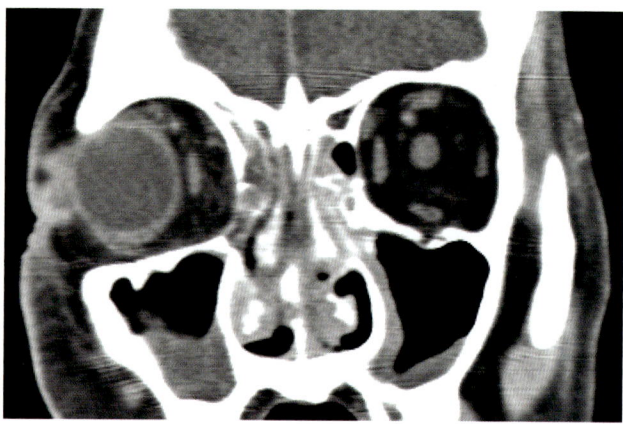

Right-eye proptosis and maxillary sinusitis

AR 19

Otolaryngology and ophthalmology are consulted. In the meantime, what would you give her?

A. IV vancomycin and cefepime
B. IV vancomycin, cefepime, and metronidazole
C. PO posaconazole
D. IV itraconazole
E. Liposomal amphotericin B

Answer:_____

Mucormycosis

- Microbiology
  - Ubiquitous: *Rhizopus*, *Mucor*, and *Rhizomucor*
- Epidemiology
  - Prolonged neutropenia, immunosuppressed, DKA
  - Deferoxamine-iron chelation promotes growth
  - Predisposed by prior voriconazole administration
- Clinical manifestations
  - Rhinocerebral
  - Pulmonary
- Diagnosis
  - Broad nonseptate hyphae, 90° angle branching
  - Fragile, often culture negative

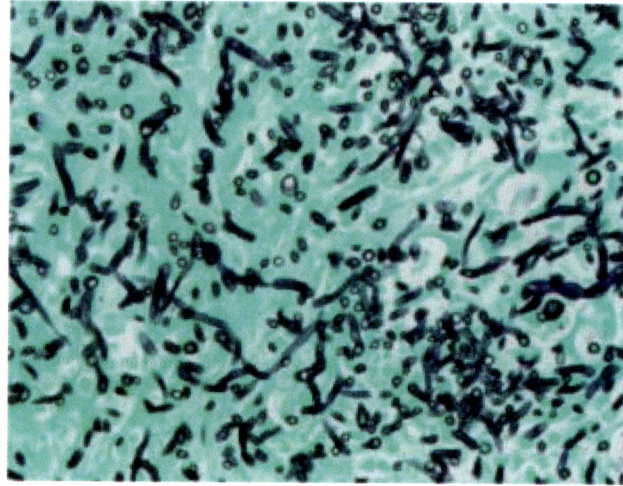

Rhinocerebral Mucormycosis
- Initial presentation
  - Unilateral headache, stuffiness, epistaxis
- Progression
  - Periorbital swelling, proptosis, ophthalmoplegia, blindness, stroke
- Images show bone destruction
- Treatment
  - Correct predispositions
  - Debridement
  - **Liposomal amphotericin B**
    - Posaconazole if not tolerated

Case 19 — Key Points
- Recognize the clinical settings in which mucormycosis occurs
- Recognize the need for emergent surgical intervention
- Know the initial and alternative therapy for mucormycosis

Case 20 — History and Physical
Hx: A 35-year-old man presents with a 10-day history of sudden onset of watery diarrhea. Five days ago, he noted RUQ pain worse with eating and a temperature of 100.9°F (38.3°C). He was found to be HIV (+) 3 years ago but is not currently on antiretrovirals. He has not been on any antibacterial drugs.

PE: T 101.3°F (38.5°C), BP 90/64 mmHg, HR 120 beats/minute, RR 12 breaths/minute

Orthostatic; dry mucous membranes;

Abdomen: RUQ tenderness and Murphy sign (+)

Case 20 — Labs and Imaging
Labs:

Hgb 10.3

WBC 4.3×10^3/mm^3: 86% P; 6% L

Pl 129,000 cells/mm^3

Lytes, creat, lipase normal

AST 44 U/L, ALT 61 U/L, ALP 211 U/L (20–70)

RUQ U/S:

Thickening of gallbladder wall;

No stones, pericholecystic fluid, bile duct dilation

AR 20
Which of the following tests on his stool is most likely to reveal the causative agent of his symptoms?

A. Stool for bacterial culture
B. Stool for viral culture
C. Stool for ova and parasites
D. Stool for PCR testing
E. Stool for *Clostridioides difficile* toxin gene assay

Answer:_____

Opportunistic Parasites

	Cryptosporidiosis	*Cystoisospora*	*Cyclospora*	Microsporidiosis
Organism	*C. parvum*	*C. belli*	*C. cayetanensis*	*Enterocytozoon* spp.
Stain	Acid fast	Acid fast	Acid fast	Trichrome
Treatment	Nitazoxanide	TMP/SMX (quinolone)	TMP/SMX (quinolone)	Albendazole

1) All cause watery diarrhea and may cause acalculous cholecystitis
2) Acid fast and trichrome stains of lower yield than monoclonal antibody staining; **PCR assay gold standard**
3) *Cystoisospora* causes eosinophilia

Case 20 — Key Points
- Recognize the clinical presentation of opportunistic parasites that cause diarrhea and acalculous cholecystitis in HIV-infected patients
- Know the methods of diagnosing these infections
- Know the pathogen-specific treatment of these infections

Case 21 — History and Physical
Hx: A 34-year-old woman is brought in by her family after she suffered a generalized tonic-clonic seizure 2 hours ago at home. She has never had a prior seizure and is otherwise healthy. She emigrated from Mexico to Chicago 9 years ago.

PE: VS normal

Slightly confused without focal neurologic deficit;

Rest of the exam normal

Case 21 — CT Head

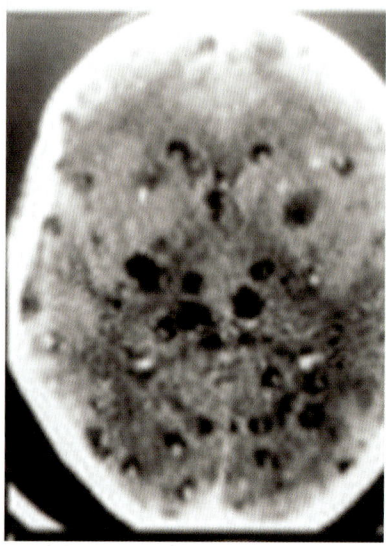

AR 21A
Which test would you do next?

A. Serum antibody assay
B. CSF antibody assay
C. Brain biopsy
D. Stool for ova and parasites
E. No test is needed prior to treatment.

Answer:_____

AR 21B
In addition to antiseizure medication, what additional treatment would you give her?

A. Praziquantel
B. Praziquantel and glucocorticoids
C. Albendazole
D. Albendazole and glucocorticoids
E. Praziquantel, albendazole, and glucocorticoids

Answer:_____

T. solium and Neurocysticercosis[43]
- Pathogenesis and diagnosis
  - **Tapeworm** (*Taenia solium*)
    - From ingesting **cysts** in undercooked pork → excyst → tapeworm
    - Dx: **eggs** shed in stool
  - **Neurocysticercosis**
    - From ingesting **eggs** from human feces → forms **cysts** in brain and muscle
    - Dx: imaging (serology)
- Clinical manifestations
  - **Tapeworm**
    - Usually none
  - **Neurocysticercosis**
    - Intraparenchymal: seizures
    - Extraparenchymal: hydrocephalus
- Treatment
  - **Tapeworm:** praziquantel 1 dose
  - **Neurocysticercosis:**
    - 1–2 cysts: albendazole for 10–14 days + steroids
    - > 2 cysts: add praziquantel for 10–14 days

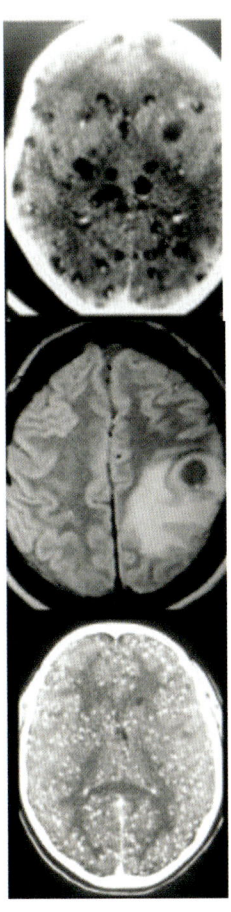

Combination Therapy of Neurocysticercosis[44]
- **The Study**
  - Randomized to 3 groups, Rx for 10 days
    - Albendazole standard (15 mg/kg/days)
    - Albendazole high (22.5 mg/kg/days)
    - Albendazole standard + praziquantel 50 mg/kg/days
- <u>Outcome</u> = Cyst resolution at 6 months

	Albendazole Standard Dose	Albendazole High Dose	Albendazole + Praziquantel
All Patients	15/41 (14%)	20/38 (53%)	25/39 (64%)*
1–2 Cysts	14/20 (70%)	15/18 (83%)	12/20 (60%)
> 2 Cysts	1/21 (5%)	5/20 (25%)	13/19 (68%)**

*p = 0.14 vs. albendazole standard dose
**p < 0.0001 vs. other two groups

Case 21 — Key Points
- Recognize the clinical presentation of neurocysticercosis in a patient from an endemic area
- Know that neuroimaging, when classic, is diagnostic of neurocysticercosis
- Know the indications for treatment and the drugs of choice for neurocysticercosis based on the number of cysts

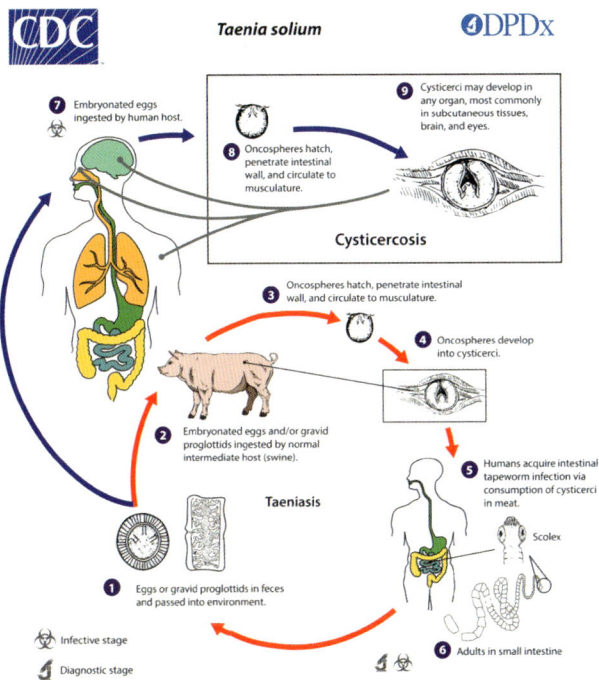

Case 22 — History and Physical

Hx: A 22-year-old man presents to your clinic with a painful, itchy eruption on his penis for 3 days. He has an unmeasured fever, body aches, headache, and burning with urination for 1 day. He has a new female sex partner who has a history of gonorrhea in the past. He has no history of sexually transmitted infections.

PE:

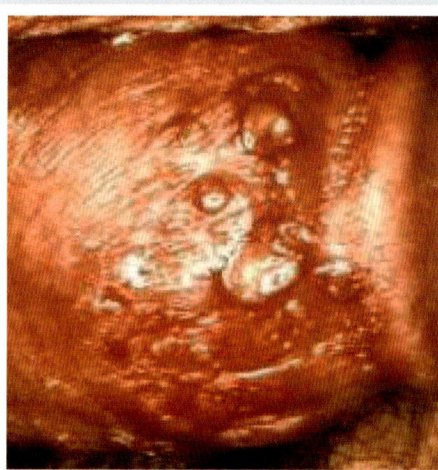

AR 22
What would you do next?

A. Send vesicular fluid for PCR assay and await results.
B. Send vesicular fluid for PCR assay; start valacyclovir.
C. No assay needed; start valacyclovir.
D. No assay needed; no antiviral treatment indicated.

Answer:_____

Why Do a PCR Assay for Clinically Suspected Genital HSV?

1) Distinction between HSV-1 and HSV-2 informs discussion of relapse potential
2) Definitive diagnosis assists psychosocial and psychosexual discussions
3) Incorrect diagnosis of HSV (false-positive clinical diagnosis) leads to unnecessary treatment
4) Lesions may be atypical, failure to diagnose (false-negative clinical diagnosis) has public health and pregnancy ramifications

Herpes Simplex Treatment

- Primary infection
  - Who to treat
    - **Lesions ≤ 72 hours**
    - Immunocompromised
  - How long to treat
    - 7–10 days
- Recurrences
  - Who to treat
    - **Lesions ≤ 48 hours**
    - Severe symptoms
  - How long to treat
    - 5 days
- Suppressive Rx for recurrent
  - Who to treat
    - **≥ 6× per year**
    - Erythema multiforme, eczema herpeticum, aseptic meningitis
  - How to treat
    - Valacyclovir 500 mg q day

Case 22 — Key Points

- Recognize primary genital herpes simplex infection
- Recognize the utility of culture or PCR to identify which serotype is present
- Know the clinical scenarios in which treatment of genital herpes is of benefit
- Know when to give suppressive therapy and what to give

Case 23 — History and Physical

Hx: A 30-year-old undomiciled woman presents to the ED with a 5-day history of rash and pain on her right side above her right hip. She intermittently comes to your student-run free clinic. She has been a sex worker, which led to HIV antibody testing 2 months ago; it was negative. She denies any shortness of breath, chest pain, abdominal pain, nausea, or vomiting. She has no significant past medical history.

PE: VS normal

Neuro, lung, heart abdominal exam normal;

Skin exam

Case 23 — Skin Exam

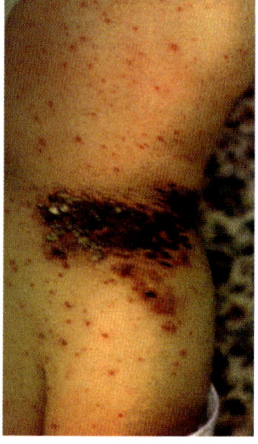

AR 23
What would you do next?

A. Start high-dose acyclovir.
B. Start high-dose acyclovir and prednisone.
C. Start high-dose acyclovir, prednisone, and amitriptyline.
D. Observe without antiviral therapy.

Answer:_____

Varicella-Zoster Virus (VZV)
- Treatment
  - Immunocompetent
    - **If > 50 years of age and ≤ 72 hours**
    - Disseminated
      - > 3 dermatomes, or
      - > 30 lesions outside of primary dermatomes
  - Immunocompromised: all
  - **Steroids and TCAs have no role**
- Prevention
  - **Recombinant vaccine is superior to live attenuated vaccine and safe in immunocompromised**

Zoster Vaccine Trials, Persons ≥ 50 Years of Age
- Live Vaccine Trials[45][46]

Outcome	Vaccine	Placebo	Efficacy
Zoster	345/30,465 (1.13%)	741/30,475 (2.43%)	53.5%
PHN	27/19,254 (.014%)	80/19,247 (0.41%)	66.1%

- Recombinant Vaccine Trials[47][48]

Outcome	Vaccine	Placebo	Efficacy
Zoster	25/8,250 (0.30%)	284/8,346 (3.40%)	91.3%
PHN	4/13,881 (.029%)	46/14,035 (3.28%)	91.2%

Recombinant Vaccine Administration
- Indications
  - **> 50 years of age**
  - **Regardless of history of chickenpox or zoster**
- Dosing
  - 0.5 mL IM
  - **2 doses: 0 and 2–6 months later**
  - Wait at least 8 weeks after live vaccine
  - Do not give if active zoster

Case 23 — Key Points
- Make a clinical diagnosis of herpes zoster
- Recognize disseminated herpes zoster in an immunocompetent host
- Know when antiviral treatment for herpes zoster is beneficial
- Know that glucocorticoids and tricyclic antidepressants are not useful in acute zoster
- Know the indications for zoster vaccine and which one to use

Case 24 — History and Physical
Hx: An 18-year-old high school student is seen in the student health center with 3 days of a sore throat, fever of 102.2°F (39.0°C), and fatigue. She is otherwise healthy and has had all required immunizations. Her 2 older brothers and her parents are well at home. She has had 2 boyfriends in the last 18 months but denies sexual intercourse with either of them. Her only medication is an oral contraceptive.

PE: T 101.8°F (38.8°C), BP 110/75 mmHg, HR 110 beats/minute, RR 12 breaths/minute

Throat; posterior cervical adenopathy;

Palpable spleen tip

Case 24 — Throat Exam

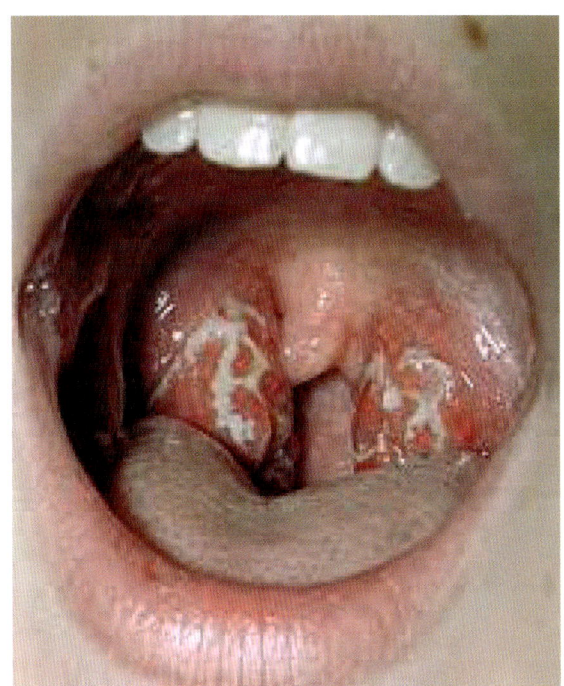

Case 24 — Labs
CBC: Hgb 15.1 g/dL; WBC 14,800 cells/mm³: P 35%, L 50% (12% atypical), M 10% Pl 150,000 cells/mm³

Group A strep rapid Ag (–)

Heterophile antibody (–)

AR 24
Which of the following is likely to make an etiologic diagnosis?

A. EBV IgM capsid antibody
B. CMV IgM antibody
C. Toxoplasma IgM antibody
D. HIV antibody
E. HIV viral load

Answer:_____

Exudative Pharyngitis

- Bacterial
  - *Streptococcus* group A, C, G
  - *Arcanobacterium haemolyticum*
  - Vincent angina
  - *Neisseria gonorrhoeae*
  - *Corynebacterium diphtheriae*
  - *Yersinia enterocolitica*
  - *Francisella tularensis*
- Viral
  - Adenovirus (Types 3, 4, 7, 14, 21)
  - Epstein-Barr virus
  - Herpes simplex virus

Epstein-Barr Virus (EBV) Diagnosis

Heterophile Antibodies		IgM Capsid Antibody	
Week	Sensitivity	Week	Sensitivity
1	75%	1	97%
2	90%		
3	95%		

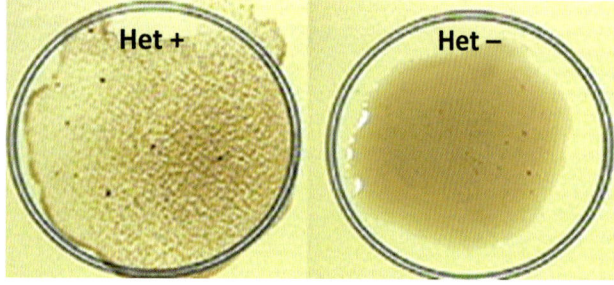

Case 24 — Key Points

- Recognize the clinical presentation of acute EBV infection (acute mononucleosis) in an adolescent
- Know the operating characteristics of heterophile antibody testing in the setting of acute mononucleosis
- Know the likely pathogens that cause heterophile antibody-negative acute mononucleosis
- Know that EBV is the most common cause of heterophile antibody-negative acute mononucleosis with exudative pharyngitis

Case 25 — History and Physical

Hx: A 24-year-old woman presents with progressive dyspnea on exertion over the last 3 days. She has Hb SS sickle cell disease and has about 1 pain crisis per year. She has had a low-grade fever and bilateral small joint pains for about 1 week. She denies rash, cough, or chest pain.

PE: T 101.3°F (38.5°C), BP 100/68 mmHg, HR 120 beats/minute, RR 22 breaths/minute

Alert and slightly short of breath at rest;

Conjunctiva pale; lungs clear;

Heart with 2/6 SEM over pulmonic area;

Abdomen benign, no hepatosplenomegaly;

Fingers, wrists, and ankles with pain on ROM, no swelling

Case 25 — Labs and Imaging

CBC: Hgb 4.2 g/dL; MCV 84 μm³; corrected retic index = 0.3%

WBC 4,800 cells/mm³: P 75%, L 12%, M 5%

Pl 150,000 cells/mm³

Chest x-ray normal

Bone marrow aspiration:

Red cell arrest

Normal white cell and platelet maturation

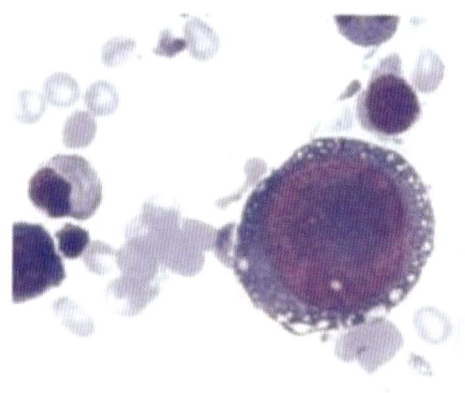

Bone marrow aspiration

AR 25A
What other testing would you do?

A. Bone marrow culture
B. Chest CT
C. *Borrelia* serologies
D. Fungal serologies
E. Pregnancy test

Answer:_____

AR 25B
In addition to PRBC transfusions, what else would you administer?

A. Intravenous immunoglobulin
B. Acyclovir
C. Ganciclovir
D. Ribavirin
E. Nothing

Answer:_____

Parvovirus — Arthritis and Rash

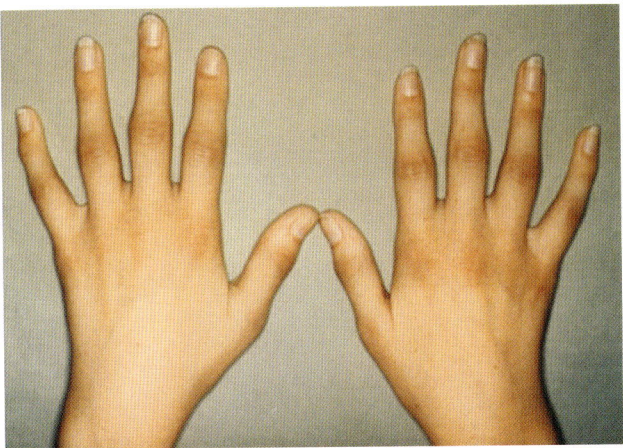

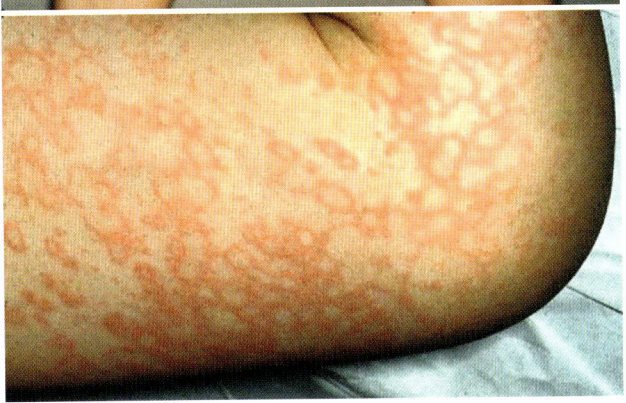

Parvovirus B19 — Vulnerable Hosts
- <u>Pregnant women</u>
  - Fetal loss
  - Hydrops fetalis
- <u>Hemoglobinopathies</u>
  - **Self-limited** aplastic anemia
  - Support with transfusions
- <u>Immunosuppressed</u> (HIV, Txpl, CVI)
  - **Prolonged** aplastic anemia
  - Treat with intravenous immunoglobulin

Case 25 — Key Points
- Recognize the clinical manifestations of acute parvovirus infection
- Recognize the need for pregnancy testing in acute parvovirus infection
- Recognize hosts that are susceptible to aplastic anemia and how to treat them

Case 26 — History and Physical

Hx: A 27-year-old man presents with fever and severe headache and myalgias for 1 day. He is a medical student who returned 4 days ago from a trip to the Dominican Republic as part of the school's international medicine program. He took mefloquine for malaria prophylaxis.

PE: T 103.1°F (39.5°C), BP 90/68 mmHg, HR 90 beats/minute, RR 20 breaths/minute

Alert but in pain from his head and muscle aches;

Neck supple;

Lungs, heart, and abdomen benign;

Fine petechial rash all over

Case 26 — Leg Rash

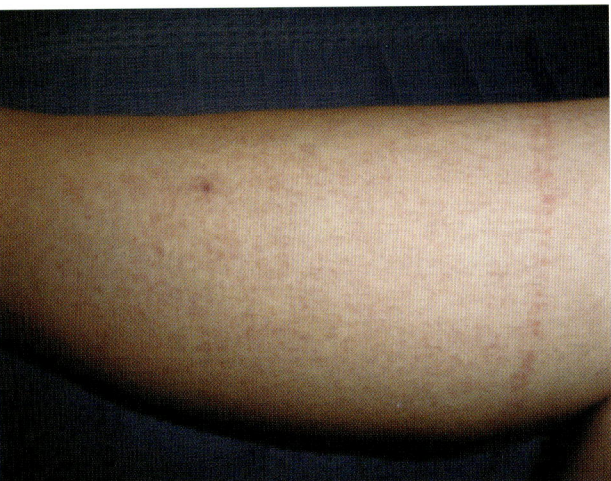

Case 26 — Labs

CBC: Hgb 16.1 g/dL; WBC 2.8×10^3/mm^3: P 82%, bands 8%, M 5% Pl 28,000 cells/mm^3

Creat 2.4 mg/dL

AST 85 U/L, ALT 92 U/L, ALP nl, T bili 1.1 mg/dL

U/A: 2+ protein, RBC 8 cells/HPF, WBC 2 cells/HPF

AR 26

What test is likely to confirm your diagnosis?

A. Skin biopsy for rickettsial fluorescent Ab
B. Blood malarial smear
C. Blood for bacterial culture
D. Blood for viral culture
E. Blood for viral serology

Answer:_____

Dengue Fever

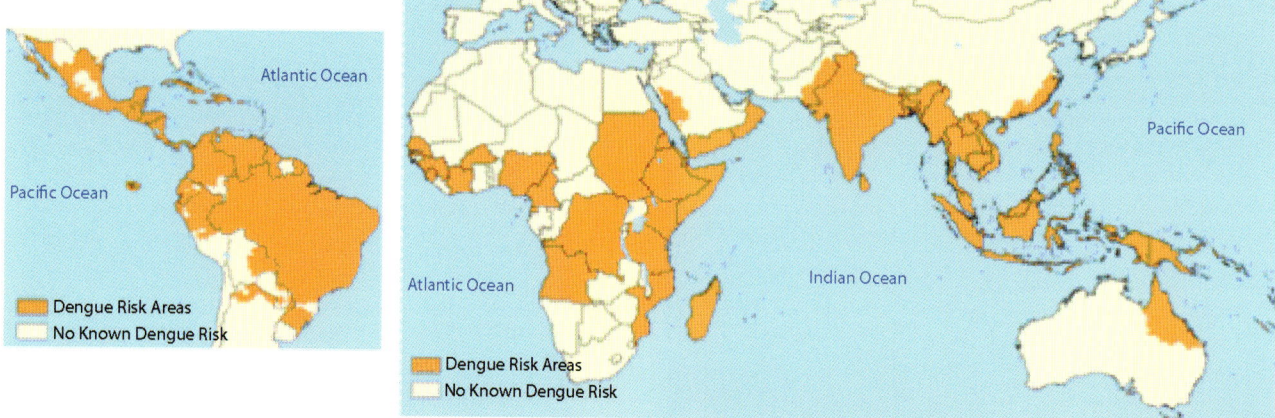

Dengue Risk Areas
No Known Dengue Risk

- Microbiology
  - Most common mosquito-borne viral disease (*Aedes* mosquito)
  - 4 serotypes → lifetime immunity
  - Disease is worse if immune to another serotype
- Classic dengue fever (4- to 7-day incubation)
  - **Severe HA, muscle and joint pains, fever**
  - Hemorrhagic manifestations in 10–20%
  - Self-limited ~ 7 days
- Dengue hemorrhagic fever
  - **Capillary leak syndrome: multiple sites with shock**
- Diagnosis
  - **Serology**
  - PCR (through CDC)
- Treatment
  - Support fluid status
  - Platelets only if < 10,000 and active bleed
- Prevention
  - Live attenuated CYD-TDV (Dengvaxia) only if **seropositive and ages 9–16.**

Case 26 — Key Points
- Recognize the classic presentation of dengue fever in a person who has recently visited an endemic area
- Know the diagnostic test of choice for dengue fever
- Know the treatment of dengue
- Be aware of the dengue vaccine and its limited indications

Case 27 — History and Physical

Hx: A 33-year-old man presents to your office in December with a 4-day history of acute onset of fever and cough. He denies shortness of breath or pleuritic chest pain. He is an otherwise healthy math teacher at a local high school. Influenza H1N1 has been diagnosed in 3 of his students.

PE: T 101.5°F (38.6°C), BP 110/78 mmHg, HR 106 beats/minute, RR 20 breaths/minute

Alert and oriented;

Lung and heart exams normal

Case 27 — Labs and Imaging

CBC: Hgb 15.1 g/dL; WBC 8,800 cells/mm³:
P 74%, L 15%, M 4%
Pl 328,000 cells/mm³

Chest x-ray normal

AR 27
What would you do now?

A. Nasopharyngeal swab for rapid Ag testing for influenza
B. Nasopharyngeal swab for PCR testing for influenza
C. No testing; treat with oseltamivir.
D. Neither test nor treat with oseltamivir.

Answer:_____

Seasonal Influenza[49]
- Epidemiology and pathogenesis
  - Highly contagious, winter months in North America
  - 3–11% incidence/season
- Clinical manifestations
  - **Acute fever and cough during seasonal disease (80% PPV)**
- Testing
  - Immunoassays: 60% sens; 98% spec
  - **Nucleic acid amplification: > 90% sens and spec**
- Who to test with nasopharyngeal swab
  - Immunocompromised
  - Immunocompetent with exacerbation of comorbidity
  - Complicated infection (e.g., pneumonia)
  - Inpatients with acute febrile respiratory disease

IDSA 2019

Influenza Treatment and Prevention

When and who to treat

- **Regardless of duration**
  - **Hospitalized**
  - LRTI
  - At risk for severe disease
    - LTCF residents
    - ≥ 65 years of age
    - Pregnant
    - COPD, HF, CA, CKD, CLD
    - DM
    - Sickle cell disease
    - Immunosuppressed
    - Trouble with secretions
    - Native American, Alaskan
    - BMI ≥ 40
- **Within 48 hours**
  - **All others**

How to treat

- Neuraminidase inhibitor
  - **Oseltamivir** PO × 5 days
  - Zanamivir inhaler × 5 days
  - Peramivir IV × 1
- Endonuclease inhibitor
  - Baloxivir PO × 1
- Influenza vaccine
  - Annually > 6 months old[50]
  - Inactivated or live
    - **High-dose vaccine (4-fold)**
    - **≥ 65 years of age**

Case 27 — Key Points

- Recognize an influenza-like illness in the setting of an influenza epidemic
- Know the operating characteristics of clinical impression and various diagnostic tests for influenza
- Know in which clinical setting specific tests for influenza virus are useful
- Know who to treat for influenza and what to give

Case 28 — History and Physical

Hx: A 28-year-old woman comes to you because she tested (+) for HIV at your STI clinic. She has been a sex worker for 8 years and had never been tested before.

She has unintentionally lost 15 pounds over the last 2 years and currently weighs 100 pounds.

PE: VS normal

Exam completely normal

Case 28 — Labs

CBC: Hgb 9.1 g/dL, MCV 88 μm^3;
WBC 3,800 cells/mm^3: P 87%, L 5%, M 4%
Pl 178,000 cells/mm^3

CD4 count 38 cells/mm^3

Interferon-γ release assay (−)

Chest x-ray normal

AR 28A

If genotypic sensitivity testing permits, which antiretroviral therapy would you start?

A. 3 NRTIs
B. 2 NRTIs and an integrase inhibitor
C. An NRTI, an rPI, and an NNRTI
D. An NRTI, an rPI, and an integrase inhibitor

Answer:_____

Antiretroviral Drugs 2022

- NRTIs
  - **Abacavir**
  - Didanosine
  - **Emtricitabine**
  - **Lamivudine**
  - Stavudine
  - **Tenofovir**
  - Zidovudine
- NNRTIs
  - Delavirdine
  - Efavirenz
  - Etravirine
  - Nevirapine
  - Rilpivirine (IM)
  - Doravirine

NRTIs = nucleoside/nucleotide reverse transcriptase inhibitors

NNRTIs = nonnucleoside reverse transcriptase inhibitors

- Protease inhibitors (PIs)
  - Atazanavir
  - Darunavir
  - Fosamprenavir
  - Indinavir
  - Lopinavir
  - Nelfinavir
  - Ritonavir
  - Saquinavir
  - Tipranavir
- Fusion inhibitor
  - Enfuvirtide
- Attachment inhibitor
  - Fostemsavir
- Post-attachment inhibitor
  - Ibalizumab
- CCR5 antagonist
  - Maraviroc
- Integrase inhibitors
  - Cabotegravir (IM)
  - Elvitegravir
  - **Dolutegravir**
  - **Raltegravir**
  - **Bictegravir**

Antiretroviral Fixed-Dose Combinations 2022
- Abacavir-lamivudine
- Abacavir-lamivudine-zidovudine
- Efavirenz-tenofovir-emtricitabine
- Elvitegravir-cobicistat-tenofovir-emtricitabine
- **Tenofovir-emtricitabine**
- Rilpivirine-emtricitabine-tenofovir
- Zidovudine-lamivudine
- **Dolutegravir-abacavir-lamivudine**
- Emtricitabine-rilpivirine-tenofovir
- Doravine-lamivudine-tenofovir
- Bictegravir-emtricitabine-tenofovir
- Darunavir-cobicistat-emtricitabine-tenofovir
- **Dolutegravir-lamivudine**
- Dolutegravir-rilpivirine
- Cabotegravir-rilpivirine

Treatment of HIV Infection[51]
- Who to treat
  - Everyone
- Initial genotypic resistance testing
  - Everyone
- What to start
  - An INSTI and 1 or 2 NRTIs
    - **Bictegravir + tenofovir + emtricitabine**
    - **Dolutegravir + abacavir + lamivudine**
    - **Dolutegravir + (emtricitabine or lamivudine) + tenofovir**
    - **Dolutegravir + lamivudine**
- Scenarios that need attention
  - Prior to abacavir (test for HLA B*5701)
  - Bictegravir has insufficient data to use in pregnancy
  - The last regimen should be avoided if HBV (+), or VL > 500,000, or genotypic testing not back yet, or opportunistic infection

AR 28B

What antimicrobials should be given to prevent opportunistic infections?

A. TMP/SMX
B. TMP/SMX and azithromycin
C. TMP/SMX, azithromycin, and fluconazole
D. TMP/SMX, azithromycin, and valganciclovir

Answer:_____

HIV — 1° Prophylaxis of Opportunistic Infections[52]

Infection	Trigger	Regimen
Pneumocystosis	CD4 < 200	TMP/SMX DS daily or tiw
Toxoplasmosis	CD4 < 100 + serology	TMP/SMX DS daily
MAC	None	None
Tuberculosis	TST > 5 mm or IGRA (+)	INH × 9 months

HIV Preexposure Prophylaxis (PrEP)[53]
- **What to use**
  - Counseling!
  - Tenofovir-emtricitabine q day
    - Give initial 30-day supply, then 90-day supplies
  - Cabotegravir IM q 8 weeks appears equally efficacious
  - Check HIV prior to renewing
- **Who to give it to**
  - MSM
  - Transgender
  - No condom use
  - Sex workers
  - Infected partner(s) or multiple partners
  - Recent STI
  - Incarcerated
  - Sharing injection drug needles/syringes

HCW Postexposure Prophylaxis
- **If the answer to these 2 questions is "yes," then give postexposure prophylaxis:**
  1) Was the **fluid bloody?**
  2) Was the **skin integrity compromised?**
- What to give?
  - If known HIV (+) source, base on resistance if known
  - **Dolutegravir + tenofovir + emtricitabine**
  - Test for seroconversion at 0, 6, and 12 weeks

Other Postexposure Prophylaxis[54]
- Who to give it to:
  - **Mucosal or blood contact**
  - **Occurred in < 72 hours**
- What to give:
  - Raltegravir + emtricitabine + tenofovir + × 4 weeks
  - Can discontinue if source is HIV (−)
- How to follow:
  - Test for HIV infection at 3 months

AR 28C

Her brother has accompanied her and asks if he should be tested. He is 16 and has not been sexually active. He denies IVDU.

What HIV screening, if any, should you do?

A. No testing is indicated.
B. Test him once now.
C. Test him once now; repeat in 3–5 years.
D. Test him once now; repeat every year.

Answer:_____

HIV — Screening[55]
- General recommendations
  - All persons 15–65 years of age at least once
    - Older and younger if at risk
  - All pregnant women, each pregnancy

- Risk stratification for repeat testing
  - High risk
    - IVDU, MSM, STI diagnosis, STI testing
    - **Repeat every 3–12 months**
  - Risk
    - Unprotected intercourse, partners at risk, sex for drugs/money
    - **Repeat every 3–5 years**
  - No risk
    - Not sexually active, monogamous (–) partner
    - **No need to repeat (unless pregnant)**

Acute Retroviral Syndrome
- Epidemiology
  - Occurs in ~ 90% of new HIV infections
  - Incubation = 2–4 weeks, lasts 2–4 weeks
- Clinical manifestations (> 50% occurrence)
  - Fever, LNs pharyngitis, rash, myalgia/arthralgia
- Diagnosis
  - **HIV antibody is negative**
  - **Viral detection via p24 assay or PCR**
- Treatment
  - **Initiate antiretroviral therapy**

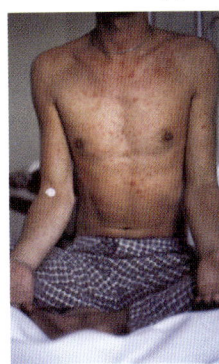

[56]

HIV Infection Assays

Assay	Days to Positivity
HIV IgG Ab	25–35
HIV IgM Ab	20–30
HIV p24 Ag	15–20
HIV PCR (50 copy cutoff)	10–15
HIV PCR (1–5 copy cutoff)	5

Diagnosing HIV Infection[57]

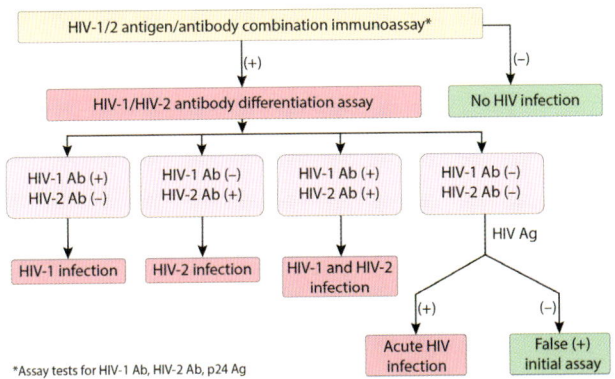

Case 28 — Key Points
- Know when to treat antiretroviral-naïve HIV-infected persons
- Know which regimens are recommended
- Know the groups that may benefit from preexposure and prophylaxis
- Know the approach to a needlestick sustained by a health care worker
- Know who should be screened for HIV and how often
- Recognize the acute retroviral syndrome

Case 29 — History and Physical
Hx: A 34-year-old man presents to the ED with 2 weeks of slowly worsening shortness of breath, low-grade fever, and cough. He has had HIV infection for 12 years and has intermittently been on antiretrovirals. He had Stevens-Johnson syndrome after receiving TMP/SMX 10 years ago for a prior pneumonia.

PE: T 100.2°F (37.9°C), BP 128/78 mmHg, HR 94 beats/minute, RR 20 breaths/minute

Alert, oriented, and in moderate respiratory distress; lungs with bilateral diffuse crackles, no signs of consolidation;

Rest of the exam normal

Case 29 — Labs and Imaging
CBC: Hb 9.8 g/dL

WBC 7,600 cells/mm^3: 88% P, 6% L

Pl 178,000 cells/mm^3

ABG on room air: pO$_2$ 59 mmHg, pCO$_2$ 20 mmHg, pH 7.56

Chest x-ray:

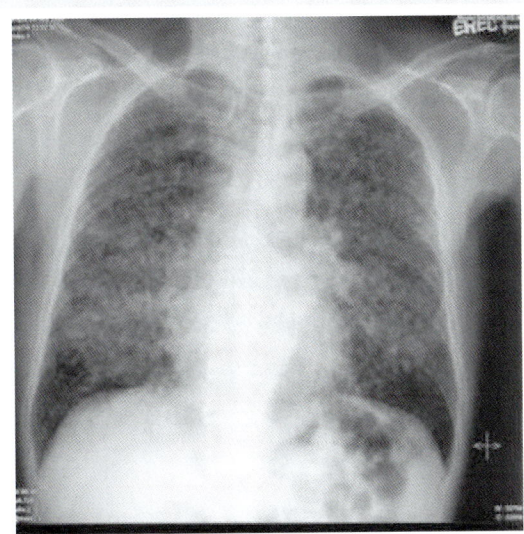

Case 29 — Induced Sputum

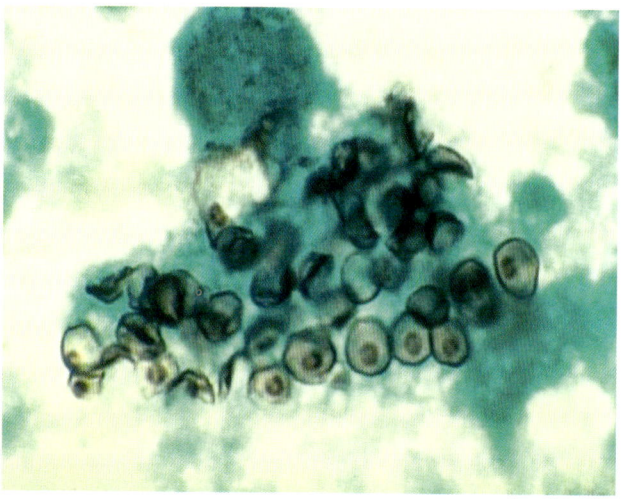

AR 29

In addition to oxygen, what antibiotic would you give?

A. Atovaquone
B. Clindamycin
C. Clindamycin, primaquine, and prednisone
D. Pentamidine and prednisone

Answer:_____

Pneumocystis jiroveci — An Odd Bug
- Looks like a protozoa
- Genetically a fungus
- Killed by antibacterials and antiprotozoal agents, but not antifungals

Severity of *Pneumocystis* Pneumonia
(Determines Antibiotic and Need for Steroids)[58]

Severity	pO₂	A-a Gradient
Mild	> 70 mmHg	< 35 mmHg
Moderate	60–70 mmHg	35–45 mmHg
Severe	< 60 mmHg	> 45 mmHg

Treatment of *Pneumocystis* Pneumonia[59]
- Mild to moderate
  - **TMP/SMX 2 DS bid × 21 days**
  - 2nd line
    - Atovaquone
    - Clindamycin + primaquine
- Severe
  - **TMP/SMX IV 5 mg/kg q 8 hours**
  - 2nd line
    - **Clindamycin and primaquine**
  - 3rd line
    - **Pentamidine**
- **Steroids**
  - If P_aO_2 is < 70 mmHg, or A-a gradient > 35

Case 29 — Key Points
- Know the clinical presentation of *Pneumocystis jiroveci* pneumonia (PJP)
- Know the appropriate treatment for PJP based on severity and drug allergies
- Know the indications for adjunctive glucocorticoids in PJP

Case 30 — History and Physical
Hx: A 68-year-old man comes to the ED with fever for 5 days and no other symptoms. He has a past history of HTN, Type 2 DM, and asymptomatic aortic stenosis.

PE: T 101.1°F (38.4°C), BP 158/98 mmHg, HR 98 beats/minute, RR 16 breaths/minute

Alert and oriented; HEENT normal; heart PMI sustained, 3/6 SEM radiating to carotids; abdomen benign; lungs clear;

Extremities show an open ulcer of right heel, nonfoul exudate, does not probe to bone;

Skin otherwise normal

Case 30 — Labs, Imaging, and Course
Labs

CBC:
WBC 8.8 × 10³/mm³: 84% P, no bands
Hgb 10.2 g/dL, MCV 86 μm³
Pl 298,000 cells/mm³

Images
X-ray right foot: no osteomyelitis or gas in tissues

Chest x-ray: cardiomegaly, no pulmonary infiltrates

Course
Started on vancomycin and piperacillin-tazobactam

Day 2: T 100.8°F (38.2°C); 3 of 3 blood cultures with gram-positive cocci in clusters

AR 30A
What would you do next?

A. MRI of right heel
B. CT head
C. Lumbar puncture
D. Transthoracic echo
E. Transesophageal echo

Answer:_____

Major Criteria for Infective Endocarditis (IE)
(Need 2 major; 1 major + 3 minor; 5 minor)[60]
- Positive blood culture for endocarditis
  - <u>**Typical organism in ≥ 2 BCs, or**</u>
    - Viridans strep, *S. bovis*, HACEK, *S. aureus*, **or**
    - *Enterococcus*, community-acquired, no 1° focus
  - <u>**Persistent bacteremia, or**</u>
    - ≥ 2 BC, > 12° apart, **or** 3/3 **or** > 50% of > 3, > 1° apart
  - <u>One BC for *Coxiella burnetii* or antiphase IgG Ab > 1:800</u>
- <u>**Evidence of endocardial involvement**</u>
  - <u>**Positive echocardiogram, or**</u>
    - Oscillating mass (unexplained) on valve, or supporting structure or in path of regurgitant jet, or implanted device, **or**
    - Abscess, **or**
    - New prosthetic dehiscence
  - <u>**New valvular regurgitation**</u>

HACEK to AACEK
- *Haemophilus aphrophilus* → ***Aggregatibacter aphrophilus***
- *Actinobacillus actinomycetemcomitans* → ***Aggregatibacter actinomycetemcomitans***
- *Cardiobacterium hominis*
- *Eikenella corrodens*
- *Kingella kingae*
- <u>**Characteristics they share**</u>
  - Take longer to grow in lab
  - Cause large vegetations and higher embolic risk
  - Resistance to penicillin and ampicillin, susceptible to ceftriaxone which is the drug of choice

Minor Criteria for IE
(Need 2 major; 1 major + 3 minor; 5 minor)[61][62]
- <u>Predisposition</u>
  - Endocardial disease or IVDU
- <u>Temperature > 100.4°F (38.0°C)</u>
- <u>Vascular phenomena (1 of):</u>
  - Major arterial embolus, septic pulmonary emboli, mycotic aneurysms, intracranial bleed, conjunctival hemorrhages, Janeway lesions (Not petechiae/splinters)
- <u>Immunologic phenomena (1 of):</u>
  - Glomerulonephritis, Osler's, Roth's, (+) RhF
- <u>Microbiologic evidence</u>
  - BC (+) yet not meeting major criteria
  - Seropositive: *Brucella, Chlamydia, Coxiella, Legionella, Bartonella*

Approach to the Diagnostic Use of Echocardiography[63]

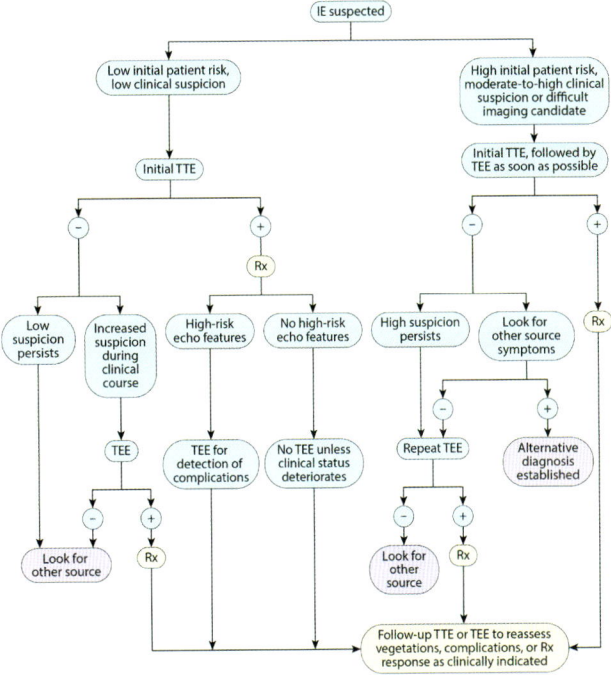

Indications for TEE in IE[64]
- TTE is a poor study
- Suspected or known IE and TTE (−)
- Suspected or known complications of IE
  - Abscess
  - Perforation
  - Papillary muscle rupture
- Intravascular device leads

Case 30 — Continued
Blood cultures grow methicillin-sensitive *S. aureus*.

Echocardiogram shows a 5-mm vegetation on the left aortic valve cusp.

AR 30B
What antibiotic(s) would you give?

A. Nafcillin + gentamicin × 2 weeks
B. Nafcillin × 4 weeks
C. Vancomycin × 4 weeks
D. Nafcillin × 6 weeks

Answer:_____

Antibiotic Therapy of Endocarditis[65]
- Bactericidal drugs
  - β-Lactam, vancomycin, daptomycin
- Intravenous
- Maximum dose
- Durations
  - 2 weeks:
    - Viridans strep (β-lactam + AG)
    - R-sided *S. aureus* (β-lactam + AG)
  - **6 weeks: L-sided *S. aureus***
  - 4–6 weeks: all others

Indications for Surgery in NVE[66]
- **Class I**
  - Heart failure from valve disease
  - Heart block, abscess, perforating lesion
  - BC (+) > 5–7 days
  - Fungi, VRE, MDR-GNB
- **Class II**
  - Recurrent emboli
  - Persistent or increasing vegetation
  - Vegetations > 10 mm and
    - Severe valve regurgitation
    - Vegetation is mobile

Cardiac Conditions Requiring Endocarditis Prophylaxis against Viridans Streptococci[67]
- **Prosthetic material (valves, rings, clips, LVAD)**
- **Prior infective endocarditis**
- Congenital heart disease
  - Unrepaired cyanotic disease
  - Repaired cyanotic disease with prosthesis < 6 months
  - Repaired cyanotic disease with residual defects
- Cardiac transplant that develops valvulopathy

Procedures Requiring Endocarditis Prophylaxis[68]
- **Dental procedures if**:
  - Manipulation of gingiva or periapical
  - Perforation of oral mucosa
- **Respiratory procedures if**:
  - Cutting mucosa
  - Tonsillectomy, bronch and incision

Antibiotic Regimens for Prophylaxis of IE[69]

Penicillin Allergy?	Route	Drug and Dose (Single Dose 30–60 Minutes Prior)
No	Oral	Amoxicillin 2 g
	Parenteral	Ampicillin 2 g Cefazolin 1 g Ceftriaxone 1 g
Yes	Oral	Cephalexin 2 g Azithromycin 500 mg Clarithromycin 500 mg ~~Clindamycin 600 mg~~
	Parenteral	Cefazolin 1 g Ceftriaxone 1 g ~~Clindamycin 600 mg~~

*Clindamycin no longer recommended due to increased resistance

Case 30 — Key Points
- Recognize the potential for endocarditis when there is high-grade bacteremia with a typical endocarditis pathogen
- Review the diagnostic criteria for endocarditis
- Know that TTE is the preferred initial echo but also when TEE is indicated
- Describe the approach to the therapy of endocarditis
- Know the current recommendations for prophylaxis of endocarditis

Case 31 — History and Physical
Hx: A 48-year-old man presents to the Emergency Department with a 2-day history of fever and productive cough. He has a history of hypertension and Type 2 diabetes.

PE: T 101.3°F (39.5°C), PR 100, BP 136/84, RR 18, O$_2$ sat 97%; no acute distress; bronchial breath sounds right anterior chest

Labs: glucose 165, creat 0.9, BUN 20, Hct 47

Chest x-ray as shown

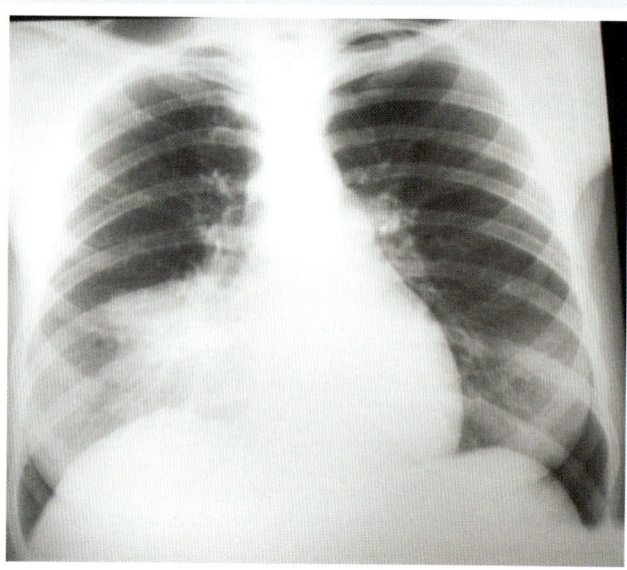

AR 31
Which of the following is the best treatment?

A. Outpatient treatment with doxycycline
B. Outpatient treatment with levofloxacin
C. Inpatient treatment with ceftriaxone and azithromycin
D. Inpatient treatment with ceftriaxone and levofloxacin

Answer:_____

Empiric Rx of Community-Acquired Pneumonia

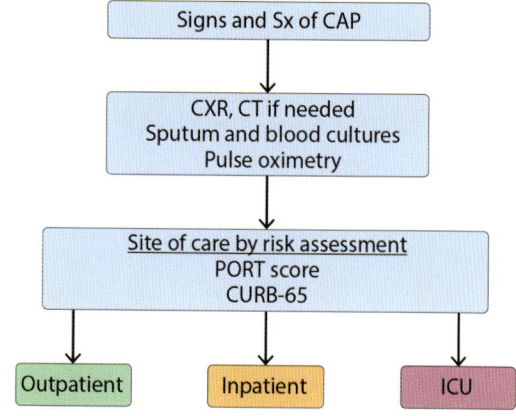

Signs and Sx of CAP
↓
CXR, CT if needed
Sputum and blood cultures
Pulse oximetry
↓
Site of care by risk assessment
PORT score
CURB-65
↓
Outpatient | Inpatient | ICU

Patient Outcomes Research Team (PORT)[70]
- Pneumonia Severity Index (PSI) retrospective analysis of 38,039 patients with community-acquired pneumonia (CAP)
- **Class 1 patients**
  - < 50 years old, and <u>no comorbid conditions</u>:
    - Neoplastic disease
    - Liver disease
    - Heart failure
    - Cerebrovascular disease
    - Renal disease
  - <u>None of these on PE</u>:
    - Altered mental status
    - Pulse ≥ 125 beats/minute
    - Respiratory rate ≥ 30 breaths/minute
    - Systolic BP < 90 mmHg
    - Temp < 95.0°F (35.0°C) or ≥ 104.0°F (40.0°C)

Patient Outcomes Research Team (PORT)[71]
- Pneumonia Severity Index (PSI) retrospective analysis of 38,039 patients with CAP
- **Scoring for Classes 2–5**

Demographics	Points Given
Male	Age in years
Female	Age − 10
NH resident	Age + 10
Comorbid Illness	
Neoplastic disease	+ 30
Liver disease	+ 20
Heart failure	+ 1
Cerebrovascular disease	+ 10
Renal disease	+ 10
Physical Exam	
Altered mental status	+ 20
RR ≥ 30 breaths/minute	+ 20
Systolic BP < 90 mmHg	+ 20
Temp < 95.0°F or ≥ 104.0°F	+ 15
Pulse ≥ 125 beats/minute	+ 10
Labs and Imaging	
pH < 7.35	+ 30
BUN ≥ 30 mg/dL	+ 20
Na^+ < 130 mEq/L	+ 20
Glucose ≥ 250 mg/dL	+ 10
Hct < 30%	+ 10
P_aO_2 < 60 mmHg, O_2 sat < 90%	+ 10
Pleural effusion	+ 10

Patient Outcomes Research Team (PORT)[72]
- Pneumonia Severity Index (PSI) retrospective analysis of 38,039 patients with CAP

Risk Class	Points	Mortality	Site of Care
1	N/A	0.1%	Outpatient
2	< 70	0.6%	Outpatient
3	71–90	2.8%	Observation
4	91–130	8.2%	Inpatient
5	> 130	29.2%	Inpatient/ICU
Total	N/A	10.6%	All

BTS Criteria of Severity — CURB-65[73]
- Cohort of 1,068; multivariate analysis
- Factors increasing risk of death:
  - **C**onfusion
    - Mini-Mental exam, or
    - Disorientation
  - **U**remia (BUN > 20 mg/dL)
  - **R**R > 30
  - **B**lood pressure
    - < 90 systolic, or
    - ≤ 60 diastolic
  - **65** years of age or older

# of Factors	30-day M	Site of Care
0	0.7%	Outpatient
1	2.1%	Outpatient
2	9.2%	Inpatient
3	14.5%	ICU
4	40.0%	ICU
5	57.0%	ICU

This Patient's Severity Scores
- PORT/PSI
  - He is Class 1
  - Even if calculated
    - Age 48 = 48 points
- CURB-65
  - Has 0 factors

Outpatient Rx of Non-Severe CAP[74]

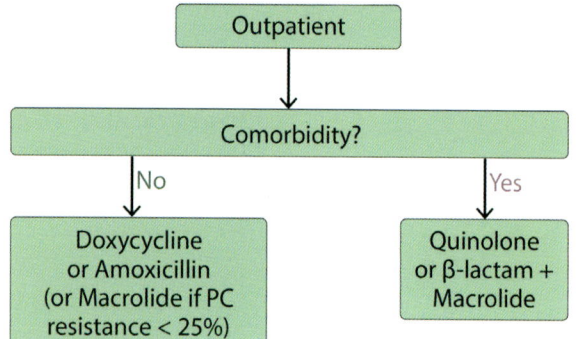

- **Comorbidities**
  - Organ disease
    - Heart, lung, liver, renal
  - Diabetes
  - Alcoholism
  - Cancer
  - Asplenia
- **Acceptable β-lactams**
  - Amox/Clav, cefuroxime, cefpodoxime
- **Acceptable quinolones**
  - Levofloxacin, gemifloxacin, moxifloxacin

Inpatient Rx of CAP[75]

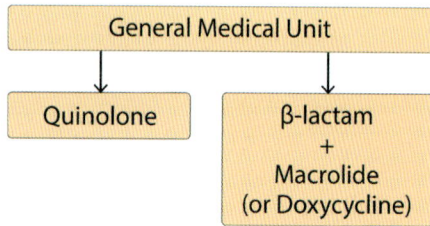

- **Acceptable β-lactams**
  - Ampicillin/Sulbactam
  - Cefotaxime
  - Ceftriaxone
  - Ceftaroline
- **Acceptable quinolones**
  - Levofloxacin
  - Moxifloxacin
- **If history of MRSA**
  - Add vancomycin or linezolid
- **If history of *P. aeruginosa***
  - Use anti-Ps β-lactam

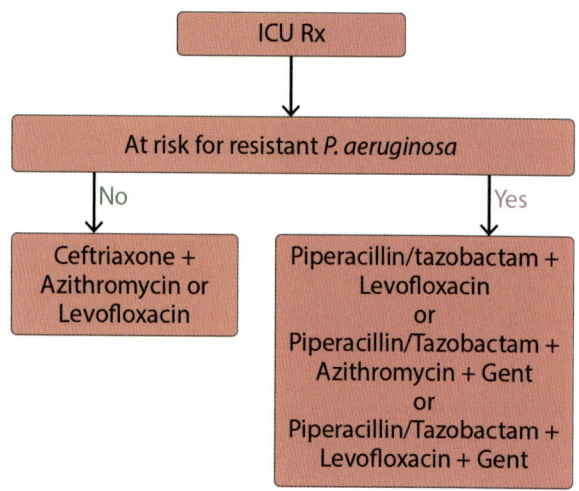

[76]
- *P. aeruginosa* risk factors
  - Severe structural lung disease
  - Recent antibiotics
  - Recent hospitalization

IDSA / ATS Updates on CAP 2019 — Testing and Site of Care[77]
- When to do sputum and blood cultures
  - Inpatient and severe CAP
  - Suspicion of MRSA or *P. aeruginosa*
  - Was an inpatient ≤ 90 days ago, got IV Ab
- When to do urine Ag testing
  - *S. pneumoniae*: if severe
  - *Legionella*: if severe, outbreak, or travel
- When to test for influenza
  - If it is in the community (NAAT preferred)
- Should we use procalcitonin?
  - Not to decide to give antibiotics
- How to determine admission
  - PSI preferred over CURB-65
- Determining ICU admission
  - Use IDSA/ATS severe pneumonia definitions
- Follow-up chest x-ray
  - Not needed if they have improved in 5–7 days
- Duration of treatment
  - ≥ 5 days

Definition of Severe CAP — 1 Major or ≥ 3 Minor Criteria
- Major
  - Septic shock
  - Ventilator
- Minor
  - RR ≥ 30 breaths/minute
  - Temp ≤ 98.6°F (36.0°C)
  - P_aO_2/F_iO_2 ≤ 250
  - Multilobe
  - Altered mental status
  - BUN ≥ 20
  - WBC < 4.0
  - Platelets < 100,000
  - Shock responsive to IV fluids

Case 31 — Key Points
- Recognize how to risk stratify patients with community-acquired pneumonia (CAP)
- Use risk stratification to determine the site of care for CAP
- Prescribe appropriate antibiotics for CAP based on site of care
- Be aware of the most recent IDSA/ATS recommendations for the management of CAP

Case 32 — History and Physical
Hx: You are consulted from the psychiatry service to evaluate a patient with a urinary tract infection. She is a 44-year-old woman admitted with suicidal ideation. She admits to recent use of crack cocaine. A urinalysis and drug screen were sent as part of her admission labs. She denies dysuria, frequency, or urgency. She has no other medical problems.

PE: VS normal

Physical exam normal

Case 32 — Labs
Urine toxicology
(+) for cocaine and cannabinoids

Urinalysis
pH 5.5; protein negative
Glucose negative
Leukocyte esterase 2+
Nitrites 3+
WBC 25 × 10³/mm³
RBC 3 cells/mm³
Bacteria moderate

Urine culture
> 10⁵ *E. coli*
Pregnancy test negative

AR 32
What would you recommend to the psych service?

A. Trimethoprim/Sulfamethoxazole × 3 days
B. Levofloxacin × 3 days
C. Nitrofurantoin × 5 days
D. Fosfomycin × 1
E. No treatment at this time

Answer:_____

Treatment of Asymptomatic Bacteriuria*[78]

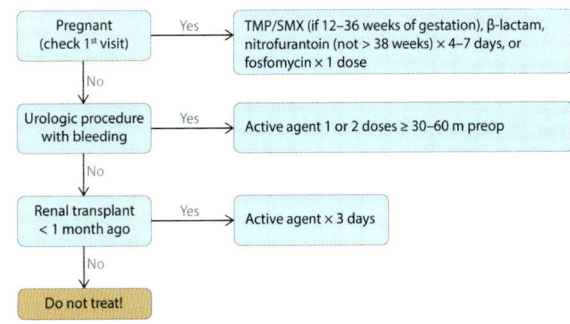

≥ 10⁵ organisms/mL; pyuria irrelevant
IDSA 2019

Case 32 — Key Points
- Recognize asymptomatic bacteriuria
- Know the few indications to treat asymptomatic bacteriuria
- Know what regimens to use when treatment is indicated

Case 33 — History and Physical
Hx: A 28-year-old woman calls your office with dysuria and urinary frequency × 2 days. She denies fever, abdominal pain, or flank pain. She is an established patient of yours. She has never had a urinary tract infection before. She is sexually active only with her husband of 7 years.

According to the microbiology lab of the hospital in your community, 25% of *E. coli* are resistant to TMP/SMX.

AR 33
What do you recommend to her?

A. TMP/SMX × 3 days
B. Levofloxacin × 3 days
C. Nitrofurantoin × 5 days
D. Fosfomycin × 1
E. Come in for a culture prior to treatment.

Answer:_____

Complicated vs. Uncomplicated UTIs
- Definition of complicated UTI
  - Diabetes mellitus
  - Immunocompromised
  - Structural anomaly
  - Foreign body
  - Resistant organism
  - Male
- All others are uncomplicated

Treatment of Symptomatic UTIs[79]

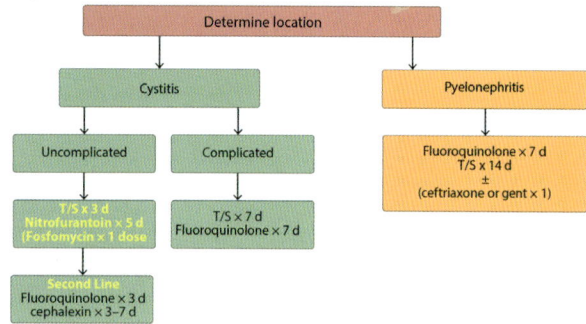

Caveats about Antibiotics for UTIs
- Trimethoprim/Sulfamethoxazole
  - No allergy, no antibiotics or inpatient × 90 days, TMP/SMX resistance ≤ 20%
- Nitrofurantoin
  - No suspicion of pyelonephritis
- Fosfomycin use
  - No suspicion of pyelonephritis, less efficacy
- Ceftriaxone or AG use
  - If quinolone resistance ≥ 10%
- β-Lactams
  - Routinely less effective than other agents

FDA Warnings — Fluoroquinolones[80]
- Side effects
  - Tendinopathy, tendon rupture
  - Myopathy
  - Neuropathy
  - Arthropathy
  - CNS: insomnia, mood alteration, dizzy
  - Hypoglycemia
  - Aortic aneurysms and rupture
- Only use if no alternative for Rx of:
  - Acute sinusitis, exacerbation of COPD, uncomplicated UTI

Case 33 — Key Points
- Know what constitutes a complicated urinary tract infection
- Know the antibiotics recommended to treat uncomplicated and complicated cystitis
- Know how to use local antibiotic susceptibilities to determine empiric treatment
- Remember the FDA warnings about quinolone use as 1st line drugs

Case 34 — History, Physical, and Hospital Course
Hx: A 44-year-old man is admitted to the general medicine floor with fever, cough for 2 days and shortness of breath for 1 day. He received an initial COVID-19 vaccine 2 months ago, but had a fever and myalgias afterward and did not seek out another dose.

PE: T 102.2°F (39.0°C), BP 128/78, HR 100, RR 24. O_2 sat 92% on room air. Lungs show diffuse bilateral crackles.

Hospital Course: He is placed on 4 L of O_2 and the pO_2 rises to 95%. COVID-19 nasal PCR is (+) and he is started on remdesivir. CXR is as shown. Overnight his O_2 sat drops to 85% on high-flow oxygen. He is transferred to the ICU and intubated.

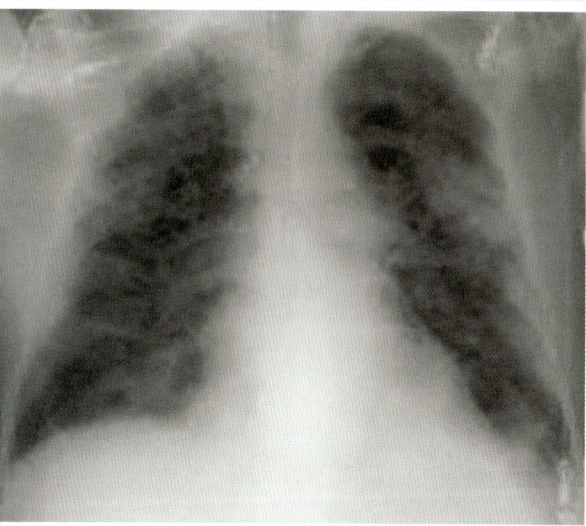

AR 34
In addition to dexamethasone what COVID-19 therapy would you give now?

A. Continue remdesivir
B. Continue remdesivir and start tocilizumab
C. Discontinue remdesivir and start bamlanivimab + etesevimab
D. Discontinue remdesivir and start tocilizumab
E. Discontinue remdesivir and start baricitinib and tocilizumab

Answer:_____

COVID-19 Drugs (FDA approved or EUA)
Mechanisms of Action
- **IL-6 receptor antagonists**
  - Tocilizumab
- **RNA polymerase inhibitors**
  - Remdesivir
- **Spike protein monoclonal antibodies combinations**
  - Casirivimab/Imdevimab
  - Bamlanivimab/Etesevimab
- **Janus kinase inhibitors**
  - Baricitinib

Drugs to Treat COVID-19*[81]

Drug	Postexposure prophylaxis	Ambulatory	Hospital pO₂ > 94%	Hospital pO₂ ≤ 94%	Hospital ICU
Bamlanivimab/ Etesevimab	Suggested†	Suggested†			
Casirivimab/Imdevimab		Suggested†			
Sotrovimab		Suggested			
Nirmatrelvir + Ritonavir		Suggested			
Molnupiravir		Alternative			
Remdesivir				Suggested	
Baricitinib				Suggested	
Tocilizumab				Suggested	Suggested
Dexamethasone				Suggested	Recommended

*FDA approved or emergency use authorization; dexamethasone is off label
†Not effective against omicron variant

COVID–19 Vaccines

Developer	Name	Age	Initial	Booster	Adverse
Pfizer	BNT162b2	≥ 5 yo	0 + 21d	5 months	Anaphylaxis, myocarditis, pericarditis
Moderna	mRNA-1273	≥ 18 yo	0 + 28d	5 months	Anaphylaxis, myocarditis, pericarditis
Janssen (Johnson & Johnson)	Ad26.COV2.S	≥ 18 yo	0	2 months	Central venous thrombosis, Guillain Barré

A combination of two monoclonal antibodies, tixagevimab and cilgavimab, is recommended for individuals who have severe reactions to vaccination that prevents them from being fully vaccinated or immunocompromising illness that may prevent them from a protective immune response to the vaccine.

COVID-19 — Vaccine Efficacies Initial Trials

Manufacturer	N	Symptomatic P/V* (efficacy)	Severe Disease P/V* (efficacy)
Pfizer	43,448	162/8 (95.0%)	9/1 (89%)
Moderna	30,420	185/11 (94.1%)	30/0 (100%)
Janssen	39,321	348/116 (67.7%)	16/3 (81.2%)
TOTAL	113,189	695/135 (80.6%)	55/4 (92.7%)

*P/V = placebo/vaccine

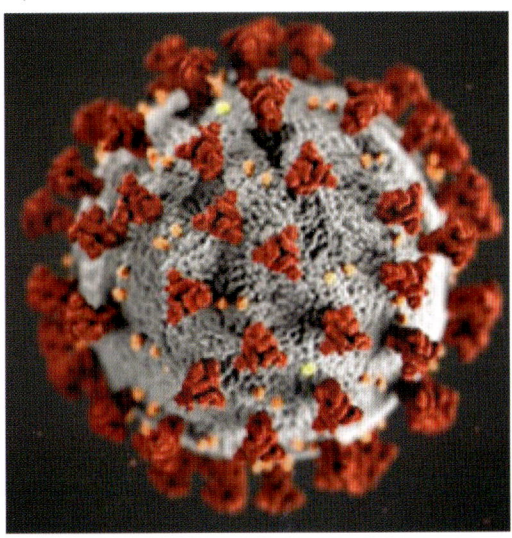

COVID-19
- **Clinical manifestations**
  - Incubation period 12 days in 98% (usually 4–5d)
  - Asymptomatic in 30–90%
  - Symptoms: cough (50%), fever (40%), headache (35%), SOB (30%), sore throat (20%), diarrhea (20%), emesis (10%)
  - Disease severity
    - Mild (80%)
    - Severe, requiring hospitalization (15%)
    - Critical, requiring ICU (5%)
- **Diagnosis**
  - PCR nasal swab, saliva testing
  - False negatives early

Case 34 — Key Points
- Recognize the rapidity with which patients with COVID can deteriorate and appropriately escalate care and adjust treatment
- Know the currently FDA approved and Emergency Use Authorization approved COVID-19 therapies
- Know the specific indications for these drugs related to the spectrum of severity of COVID-19
- Understand the indications, dosing, and efficacy of COVID vaccines

AUDIENCE RESPONSE ANSWERS

Audience Response 1
E. Switch to penicillin and clindamycin.

AR 2
E. Obtain a bone biopsy for culture prior to antibiotics.

AR 3
D. Start fidaxomicin PO.

AR 4
A. Progressive multifocal leukoencephalopathy

AR 5A
B. Start cefepime.

AR 5B
B. Start IV voriconazole.

AR 6A
E. Peripheral smear of blood

AR 6B
D. Azithromycin and atovaquone

AR 6C
E. Peripheral smear of blood

AR 6D
A. Doxycycline

AR 7A
C. *Coccidioides immitis*

AR 7B
D. None

AR 8A
C. Dexamethasone

AR 8B
B. Vancomycin and ceftriaxone

AR 8C
A. Ceftriaxone alone

AR 8D
A. Her roommates

AR 9
C. Doxycycline PO

AR 10A
A. Swab for rapid antigen testing for group A strep prior to treatment.

AR 10B
D. No further testing; prescribe no antibiotics.

AR 11
E. An equine antitoxin

AR 12
D. Start ceftriaxone 500 mg IM plus doxycycline 100 mg bid x 7 days.

AR 13
C. Perform a lumbar puncture prior to treatment.

AR 14
A. Start metronidazole 500 mg bid × 7 days.

AR 15A
D. No antibiotic therapy

AR 15B
D. No antibiotic therapy

AR 15C
D. No antibiotic therapy

AR 16A
D. No tetanus prevention is needed.

AR 16B
D. Amoxicillin/Clavulanate

AR 16C
D. Observe dog for 10 days.

AR 17
C. Treat for Lyme disease without performing serology.

AR 18A
D. Fungal culture

AR 18B
C. Mycobacterial culture

AR 19
E. Liposomal amphotericin B

AR 20
D. Stool for PCR testing

AR 21A
E. No test is needed prior to treatment.

AR 21B
E. Praziquantel, albendazole, and glucocorticoids

AR 22
B. Send vesicular fluid for PCR assay; start valacyclovir.

AR 23
A. Start high-dose acyclovir.

AR 24
A. EBV IgM capsid antibody

AR 25A
E. Pregnancy test

AR 25B
E. Nothing

AR 26
E. Blood for viral serology

AR 27
D. Neither test nor treat with oseltamivir.

AR 28A
B. 2 NRTIs and an integrase inhibitor

AR 28B
A. TMP/SMX

AR 28C
B. Test him once now.

AR 29
C. Clindamycin, primaquine, and prednisone

AR 30A
D. Transthoracic echo

AR 30B
D. Nafcillin × 6 weeks

AR 31
B. Outpatient treatment with levofloxacin

AR 32
E. No treatment at this time

AR 33
C. Nitrofurantoin × 5 days

AR 34
D. Discontinue remdesivir and start tocilizumab

ENDNOTES

[1] Sonneville E. *Clin Infect Dis*. 2006;42:57–62.

[2] Dinh MT. *Clin Infect Dis*. 2008;47:519–527.

[3] Zar FA. *Clin Infect Dis*. 2007;45:302–307.

[4] NEJM 364:422-431, 2011.

[5] Lancet Infect Dis 12:281-9, 2012.

[6] J Infect Chemother 24:744-52, 2018.

[7] Lancet Infect Dis 18:296-307.

[8] Johnson S: Clinical Practice Guideline by the Infectious Diseases. Society of America (IDSA) and Society for Healthcare. Epidemiology of America (SHEA): 2021 Focused Update Guidelines on Management of Clostridioides difficile Infection in Adults .

[9] Johnson S: Clinical Practice Guideline by the Infectious Diseases. Society of America (IDSA) and Society for Healthcare. Epidemiology of America (SHEA): 2021 Focused Update Guidelines on Management of Clostridioides difficile Infection in Adults .

[10] Wilcox MH: NEJM 376:305-317, 2017

[11] Johnson S: Clinical Practice Guideline by the Infectious Diseases. Society of America (IDSA) and Society for Healthcare. Epidemiology of America (SHEA): 2021 Focused Update Guidelines on Management of Clostridioides difficile Infection in Adults

[12] Freifeld, et al. Clinical practice guideline for the use of antimicrobial agents in neutropenic patients with cancer: 2010 update by the Infectious Diseases Society of America. *Clin Infect Dis*. 011;52(4): e56–e93.

[13] CDC. 2012 Data Archive.

[14] CDC

[15] CDC

[16] IDSA. *Clin Infect Dis*. 2016

[17] J. Hopkins Hosp Reports 1.269.1896.

[18] Chapman SW. *CID*. 2008;46:1801–1812.

[19] Wheat J: *Clin Infect Dis* 2007; 45:807–25

[20] de Gans J: *NEJM* 347:1549–56, 2002.

[21] Thigpen MC, et al. *N Engl J Med*. 2011;364:2016–2025.

[22] Quigliarello VJ. *NEJM*. 1997;336:708–716.

Van de Beek D. *NEJM*. 2006;354:44–53.

[23] https://www.cdc.gov/mmwr/volumes/69/rr/rr6909a1.htm

[24] Stevens DL. *CID*. 2014;59:147.

[25] Stevens DL. *CID*. 2014;59:147.

[26] Talan DA: *N Engl J Med* 2016;374:823-32

[27] Stevens DL. *CID*. 2014;59:147.

[28] STI Treatment Guidelines, 2021. *MMWR* 2021 70(4) 1-192.

[29] STI Treatment Guidelines, 2021. *MMWR* 2021 70(4) 1-192.

[30] STI Treatment Guidelines, 2021. *MMWR* 2021 70(4) 1-192.

[31] STI Treatment Guidelines, 2021. *MMWR* 2021 70(4) 1-192.

[32] STI Treatment Guidelines, 2021. *MMWR* 2021 70(4) 1-192.

[33] STI Treatment Guidelines, 2021. *MMWR* 2021 70(4) 1-192.

[34] STI Treatment Guidelines, 2021. *MMWR* 2021 70(4) 1-192.

[35] Molgarrd-Nielsen D. *JAMA*. 315:58–57, 2016.

[36] DuPont H. *JID*. 1989; 159:1126–1128.

[37] Sirinavin S and Garner P. *Cochrane Database Syst Rev*. 2000; (2):CD001167.

[38] Wong CS. *Clin Infect Dis*. 2012; 55:33–41.

[39] CDC 2019

[40] CDC 2019.

[41] IDSA 2020. DOI: 10.1093/cid/ciaa1215

[42] IDSA 2020. DOI: 10.1093/cid/ciaa1215

[43] White AC: *Clin Infect Dis*. 2018;66:1159-63

[44] Garcia HH. Lancet *Infect Dis*. 2014;14:687-95.

[45] *NEJM*. 2005;352:2271–84.

[46] *Clin Infect Dis*. 2012;54:922–8

[47] *NEJM*. 2015;372:2087–96.

[48] *NEJM*. 2016;375:1019–32

[49] IDSA: *Clin Infect Dis* 2019; 68:895-902.

[50] International Antiviral Society–USA Panel. *JAMA*. 2018; 320(4):379-349.

[53] https://clinicalinfo.hiv.gov/en/guidelines

[52] https://clinicalinfo.hiv.gov/en/guidelines

[53] Antiretroviral Drugs for Treatment and Prevention of HIV. JAMA 2020 324(16), 1651.

[54] International Antiviral Society–USA Panel. *JAMA*. 312:390-409, 2014.

[55] USPSTF. *Annals Intern Med.* 2013;159:51–60.

International Antiviral Society–USA Panel.

JAMA. 2014;312:390–409.

CDC. *MMWR* 66:830, 2017.

[56] Photo courtesy of Fred Zar, MD

[57] cdc.gov/hiv/pdf/hivtestingalgorithmrecommendation-final. pdf June 24, 2014.

[58] https://clinicalinfo.hiv.gov/en/guidelines/adult-and-adolescent-opportunistic-infection/whats-new-guidelines

[59] https://clinicalinfo.hiv.gov/en/guidelines/adult-and-adolescent-opportunistic-infection/whats-new-guidelines

[60] Durack DT, et al. *Am J Med.* 1994; 96:200–209. Li JS, et al. *CID*. 2000; 30(4):633–638.

[61] Durack DT, et al. *Am J Med.* 1994; 96:200–209.

[62] Li JS, et al. *CID*. 2000; 30:633–638.

[63] Baddour L, et al. American Heart Association Guidelines. *Circulation*. 2015; 132:1435–1486.

[64] Baddour L, et al. American Heart Association Guidelines. *Circulation*. 2015; 132:1435–1486.

[65] Baddour L, et al. American Heart Association Guidelines. Circulation. 2015; 132:1435–1486.

[66] Baddour L, et al. American Heart Association Guidelines. *Circulation*. 2015; 132:1435–1486.

[67] Circulation. 2021;143:e963–e978. DOI: 10.1161/ CIR.0000000000000969

[68] Circulation. 2021;143:e963–e978. DOI: 10.1161/ CIR.0000000000000969

[69] Circulation. 2021;143:e963–e978. DOI: 10.1161/ CIR.0000000000000969

[70] Neill AM: Thorax 51:1010–6, 1996.

[71] Fine MJ: *NEJM* 336:243–50, 1997.

[72] Fine MJ: *NEJM* 336:243–50, 1997.

[73] Neill AM: Thorax 51:1010–6, 1996.

[74] Metlay JP: American Thoracic Society Documents 200:e45–e67, 2019

[75] Metlay JP: American Thoracic Society Documents 200:e45–e67, 2019

[76] Metlay JP: American Thoracic Society Documents 200:e45–e67, 2019

[77] Metlay JP: American Thoracic Society Documents 200:e45–e67, 2019

[78] IDSA: *Clin Infect Dis* 68:83-110, 2019.

[79] Gupta K, et al. *CID*. 2011; 52:561–564.

[80] FDA: Posted December 20, 2018.

[81] https://www.idsociety.org/COVID19guidelines.

MedStudy

INTERNAL MEDICINE REVIEW

Nephrology

Presented by

Manish Suneja, MD

TABLE OF CONTENTS

Nephrology Topics

- Acute Kidney Injury
- Glomerular Disorders (Nephritic Syndrome)
- Glomerular Disorders (Nephrotic Syndrome)
- Nephrolithiasis
- Metabolic Acid-Base Disorders with Special Attention to RTA
- Hypertension (Including Secondary Hypertension)
- Hyponatremia and Hypernatremia (Disorders of Water Homeostasis)
- Electrolyte and Mineral Disorders
- Chronic Kidney Disease
- Polycystic Kidney Disease

ACUTE KIDNEY INJURY (AKI)

- Sudden loss of renal function over hours to days
- Commonly **reflected by rise in creatinine and/or decrease in urine output**
- KDIGO 2012 (Kidney Disease Improving Global Outcomes) definition — any 1 of the following:
  - **Increase in serum creatinine by 0.3 mg/dL**
  - **1.5-fold increase over baseline in past 7 days**
  - **Oliguria (urine output < 0.5 mL/kg/hr) for at least 6 hours**

Classification of the Etiologies of Acute Kidney Injury (AKI)

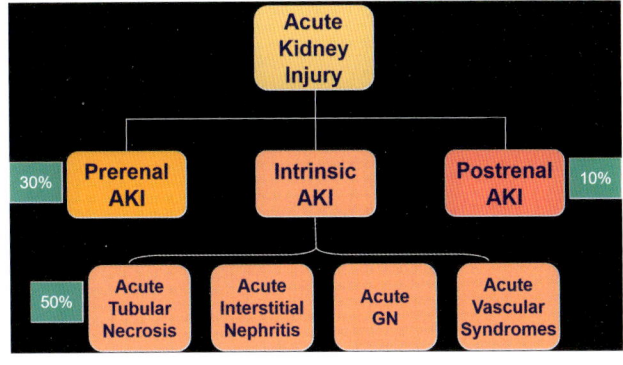

Prerenal AKI

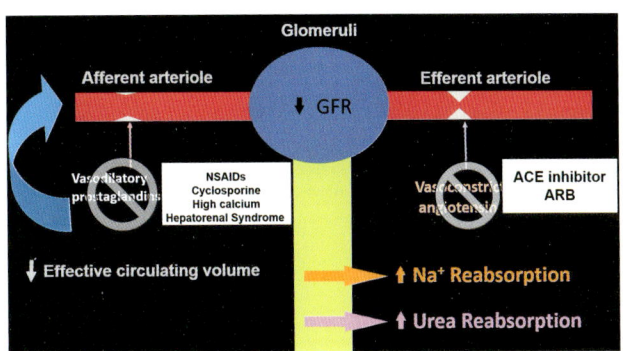

Urine Indices in AKI

	Prerenal	Intrinsic ATN
U$_{Osm}$	> 500	< 350
Na$^+$ (mEq/L)	< 20	> 40
Bun/Cr (mg/dL)	> 20:1	< 10:1
FE$_{Na}$	< 1%	> 2%
FE$_{Urea}$	**< 35%**	**> 55%**
U/P Cr	> 40	< 20
Sediment	**Bland**	**Muddy brown, granular casts**

→ Useful marker when someone is on diuretics

→ Trumps all of the urine indices
ATN*

*Pearl

Acute Tubular Necrosis

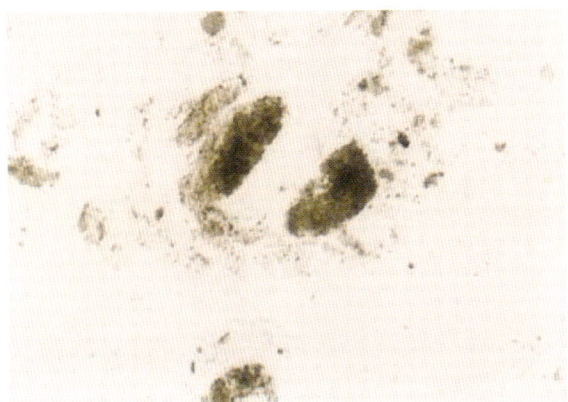

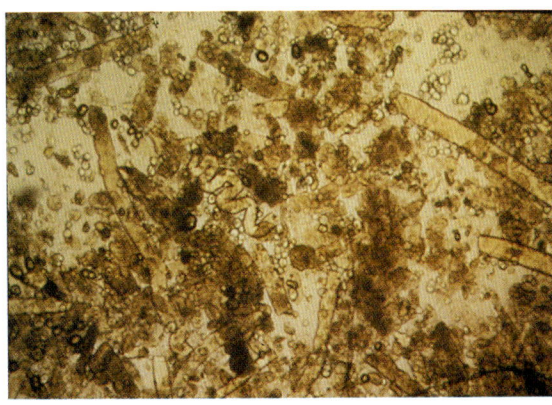

Pigmented granular ("muddy brown") casts. Marker of acute tubular necrosis.

Acute Tubular Necrosis
- **Ischemic**: prerenal → ATN
- **Nephrotoxic**
  - Endogenous
    - Free myoglobin (**rhabdomyolysis**: cocaine, statins, trauma and electrolytes → **low phosphorus and low K$^+$**)
    - Free hemoglobin (intravascular hemolysis)
  - Exogenous
    - Contrast
    - Drugs (**gentamicin**, amphotericin, cisplatin)
    - **Osmotic nephropathy**: <u>sucrose</u>/<u>mannitol</u>/ <u>dextran, especially in patients with underlying chronic kidney disease</u>

ATN — Rhabdo vs. Hemolysis
Pearl[1]: <u>Heme+ on dipstick but no RBC on micro</u>
<u>Differential Diagnosis</u>
↓
1) **Myoglobinuria (rhabdo)** → **check CPK/aldolase**
2) **Hemoglobinuria (hemolytic anemia)** → **peripheral blood smear/LDH/haptoglobin/indirect bilirubin**
- **Treatment**
  - **Early aggressive hydration with isotonic saline**
    - May need > 10 L IVF to achieve euvolemia
  - Urine alkalinization — pH > 6.5
  - Keep UO 250–300 mL/hr

Acute Interstitial Nephritis — Drugs vs. Inflammatory Condition
- Acute kidney injury due to lymphocytic infiltration of the interstitium
- #1 cause: <u>drugs</u>; #1 drug = <u>PPI/NSAIDs/antibiotics</u>
- Nondrug causes (**pearl → exams like Sjögren's and sarcoidosis**)
- U/A → **WBC or WBC cast in urine with no evidence of infection**
- <u>Eosinophils in the urine on Wright or Hansel stain</u>
- Classic triad (**seen in only 10%**)
  - Fever
  - Rash
  - Eosinophilia
- **Tx: discontinue medication, PO steroids (early within 2 weeks)**

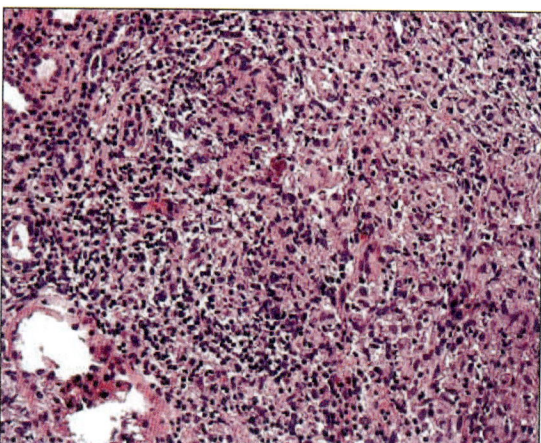

Clinical Features of <u>PPI-Associated AIN</u>[2]

Finding	Frequency
Pyuria	72%
Fatigue and nausea	39%
Eosinophilia	33%
Weakness	22%
Fever	10%
Rash	< 10%

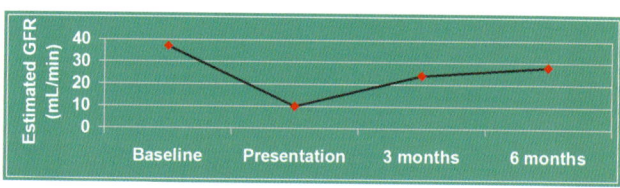

AKI after Arterial Catheterization[3]
- **Postcontrast**
  - AKI within 24–48 hours
  - Prevention with **hydration pre- and postprocedure**
  - **Lowest possible volume** of contrast
  - **Low or isoosmolar contrast** agent
  - Possible benefit from *N*-acetylcysteine (1,200 mg bid dose) though recent metaanalysis negative

Bottom line → hydration with normal saline

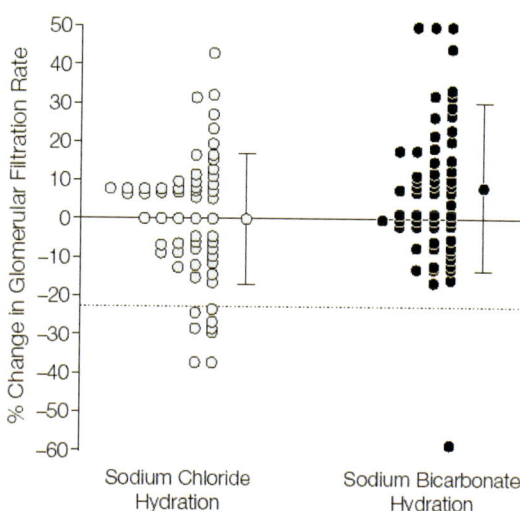

- **Atheroembolic disease**: If not recovering by Day 5 postcontrast, must consider atheroembolic disease (**pearl**)
  - **Hollenhorst plaque, livedo reticularis, and peripheral emboli**
  - **Eosinophiluria/eosinophilia, low complement,** high amylase
  - **Step ladder worsening** of kidney function over weeks to months
  - Tx
    - Consider stopping anticoagulation (if not a strong indication)
    - **Statins?** Otherwise supportive care

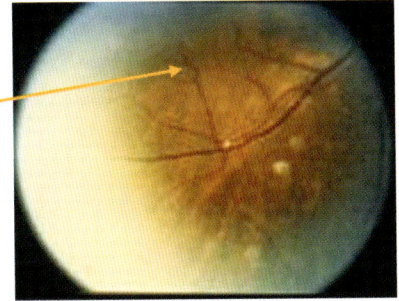

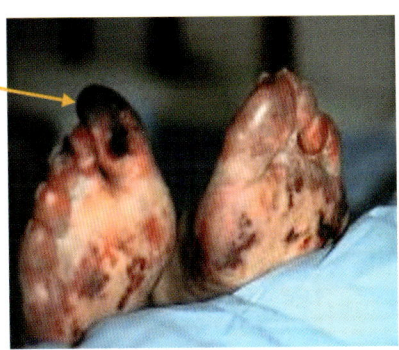

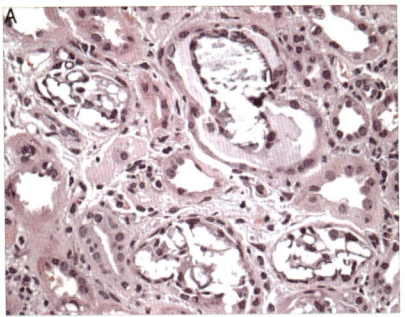

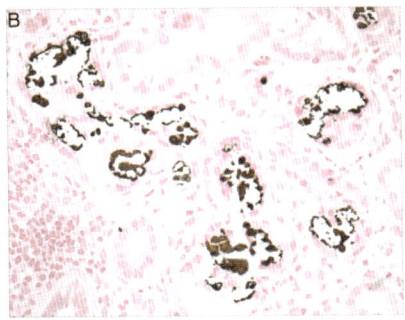

Audience Response 1

51-year-old Caucasian female with AKI, h/o hypertension, hypercholesterolemia, and Type 2 diabetes mellitus

Medications: lisinopril, hydrochlorothiazide, glipizide

2 weeks prior admitted to another hospital because of weakness

Laboratory test 2 weeks earlier: SCr 1.4 mg/dL, eGFR 42 mL/min/m^2, hemoglobin 10.1 g/dL, and hematocrit 30%; and she underwent a colonoscopy

She now presents with SCr of 6.3 mg/dL, K$^+$ 5.3 mEq/L, and phos 11.2 mg/dL

What's the etiology of her AKI?

A. Acute tubular necrosis
B. Acute interstitial nephritis
C. Vasculitis
D. Acute phosphate nephropathy

Answer:_____

- Develops within days after exposure (to an oral sodium phosphate bowel preparation or enema)
- Generally recognized only when lab studies are performed at some later time
- Risk factor → **CKD and diabetes (older age)**
- **Diagnosis suggested by AKI with a recent history of receiving bowel purgatives containing sodium phosphate**
- **Hyperphosphatemia is out of proportion to the degree of kidney injury, and urinalysis has minimal findings***

Some Other Important Stuff!!
- **Abdominal Compartment Syndrome***

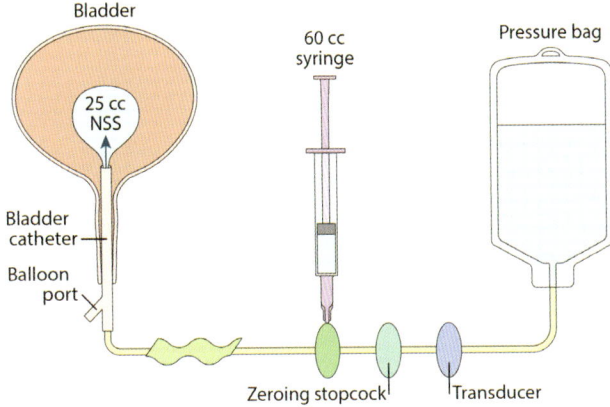

- Diagnosis → sustained IAP > 20 mmHg with AKI (often looks prerenal)
- Pathophysiology → decreased renal perfusion from increased renal vein pressure
- Treatment → decompressive laparotomy (trauma) or high-volume paracentesis (massive ascites)

Abnormal Urinalysis (Pearls)
- Cells
  - RBCs
    - **Dipstick blood+, no RBCs: rhabdo- or hemolysis***
    - **RBC casts or dysmorphic RBCs** = Glomerulonephritis
  - WBCs
    - **Sterile pyuria: interstitial nephritis vs. tuberculosis***
  - Eosinophils
    - **Drug-induced interstitial nephritis***, atheroembolic disease

AR 2

A 77-year-old man presents with nausea, vomiting, and general malaise; 10 cc urine output in the last 2 days.

PMH: hyperlipidemia, HTN, T2DM, cigarettes × 40 years

Exam: pale and stuporous; BP 170/70 mmHg, HR 88 bpm

Loud carotid bruits; faint systolic ejection murmur

Clear lungs

Obese abdomen that is soft and without peritoneal signs

Labs: BG 142 mg/dL; K$^+$ 5.4 mEq/L; Cr 6.4 mg/dL; BUN 165 mg/dL

Urinalysis: bland

Which of the following is the next best step in management?

A. Order ANCA and anti-GBM antibodies.
B. Insert a temporary pacemaker in case hyperkalemia worsens.
C. Obtain a CT of the abdomen and pelvis with contrast.
D. Place a Foley catheter in the bladder.
E. Place a temporary dual lumen dialysis catheter.

Answer:_____

GLOMERULAR DISORDERS

Proteinuria
- **Normal**
  - 24-hour urine = < 150 mg/day
  - "Spot" urine protein/creatinine ratio: < 200 mg/g (0.2) roughly equivalent to 24-hour sample
- **Glomerular disorders:** if spot protein:creatinine ratio > 1.0–2.0 or 24-hour urine > 1.0–2.0 g/24 hours
- **Tubulointerstitial disease:** > normal but < glomerular
  - If spot protein:creatinine ratio < 1.0 or 24-hour urine < 1.0 g/24 hours

NEPHRITIC SYNDROME

Nephritic vs. Nephrotic

	Nephrotic	Nephritic
Proteinuria	> 3.5 g	< 1–2 g
RBCs	Minor, if any	Significant
Casts	Fatty casts, lipid droplets	**Dysmorphic RBC or RBC casts**

Nephritic Syndrome — Features

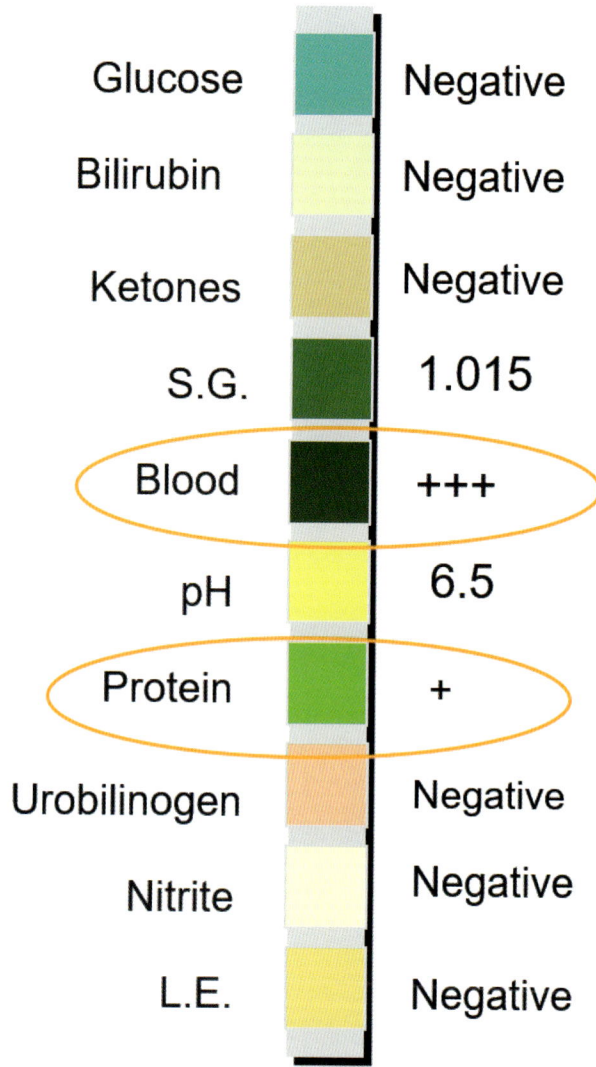

- **Glomerular hematuria** (main feature RBC cast or dysmorphic RBC)
- Proteinuria (0.5–2 g/24 hours)
- **Azotemia (elevated BUN/creatinine)**
- Hypertension and edema
- Hematuria (main feature RBC cast [A] or dysmorphic RBC [B])
- Proteinuria (1–2 g/24 hours)
- Hypertension and edema
- Azotemia (elevated BUN/creatinine)

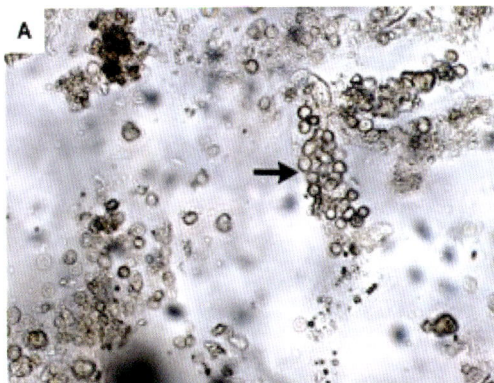

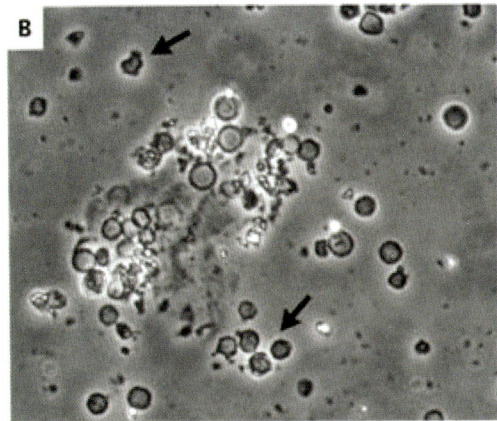

Urine Sediment in Nephritic Syndromes

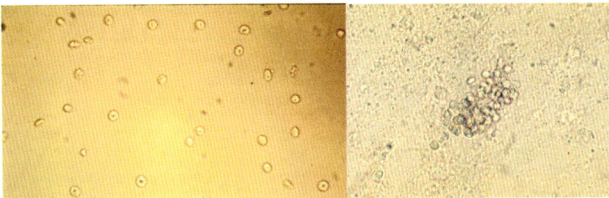

Hematuria: 1–3+

- Proteinuria: mild (< 1–2 g)

Glomerulonephritis / RPGN

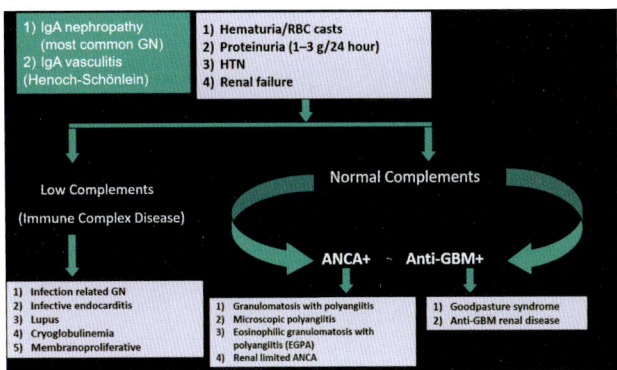

Acute Infection-Related Glomerulonephritis (IRGN)

- Usually occurs in children; poststreptococcal GN is the most common cause of IRGN (a.k.a. postinfectious GN [PIGN])
- Occurs after a streptococcal **pharyngitis or impetigo**
- Latent period: Acute onset of gross hematuria **(cola-colored)** or microscopic hematuria occurs 7–10 days after pharyngitis and up to 30 days after skin infection
- Caused by group A β-hemolytic streptococci, particularly nephritogenic strains (also staph)

Pearl:
Nephritic syndrome after (skin infection or URI)
Decreased complement level (especially C3)
Increased ASO titer

IgA Nephropathy — Berger's (Immune Complex Disease With Normal Serum Complements)*

- IgA nephropathy is the **most common primary GN** worldwide; IgA reacts to unidentified antigens
- Episodes of **gross hematuria are precipitated by flu-like illness**, exercise
- Urinary protein excretion usually subnephrotic
- Diagnosis is made clinically or on percutaneous renal biopsy
- **IgA vasculitis is the systemic form affecting skin, GI tract, joints, kidneys**

Pearl: IgA vasculitis

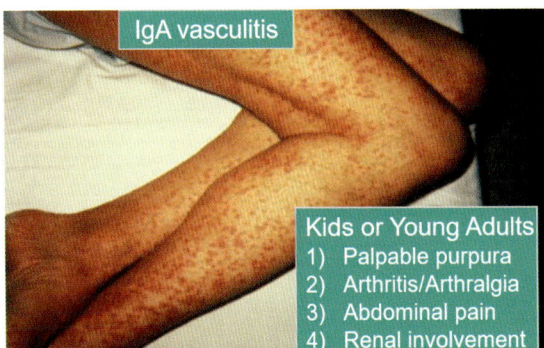

Cryoglobulinemic GN

- **"Cryoglobulins"** is a generic term given to immunoglobulins that precipitate on cooling and resolubilize on warming
- 3 types
  - Type 1 — Monoclonal Ig (usually IgM)
  - **Type 2** — Monoclonal Ig directed against Fc portion of polyclonal Ig **(hepatitis C)**
  - Type 3 — Polyclonal Ig directed against Fc portion of polyclonal Ig

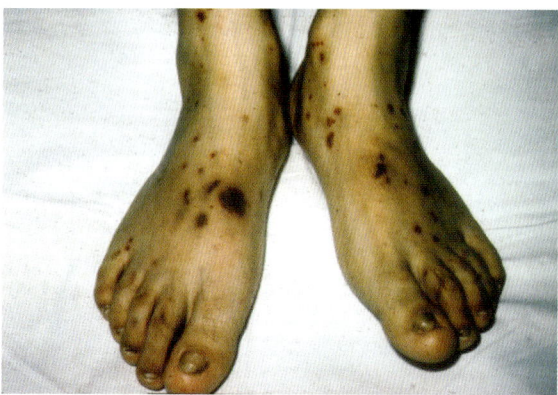

Pearl
Purpuric Rash
Pseudo-Raynaud's
C4 is depressed, whereas C3 levels are low normal. Renal disease may improve with Tx of hepatitis C.

Lupus Nephritis

- SLE is a multisystem autoimmune disease with antibodies directed against a wide variety of cellular components
- Predominantly affects young women
- Various organ systems are involved like skin, joints, serous membranes, heart, neurologic, blood, and the kidneys
- **Type 4 lupus nephritis (diffuse proliferative): most common and most worrisome, whereas Type 5 results in nephrotic syndrome/membranous changes**
- **ANA, Anti-dsDNA, depressed complement level (both C3 and C4)**

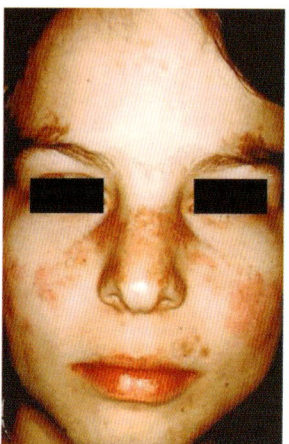

Tx
**Induction → MMF/cyclophosphamide + steroids
Maintenance → MMF/azathioprine**

Membranoproliferative GN (MPGN)

- Group of disorders generally presenting with proteinuria, hematuria, and hypertension
- Generally associated with **hepatitis C** and **hepatitis B (clue risk factors or elevated liver enzymes)***
- Can present as both **nephrotic** and **nephritic** syndromes
- **Low C3 level is seen in up to 70% of patients**
- Biopsy diagnosis

!!! New — Problems with alternate complement pathway: **C3 glomerulopathy**

Glomerular Disorders Associated with Low Complement Levels

- IRGN
- Lupus nephritis
- Infective endocarditis
- Membranoproliferative GN (MPGN)
  - Hepatitis B
  - Hepatitis C
- Cryoglobulinemia-associated GN

Nephritis with Normal Complements — ANCA Vasculitis and Anti-GBM

- Granulomatosis with polyangiitis
  - **URTI (sinusitis, epistaxis)**
  - LRTI (infiltrates, cavitary lesions, DAH, consolidation)
  - **c-ANCA → anti-PR3**
- Microscopic polyangiitis
  - Pulmonary hemorrhage
  - **Mononeuritis multiplex**
  - Cutaneous small vessel vasculitis (palpable purpura)
  - **p-ANCA → anti-MPO**
- Eosinophilic granulomatosis with polyangiitis (EGPA)
  - **Asthma/Atopy**
  - **Mononeuritis multiplex**
  - **Eosinophilia**

How to Remember All This?

- Look for clues in history and lab results
- Place the case in a broad category like nephrotic syndrome, **nephritic syndrome**
- **Narrow differential based on complement levels**
- **Renal-pulmonary syndrome** — look at the nephritic syndrome table
- Look for key features

AR 3

A 19-year-old male:

Tea-colored urine × 1 day

H/O rhinorrhea and a cough × 2 days

PE: BP 138/92 mmHg; normal exam

U/A: TNTC RBCs, 2+ protein

ASO titer positive, C3/C4 normal, Cr normal

Which of the following is the most likely diagnosis?

A. IRGN
B. Endocarditis
C. Poststreptococcal glomerulonephritis
D. Lupus nephritis
E. IgA nephropathy

Answer:_____

NEPHROTIC SYNDROME

Nephritic vs. Nephrotic

	Nephritic	Nephrotic
Proteinuria	< 1–2 g	> 3.5 g
RBCs	Significant	Minor, if any
Casts	Dysmorphic RBC or RBC casts	**Fatty casts, lipid droplets**

Nephrotic Syndrome — Features

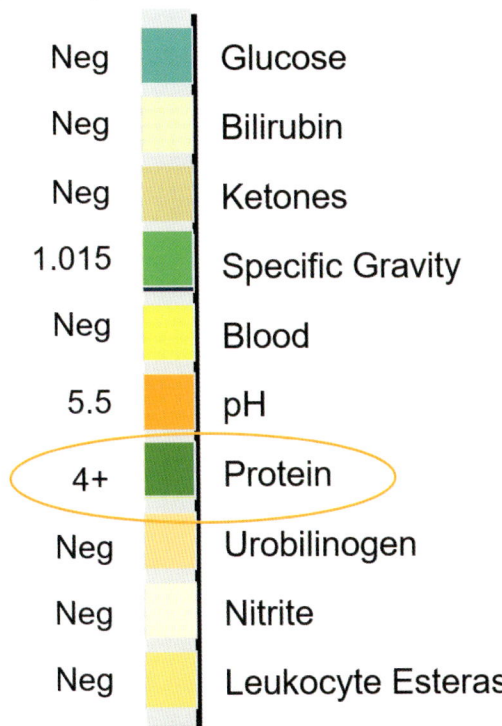

Neg	Glucose
Neg	Bilirubin
Neg	Ketones
1.015	Specific Gravity
Neg	Blood
5.5	pH
4+	Protein
Neg	Urobilinogen
Neg	Nitrite
Neg	Leukocyte Esterase

- Proteinuria > 3.5 g/24 hours
- Edema
- Hypoalbuminemia
- Hyperlipidemia
- Lipiduria

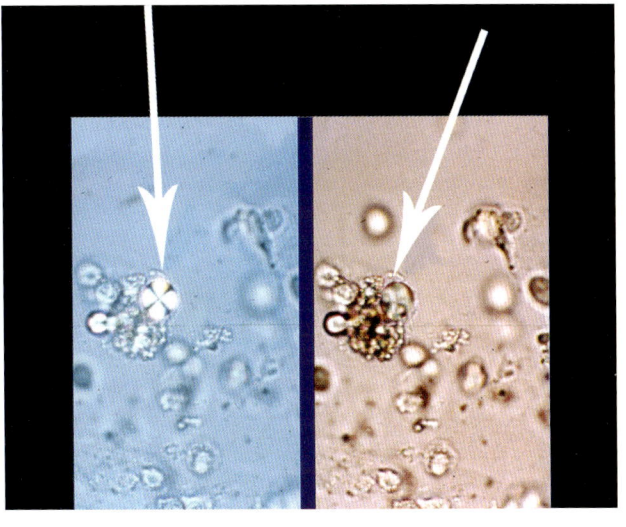

- HTN

Hypercoagulable
Urinary loss of antithrombin (AT) and plasminogen
hemoconcentration

Nephrotic Syndrome — Histologic Classification
- Minimal change disease
- Membranous glomerulopathy
- Focal segmental glomerulosclerosis (FSGS)
- Membranoproliferative GN

Minimal Change Disease — Clinical Clues and Features
- **Most common in children/young adults (sudden onset of severe nephrosis)**
- Patient usually normotensive, nephrotic sediment, normal renal function
- **Secondary etiologies**
  - Idiopathic
  - Drugs — **NSAIDs**
  - Toxins — Mercury, lead
  - Tumors — **Hodgkin lymphoma (HL)**
- **Rx: steroids; adults may require cytotoxics**

Focal Segmental Glomerulosclerosis — Clinical Clues and Features
- Most common primary renal disease in **African Americans**
- Patient usually hypertensive; usually progresses to ESRD over 5–20 years
- **Primary (idiopathic)**
- **Secondary etiologies**
  - Familial — **gene mutations (APOL1)**
  - Drugs — intravenous heroin, pamidronate
  - Infections — **HIV (collapsing FSGS)*, parvovirus**
  - Adaptive — reflux nephropathy, **obesity**
- **Rx: ACEIs/ARBs, steroids**

Membranous Nephropathy — Clinical Clues and Features
- Most common cause of idiopathic nephrotic syndrome in **Caucasian adults**
- Heavy proteinuria is common; hypertension and azotemia develop as disease progresses
- **Increased incidence of renal vein thrombosis; (flank pain/hematuria/high LDH)***
- **Idiopathic → anti-PLA2R antibodies in 70% cases (phospholipase A2 receptor)***
- **Secondary etiologies**
  - Drugs — NSAIDs, gold, penicillamine
  - Infections — hepatitis B/C, syphilis
  - Tumors — **carcinoma***
  - Immunologic — SLE
- **Rx: ACEI ± immunomodulation**

Nephrotic Syndrome — Systemic Disease: Diabetic Nephropathy
- **Most common cause of nephrotic syndrome in adults**
- Leading cause of ESRD in USA
- 30% of patients with Type 1 and 20% of patients with Type 2 DM develop diabetic nephropathy
  - **Initially microalbuminuria** followed by heavy proteinuria and decline in renal function
- Diagnosis usually made on clinical grounds (unless no retinopathy present)
  - Up to 30% without retinopathy might have another etiology for their nephrotic syndrome
    Drug of choice → ARB/ACEI

Nephrotic Syndrome — Systemic Disease: Amyloidosis / Multiple Myeloma
- **Amyloid**: biochemical forms
  - Amyloid AL — immunoglobulin origin → MM
  - Amyloid AA — inflammatory states
- **Multiple myeloma (<u>very</u> important to recognize these <u>clues</u>)***
  - **Renal failure with hypercalcemia**
  - **<u>Discrepancy in urine dipstick and urine protein/Cr ratio</u>**
  - **Low anion gap**
  - **Total protein to albumin ratio > 2:1**
  - **Back pain in older adults**

Nephrotic Syndrome

	Primary	Secondary
Minimal change disease **(Clue: young adults/ kids)**		**NSAIDs** Lymphoma
Focal segmental glomerulosclerosis **(Clue: African Americans)**		**Genetic (*APOL1* & *MYH9* in AA)** HIV Heroin Obesity
Membranous glomerulopathy **(Clue: adults — cancer?)**	Presence of PLA2R antibodies	**Solid tumors** SLE (lupus nephritis)
Membranoproliferative GN **(Clue: low complements)**		**Hepatitis C**
Primary = de novo renal disease = Idiopathic		

How to Remember All This?
- **Summary Principles**
  - Look for clues in history and lab results
  - Place the case in a broad category like **nephrotic syndrome**, nephritic syndrome, etc.
  - Just remember **key features**

AR 4
An 84-year-old man with T2DM and HTN:

Severe lower back pain and increasing confusion

3-month history of 20-lb weight loss

Exam: frail and generally decompensated with normal vital signs and point tenderness over L3

Labs: Na^+ 139 mEq/L, K^+ 5.9 mEq/L, Cl^- 115 mEq/L, HCO_3^- 18 mEq/L, albumin 2.5 g/dL, total protein 8 g/dL

BUN 68 mg/dL, Cr 3.6 mg/dL, Ca^{2+} 11.1 mg/dL, BG 145 mg/dL

U/A 1.020, pH 6.0, 2 RBCs/HPF, trace protein

24-hour urine: clearance 18 cc/m; urine protein 5.5 g

Which of the following is the most appropriate next step in patient care?

A. PSA
B. Colonoscopy
C. Complement levels
D. Urine and serum electrophoresis
E. Urine Hansel stain for eosinophils

Answer:_____

AR 5
A 64-year-old male PMH HTN, hyperlipidemia, OA:

New-onset lower extremity edema

Recent history: fatigue/tiredness; weight loss 5 lb

Meds: acetaminophen, metoprolol, simvastatin

Exam: BP 122/74 mmHg, HR 82 bpm

Fundi not visible, abdomen is slightly obese; 3+ pitting edema of the lower extremities to mid-calf

Fasting BMP: Cr 1.1 mg/dL, albumin 2.1 g/dL, total cholesterol is 314 mg/dL, fasting glucose is 98 mg/dL

U/A: 4+ protein, micro shows fat droplets

Urine protein to Cr ratio is 7.5

Hemoglobin is 9.8 g/dL, and stool occult is positive

What is the most likely diagnosis?

A. FSGS (focal segmental glomerulosclerosis)
B. Minimal change disease
C. Amyloidosis
D. Membranous nephropathy
E. Membranoproliferative glomerulonephritis

Answer:_____

NEPHROLITHIASIS

Renal Stones

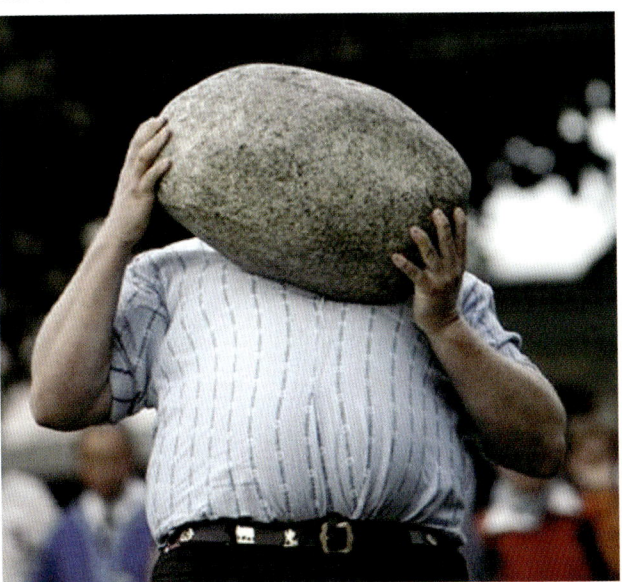

World's largest kidney stone!

Nephrolithiasis → The Afflicted
- Prevalence
  - Estimated **12% of men** and **6% of women** will develop a stone during lifetime
- Recurrence
  - **30–50% will have recurrence** within 5 years
  - However, treatment can **reduce this risk by up to 50%**
  - ~ 80% contain calcium, with calcium oxalate the <u>most common</u>

Types of Stones
- Basically 2 types
  1) **Calcium based**
     - **Calcium oxalate ~ 70% (most common)**
     - Calcium phosphate — 10% **(think distal RTA)**
  2) **Everything else**
     - **Uric acid — ~ 10%**
     - Struvite — ~ 10% **(urease splitting organisms)***
     - Cysteine — 1%
     - Drug induced

Drugs Associated with Stones
- **Triamterene**
- **Indinavir**
- Sulfonamides
- Acetazolamide
- Ascorbic acid/Vitamin C
- Chemotherapy (increased urate load)

Urinary Risk Factors
- **Increase in promoters or decrease in inhibitors!**
  - **High (promoters)**
    - High urine calcium (hypercalciuria)
    - High urine oxalate (hyperoxaluria)
    - High urine uric acid (hyperuricosuria)
  - **Low (inhibitors)**
    - Low urine citrate (hypocitraturia)
    - Low urine volume (very important in all stone formers)

Risk Factors for Calcium Oxalate Stone
- **Hypercalciuria → most important**
- **Hyperoxaluria**
- Hyperuricosuria
- Hypocitraturia
- Low urine volume (common to all stones)

Risk Factor — Idiopathic Hypercalciuria

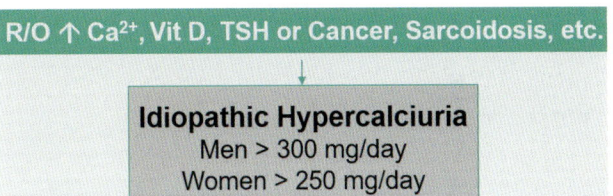

R/O ↑ Ca^{2+}, Vit D, TSH or Cancer, Sarcoidosis, etc.

Idiopathic Hypercalciuria
Men > 300 mg/day
Women > 250 mg/day

- Treatment
  - Anticalciuric diuretics (thiazides)
    - **HCTZ**
    - **Chlorthalidone**
    - **Indapamide**
- Diet
  - Reduce animal protein
  - Reduce Na^+
  - Reduce sucrose and fructose

Risk Factor — Hyperoxaluria

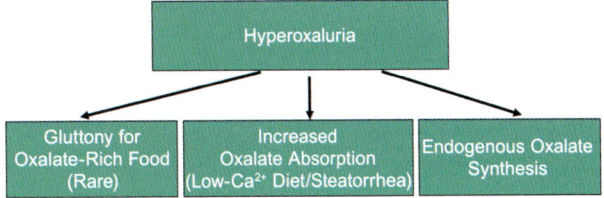

Hyperoxaluria

| Gluttony for Oxalate-Rich Food (Rare) | Increased Oxalate Absorption (Low-Ca^{2+} Diet/Steatorrhea) | Endogenous Oxalate Synthesis |

Current Understanding → Oxalate

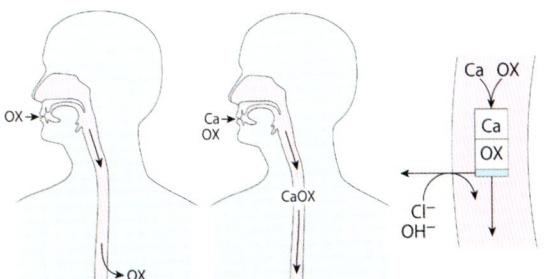

Treatment of Idiopathic Hyperoxaluria
- Diet
  - Reduce oxalate-containing food (spinach, rhubarb, beet roots, nuts)
  - Avoid low-calcium diet

Calcium and the Risk of Symptomatic Kidney Stones in Males[4]

	Group 1	Group 2	Group 3	Group 4	Group 5
Calcium intake (mg)	< 605	605–722	723–848	849–1,049	> 1,050
Incidence/100,000 person/year	435	310	279	266	243
Multivariate RR (95% CI)	1.0	0.74 (0.57–0.97)	0.68 (0.52–0.90)	0.68 (0.51–0.90)	0.66 (0.49–0.90)

$p = 0.018$ for trend

Risk Factors for Uric Acid Stone!! (Becoming More Common with Diabetes and Obesity)
- **Acidic urine pH***
- Hyperuricosuria
- Low urine volume

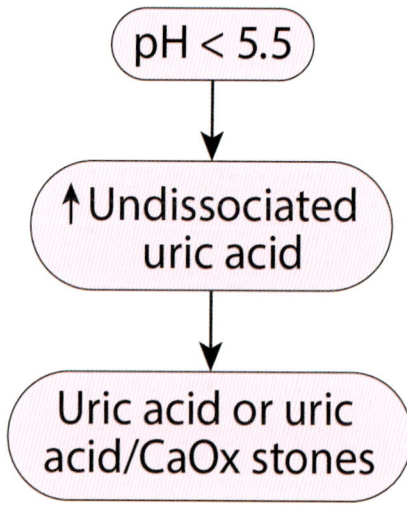

$$pKa = 5.5$$

$$H^+ + urate \rightleftharpoons Uric\ acid$$

pH < 5.5

↑Undissociated uric acid

Uric acid or uric acid/CaOx stones

Prevention and Tx of IUAN
- **Increase urine pH above > 6**
  - **Potassium citrate 20–30 mEq 2–3 times daily**
- Allopurinol
  - If urine UA level is increased
- Improve the metabolic risk factors

Medical Treatment of Nephrolithiasis
- **Thiazides:** ↑ renal tubular calcium absorption Rx for hypercalciuria
- **Potassium citrate:** Rx for hypocitraturia

Dietary Prescription
- **Urinary volume → Increase fluid intake to maintain a urine volume > 2 L (fluids: 2.5–3 liters/day)**
- **High urine calcium →**
  1) Reduce nondairy animal protein intake (5 servings of meat/week)
  2) Reduce sodium intake (< 2.4 g/day)
  3) Reduce sucrose and fructose intake
- **High urine oxalate →**
  1) Avoid high-oxalate foods
  2) **Adequate dietary calcium (> 700 mg at least)**
  3) Avoid vitamin C supplements
- **High urine uric acid →** reduce purine intake
- **Low urine citrate →**
  1) Increase fruit and vegetable intake (phytates)
  2) Reduce nondairy animal protein intake

Stones — Key Points*
- Calcium oxalate (**1° HPT**, idiopathic hypercalciuria, low urine citrate, hyperoxaluria) **most common**
- Calcium phosphate (**distal renal tubular acidosis**)
- Uric acid 10% (**low urine pH** and hyperuricosuria: associated with gout, chronic diarrhea, ileostomy) → **Radiolucent → Tx: increase the urine pH**
- Struvite — magnesium ammonium phosphate (**infection with bacteria** that express urease) → Staghorn calculi
- Cystine (cystinuria) — **hexagonal**

ACID-BASE DISORDERS

METABOLIC ACIDOSIS

Metabolic Acid-Base Disorders
- **Metabolic acidosis**
  - High anion gap (HAGMA)
  - Normal anion gap metabolic acidosis (NAGMA; a.k.a. non–anion gap metabolic acidosis)
    - **Pearl: On exams NAGMA = either RTA or diarrhea**
- **Metabolic alkalosis**

The Henderson-Hasselbalch Formula Is the Mantra of Acid-Base Physiology

The Mantra

$$pH = pKa + \log \frac{[HCO_3^-]}{[CO_2]}$$

$$pH \propto \frac{[HCO_3^-]}{[CO_2]}$$

$$Acidity = \frac{Bicarbonate}{Carbon\ Dioxide}$$

$$A = {}^{B}/_{CD}$$

There Are 4 Primary Ways That pH Can Change

1) **Increase** in HCO_3^- **increases** pH: metabolic alkalosis

$$\uparrow pH \propto \frac{\uparrow[HCO_3^-]}{[CO_2]}$$

2) **Decrease** in HCO_3^- **decreases** pH: metabolic acidosis

$$\downarrow pH \propto \frac{\downarrow[HCO_3^-]}{[CO_2]}$$

3) **Increase** in pCO_2 **decreases** pH: respiratory acidosis

$$\downarrow pH \propto \frac{[HCO_3^-]}{\uparrow[CO_2]}$$

4) **Decrease** in pCO_2 **increases** pH: respiratory alkalosis

$$\uparrow pH \propto \frac{[HCO_3^-]}{\downarrow[CO_2]}$$

Simple Acid-Base Disorders

	Primary Process	Compensation
Metabolic acidosis	$\downarrow [HCO_3^-]$	$\downarrow pCO_2$
Metabolic alkalosis	$\uparrow [HCO_3^-]$	$\uparrow pCO_2$
Respiratory acidosis	$\uparrow pCO_2$	$\uparrow [HCO_3^-]$
Respiratory alkalosis	$\downarrow pCO_2$	$\downarrow [HCO_3^-]$

Causes of HAGMA
- **MUDPILES**
  - **M**ethanol (increased osmol gap)
  - **U**remia
  - **D**iabetic ketoacidosis
  - **P**araldehyde → replaced with **P**ropylene glycol
  - **I**soniazid, iron (very uncommon)
  - **L**actate
  - **E**thylene glycol (increased osmol gap)
  - **S**alicylates (respiratory alkalosis → mixed resp alkalosis + HAGMA)
- **Mnemonic for the 21st century: GOLDMARK***
  - **G**lycols (ethylene and propylene)
  - **O**xoproline
  - **L**-lactate
  - **D**-lactate
  - **M**ethanol
  - **A**spirin
  - **R**enal failure
  - **K**etoacidosis

If You Do Not Like Mnemonics!!!

Type	Increased Anions
Diabetic **ketoacidosis**	β-Hydroxybutyrate, acetoacetate
Alcoholic **ketoacidosis**	β-Hydroxybutyrate, acetoacetate, lactate
Starvation **ketoacidosis**	β-Hydroxybutyrate
Lactic acidosis	Lactate
Renal failure	Phosphate, sulfate, organic anions
Toxins	
Methanol (osmol gap + eye)	Formate, lactate
Ethylene glycol (osmol gap + oxalate)	Oxalate, glycolate
Salicylates (+respiratory alkalosis)	Salicylates
Propylene glycol	Lactate

Possible RTA?

RTA should be suspected
↓
Metabolic **acidosis**+
Hyperchloremia+
Normal plasma anion gap
(In a patient without evidence of gastrointestinal HCO_3^- losses)

Urine Anion Gap
- Urine AG = urine (Na⁺ + K⁺ − Cl⁻)
  The urine AG is **negative** in patients
  with a normal AG metabolic acidosis

  ↓

  This is secondary to an appropriate **increase in urinary ammonium** (unmeasured cation) in order to excrete the excess acid.

Urine Anion Gap — NAGMA
- Urine AG = Urine (Na⁺ + K⁺ − Cl⁻)
- Type 1 (distal) RTA: **Urine AG is positive** (unable to excrete ammonium normally; it is also positive in Type 4)
- Diarrhea: **Urine AG is negative**

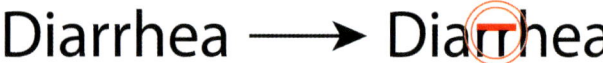

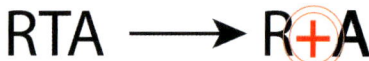

Types of RTA
- **Pearl: Exams like Sjögren syndrome + distal RTA**
- **Proximal RTA (Type 2) — hypokalemia**
  - Isolated bicarbonate defect
  - **Urine anion gap → negative**
  - Fanconi syndrome (**multiple myeloma**), drugs
- **Distal RTA (Type 1) — hypokalemia**
  - Classic type (**Sjögren syndrome**) or **SLE**
  - **Urine anion gap → positive**
  - **Associated with stones and nephrocalcinosis (hypercalciuria → calcium phosphate)**
- **RTA Type 4 (low renin/low aldosterone) — hyperkalemia (diabetes, HIV, obstruction)**
  - **Urine anion gap → positive**

AR 6

A 26-year-old Caucasian female is referred for further evaluation of hypokalemia and acidosis. She was in her usual state of excellent health until 4 months ago when she developed dry mouth and muscle weakness. She was found to have a serum potassium of 2.8 mEq/L and a bicarbonate level of 15 mEq/L during her lab check.

She was treated with oral potassium and bicarbonate supplements, and then she stopped taking these medications. Six weeks later, she developed myalgias and collapsed due to profound weakness. She was found to have a serum bicarbonate level of 14 mEq/L and a serum potassium of 2.0 mEq/L.

ABG: pH 7.29, pCO_2 30 mmHg, pO_2 100 mmHg

Urine K⁺ 46 mEq/L, urine Na⁺ 36 mEq/L, urine Cl⁻ 42 mEq/L, urine Osm 580 mOsm/kg

U/A: pH 6.8, no casts

Which of the following is the correct diagnosis?

A. Type 4 RTA
B. Diarrhea
C. Type 1 RTA (distal RTA)
D. Renal tubular alkalosis
E. Type 2 RTA (proximal RTA)

Answer:_____

METABOLIC ALKALOSIS

Metabolic Alkalosis (Exams Like Metabolic Alkalosis and Urine Chloride)*

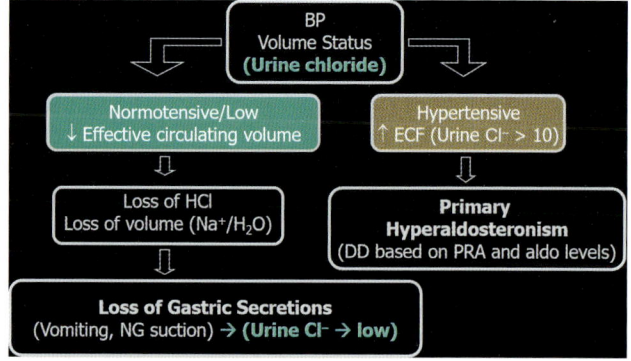

Clues to Acid-Base Disorders*
- Normal ABGs and ↑ AG = **mixed metabolic acidosis/alkalosis**
- Low AG (< 8) = **hypoalbuminemia, paraproteinemia,** hypercalcemia/magnesemia, lithium intoxication
- Osmol gap > 10 = **methanol (blindness), ethanol, ethylene glycol (oxalate crystals)**
- Isopropyl alcohol **osmol gap without acidosis**

HYPERTENSION (HTN)

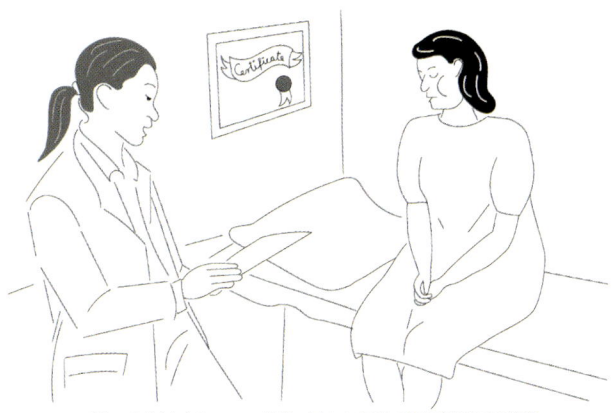

"The only diet shake I recommend is the shake your booty makes when you exercise."

CLASSIFICATION

HTN — JNC 8

- Classification of BP **(JNC 7): definition not addressed in JNC 8**
  - Normal = < 120/80 mmHg
  - Prehypertension: 120–130/80–89 mmHg
  - HTN, Stage 1: 140–159/90–99 mmHg
  - HTN, Stage 2: > 160/100 mmHg
- **Goals of treatment:** Threshold for pharmacologic treatment was defined in JNC 8 based on **age, diabetes, and chronic kidney disease**
  - General population < 60 years of age → < 140/90 mmHg
  - General population **> 60 years of age → < 150/90 mmHg**
  - All ages, no CKD, diabetes + → < 140/90 mmHg
  - All ages CKD+, with/without diabetes → < 140/90 mmHg

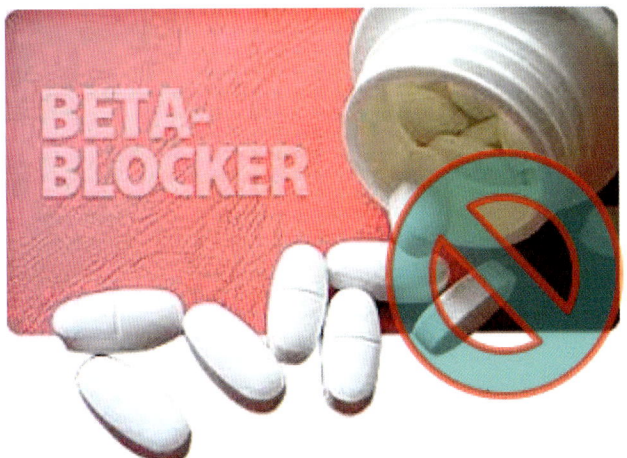

TREATMENT OF HTN

JNC 8 — Treatment of HTN (ACC / AHA 2017 Similar Recommendations)
- **Treatment (lifestyle interventions for all)**
- **Drug therapy**
  - Recommendation based on **CKD and race**
    1) **CKD (regardless of race or diabetes, population > 18 years):** Treatment should include **ACEI or ARB**
    2) **Race** (General population < 60 or > 60 years and diabetic without CKD)
       - **Black** (including those with diabetes): **thiazide or CCB**
       - **Nonblack** (including those with diabetes): **ACEI or ARB, CCB, or thiazide diuretics**
         Can begin with 2 drugs:
         - SBP > 20 mmHg above goal
         - DBP > 10 mmHg above goal

ACC / AHA Guidelines 2017 — Categories of BP Heavily Influenced by SPRINT

BP Category	SBP		DBP
Normal	< 120 mmHg	and	< 80 mmHg
Elevated	120–129 mmHg	and	< 80 mmHg
Hypertension			
Stage 1	130–139 mmHg	or	80–90 mmHg
Stage 2	≥ 140 mmHg	or	≥ 90 mmHg

ACC / AHA Guidelines 2017 — BP Threshold and Goals for Pharmacological Rx

Clinical Condition(s)	BP Threshold (mmHg)	BP Goal (mmHg)
General		
Clinical CVD or 10-yr ASCVD risk ≥ 10%	≥ 130/80	< 130/80
No clinical CVD and 10-yr ASCVD risk < 10%	≥ 140/90	< 130/80
Older persons (≥ 65 years of age; noninstitutionalized, ambulatory, community-living adults)	≥ 130 (SBP)	< 130 (SBP)
Specific Comorbidities		
Diabetes mellitus	≥ 130/80	< 130/80
Chronic kidney disease	≥ 130/80	< 130/80
Chronic kidney disease after renal transplantation	≥ 130/80	< 130/80
Heart failure	≥ 130/80	< 130/80
Stable ischemic heart disease	≥ 130/80	< 130/80
Secondary stroke prevention	≥ 140/90	< 130/80
Secondary stroke prevention (lacunar)	≥ 130/80	< 130/80
Peripheral arterial disease	≥ 130/80	< 130/80

- Compelling indication:*
  - **Stable ischemic heart disease:**
    - 1st line → **β-blockers/ACEI/ARBs**
    - 2nd line → **dihydropyridine calcium channel blockers**
  - **Chronic kidney disease: 1st-line ACEI and 2nd-line ARBs**

Hypertension in Older Adults
- **JNC 8**
  - **Rx of patients > 60 years of age**
  - Threshold for pharmacologic **treatment (> 150/90 mmHg)** strong recommendation — Grade A ... **questions raised by SPRINT**
- **ACC/AHA 2017**
  - Adults > 65 who are noninstitutionalized ambulatory community dwelling: **goal SBP < 130**
  - If presence of high comorbidity and limited life expectancy: clinical judgment
- Evaluate for secondary cause, if new diagnosis after 65 years of age

Antihypertensive Diuretic
- **Chlorthalidone** recommended over hydrochlorothiazide
  - HCTZ less potent and shorter acting
  - Problems: lack of fixed-dose combinations and no 12.5-mg tablet, more likely to induce hypokalemia
- Loop diuretics for **HF and CKD**

ARB + ACEI (Do Not Use Together)
- > 2× risk
  - Acute kidney injury
  - Hyperkalemia
  - ONTARGET (negative study: Rx to prevent vascular events in patients with CAD/DM)
- Previous indication for combination was persistence of proteinuria > 1 g following trial on ARB or ACEI
  - **Lancet retracted the COOPERATE trial in 2009**
  - Would recommend adding nondihydropyridine CCB (diltiazem) or spironolactone

SECONDARY HTN

Indicators of Secondary HTN
- Abrupt or accelerated
- Onset < 30 years or > 65 years
- Malignant/accelerated/resistant HTN
- Systolic-diastolic epigastric or renal bruits
- **Hypokalemia with metabolic alkalosis**

Common Causes of Secondary HTN
- **Structural**
  - Coarctation of aorta (UE BP > LE BP)
- **Renal**
  - Chronic kidney disease
- **Renovascular**
  - Renal artery stenosis (atherosclerosis vs. FMD → young females)
- **Endocrine**
  - Adrenal
    - **Primary aldosteronism (very important — know the work up)**
    - **Cushing syndrome (cortisol acts like aldosterone)**
    - Pheochromocytoma
  - Thyroid disorders/parathyroid disorders
- **Medication (important cause of resistant HTN)**
  - Pseudoephedrine
  - NSAIDs
  - Herbals
  - Excessive salt intake
- **Sleep apnea (important cause of resistant HTN)**

Hypokalemic Hypertensive

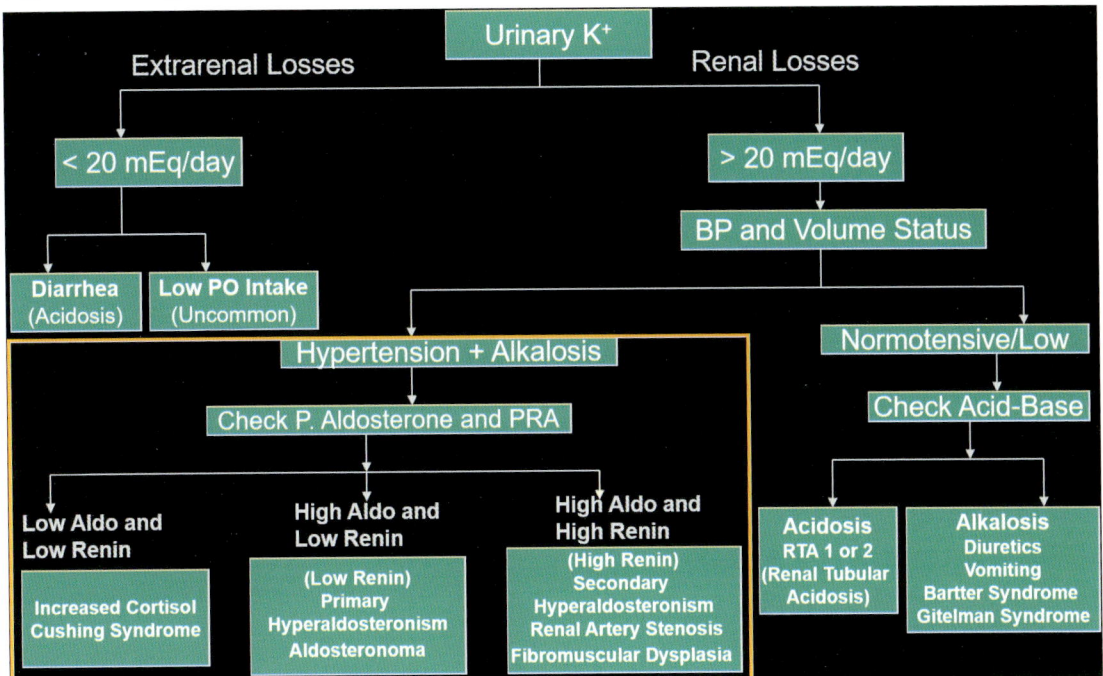

- If you have no idea what I'm talking about …
- If "hyperreninemic" and "hyperaldo" sounds like gibberish to you …
- When you see a <u>hypertensive patient with hypokalemia</u>, think:
  PAC:PRA!
- If you're in practice: **Get help!**

Primary Aldosteronism

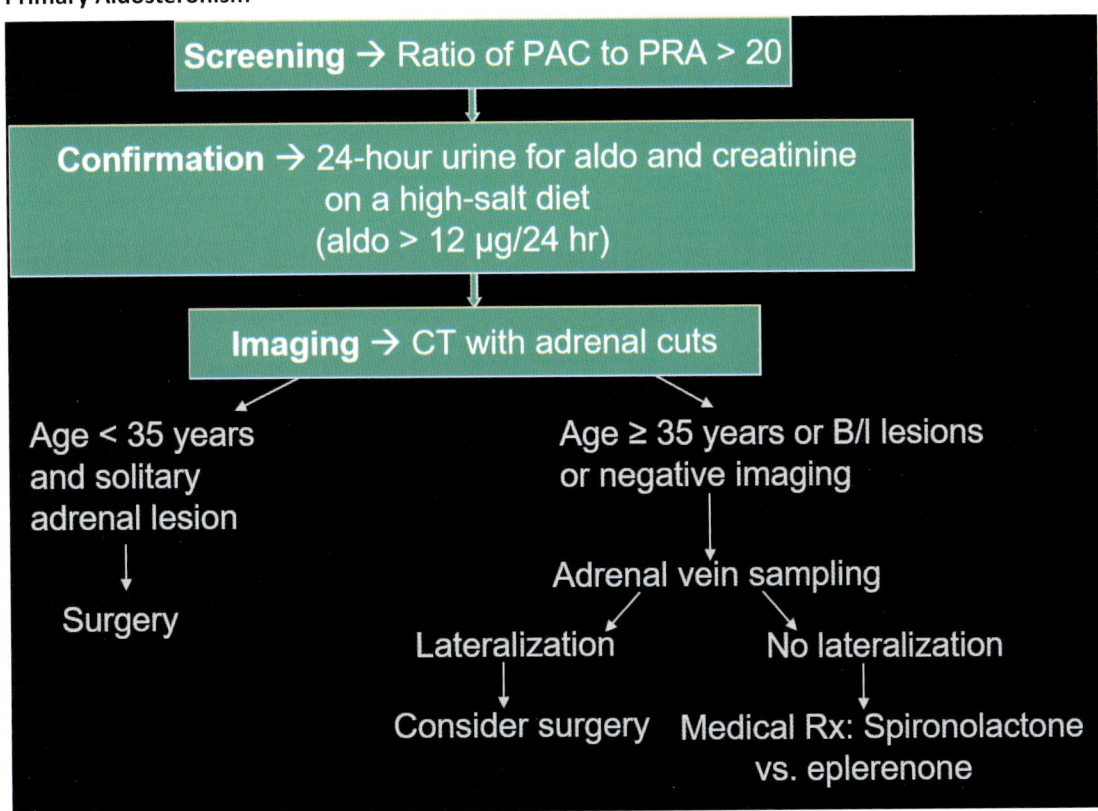

AR 7

A 22-year-old woman referred from GYN for BP eval:

Previous BPs 149/92 mmHg and 154/95 mmHg

Review of systems negative

No family history of HTN

PE: 155/94 mmHg, HR 86 bpm, afebrile, RR 14 breaths/min

Examination normal

Na⁺ 142 mEq/L, K⁺ 2.9 mEq/L, Cl⁻ 104 mEq/L, HCO₃⁻ 32 mEq/L, BUN 10 mg/dL, Cr 0.6 mg/dL, BG 102 mg/dL

CBC normal

Which of the following is the most appropriate next step in her management?

A. CT scan of the adrenals
B. Ratio of plasma aldosterone concentration to plasma renin activity
C. Helical CT of the renal vasculature
D. Morning cortisol level
E. Captopril renal scintigraphy

Answer:_____

AR 8

Based on the last question, which of the following is the most likely diagnosis if both PRA and plasma aldosterone levels returned high?

A. Renal artery stenosis
B. Fibromuscular dysplasia
C. Primary aldosteronism (adrenal adenoma)
D. Bilateral adrenal hyperplasia
E. Cushing syndrome

Answer:_____

DISORDERS OF HOMEOSTASIS

Hyponatremia and Hypernatremia (Disorders of Water Homeostasis)

Hypernatremia → [Na⁺] > 145 mEq/L

and

Hyponatremia → [Na⁺] < 135 mEq/L

**Represent
disorders of water homeostasis
(or the concentration of serum Na⁺)**

$$P_{Osm} = 2[Na^+] + BG/18 + BUN/2.8$$

ADH Regulates Water Balance

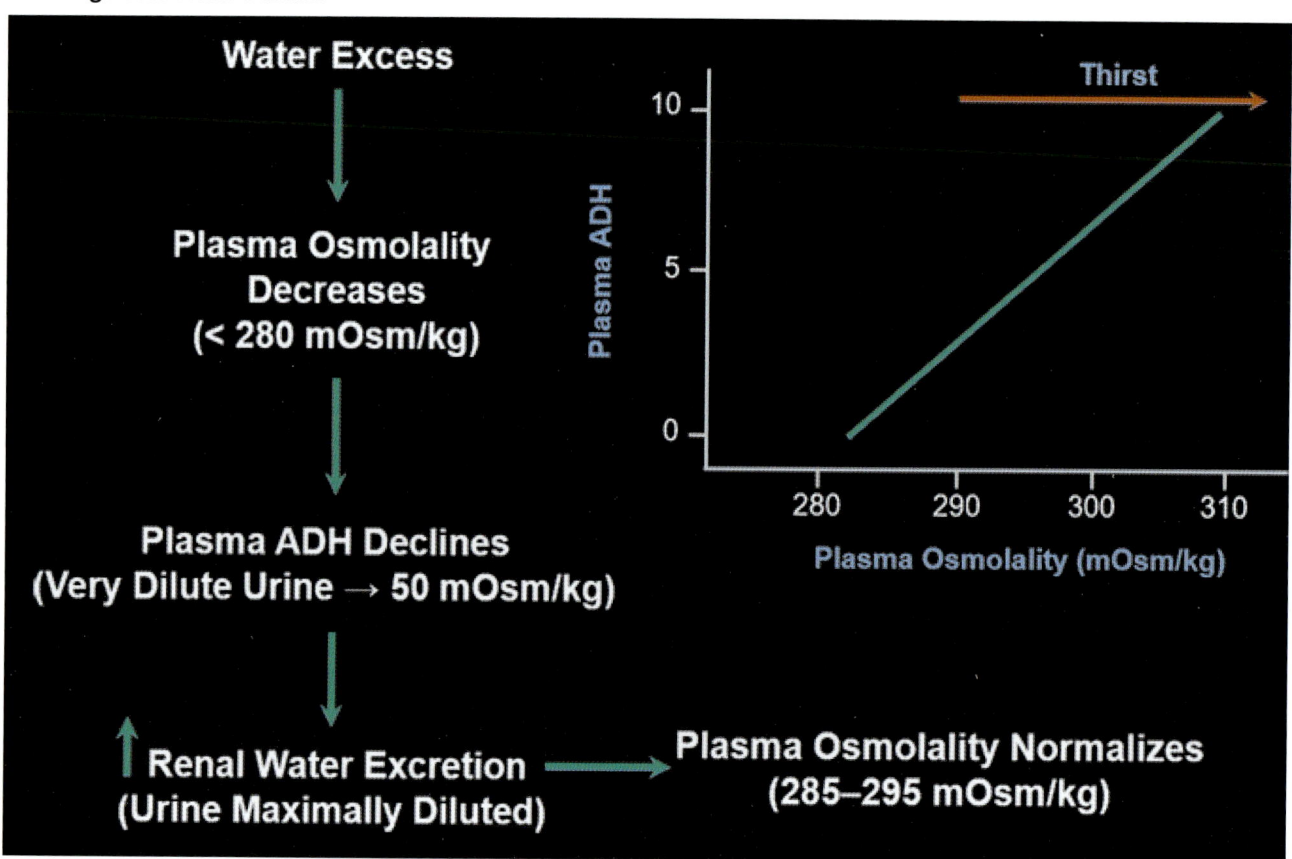

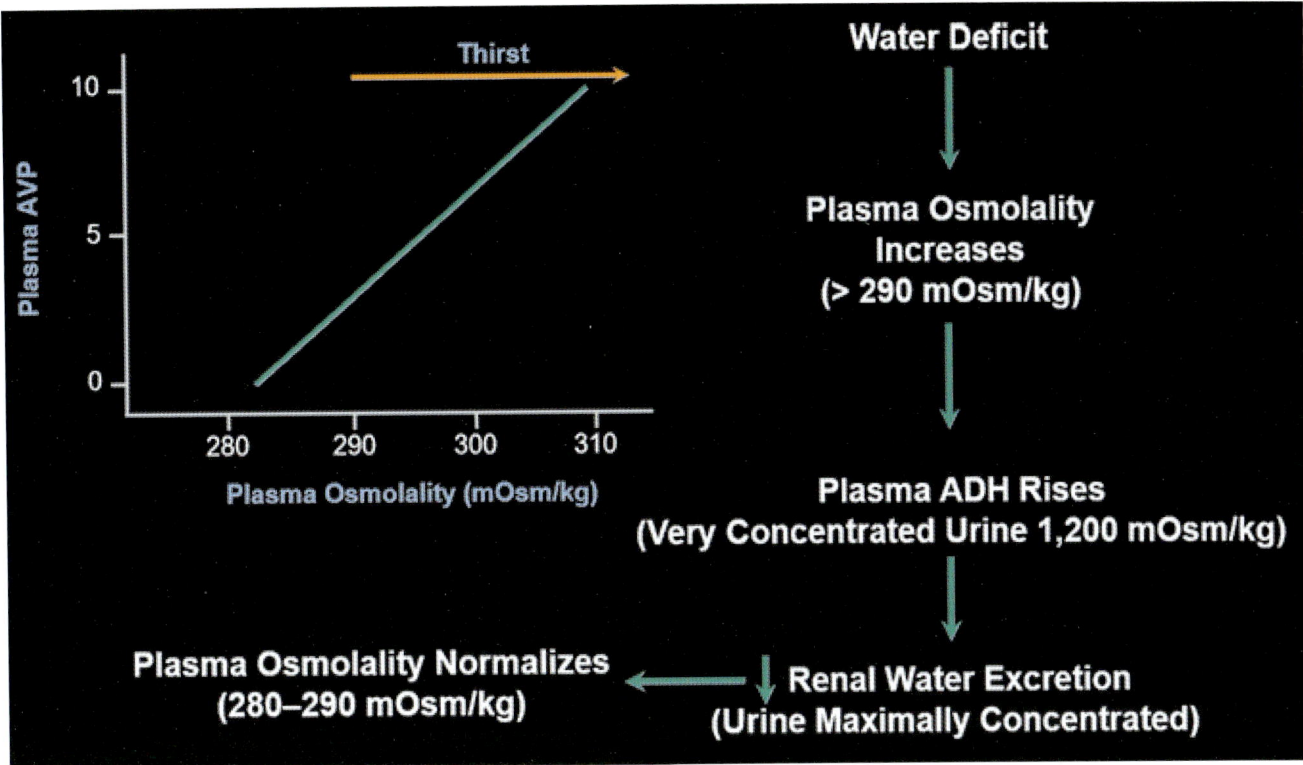

Physiological Stimuli for ADH Release
- Elevated plasma osmolality
- Decreased effective arterial blood volume
  - Hypotension
  - Hypovolemia
- Endogenous stimuli
  - Nausea
  - Pain

HYPONATREMIA

How Does Hyponatremia Develop?
- **Physiology**
  - **Huge water intake** with normal water excretion (i.e., psychogenic polydipsia)

    or
  - Normal water intake with **impaired water excretion** (common)
- **Factors causing impaired water excretion**
  1) **High ADH**
     - Promotes water reabsorption in collecting duct
  2) **Low EABV**
     - Enhances ADH secretion
     - promotes proximal fluid reabsorption resulting in decreased distal delivery

Water Intake > Water Excretion
Must have water intake!

Approach to Hyponatremia
- **Measure plasma osmolality → need to know P_{Osm}**
  - When low, defines true hypoosmolar state or clinical hyponatremia
  - If high → plasma glucose; if normal → protein and lipids
- **Assess volume status → need to know volume status**
  - Clinical parameters: **orthostatics, JVD, S_3 gallop, lung exam/pedal edema, skin turgor**
  - Objective assessment of volume status: $U_{Na} < 20$, Fe_{Na} and $Fe_{Urea} < 35$ consistent with hypovolemic state
- **Urine osmolality and urine sodium → need U_{Na}, U_{Osm}**
  - Urine osmolality → presence of ADH
  - Urine Na^+ → if low, suggest volume depletion

Approach to Differential Diagnosis — Hyponatremia

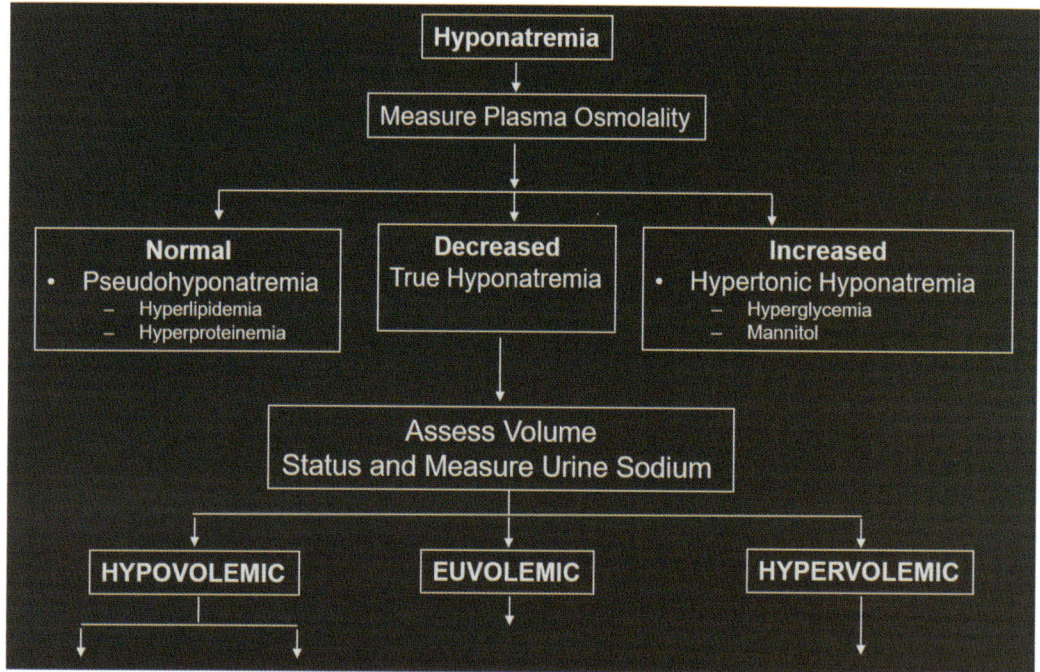

Hyponatremia — Further Investigation

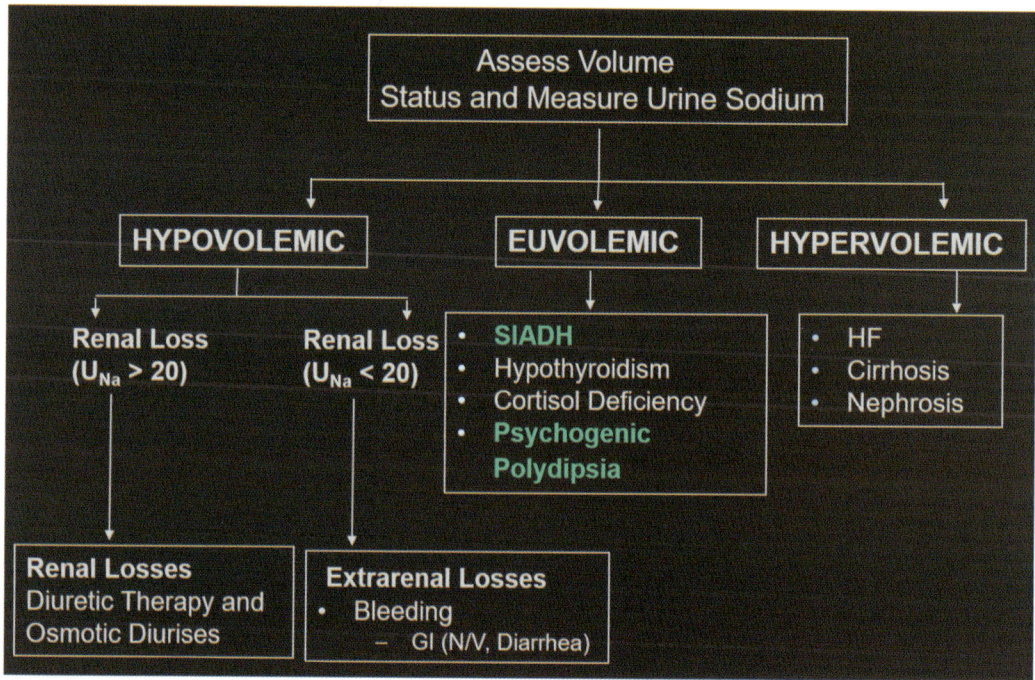

SIADH

- **Diagnosis**
  - Hypoosmotic hyponatremia
    1) In a euvolemic patient **(no suggestion of volume depletion and urine Na$^+$ > 20)***
    2) An inappropriately concentrated urine **(high urine osmolality suggesting presence of ADH)**
    3) **Cortisol deficiency and thyroid disease needs to be ruled out***

Inappropriate Stimuli for ADH Release
- **SIADH**
  - Drugs (e.g., SSRI, phenothiazines, cyclophosphamide)
  - Pulmonary diseases
  - CNS disease
  - Malignancies (small cell cancer)

A Prudent Approach to the Treatment of Hyponatremia
Symptomatic Hyponatremia
(Acute — duration < 48 hours)
1) Risk for complication of **cerebral edema greater than risk of treatment of complication**
2) Treat with hypertonic NaCl: **3% NaCl (1 mL/kg/hr) until convulsions subside**

Symptomatic hyponatremia
(chronic or unknown duration)
1) Do not increase serum sodium by **more than 8 mEq/day** (if the serum sodium increases too rapidly, interrupt the increase by starting hypotonic fluids and/or desmopressin [DDAVP] 4 mcg SC)*
2) **Long term**
   A) H_2O restriction
   B) Oral urea / Sodium chloride tablets
   C) Demeclocycline 300–600 mg bid
   D) V_2 receptor antagonist → aquaretics (tolvaptan)

Points to Remember!!!
- In evaluating patients with **hyponatremia**
  - 1st determine the **osmolarity**
  - If patient is hypoosmolar, then assess the **volume status**
  - Differential depends on the volume status

HYPERNATREMIA

How Does Hypernatremia Develop?
- **Physiology**
  - Plasma osmolality increase stimulates ADH secretion and thirst, which results in decreased water excretion (ADH) and increased water intake (thirst)
    - → **Absence of hypernatremia in normal subjects**
  - For persistent hypernatremia:
    - There should be either a **defect in thirst mechanism**
      or
    - **Access to free water is restricted** (older patients with confusion, or infants)

Points to Remember!!!*
- In evaluating patients with **hypernatremia**
  - Remember both ADH secretion and thirst are necessary physiologic responses to defend against the development of hypernatremia
  - **If urine osmolality is high → water deprivation** (access to water) or thirst problems (hypodipsic)
  - **If urine osmolality is low → central or nephrogenic diabetes insipidus**

Central Diabetes Insipidus
- Etiologies
  - Idiopathic
  - Tumor or infiltration (e.g., sarcoid, histiocytosis, TB)
  - Surgery or trauma
  - CVA
- With water restriction
  - **Will respond to ADH administration**
- Treatment
  - **Desmopressin** is primary therapy

Nephrogenic Diabetes Insipidus
- Collecting tubule does not respond to ADH → polydipsia
- Etiologies
  - Hereditary: X-linked defect in V2 receptor gene
  - Drugs: **lithium,** demeclocycline, Ampho B
  - **Hypercalcemia,** hypokalemia, **Sjögren's**
- Rx: **thiazide diuretics**
  - Cause volume depletion and increase proximal water absorption, so little is delivered to distal tubules

Evaluation of Polyuria (Urine Output Exceeding 3 L per Day)

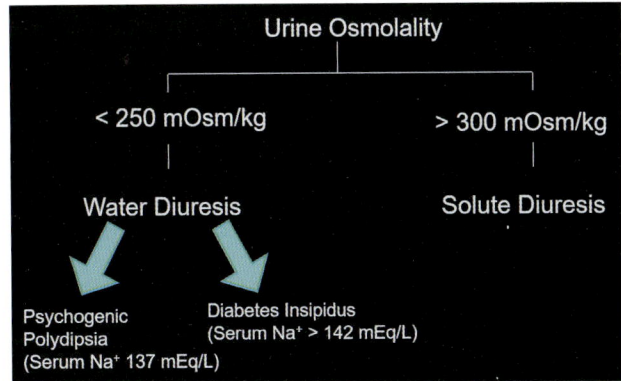

AR 9
A 76-year-old male smoker:

Admitted with 3 weeks of falling and dizziness

Lost 20 lb in the past 6 months

Exam: BP 120/80 mmHg, HR 85 bpm (lying and standing)

Chest: end-expiratory wheezes

Na^+ 116 mEq/L, S_{Osm} 241 mOsm/kg, Urine Na^+ 25 mEq/L, U_{Osm} 673 mOsm/kg

TSH normal; cortisol is normal

Which of the following is the most likely diagnosis?

A. Central diabetes insipidus
B. Nephrogenic diabetes insipidus
C. Beer potomania
D. SIADH
E. Volume depletion

Answer:_____

POTASSIUM DISORDERS

Electrolyte and Mineral Disorders
- **Hypokalemia and Hyperkalemia**
- **Calcium Homeostasis**
- **Hypomagnesemia**

HYPOKALEMIA

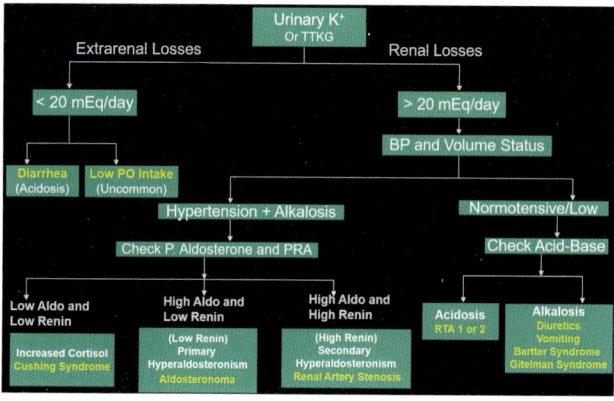

- Management issue: <u>AMI</u>
  - GISSI-2 study, 1998
    - 2× increased risk of <u>ventricular fibrillation</u> when K⁺ < 3.6 mEq/L
    - Recommendation: keep <u>K⁺ > 4.0 mEq/L</u> and <u>Mg²⁺ > 2.0 mEq/L</u> in patients post-MI

HYPERKALEMIA

Hyperkalemia — Inhibitors of the Renin-Angiotensin-Aldosterone System

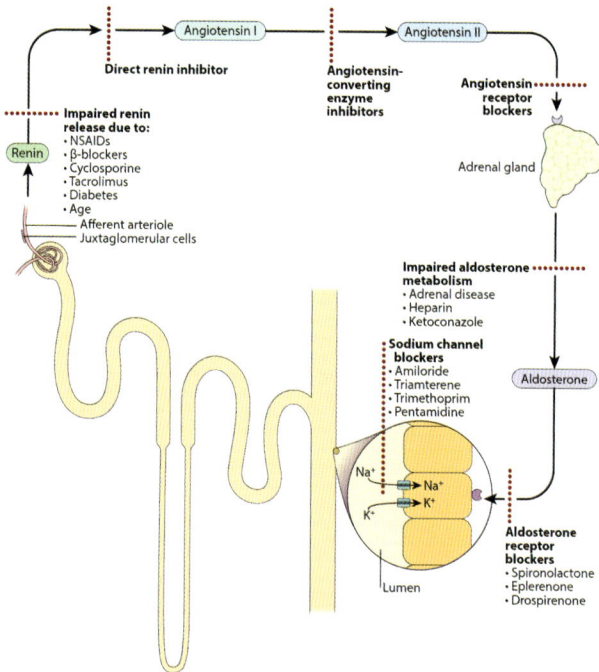

Acute Hyperkalemia

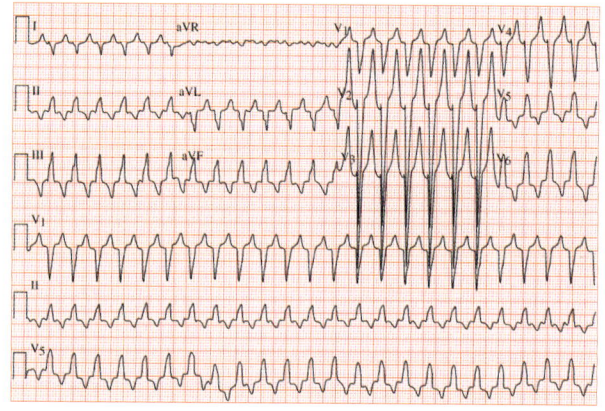

- **ECG Changes**
  - <u>Peaked T waves</u>
  - <u>Widened QRS</u>
  - Loss of P waves
  - Bradyarrhythmias

Hyperkalemia — Treatment

- Treatment is **urgent if K+ > 7 mEq/L**
1) **Cardioprotection (1st thing to do if ECG changes present)**
   - Calcium gluconate for membrane stabilization
   - ECG monitor
2) **Redistribution**
   - Glucose + insulin
   - Bicarbonate
   - β-Adrenergic agonist (albuterol inhaled)
3) **Loss**
   - Cation-exchange resins (newer agents preferred)
     - Patiromer: 8.4 g once daily (Veltassa)
     - Zirconium cyclosilicate: 10 g tid for 8 hours (Lokelma)
     - Avoid sodium polystyrene sulfate (Kalexate, Kayexalate, Kionex)
   - Diuretics (furosemide)
   - Dialysis

CALCIUM, PHOSPHORUS, AND MAGNESIUM DISORDERS

Causes of Hypercalcemia

(1st test → parathyroid hormone [PTH])*

- Malignancy → **low PTH**
  - Multiple myeloma: IL6
  - Lymphomas: increased production of 1,25 hydroxy vitamin D
  - Solid tumors (e.g., squamous cell cancer, lung cancer): PTH-related peptide
- Granulomatous disease including fungal infections → **low PTH**
- Milk alkali syndrome or excessive calcium and vitamin D intake → **low PTH**
- Primary hyperparathyroidism → **high PTH**
  - Asymptomatic
  - **Bones** (osteoporosis/osteopenia)
  - **Stones** (calcium oxalate)
  - **Moans** (constipation)
  - **Groans** (weakness & fatigue)
  - Osteitis fibrosa cystica: subperiosteal bone resorption radial middle phalanges
- Familial hypocalciuric hypercalcemia (FHH) → **high PTH**

Primary Hyperparathyroidism

- Diagnosis is simple
  - **High Ca^{2+} and low phos**
  - Normal or ↑ PTH
    - Clearly inappropriate if the Ca^{2+} is high
    - Be aware: Even normal PTH is inappropriate!*
  - High urine calcium increases the risk of stones* **(Pearl: distinguishes it from FHH)**

Familial Hypocalciuric Hypercalcemia (FHH)

- Common distractor on exams when primary hyperparathyroidism is the correct answer*
- Autosomal dominant (defect in **calcium-sensing receptor**)
- No clinical features of hypercalcemia
  - Ca^{2+} with normal or ↑ PTH
  - > 99% urine calcium absorption **(These patients are hypocalciuric)*** in contrast to hypercalciuria with primary hyperparathyroidism
- No treatment

Primary vs. Secondary Hyperparathyroidism

- Both have **increased PTH (p**hosphate-**t**rashing **h**ormone) **levels**
- Primary occurs when PTH is **inappropriately** released → high calcium and low phosphorus
- Secondary occurs when **calcium is low/normal** in CKD and **phosphorus is high**
- ****Look at the clinical case; is CKD present or not? Pearl: hyperphosphatemia → secondary due to CKD****

Calcium Management Issues

- Hypercalcemia
  - *Saline: 1st (loop diuretics are out)
  - Calcitonin (1st 48°)
  - *Bisphosphonates
    - Pamidronate
    - Etidronate
    - Zoledronic acid
    - Do not forget about jaw osteonecrosis
  - Steroids
- Hypocalcemia
  - Always check Mg^{2+}
  - Long QT

AR 11

A 55-year-old female:

PMH squamous cell lung cancer 2 years ago

Doing fine

Exam normal

Calcium 11.4 mg/dL (9–10.5)

Calcium over previous 3 years 9.0–10.0 mg/dL

PO$_4$ 2.1 mg/dL

Alkaline phosphatase (ALP)

180 U/L (36–92)

Cr 1.2 mg/dL

PTH 108 pg/mL (10–60)

Which of the following is the most likely cause of her hypercalcemia?

A. Hypercalcemia of malignancy
B. Vitamin D deficiency
C. Primary hyperparathyroidism
D. Osteoporosis
E. Familial hypocalciuric hypercalcemia

Answer:_____

Hypomagnesemia

- Etiologies
  - Diarrhea
  - Drugs: thiazides, aminoglycosides, penicillins
  - Alcohol abuse
  - **New: chronic use of proton pump inhibitors!**
    - <u>Sometimes refractory to supplementation unless discontinue the PPI!</u>
- Treatment: magnesium sulfate PO or IV

CHRONIC KIDNEY DISEASE (CKD)

- Structural/Functional kidney abnormalities × 3 months
  or
- Decreased GFR, with or without evidence of kidney damage

NKF KDOQI CKD Staging Classification

Stage	Description	GFR (mL/min/1.73 m²)
1	Chronic kidney damage with normal or ↑ GFR	> 90
2	Mild ↓ GFR	60–89*
3	3a: Moderate ↓ GFR	45–59
	3b: Moderate ↓ GFR	30–44
4	Severe ↓ GFR	15–29
5	Kidney failure	< 15 or dialysis

CKD and CHD

- Substantial increase in CHD risk
  - RFs: HTN, DM, metabolic risk
  - Increase in CHD even without these RFs
- Know that the risk of death from CHD is higher than progression to dialysis in patients with CKD
- ? Coronary artery calcification related to increased calcium phosphate product

CKD — Miscellaneous Management

- **ACEI/ARBs:** Okay if creatinine ↑ up to 30% over baseline if stabilizes within 4 months; do not discontinue! **Reduce proteinuria — Do not use ACEI and ARB together**
  - **Blood pressure goal < 130/80 mmHg (KDIGO 2021 suggests that systolic BP in CKD < 120/80 mmHg when a standardized office BP is measured)***
- NaHCO₃: **Treat acidosis** to maintain **HCO₃⁻ > 22 mEq/L** (slows progression and improves nutrition in Stage 4)
- **Secondary hyperparathyroidism** and CKD-associated bone and mineral disease
  - **Inability to excrete PO₄ → ↑ PO₄ → ↑ PTH ← ↓ 1,25 vitamin D**
    - **1ˢᵗ →** control phosphorus level
    - **2ⁿᵈ →** start active 1,25 hydroxy vitamin D (calcitriol)

Control of Hyperphosphatemia and Secondary Hyperparathyroidism in CKD

1) **Diet:** Reduce dietary P intake (< 800 mg)
2) **Binders (1ˢᵗ):** Prevent gut absorption of P with binders
   - **Calcium based if Ca²⁺**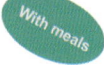
     1) Calcium acetate
     2) Calcium carbonate
   - **Noncalcium-, nonaluminum-based if normal or high serum Ca²⁺**
     1) Sevelamer (Renagel, Renvela)
     2) Lanthanum (Fosrenol)
3) **Vitamin D (2ⁿᵈ):** Prevent severe secondary hyperparathyroidism and attendant effluxes of P and Ca²⁺ from bone
   - Tx elevated PTH with vitamin D/vitamin D analogues → calcitriol

CKD — Miscellaneous Management CKD

- Do not forget **anemia recommendations**
  - Replace iron 1ˢᵗ and rule out other causes of anemia
  - Erythropoietin stimulating agents to target Hgb 10–11 mg/dL

Gadolinium and CKD*
(Nephrogenic systemic fibrosis)*

Fibrosing disorder (thickening and hardening of skin and fibrosis in organs) related exposure to gadolinium containing agents in patients with reduced kidney function

- **FDA recommend avoidance in CKD with GFR < 30 mL/min/1.73 m², ESRD and acute kidney injury**
- American College of Radiology states to avoid it for patients with GFR of < 44 mL/min/1.73 m²

POLYCYSTIC KIDNEY DISEASE (PKD)

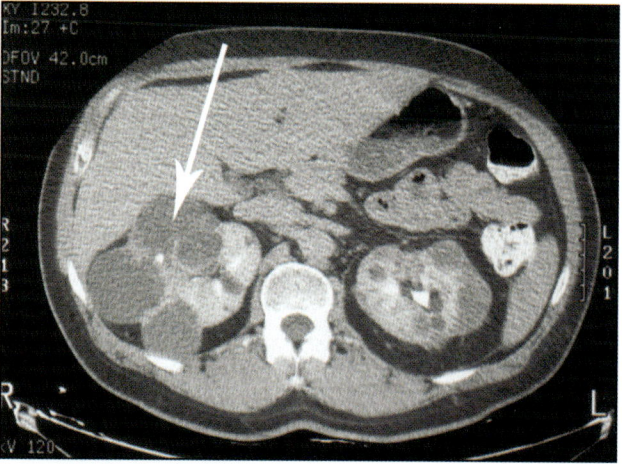

Complications of PCKD

- Renal failure, hypertension
- Hemorrhage into cysts
- Infected cysts → **use ciprofloxacin**
- <u>40% of patients have cysts in liver</u>
- High risk for stones
- <u>Association with cerebral aneurysms* →</u> **<u>Do not screen unless h/o aneurysms in 1ˢᵗ-degree relative or high-risk occupation</u>**

AUDIENCE RESPONSE ANSWERS

Audience Response 1
D. Acute phosphate nephropathy

AR 2
D. Place a Foley catheter in the bladder.

AR 3
E. IgA nephropathy

AR 4
D. Urine and serum electrophoresis

AR 5
D. Membranous nephropathy

AR 6
C. Type 1 RTA (distal RTA)

AR 7
B. Ratio of plasma aldosterone concentration to plasma renin activity

AR 8
B. Fibromuscular dysplasia

AR 9
D. SIADH

AR 10
A. High urine osmolality and high urine Na^+

AR 11
C. Primary hyperparathyroidism

ENDNOTES

[1]   Ron D, et al. Prevention of acute renal failure in traumatic rhabdomyolysis. *Arch Intern Med.* 1984 Feb;144(2):277–280.

[2]   Geevasinga N, et al. *Clin Gastroenterol Hepatol.* 2006;4:597–604

[3]   Merten GJ, et al. Prevention of contrast-induced nephropathy with sodium bicarbonate: A randomized controlled trial. *JAMA.* 2004 May 19;291(19):2328–2334.

[4]   Curhan GC, et al. A prospective study of dietary calcium and other nutrients and the risk of symptomatic kidney stone. *NEJM.* 1993;328:833–838.

NEPHROLOGY

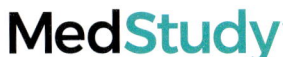

INTERNAL MEDICINE REVIEW

Neurology

Presented by

Robert Kowalski, MD, MS

TABLE OF CONTENTS

Why We Moved Some Slide Information to the Audience Response Answers Page

At MedStudy, we do all we can to optimize your self-testing and learning.

In this presentation, the speaker will give some extra information after their AR questions to help explain the correct and incorrect answers. To keep from interfering with your self-testing, we've moved that explanatory text to the Audience Response Answers page(s) at the end of the section.

Be assured, all the content on the slides is in your syllabus—so you can focus on the teaching instead of taking detailed notes.

Outline of Major Topics
- Neuromuscular Junction Disease
- Peripheral Nerve and Back Pain
- Muscle Disease
- Motor Neuron Disease
- Vertigo
- Movement Disorders
- Headache
- Epilepsy
- Stroke
- Dementia
- Multiple Sclerosis

DISEASES OF THE NEUROMUSCULAR JUNCTION

MYASTHENIA GRAVIS (MG)

Audience Response 1

A 33-year-old female presents with ptosis of the left eye. On exam, she has a dysconjugate gaze that worsens with fatigue and has weakness of her proximal arms and legs.

Her sensation is normal.

Reflexes are 2+.

No dysmetria

No ataxia

Audience Response 1[1]

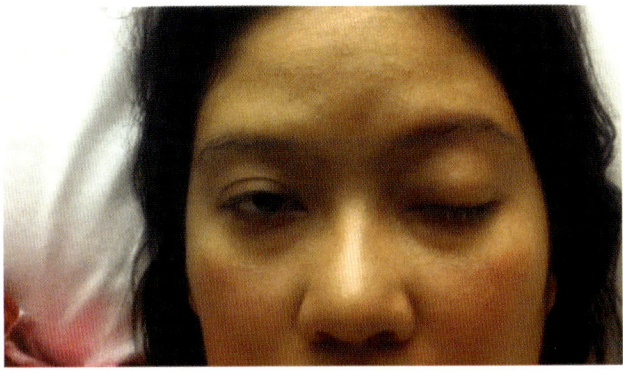

Which test is most likely to be abnormal in this patient?

A. MRI brain
B. CT chest
C. CT abdomen
D. MRI cervical spine

Answer:_____

Myasthenia Gravis
- Clinical features: ocular, bulbar, or proximal weakness (fatigable)
- Evaluation
    - AChR Ab (binding, blocking, modulating); if negative, test MUSK Ab
    - EMG (decrement)
    - CT chest or MRI to rule out thymoma (15%)
- Treatment
    - Anticholinesterase therapy: pyridostigmine
    - Corticosteroids
    - Plasmapheresis or IVIG (crisis)
    - Surgery (thymectomy)
    - Other immunosuppressants (e.g., azathioprine, mycophenolate)

Rep Nerve Stim R Orb Oris

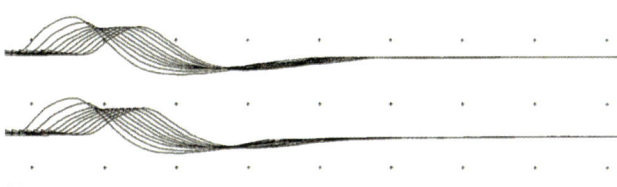

[2]

LAMBERT-EATON MYASTHENIC SYNDROME (LEMS)

Lambert-Eaton's
- Symptoms may be similar to myasthenia, except instead of fatiguing, the patient may actually get "facilitation" with exercise
- > 50% of cases paraneoplastic (mostly small cell lung cancer)
- Reflexes are hyporeflexic and there are more autonomic symptoms like dry mouth, blurred vision, constipation, impotence
- Involvement of the voltage-gated presynaptic Ca^{2+} channel antibody and <u>increment</u> on high-frequency repetitive nerve stimulation

NEUROLOGY

AR 2

A 25-year-old male presents with acute dysphagia for the past 2 days. He is found to have ophthalmoparesis, bilateral ptosis, proximal muscle weakness, and decreased reflexes. His sensation and coordination are normal. His pupils are enlarged and poorly reactive.

Pre- and post-10-second exercise of thumb, demonstrating increment:

Motor NCS R Median – APB

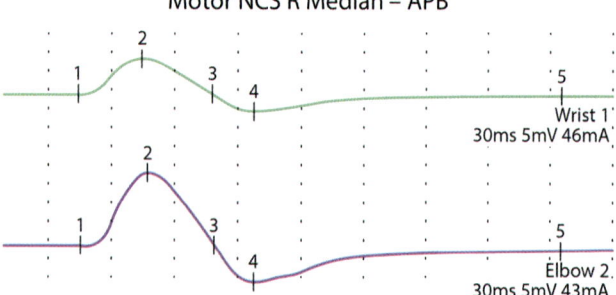

Wrist 1
30ms 5mV 46mA

Elbow 2
30ms 5mV 43mA

[3]

Which is the most likely diagnosis?

A. Myasthenia gravis
B. Lambert-Eaton myasthenic syndrome
C. Botulism
D. Ciguatoxicity
E. Hypercalcemia

Answer:_____

NEUROPATHIES

MONONEUROPATHIES

AR 3

A 44-year-old female presents with a 2-month history of waking up at night with her whole right hand tingling. She has pain in the wrist at times but no pain elsewhere.

PMH of HTN and hypothyroid

Medications include HCTZ and levothyroxine.

On neuro exam, AAO × 3

CN intact

There is decreased sensation over digits 1–3 on the right.

Muscle bulk and strength are normal.

2+ reflexes

No dysmetria

No ataxia

What is your best next step in management?

A. Night splints
B. MRI cervical spine
C. Steroid taper
D. Steroid injection
E. Orthopedic hand surgeon referral

Answer:_____

Focal Neuropathy

Disorder	Associations
Median neuropathy — carpal tunnel	Sensory involvement of first 1–3 digits; nocturnal symptoms; Tinel sign and Phalen test; more severe cases with weakness ± atrophy of thenar eminence; EMG helpful to localize and grade cases; for milder cases, bracing at night initially; steroid injection as an intermediate option; for more significant cases, surgery
Ulnar neuropathy	Most commonly across the elbow; medial hand sensory loss; more severe cases with interossei weakness and atrophy; EMG helpful to localize and grade cases; milder cases, avoid resting elbow precariously; more significant cases, consider surgery
Radial neuropathy	Think "Saturday night palsy"; wrist drop — compression across the spiral groove; EMG helpful to localize; supportive care; typically excellent recovery
Femoral neuropathy	Weakness of knee extension and hip flexion; absent patellar reflex; think about a case of retroperitoneal hematoma
Peroneal neuropathy	Think compressive across the fibular head; foot drop with poor eversion but retained inversion and plantarflexion; EMG helpful to localize; supportive care — AFO; low-weight patients, frequently crossing legs or resting leg against fibular head region

Localization

L3–4	Absent patellar reflex	Knee extension weakness
L5	------------------------	Dorsiflexion weakness; both inversion and eversion weakness; decreased sensation dorsum of foot
S1	Absent ankle reflex	Plantarflexion weakness; decreased sensation bottom of foot

POLYNEUROPATHIES

AR 4

A 35-year-old male presents with back pain radiating down his right leg for the past week and a half.

No PMH

On exam: CN intact

Motor 5/5

Straight-leg raising test elicits radiating pain. He gets tingling on the bottom of his foot.

His ankle reflex is absent asymmetrically on the right.

What is the most appropriate statement and plan at this point?

A. Lumbar strain; provide conservative treatment.
B. S1 radiculopathy; provide conservative treatment.
C. L5 radiculopathy; provide conservative treatment.
D. S1 radiculopathy; confirm with MRI L spine.
E. L5 radiculopathy; confirm with MRI L spine.

Answer:_____

Guillain-Barré Syndrome (GBS)
- Antecedent viral URI prodrome or history of diarrhea (*Campylobacter*)
- Ascending, symmetric, paralysis (proximal and distal involvement) with areflexia, back pain, some sensory involvement
- Monitor closely for respiratory failure and for autonomic dysfunction
- CSF
  - Cytoalbuminologic dissociation (elevated protein with normal WBC)
- Miller-Fisher variant — axonal variant with areflexia, ataxia, and ophthalmoplegia; associated with anti-GQ1b (ganglioside) antibodies

GBS — AAN Practice Parameter 2003
- IVIG and plasmapheresis are equivalent
- For ambulant patients within 2 weeks of onset of symptoms or nonambulant patients within 4 weeks of symptoms, proceed with plasmapheresis
- For patients requiring an ambulation aid, IVIG started within 2–4 weeks from onset of symptoms
- Corticosteroids not proven efficacious
- IVIG followed by PE or vice versa provides no additional benefit

CIDP
- Autoimmune neuropathy with > 8 weeks of progression or relapsing
- Proximal and distal muscle weakness on exam with more diffuse rather than length-dependent areflexia
- Demyelinating features, especially conduction blocks on EMG
- Elevated CSF protein
- Treatment: IVIG, steroids, apheresis, steroid-sparing agents (e.g., azathioprine, mycophenolate)

General Metabolic Neuropathy Workup

	General Neuropathy Screen
OGTT	Diabetes or impaired glucose tolerance most common cause; OGTT more sensitive than A1c
B$_{12}$	If borderline low (i.e., < 350), still check methylmalonic acid
TSH	Associations with thyroid — carpal tunnel, neuropathy, myopathy
Serum Immunofixation	MGUS, but also could hint toward hematological conditions, such as multiple myeloma, amyloid, or Waldenström's
Idiopathic	1/3, sensory predominant, pain
Toxic	Temporally linked with exposure, coasting; chemo, HIV meds, alcohol on the top of the list; lead — wrist drop

MYOPATHIES

Inflammatory Myopathy
- Subacute weakness, elevated CK
- Dermatomyositis: rash and myopathy; path — perifascicular atrophy
- Polymyositis: path — inflammation invading nonnecrotic muscle fibers
- **Dermatomyositis and polymyositis — also rule out underlying malignancy**
- Inclusion body myositis: does not respond well to immunomodulation, finger flexor and knee extensor weakness; path — vacuoles, amyloid
- Treatment options: steroid, IVIG, methotrexate, rituximab, azathioprine, mycophenolate

Dermatomyositis

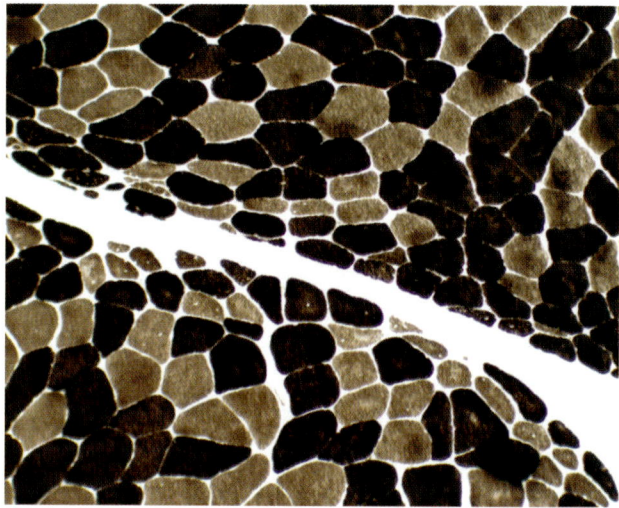

Perifascicular atrophy on biopsy

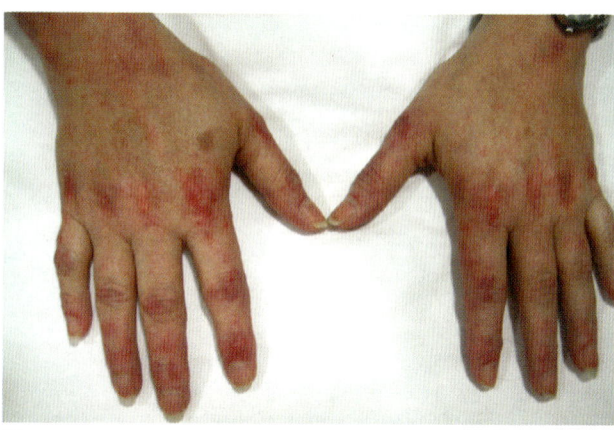

[4]

Gottron papules on skin

AR 5

A 67-year-old presents with a 5-month history of progressive weakness. It began with a right foot drop but has been progressing slowly to other limbs as well.

He has atrophy of associated muscles of weakness with some fasciculations.

DTRs are 3+ throughout with upgoing plantars bilaterally.

He has normal sensation.

No ataxia; no dysmetria

Which is the best medication management choice?

A. Prednisone
B. Azathioprine
C. Pyridostigmine
D. Creatine
E. Riluzole

Answer:_____

Motor Neuron Disease

- Amyotrophic lateral sclerosis (a.k.a. Lou Gehrig disease)
- Most common anterior horn cell disease (motor neuron disease)
- Hallmark — simultaneous upper and lower motor neuron signs
- Tongue fasciculations
- Progressive disease with pseudobulbar affect
- Prognosis — 3–5 years with variance
- Riluzole, edaravone (approved in 2017)
- Differential includes B_{12} deficiency, cervical myelopathy, syringomyelia

DIZZINESS AND VERTIGO

AR 6

A 47-year-old male presents with vertigo to your office. This has been going on for 1 week. He describes multiple discrete bouts of an intense room-spinning sensation multiple times per day. The attacks last about 15 seconds at a time and are generally triggered by standing up or looking to the left.

PMH: lupus

Medications: hydroxychloroquine

Neurologic exam demonstrates no dysmetria or ataxia.

Which treatment is the most likely to be effective in this patient?

A. Salt restriction
B. Prednisone
C. Canalith repositioning
D. Aspirin

Answer:_____

Vertigo

- "Central" concern — nystagmus in all directions, vertically, or does not extinguish; focal deficits; CN abnormalities; etiologies: brainstem/cerebellar disease

	Peripheral Vertigo
BPPV	Brief, generally seconds of positional vertigo; Dix-Hallpike maneuver; Tx — Epley maneuver
Labyrinthitis / Neuronitis	Acute, significant vertigo, N/V lasting a couple days, with slow resolution to normal over a few days to a few weeks
Ménière's	Episodes generally lasting hours; hearing loss, tinnitus, aural fullness
Acoustic Neuroma	Hearing loss, tinnitus, unsteadiness/tilting/veering

PARKINSON DISEASE (PD)

AR 7

A 73-year-old female presents with tremor, which has been progressively worse over the past 6 months. On exam, you notice some mild increased tone of the extremities and decreased arm swing during the gait evaluation; the rest of the exam is nonfocal. The patient states that she has a tremor of the head, but you just notice a chin tremor on exam.

PMH: HTN, diabetes, hyperlipidemia, osteoarthritis, MI

Family history: cancer and heart disease; no family history of tremor

Characteristics of the tremor are outlined in the upcoming video.

VIDEO

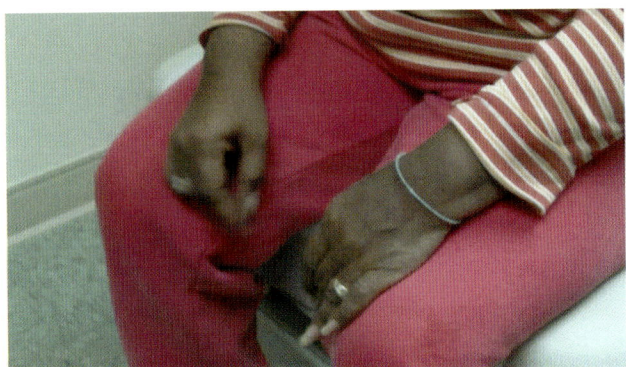

Which would be the most effective medication for this patient?

A. Propranolol
B. Primidone
C. Clonazepam
D. Carbidopa/Levodopa

Answer:_____

Parkinson Disease

- Rest tremor, bradykinesia, postural instability, and rigidity
- Responds very well early to dopaminergic therapy
- **Differentiate from benign essential tremor (postural tremor of hands or head-nodding tremor with family Hx or improved with alcohol as clues; Tx with propranolol or primidone); no other parkinsonian cardinal features with essential tremor**
- Drug induced (consider neuroleptics and medications such as metoclopramide)

Movement Disorders

- If the parkinsonian symptoms do not seem to respond to dopaminergic medications, then it might be a "Parkinson-plus" syndrome

Progressive Supranuclear Palsy (PSP)	Multiple System Atrophy (MSA)	Corticobasal Degeneration (CBD)
Vertical gaze palsy	Significant autonomic dysfunction	Alien hand phenomenon
Early falls	Cerebellar/ Brainstem atrophy	Cortical sensory loss
	Ataxia	

- Consider NPH if presenting with cognitive dysfunction, incontinence, and gait apraxia

OTHER MOVEMENT DISORDERS

Other Considerations

Neuroleptic Malignant Syndrome	Serotonin Syndrome
Rigidity	**Hyperreflexia, tremor, clonus**
Triggers — neuroleptics, antiemetics, and rapid withdrawal of antiparkinsonian medication	Triggers — combinations of SSRIs, MAOIs, TCAs, SNRIs, tramadol, dextromethorphan, cocaine, amphetamines, triptans
Tx — supportive care, address offending agent; consider dantrolene, bromocriptine, amantadine, ECT as options	Tx — discontinue offending agents, supportive care, cyproheptadine

- Restless leg syndrome — check iron, ferritin, and TIBC

NEUROLOGY

AR 8

A 26-year-old male presents to the ED with a severe, ongoing retroorbital, stabbing headache × 40 minutes. He has awakened from sleep at 2 a.m. × 5 days with similar headaches lasting about 1 hour. He had similar episodes for about 3 weeks last year. Medical history and family history are negative.

Meds: multivitamin

On neurologic exam, there are no deficits.

No papilledema

No nuchal rigidity

Which of the following is the most appropriate next step in patient care?

A. 100% high-flow oxygen through a mask
B. Propranolol
C. Prednisone taper
D. Verapamil daily
E. Lumbar puncture
F. Trial of indomethacin

Answer:_____

Primary Headaches

	Quality / Associations	Location	Timing
Tension Headache	Dull, band-like, mild to moderate	Bilateral	May be indolent
Migraine Headache	Pounding, throbbing Nausea Photo-/Phonophobia	Unilateral or bilateral	4–72 hours
Cluster	Boring/Stabs Male Autonomic features Alcohol triggers	Unilateral Retroorbital	15–180 minutes Circadian rhythm May awaken out of sleep
Trigeminal Neuralgia	Lancinating	V2/V3 most common	Brief, seconds

Secondary Headaches

Idiopathic Intracranial Hypertension	Young, obese female, TVO, visual loss, diplopia, pulsatile tinnitus, papilledema; associated with high vit A, tetracyclines, GH, Behçet's, lupus, PCOS; Tx — acetazolamide, furosemide, ONF, shunt
Intracranial Hypotension	Postural headache, post LP, diffuse dural enhancement, low-lying Crb tonsils; Tx — fluid, IV caffeine, blood patch
Cerebral Venous Thrombosis	Headache with increased ICP, altered LOC, focal deficits, visual change, seizures; peripartum/hypercoagulable; Tx — anticoagulation
Carotid Dissection	Cervical pain radiating to eye, trauma/chiropractor, Horner's, stroke in the young; Tx — antiplatelet or anticoagulation
Temporal Arteritis	Age > 55, visual loss, high ESR, jaw claudication, temporal tenderness, PMR, temporal artery Bx; Tx — high-dose steroids

Subarachnoid Hemorrhage

- Ottawa Rules 2013 *JAMA* — no concern if:
  - Younger than 40 years of age
  - No thunderclap onset or onset with exertion
  - No witnessed LOC
  - No neck pain/meningismus
- Evaluate for SAH with CT and LP if needed
- If present, evaluate for underlying aneurysm, Tx vasospasm (days 4–14); address hyponatremia

SEIZURES

AR 9

A 34-year-old male comes to the ED due to severe pain radiating from the flank to the groin with hematuria. He has a history of epilepsy. He has been seizure free for over 1 year.

On neurologic examination, there are no deficits.

Which seizure medication is the patient most likely taking?

A. Levetiracetam
B. Pregabalin
C. Lamotrigine
D. Gabapentin
E. Topiramate

Answer:_____

Antiseizure Medications[5]

Medication	Associations
Phenytoin	Gingival hypertrophy, chronic ataxia, osteoporosis
Carbamazepine	Hyponatremia, very cheap
Oxcarbazepine	Hyponatremia
Topiramate	Weight loss, kidney stones, paresthesias, cognitive difficulties (word-finding troubles)
Levetiracetam	Irritability/Agitation
Valproic acid	Weight gain, hair thinning, tremor, thrombocytopenia, hyperammonemia, pregnancy risk
Lamotrigine	Rash (Stevens-Johnson syndrome)
Lacosamide	Diplopia, vertigo, emesis

Seizures

- Evaluation of first seizure
  - H&P
  - BMP (Na^+, Ca^{2+}, glucose), LFTs, toxicology screen (CSF if encephalitis concern)
  - Imaging with MRI is preferred to rule out lesion
  - EEG; however, a negative EEG does not exclude the diagnosis of epilepsy
- Increased risk of recurrent seizure after first if unprovoked and:
  - EEG is abnormal
  - Prior neurological injury
  - Family history of seizures
  - Abnormal MRI
  - The risk of recurrence after 2 seizures is ~ 60% and ~ 35% after a single seizure
- Acute treatment
  - IV benzodiazepines
  - Load with phenytoin or fosphenytoin for status
  - Fosphenytoin causes less infusion site necrosis and cardiac disturbances
  - If continued status, intubate and put on barbiturate or propofol (monitor EEG for resolution)
- Chronic treatment
  - Start after ≥ 2 unprovoked seizures
  - Consider after 1 unprovoked focal seizure if EEG is abnormal or focal lesion on MRI
  - Generally, patients must be seizure free > 6 months to consider driving
- AEDs that reduce efficacy of OCPs
  - Phenytoin, phenobarbital, carbamazepine, topiramate (at ≥ 200 mg), felbamate, oxcarbazepine
  - Note that estrogen OCPs can decrease levels of lamotrigine
  - Lamotrigine can decrease levels of progestins (minipill)
- AEDs in pregnancy (AED pregnancy registry 1997–2011)
  - Malformations: valproate 9%, phenobarbital 6%, topiramate 4%, carbamazepine 3%, phenytoin 3%, levetiracetam 2.4%, lamotrigine 2%
  - Maintain a pregnant woman on monotherapy at lowest dose (avoid valproate)
- Psychogenic nonepileptic seizures (PNES)
  - PNES are not due to abnormal brain activity but are psychogenic
  - Suggestive features: forced eye closure during episode, pelvic thrusting, bilateral shaking with awareness, absence of a postictal state
  - Order video EEG monitoring if suspected
  - Note that 20% of patients with PNES also have epilepsy

Seizure vs. Syncope

Seizure	Syncope
Aura or no warning	Lightheaded, pallor, N/V, palpitations, chest pain, or no warning
Ictal phase — convulsion, tongue bite, incontinence, lasts 1–2 minutes	Ictal phase — brief; no convulsions or short convulsive syncope
Has a postictal period	No significant postictal

STROKE

ISCHEMIC STROKES

- Acute
  - ABCs
  - Neurologic exam (H&P)
  - Treat hypertension only if SBP > 220 mmHg or DBP > 120 mmHg
    - Bring down BP slowly
    - Of note, tPA candidate must have BP below 185/110 mmHg
- CT brain, coags, CBC, glucose

Ischemic Stroke — AHA / ASA 2019 Update to Guidelines[6]

- Systemic thrombolytics
  - NIHSS > 4
  - Acute ischemic stroke < 4.5 hours
  - 3–4.5 hours **(exclude if > 80 years of age, DM, and prior ischemic stroke, anticoagulation, NIHSS > 25)**
  - BP cannot be > 185/110 mmHg
  - No absolute tPA exclusion criteria
- Endovascular therapy
  - Acute ischemic stroke
  - Occlusion of the ICA or proximal MCA
  - > 18 years of age
  - NIHSS score ≥ 6
  - ASPECTS of ≥ 6
  - DAWN and DEFUSE 3 trial — extended window for mechanical thrombectomy out to 16–24 hours (large vessel occlusion)
- Antiplatelet
  - ASA, ASA + ER dipyridamole, or clopidogrel monotherapy
  - Consider clopidogrel and ASA for 90 days for intracranial stenosis
- Anticoagulation indications
  - AFib
  - STEMI/LV thrombus
  - DVT with PFO
  - Prosthetic or rheumatic valves
  - Sinus venous thrombosis
  - ? Dissection, low EF, hypercoagulable disorder
  - **No anticoagulation for embolic stroke from endocarditis**
- High-intensity statin treatment
- BP at least < 140/90 mmHg after several days of ischemic stroke
- Carotid endarterectomy/CAS (> 70%) — should be done within 2 weeks, and surgical risk should be < 6%

INTRACEREBRAL HEMORRHAGE (ICH)

Treatment — Hemorrhagic Stroke

- Supportive care acutely
  - ABCs and reverse anticoagulation
  - HOB at 30°
  - Optimize glucose, treat fever, treat seizures, monitor for ICP or hydrocephalus concern
  - Blood pressure
    - Generally, target systolic BP of about 160 mmHg or a CPP of 61–80 mmHg if concern for elevated ICP
- Surgery in intracerebral bleed
  - Cerebellar hemorrhage > 3 cm and clinical deterioration or hydrocephalus
  - Supratentorial bleed
    - Craniotomy for lobar clots > 30 mL within 1 cm of surface; best if young age; considered best with intermediate level of consciousness

Basic Stroke Localization

Dominant MCA	Contralateral face, arm > leg weakness, aphasia
Nondominant MCA	Contralateral face, arm, and leg weakness, neglect
ACA	Contralateral leg > face, arm weakness
Lacunar (internal capsule)	Contralateral face, arm, leg weakness
Thalamus	Contralateral sensory disturbance
Brainstem	"Crossed findings," cranial nerve deficits
Cerebellum	Ipsilateral dysmetria

AR 10

A 59-year-old male presents with fever and sepsis. His blood cultures are positive for *S. aureus*. On Day 2 of his hospitalization, he develops right-sided weakness and aphasia. He is found to have an acute left MCA stroke. Echo reveals a valvular vegetation consistent with endocarditis, providing a mechanism for embolic stroke.

Which is the best course of treatment?

A. Antibiotics and clopidogrel
B. Antibiotics and heparin
C. Antibiotics only
D. High-dose steroids
E. High-dose steroids and antibiotics
F. High-dose steroids and heparin

Answer:_____

DEMENTIA

- **Progressive cognitive disorder that interferes with activities of daily living and functioning**
- CNS imaging (MRI) brain on all patients vs. PET/NM scan
- Always look for "reversible" causes of symptoms like vitamin B_{12} deficiency, thyroid disease, and in suspected patients, syphilis; consider relationship with EtOH in chronic alcoholic; and HIV-associated dementia with long-standing disease
- Consider pseudodementia; i.e., is depressed (has trouble with attention, concentration, and forgetfulness) but retains ADLs, does well on office testing, and is concerned about deficits out of proportion to objective cognitive findings

Alzheimer Disease

- Memory + 1 of visuospatial, executive, language, personality dysfunction
- Amyloid and tau protein accumulation
- Acetylcholinesterase inhibitors for mild-to-moderate disease (also may consider 2,000 units daily of vitamin E)
- Memantine for moderate-to-severe disease
- MCI: not treated at this point; 10% yearly risk of transforming to dementia

Alzheimer Disease[7]

Standard Evaluation	Case-by-Case (Not Routine)
• CBC • Chemistries with LFTs • Thyroid studies • Vitamin B_{12}, folate • Depression screening • MRI brain 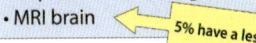 5% have a lesion	• Screening for syphilis • SPECT/PET • Genetic testing • EEG • Lumbar puncture

Dementia

Dementia Type	Associations
Multiinfarct dementia	Vascular disease on imaging, maybe stepwise decline clinically
NPH	Cognitive disease, incontinence, gait apraxia, large ventricles out of proportion to atrophy, high-volume LP for diagnosis
Lewy body disease	Fluctuating cognition, visual hallucinations, neuroleptic sensitivity, cognitive deficits within 1 year of parkinsonism
Frontotemporal dementia	Younger age (6th decade), early personality change rather than early memory loss
CJD	Rapidly progressive dementia, startle myoclonus, period sharp waves on EEG, MRI with potentially caudate/putamen/thalamus/cortical ribbon diffusion abnormality, 14-3-3 protein

Alzheimer Disease — Medication Treatment[8]

Two classes approved:	
Acetylcholinesterase inhibitors Modest effect on memory, function **No effect on progression** Side effects: GI, bradycardia, heart block	**NMDA-r antagonist** Add on mod-severe AD Rare confusion, dizziness
Donepezil　Rivastigmine　Galantamine	Memantine

MULTIPLE SCLEROSIS (MS)

AR 11

A 25-year-old female with multiple sclerosis developed worsened numbness in her legs yesterday. She has had numbness in her legs chronically from prior transverse myelitis. She has no weakness, incoordination, or visual change.

No other new symptoms.

T 100.1°F (37.8°C); WBC 11.5 cells/mcL

Urinalysis confirms a UTI.

Which of the following is the most likely to improve this patient?

A. Antibiotics
B. IV pulse of methylprednisolone for MS flare
C. Gabapentin
D. Pregabalin

Answer:_____

Multiple Sclerosis (MS)

- Females > males, 20–40 years of age
- Vitamin D deficiency increases risk
- Diagnosis
  - Must have clinical or clinical + radiologic evidence of > 1 "space" and > 1 "time"
  - Clinical
    - Most common: fatigue, weakness, spasticity, bladder dysfunction
    - Optic neuritis, diplopia (? internuclear ophthalmoplegia)
    - Paresthesias, pain, ataxia
    - Worse with increased body temp = "Uhthoff symptom"
  - Radiographic
    - MRI: CNS plaques
  - Supportive
    - LP: ↑ IgG index (90%); oligoclonal bands (> 90%)
    - Evoked potentials (75–85% sensitive)

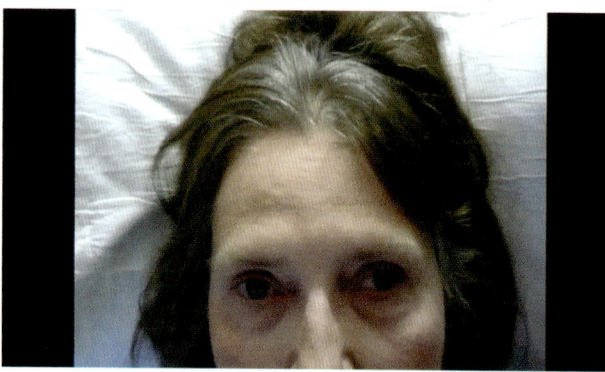

[9]

MS Treatment Issues

- Acute exacerbation
  - IV methylprednisolone
  - Look for infection (e.g., UTI) that may be causing an exacerbation or pseudoexacerbation

Chronic Disease-Modifying Medication	Injectable / Oral	Associations
Interferons	Injectable	Possible flu-like symptoms, depression, leukopenia, anemia, injection site reactions
Glatiramer acetate	Injectable	Possible side effects/ points of caution, otherwise well tolerated
Natalizumab	IV infusion	Highly effective, utilized for aggressive disease, **PML risk**
Dimethyl fumarate	Oral	Monitor absolute lymphocyte count for PML risk
Fingolimod	Oral	Zoster/Herpes, macular edema, respiratory dysfunction, tumor, **bradycardia**
Teriflunomide	Oral	Hepatotoxicity, severe teratogenicity

Neuromyelitis Optica

- NMO is characterized by longitudinally extensive myelitis and/or bilateral optic neuritis
- Confirm with aquaporin 4 antibody testing (NMO antibody)

CLINICAL PEARLS

- Practice the "essential" neurologic exam
- Know the 3 nerves of the hand and 2 in the leg
- Weakness — check for power (asthenia)
- Memory loss — function is critical
- Headaches — look in the back of the eyes
- Seizures — the history is key
- Sensory issues — use a map
- Stroke — act **FAST**
  - **F**ace (drooping)
  - **A**rm weakness
  - **S**peech slurred
  - **T**ime counts

Audience Response 1
B. CT chest

AR 2
C. Botulism
- After EMG he admitted to injecting drugs with a used needle 2 days prior to the onset of symptoms
- Foodborne, wound, and illicit drugs (i.e., black-tar heroin) are most common etiologies
- Treatment is with botulism antitoxin therapy (contact CDC)

AR 3
A. Night splints

AR 4
B. S1 radiculopathy; provide conservative treatment.

AR 5
E. Riluzole

AR 6
C. Canalith repositioning

AR 7
D. Carbidopa/Levodopa

AR 8
A. 100% high-flow oxygen through a mask

AR 9
E. Topiramate

AR 10
C. Antibiotics only

AR 11
A. Antibiotics

ENDNOTES

[1]   Source: J. Chad Hoyle, MD

[2]   Courtesy Hoyle EMG Lab

[3]   Courtesy Hoyle EMG lab

[4]   Source: Dr. Iyadurai

[5]   Review of new antiepileptic drugs from knowledge gap: Practice guideline update summary: Efficacy and tolerability of the new antiepileptic drugs II: Treatment-resistant epilepsy: Report of the Guideline Development, Dissemination, and Implementation Subcommittee of the American Academy of Neurology and the American Epilepsy Society. Neurology. 2018 Jul 10;91(2):82-90. doi: 10.1212/WNL.0000000000005756. Erratum in: Neurology. 2018 Dec 11;91(24):1117.

[6]   Powers WJ, Rabinstein AA, Ackerson T, Adeoye OM, Bambakidis NC, Becker K, Biller J, Brown M, Demaerschalk BM, Hoh B, Jauch EC, Kidwell CS, Leslie-Mazwi TM, Ovbiagele B, Scott PA, Sheth KN, Southerland AM, Summers DV, Tirschwell DL. Guidelines for the Early Management of Patients With Acute Ischemic Stroke: 2019 Update to the 2018 Guidelines for the Early Management of Acute Ischemic Stroke: A Guideline for Healthcare Professionals From the American Heart Association/American Stroke Association. Stroke. 2019 Dec;50(12):e344-e418. doi: 10.1161/STR.0000000000000211. Epub 2019 Oct 30. Erratum in: Stroke. 2019 Dec;50(12):e440-e441.

[7]   Apostolova LG. Alzheimer Disease. CONTINUUM: Lifelong Learning in Neurology. 2016;22 (2, Dementia):419-434.

[8]   Apostolova LGMDMSF. Alzheimer Disease. CONTINUUM: Lifelong Learning in Neurology. 2016; 22(2, Dementia):419-434.

[9]   Source: J. Chad Hoyle, MD

NEUROLOGY

MedStudy

INTERNAL MEDICINE REVIEW

Oncology

Presented by

Rishi Sawhney, MD

Why Some Topic Names Are Not Printed in This Section

At MedStudy, we do all we can to optimize your self-testing and learning.

In this section, the speaker has chosen to introduce topics with an Audience Response question to help you learn. In the syllabus, we've intentionally "hidden" some topic names that would give away the answers—so you can self-test more effectively. Where we've done this, instead of the topic name, you'll see an empty teal band or some extra space, but you can still find the topic on the page using the Table of Contents.

OVERVIEW

Oncology Outline
- Common Cancers — A Brief Review
- Complications of Cancer
  - Paraneoplastic
  - Direct Tumor Effects
- Cancer Therapies
- Complications of Cancer Therapy
  - Drug Side Effects
  - Tumor Lysis Syndrome
  - Febrile Neutropenia

Cancer Epidemiology
- <u>Incidence</u>
  - Females
    - Breast > Lung > Colorectal
  - Males
    - Prostate > Lung > Colorectal
- <u>Mortality</u>
  - Females
    - Lung > Breast > Colorectal
  - Males
    - Lung > Prostate > Colorectal

Common Cancers — A Brief Review
- Breast cancer
- GYN cancers
  - Cervical
  - Ovarian
  - Endometrial
- GU cancers
  - Testicular
  - Prostate
  - Bladder
  - Renal
- GI cancers
  - Esophageal
  - Gastric
  - Colorectal
- Lung, head & neck, and brain cancers

What Should I Know for Each Major Cancer Type?
- Risk factors
- Screening
- Clinical presentation
- Initial workup
- Basic approach to management

BREAST CANCER

- The most common malignancy in women
- The 2nd leading cause of cancer death in women (lung is 1st)

Breast Cancer — Risk Factors
- Personal Hx of breast cancer or benign breast disease
  - ADH, DCIS, LCIS
- Early menarche, nulliparity, late menopause
  - Anything that increases endogenous estrogen exposure can increase risk
- Increasing age
- Family history
- Inherited genetic mutations
- Moderate-heavy alcohol intake

Breast Cancer Risk
- Hereditary breast-ovarian cancer syndrome
  - Led to the description of the *BRCA1* and *BRCA2* genes
  - Together, these account for 30–50% of all **inherited** breast cancer

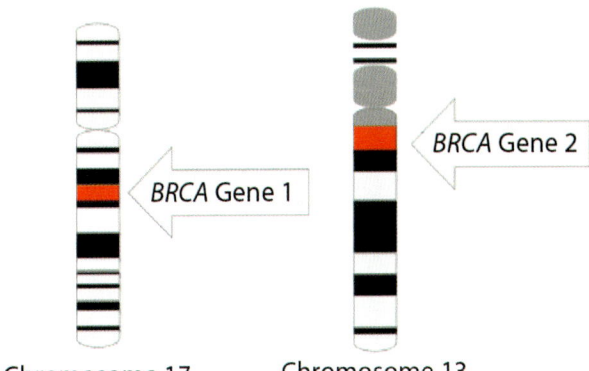

Chromosome 17   Chromosome 13

[1]

BRCA — Lifetime Cancer Risks[2]

	General Population	*BRCA1*	*BRCA2*
Breast (female)	12–14%	55–70%	45–70%
Ovarian	1%	40%	15%
Prostate	15–20%	15–20%	30–40%
Breast (male)	0.1%	1%	8%
Pancreatic	1.5%	2–4%	5%

- Think about *BRCA* when you see breast cancer:
  - At young age (i.e., < 50)
  - With multiple affected family members
  - Bilateral or multiple occurrences

ONCOLOGY

Breast Cancer — Screening

- Screening options include:
  - Breast self-exam (BSE)
  - Clinical breast exam (CBE)
  - Mammography
  - Breast MRI
- Mammography (MMG)
  - 2015 American Cancer Society
    - Age 40–44: consider MMG annually
    - Age 45–54: MMG annually
    - Age > 55: MMG every 1–2 years
  - 2016 USPSTF recommends
    - Age 40–49: consider MMG every 2 years
    - Age 50–74: MMG every 2 years
    - Age > 75: insufficient evidence

The Bottom Line …

- Focus on where guidelines agree
- Screening MMG every 1–2 years for women 50–74 years of age
- MMG has less utility (but should still be considered) for women < 50 years of age or > 74 years of age
- Breast self-exam and clinical breast exams not proven useful in preventing breast cancer

Mammography — Considerations

- Modalities
  - Film
  - Digital
  - Digital breast tomosynthesis (3D)
- Preceding COVID vaccination may cause axillary adenopathy — interpret with caution
- Decreased sensitivity with:
  - Dense breast tissue
  - Thin body habitus (BMI < 25)
  - Hormone replacement therapy (HRT)

Breast Cancer Screening — Breast MRI

- High sensitivity but limited specificity
- Use in selected high-risk women only
  - *BRCA1* or *BRCA2* positive
  - Other hereditary breast cancer syndromes including Li-Fraumeni syndrome, Cowden syndrome
  - Lifetime risk of breast cancer > 20%
  - Prior radiation to chest between 10 and 30 years of age

Breast Cancer Presentation

- Presentation is usually
  - Asymptomatic — found on screening mammogram
  - A <u>painless</u> breast mass detected by the patient
  - Asymmetric eczema — think Paget's
  - Nipple discharge
  - Nipple retraction or dimpling of the skin
  - Inflammatory cancer: "mastitis-like" picture with warmth, redness, swelling, peau d'orange — very aggressive

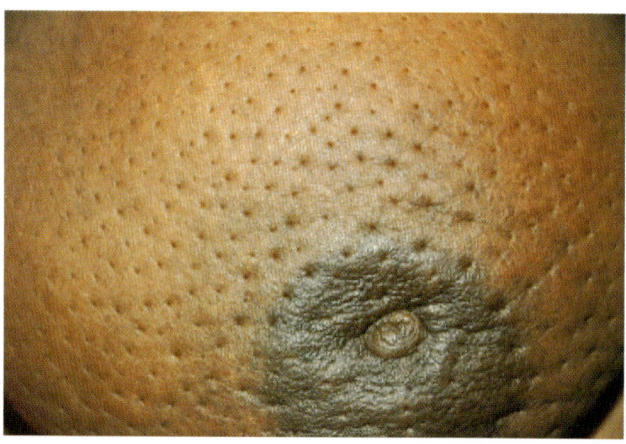

Breast Cancer — Initial Workup

- Suspicious breast finding
  - 1st — **Image** → mammogram/ultrasound ± MRI
  - 2nd — **Biopsy** → FNA/aspiration or core needle biopsy
  - 3rd — **Check receptors** → determine ER/PR and *HER2/neu* status
  - 4th — **Stage and treat**
- Palpable mass without abnormality on mammogram
  - Should biopsy

Audience Response 1

A 53-year-old postmenopausal woman finds a breast lump. Ultrasound and mammography confirm a suspicious 3-cm mass. A core biopsy is positive for infiltrating ductal carcinoma. A lumpectomy and axillary node dissection are done. The cancer is 3 cm with 2 positive axillary lymph nodes.

ER/PR receptors are negative, as is *HER2/neu*.

Which of the following should you recommend?

A. Repeat surgery with conversion to a modified radical mastectomy.
B. Local radiation therapy plus tamoxifen for 5 years
C. Adjuvant chemotherapy followed by radiation
D. Close follow-up with an exam every month
E. Local radiation therapy alone

Answer:_____

Breast Cancer — Prognosis

- Tumor size
- Lymph node status
- Distant metastasis?
- ER/PR status
- *HER2/neu* status
- Multigene assay (selected cases)
- AJCC Staging system
  - Noninvasive (carcinoma in situ)
  - Early stage (Stage I/II)
  - Locally advanced (Stage III)
  - Metastatic

Breast Cancer — General Approach to Management

- <u>Local control</u>: Remove tumor and decrease risk of locoregional recurrence
  - Lumpectomy vs. mastectomy
  - Axillary lymph node evaluation
  - Adjuvant radiotherapy
- <u>Systemic control</u>: Reduce risk of distant recurrence of disease
  - Endocrine therapy
  - Chemotherapy
  - Biologic therapy (i.e., trastuzumab)

Breast Cancer — Endocrine Therapy

- Antihormone therapy for all who are estrogen-receptor (ER) positive or progesterone-receptor (PR) positive — can reduce recurrence risk by ~ 50%!
  - Postmenopausal women — incorporate aromatase inhibitor (AI)!
    - AI × 5–10 years
    - Tamoxifen for 5 years followed by AI × 5 years
    - Tamoxifen for 2–3 years followed by AI × 5 years
  - Premenopausal women — tamoxifen × 5–10 years acceptable standard
    - Ovarian function suppression (OFS) may be added in selected situations
    - Role of AIs continues to evolve, but not effective as monotherapy here

Breast Cancer — Adjuvant Systemic Therapy

- Chemotherapy is generally considered for:
  - Node positive
  - Larger tumor size (> 1 cm)
  - Triple negative
  - *HER2* positive
  - High-risk multigene recurrence score (node negative)
- *HER2* monoclonal antibody therapy recommended for *HER2*-positive disease (combined with chemotherapy)
  - Trastuzumab
  - Pertuzumab

Breast Cancer Management — Putting It All Together

- <u>Local control</u>
  - Mastectomy = lumpectomy + radiation
  - Axillary lymph node evaluation
    - Sentinel node vs. lymph node dissection
- <u>Systemic control</u>
  - If tumor is ER/PR positive, give adjuvant endocrine therapy
    - Tamoxifen for premenopausal
    - Aromatase inhibitor for postmenopausal
  - If tumor is high risk, then give adjuvant chemotherapy
    - Node positive
    - High multigene recurrence score
    - Larger size (> 1 cm), triple negative
  - If tumor is <u>*HER2*</u> positive, give adjuvant trastuzumab

AR 2

A 64-year-old postmenopausal female presents with a 3-cm left breast mass. Needle biopsy confirms invasive ductal carcinoma. She undergoes left breast lumpectomy and axillary lymph node evaluation. Final path confirms 3.5-cm cancer, ER+, *HER2* negative, with 2 positive lymph nodes. Margins negative.

She undergoes adjuvant chemotherapy, followed by adjuvant left breast radiation. She is then placed on adjuvant endocrine therapy with letrozole.

Which of the following would represent an appropriate component of her surveillance strategy going forward?

A. Liver function studies every 6 months × 5 years
B. CT chest/abdomen/pelvis annually × 5 years
C. Bone density/DXA scan every 2 years
D. MRI plus mammogram bilateral breast annually
E. PET/CT scan annually × 5 years

Answer:_____

Breast Cancer Surveillance after Treatment (2019 NCCN and 2013 ASCO Guidelines)

- H&P every 3–6 months for 3 years; every 6–12 months for years 4 and 5, then annually
- Breast imaging — annual mammography
- Genetic counseling/testing in high-risk individuals
- Women on tamoxifen — annual GYN exams
- Women on aromatase inhibitor — monitor bone density
- Lifestyle choices — active, healthy diet, exercise, maintain healthy BMI, moderate alcohol intake
- Tests <u>not</u> to order routinely:
  - CBCs and liver function test
  - CXR, bone scan, liver ultrasound, CT
  - Tumor markers, including CA 15-3, CA 27.29, CEA
  - PET scans, breast MRIs

Pearls — Breast Cancer

- Risk factors — *BRCA1* or *2*
- Screening — where guidelines agree
- Workup of breast mass — imaging → needle biopsy → surgery
- Treat with resection (lumpectomy plus radiation **or** mastectomy) plus axillary node evaluation
- Adjuvant therapy
  - Endocrine for all ER+ cancers
    - Aromatase inhibitors — watch for osteoporosis/skeletal fracture; monitor DXA
    - Tamoxifen — watch for VTE and uterine cancer
  - Trastuzumab for all *HER2*-positive cancers
  - Chemo for "high risk" (node positive, larger tumors, high-risk genomic score)

ONCOLOGY

CERVICAL CANCER

- The 3rd most common female genital tract cancer after uterine and ovarian
- Mortality has dropped significantly with the introduction of effective screening
- Peak age is 20–30 years of age with a 2nd, later peak in the 60s
- Usually a very slow, progressive disease
- Primary risk factor
  - Human papillomavirus (HPV) infection
    - Found in > 90% of cervical cancers
    - Types 16 and 18
- Other risk factors
  - Early age at first intercourse
  - Multiple sexual partners
  - Tobacco use
  - Low socioeconomic status
- HIV

Cervical Cancer — HPV Vaccine
- Universal vaccination has had major health impact
- 9-valent vaccine targets HPV Types 16, 18
- Effective in cancer prevention!
  - Females: cervical (97–100% effective), vulvar, vaginal, anal cancers
  - Males: anal cancer and genital warts
- Recommended for individuals 9–45 years of age
  - Females — prevent cervical, vulvar, vaginal and anal cancer
  - Males — prevent anal cancer and genital warts

Cervical Cancer — Screening
- Begin
  - At age 21
- Frequency
  - Ages 21–29: Screen every 3 years with cytology alone
  - Ages 30–65: Screen every 3 years with cytology alone or every 5 years if cotesting with cytology plus HPV DNA
- Stop
  - At age 65, if patient has had adequate screening (3 consecutive negative cytology tests or 2 consecutive negative cotests within past 10 years with most recent within last 5 years), or after total hysterectomy
- Pap smear is only tool recommended for < 30 years of age; > 30 years of age, can use HPV DNA test
- Prior HPV vaccination does not change screening recommendations

AR 3
A 36-year-old woman presents with an abnormal Pap smear showing a high-grade squamous intraepithelial lesion (HSIL).

No inflammation is present. She is HPV positive, and a Pap smear 2 years prior was normal.

Which of the following is the most appropriate next step in her management?

A. Return in 6 months for repeat Pap smear.
B. Refer to GYN oncologist for hysterectomy.
C. Calculate her risk estimate for CIN-3, and then pursue colposcopy or excision if high risk.
D. Recommend HPV vaccine.
E. Refer for radiation and chemotherapy.

Answer:_____

Cervical Cancer — Pap Smear Cytology Results

Cervical Cytology	Incidence %
Negative	96
Atypical squamous cells of undetermined significance (ASCUS)	2.8
Low-grade squamous intraepithelial lesion (LSIL)	0.97
High-grade squamous intraepithelial lesion (HSIL)	0.21
Atypical glandular cells (AGCs)	0.21

Cervical Cancer — Workup of Abnormal Pap Smear
- Management based on **risk**, not results
- Determine risk of CIN 3+
  - Cytology results
  - HPV status
  - Screening history
- Management options
  - Highest risk — expedited treatment (i.e., excision/LEEP)
  - Intermediate risk — colposcopy
  - Lowest risk — surveillance

Cervical Cancer
- Most commonly presents with vaginal bleeding
- Diagnosis with colposcopy-guided biopsy
- Stage clinically, using FIGO system, CT, PET/CT
- Treatment
  - Early stage: surgery
  - More advanced disease: concurrent chemoradiation
  - Metastatic disease: chemotherapy

OVARIAN CANCER

AR 4

A 60-year-old woman presents with increasing abdominal girth and SOB. Exam reveals ascites and a pelvic ultrasound reveals a right-sided adnexal mass.

Which of the following is not correct?

A. Treatment should include TAH-BSO with omentectomy, gross tumor resection, and biopsies of all serosal surfaces.
B. There is increased risk of this malignancy with *BRCA1* and *BRCA2* mutations.
C. CA 125 should be ordered.
D. There is > 85% likelihood the mass is a germ cell tumor.
E. Most ovarian tumors are diagnosed with advanced-stage disease.

Answer:_____

Ovarian Cancer

- 4th leading cause of cancer death in women in the U.S.
- More common with advancing age
- Histology
  - Epithelial (85%) — postmenopausal women
  - Germ cell (5%) — younger women, 10–30 years of age

Ovarian Cancer — Risk Factors

- Increased risk
  - Hormonal factors
    - Nulliparity
    - Early menarche/Late menopause
    - PCOS
  - Genetic factors
    - *BRCA1* (40% lifetime risk), *BRCA2* (20% lifetime risk)
    - Lynch syndrome (LS; a.k.a. hereditary nonpolyposis colorectal cancer [HNPCC]) (12% lifetime risk)
- Decreased risk
  - Multiparity (10% decrease with each pregnancy)
  - Early menopause
  - Breastfeeding
  - OCP use

Ovarian Cancer

- Screening
  - Not recommended for standard-risk patients
  - Can be considered for high-risk patients (strong family history and/or genetic syndromes)
    - CA 125
    - Transvaginal ultrasound
- Clinical presentation
  - Most common cause of ovarian mass in postmenopausal women
  - Abdominal bloating, abdominal mass, ascites, pelvic pain
- Initial workup
  - CT chest/abdomen/pelvis
  - Tumor markers
    - CA 125, HE4 for epithelial
    - hCG, AFP for germ cell
- Treatment
  - Surgical debulking: TAH-BSO, omentectomy, node sampling with goal of optimal cytoreduction (< 1 cm residual disease)
  - Adjuvant chemotherapy
    - IV carboplatin/paclitaxel
    - Intraperitoneal chemo in selected patients
- Prognosis: depends on stage
  - 5-year overall survival:
    - 90% for Stage I disease
    - 40% for Stage III disease

ENDOMETRIAL CANCER

- Most common GYN cancer
- Present with dysfunctional uterine bleeding
- Risk factor — excess estrogen exposure (obesity, HRT)
- Histology
  - Endometrioid
  - Serous
  - Clear cell
- Treatment
  - Early stage — hysterectomy; adjuvant chemo in high risk
  - Advanced stage — palliative platinum-based chemo
- Prognosis — high cure rates with early-stage disease

PEARLS – GYN CANCERS

- Cervical cancer
  - HPV Types 16, 18
  - HPV vaccine for males/females 9–45 years of age
  - Screening — Pap smear every 3 years from age 21–30; then from age 30–65, do Pap every 3 years or Pap/HPV cotesting every 5 years
  - Workup abnormal Pap smear — colposcopy next step in most cases
- Ovarian cancer
  - Histology — epithelial in postmenopausal women; germ cell in younger women
  - Consider screening only in "high-risk" women
  - Risk factors — *BRCA*, hormonal
  - Treat with primary surgical debulking, then chemotherapy

TESTICULAR CANCER

Testicular Cancer
- Most common solid cancer in men 15–35 years of age
- Highly curable cancer; favorable prognosis in most men
- Histology
  - Germ cell tumors (95%)
    - Seminoma
    - Nonseminoma
  - Lymphoma (> 50 years of age)
- Risk factors
  - Cryptorchidism
  - Personal or family history
  - Infertility
  - HIV
- Biologic markers — AFP, hCG, and LDH
  - Staging/Prognosis
  - Monitoring for disease relapse
  - Assessing response to therapy

	AFP	hCG	LDH
Seminoma	**Never**	++	++
Nonseminoma	++	++	++

- If pathology reports seminoma, but AFP is elevated, what should you do?
  - Treat as nonseminoma!
- Diagnosis/Staging
  - Presents with painless scrotal mass
  - Check scrotal ultrasound to confirm if solid mass
  - If mass solid
    - Check tumor markers (AFP, hCG, LDH)
    - → Go straight to surgery for diagnosis
      - Radical inguinal orchiectomy
  - Do not perform percutaneous needle biopsy
  - **No** transscrotal approaches
  - CT scans for staging

- Treatment
  - Radical inguinal orchiectomy
  - Adjuvant therapy depends on stage
    - Radiation
    - Chemotherapy
    - Surveillance
  - Advanced disease
    - BEP chemotherapy
    - Surgically resect any residual masses
- Staging
- Prognosis
  - Reported 5-year overall survival:

Good-risk disease	92%
Intermediate-risk disease	80%
Poor-risk disease	48%

- Fertility preservation
  - Reproductive counseling; sperm banking
- Treatment after orchiectomy
  - Based on histology, stage, tumor markers
  - Surveillance
  - Radiation
  - Chemotherapy (BEP or EP)
- Late sequelae of therapy include:
  - Infertility
  - Second primary germ cell tumor
  - Secondary AML
  - Secondary gastrointestinal malignancies

PROSTATE CANCER

- Most common cancer and 2nd leading cause of cancer death (U.S. men)
- Lifetime risk in U.S. men: 11%
- Histology: adenocarcinoma (95%)

Prostate Cancer — Risk Factors
- Age — the most important risk factor
- Race — African Americans have increased risk
- Family history of prostate cancer
- Genetic — *BRCA1* or *2*, ATM, Lynch syndrome, and others; consider genetics evaluation if:
  - Positive family history prostate cancer
  - High-grade (Gleason score ≥ 7)
  - Metastatic prostate cancer
- Environmental
  - Intake of animal fats is associated with increased risk
  - BPH is **not** a risk factor for prostate cancer

Prostate Cancer Prevention
- Finasteride
  - 5-α-Reductase inhibitor
- Data?
  - 25% decrease in prostate cancer but ... no overall survival benefit, and ...
  - The proportion of more aggressive cancers was higher in the finasteride group
  - Finasteride toxicities: gynecomastia, decreased libido, sexual dysfunction

Prostate Cancer — Screening

- Available screening tests
  - Digital rectal exam (DRE)
  - Prostate-specific antigen (PSA)
    - Marker specific to prostate tissue
    - Normal levels increase with age
- Mortality benefit from PSA screening likely modest and must be balanced against potential harms, including risk of overdiagnosis and treatment complications
  - Randomized trials with limitations and conflicting results
- Does result in earlier diagnosis: "stage shift"
- Major guidelines now largely in agreement
- Shared decision-making regarding risks vs. benefits
  - Average risk — start at 50 years of age
  - High risk (African American race, family Hx) — start at 40–45 years of age
  - PSA ± DRE every 1–2 years
  - Life expectancy should be > 10 years
- DRE is now falling out of favor; not strongly recommended

Prostate Cancer

- Now diagnosed primarily in asymptomatic individuals after routine PSA screening
- Before the use of screening, the common presentation was:
  - Urinary obstructive symptoms
  - Back pain

AR 6

A 68-year-old man is seen for nocturia and hesitancy upon urinating. These symptoms have been present for years but have recently worsened. He has had serial prostate exams and measurements of his PSA. His last exam was 1 year ago and was consistent with BPH. His PSA was 3.5 ng/mL. Today, his PSA has risen to 10 ng/mL, and his exam is unchanged.

Evaluation that should be performed at this time includes:

A. Observation with repeat PSA in 3 months
B. Transrectal ultrasound with multiple biopsies
C. Repeat rectal exam and PSA.
D. Bone scan
E. PET/CT scan

Answer:_____

Prostate Cancer

- Diagnosis involves the same tools as screening
  - DRE
    - Usually detect a firm, hard nodule; but may just find diffuse enlargement or a normal gland
  - PSA
    - Levels > 4 ng/mL are considered abnormal (but normal levels vary with age)

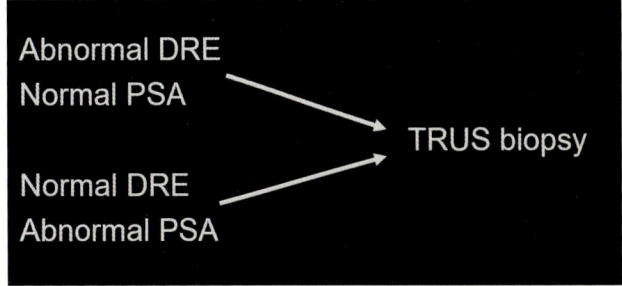

Prostate Cancer — Staging Workup

- Gleason score
- PSA
- TNM staging system
- CT/MRI abdomen/pelvis and bone scan
  - Attention to bones and pelvic lymph nodes

Prostate Cancer — Treatment

- Localized prostate cancer — options include:
  - Radical prostatectomy
  - Radiation therapy (± androgen suppression)
  - Active surveillance
- Advanced prostate cancer
  - Androgen deprivation therapy
    - Toxicities: osteoporosis, gynecomastia, sexual dysfunction, metabolic syndrome, increased risk of cardiac mortality
  - Managing castrate-resistant disease
    - Alternate endocrine therapy
    - Chemotherapy
    - Immunotherapy

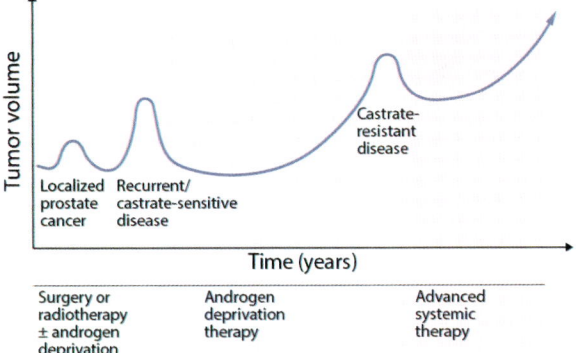

BLADDER CANCER

- 6th most common cancer in U.S.
- Histology
  - Transitional cell (90% of cases in U.S.)
  - Squamous cell more common worldwide
- Risk factors
  - Smoking
  - Medications (pioglitazone, cyclophosphamide)
  - Arsenic, aristolochic acid
  - Schistosomiasis (squamous)
- Clinical presentation
  - Painless hematuria most common
  - Urinary voiding symptoms, pelvic/flank pain
- Diagnosis
  - Cystoscopy with bladder biopsy — look for muscle invasion
  - CT scans for staging
- Treatment
  - Early stage superficial
    - TURBT, intravesical chemo
  - Early stage muscle invasive
    - Neoadjuvant chemo → radical cystectomy **or**
    - Concurrent chemoradiation
  - Metastatic disease
    - Platinum-based chemotherapy
    - PD-1 inhibitor immunotherapy

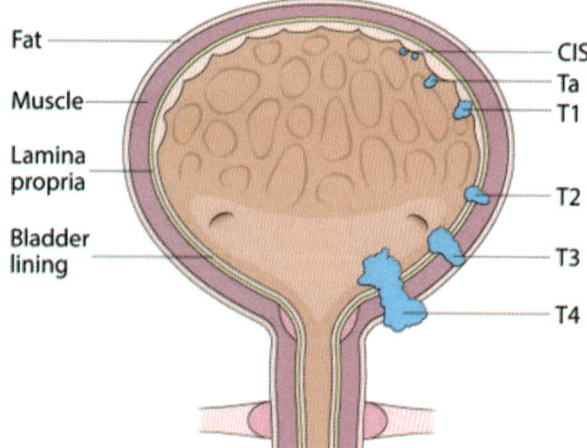

RENAL CELL CANCER

- Histology
  - Clear cell most common (70%)
  - Papillary, chromophobe, oncocytomas
- Risk factors
  - Smoking, HTN, obesity
  - Acquired polycystic kidney disease, CKD
  - Occupational exposures (asbestos, cadmium)
  - Genetic (von Hippel-Lindau syndrome, tuberous sclerosis)
- Screening — only in high-risk population; use U/S or CT
- Clinical presentation
  - Hematuria, flank pain, palpable mass
  - Paraneoplastic
    - Hypercalcemia
    - Stauffer syndrome (hepatic dysfunction without metastasis)
- Diagnosis/Staging
  - CT abdomen ± MRI, but caution regarding renal function with contrast!
  - If radiographic appearance classic → go straight to surgery
  - No percutaneous biopsy, unless no surgery planned
- Treatment
  - Early stage
  - Surgery — partial vs. radical nephrectomy
  - Nonsurgical: cryoablation, RFA
- Advanced disease
  - Checkpoint inhibitor immunotherapy
    - Nivolumab, ipilimumab
  - Tyrosine kinase inhibitors
    - Pazopanib, sunitinib
  - Surgery in selected cases
    - Cytoreductive nephrectomy
    - Metastasectomy for oligometastatic disease

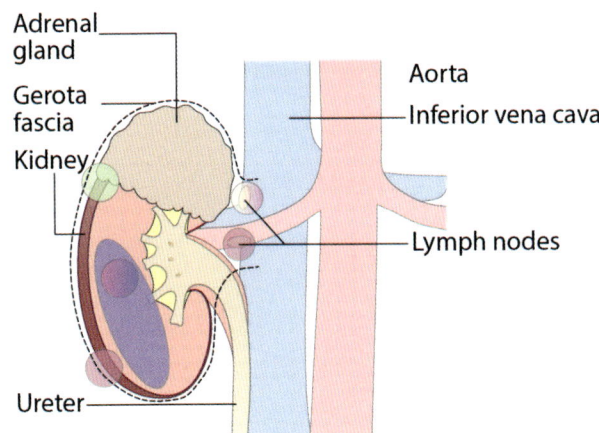

Adrenal gland
Gerota fascia
Kidney
Ureter
Aorta
Inferior vena cava
Lymph nodes

Stage I
Tumor < 7 cm in greatest dimension and limited to kidney; 5-year survival, 95%

Stage II
Tumor > 7 cm in greatest dimension and limited to kidney; 5-year survival, 88%

Stage III
Tumor in major vein or adrenal gland, tumor within Gerota fascia, or 1 regional lymph node involved; 5-year survival, 59%

Stage IV
Tumor beyond Gerota fascia or > 1 regional lymph node involved; 5-year survival, 20%

PEARLS — GU CANCERS

- Testicular cancer
  - Risk factor — cryptorchidism
  - Tumor markers — AFP only elevated in nonseminomas; hCG can be elevated in both types
  - Workup for scrotal mass — ultrasound → radical inguinal orchiectomy plus tumor markers
- Prostate cancer
  - Screening
  - Work up abnormal PSA with TRUS with biopsy
- Bladder cancer
  - Histology — transitional cell in U.S., squamous cell worldwide
  - Risk factors — carcinogens
  - Work up painless hematuria with cystoscopy; look for muscle invasion
- Kidney cancer
  - Histology — clear cell
  - Workup for solid renal mass — go straight to surgery

GASTROINTESTINAL CANCER

ESOPHAGEAL CANCER
- 2 histologic subtypes: adenocarcinoma and squamous cell
- Adenocarcinoma: **distal 1/3**; more common in **Caucasians (Barrett's), GERD, smoking**
- Squamous cell: **proximal 2/3**, caused by **smoking and alcohol**; more common in Asian countries and in African Americans

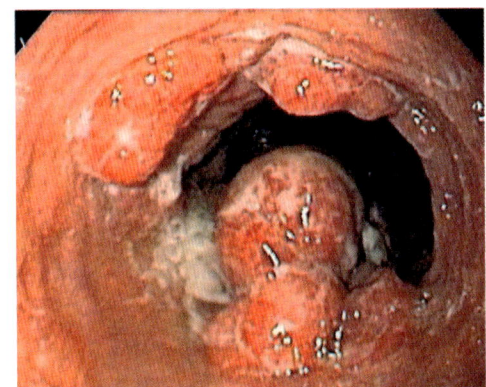

- **Localized disease:** Treat with **EMR and/or surgery ± chemo/XRT**
- **Advanced disease:** Treat with chemo ± XRT

ONCOLOGY

GASTRIC MALIGNANCIES

- 4 main tumors of the stomach:
  1) Adenocarcinoma (95%): "intestinal" or "diffuse"
  2) Lymphoma
  3) Neuroendocrine tumors (NETs)
  4) GIST (mesenchymal tumor, CD117+)
- **Adenocarcinoma** risk factors: chronic *H. pylori* infection, chronic atrophic gastritis (pernicious anemia), smoking, EtOH, nitrate/nitrites, Ménétrier disease (enlarged gastric folds), genetics (hereditary gastric cancer, Lynch syndrome, FAP)
- **Diffuse subtype** — rare, <u>linitis plastica</u>, signet ring cells, hereditary GC (E-cadherin mutation)

Gastric Adenocarcinoma

- Acanthosis nigricans = velvety dark plaques in intertriginous areas associated with diabetes and obesity
- <u>**Acanthosis nigricans**</u> in setting of malignancy is most often associated with **gastric cancer**

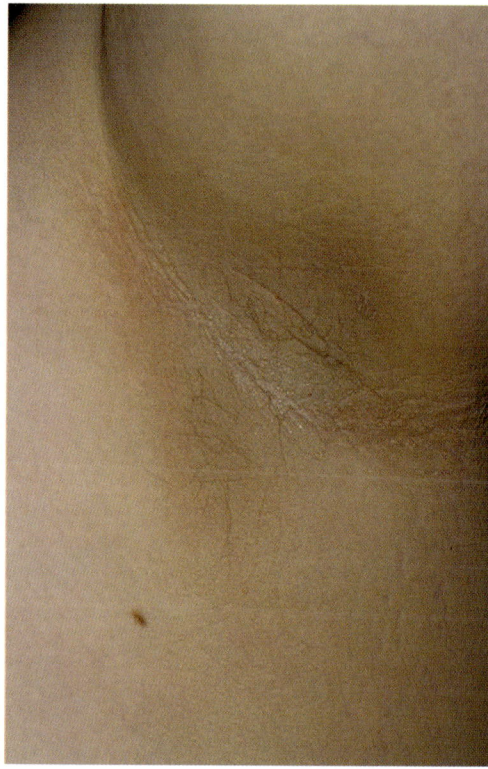

[3]

- **TNM classification** is used for staging (CT and EUS)
  - < 10% found early since they are largely asymptomatic
  - **T1N0M0** (confined to mucosa or submucosa, no lymph nodes, no mets)
- Treatment: **surgical removal of cancer and lymph nodes**; adjuvant chemoradiation prolongs survival
- Early gastric cancer sometimes can be treated with EGD with EMR (e.g., small lesion, superficial, nonulcerated)
- Prognosis (5-year survival)
  - Early stage — 85–90%
  - Metastatic — 3%

Gastric Neuroendocrine Tumors (NETs)

- Rare tumors often in setting of chronic hypergastrinemic states
- Type 1 (70–80%): **autoimmune gastritis/pernicious anemia**
- Type 2 (5%): **ZES**, as part of MEN1
- Type 3 (20%): spontaneous (**most aggressive, gastrin level usually normal**)
- Gastric NETs usually don't metastasize (but increased risk in Type 3), and they rarely cause carcinoid syndrome

COLORECTAL CANCER (CRC)

- Identified risk factors
  - Age
  - Race — African Americans (increased incidence, mortality, early onset)
  - Family history CRC
  - Genetics (e.g., Lynch syndrome, FAP, *MUTYH*, *BRCA*)
  - History of polyps
  - IBD
  - Acromegaly
  - Obesity
  - Diabetes
  - Smoking
  - EtOH
  - Diets high in calories and animal fat

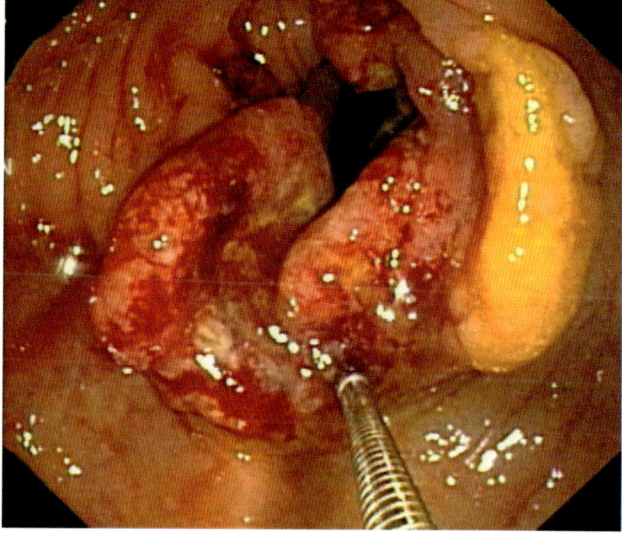

[4]

- **Diagnostic red flags for colorectal cancer**
  - Anorexia
  - Abdominal discomfort
  - Bloody/Heme+ stools
  - Unexplained weight loss
  - Change in bowel habits/Nocturnal stools
  - Iron deficiency anemia
- Lifetime risk is 6% in average-risk persons
- Rising incidence rates of early-onset CRC = take all symptoms seriously **(do not assume bleeding is from hemorrhoids!)**

Inherited CRC (Either <u>Polyposis</u> or Nonpolyposis)

- Polyposis syndromes
- Guidelines vary, but consider genetic testing for the following if > 10 <u>lifetime</u> adenomas:
  - **FAP** — AD, *APC* gene; 100s of adenomas in colon; 100% CA potential; proctocolectomy at young age; can get duodenal adenomas/CA
  - **Attenuated FAP** (AD, *APC* gene too) — fewer polyps than above, delayed-onset CRC
  - *MUTYH* **polyposis** — autosomal recessive, phenotype similar to attenuated FAP
  - **Gardner syndrome** — variant of FAP with tumors outside colon (i.e., osteomas, thyroid cancer, desmoids)

Polyposis Syndromes

- **Peutz-Jeghers syndrome**: Multiple hamartomatous polyps in small bowel but can be seen in stomach and colon as well
  - Freckles on lips/buccal mucosa
  - Intussusception common
  - Increased lifetime CA risk — CRC (39%); stomach (29%); breast (45–50%); pancreatic (11–36%); SB (13%); and multiple other sites
- **Juvenile polyposis**: Consider if at least 3–5 juvenile polyps of colon, multiple juvenile polyps throughout GI tract, polyps, and FH of JPS
  - Lifetime CRC risk is 40–50%

Inherited CRC — Nonpolyposis

- Up to 5% of CRCs are due to **Lynch syndrome** (17% if < 50 years of age): <u>historically referred to as HNPCC</u>
- Associated with 4 different mutations: *MLH1, MSH2, MSH6, PMS2*
- **3-2-1 Rule** "… the occurrence of an HNPCC-associated CA **(colorectal, endometrial, small bowel, ureter, or renal pelvis)** …"
  - In at least <u>**3**</u> relatives (one is a 1st degree relative of other two)
  - Over at least <u>**2**</u> generations
  - With at least <u>**1**</u> person diagnosed < 50 years of age
- Above Amsterdam II criteria <u>not</u> very sensitive

Lynch Syndrome

- **Universal testing guidelines**: microsatellite testing (MSI) and/or IHC testing on CRC tumor <u>regardless of age</u> — followed by genetic testing
- Genetic testing based on FH (PREMM$_5$ score — **pre**diction **m**odel for gene **m**utations); **take a good family history in your clinic!**
- LS — colonoscopy screening begins at 20–25 years of age or 2–5 years prior to the earliest CRC if diagnosed before 25 years of age
- Other cancers common, including uterine (up to 60%) and ovarian cancer: Consider TAH/BSO, decision individualized (i.e., often after child-bearing age)

CRC Screening

- Multiple different guidelines, stay up to date
- U.S. Multi-Society Task Force on CRC …
  - **1st tier tests** = colonoscopy every 10 years (assuming normal and no other risk factors) and yearly FIT
    - In sequential approach, offer colonoscopy first (much higher sensitivity for polyps than FIT and polyps can be removed)
  - **2nd tier tests** = CT colonography every 5 years, FIT-fecal DNA every 3 years, flex sig every 5–10 years
  - **3rd tier** = capsule colonoscopy
- Other guidelines: e.g., ACS, U.S. Preventative Services Task Force
- Average risk (no symptoms, no FH) screening: age 45
- Rising rates in patients < age 50: Take all symptoms and family history **very seriously**
- FH of CRC or advanced adenoma in 1st degree relative < age 60 or two 1st degree relatives with these findings at any age = colonoscopy q 5 years beginning at age 40 or 10 years before the age of diagnosis of youngest relative (whichever comes first)
- 1st degree relative diagnosed ≥ age 60 with CRC or advanced adenoma = start screening at age 40 but with intervals similar to average-risk patients
- **Colonoscopy is screening method of choice** for those with positive family history of adenomatous polyps/cancer or personal history of adenomatous polyps

CRC Stages I–IV

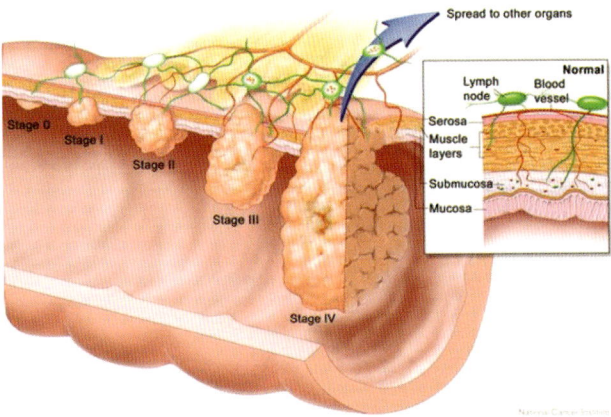

- Mucosa = epithelium (above basement membrane) + lamina propria

ONCOLOGY

CRC

- CEA useful in monitoring response to treatment, and in surveillance for relapse
- Staging: TNM
- Treatment
  - Stage I, II, III — surgery
    - Add adjuvant chemo for high-risk Stage II, and all Stage III (FOLFOX or CAPOX)
  - Stage IV — palliative systemic therapy; tumor molecular testing is key
    - 5-FU based chemo
    - VEGF antibody (bevacizumab)
    - EGFR antibody (cetuximab)
    - Immunotherapy (nivolumab, ipilimumab)
  - For localized rectal cancer, incorporate radiation as well

PANCREATIC CANCER

- Histology — adenocarcinoma most common
- Risk factors
  - Smoking, DM, family history, chronic pancreatitis
  - Peak age: 65–69 for males, 75–79 for females
- Clinical presentation
  - Jaundice, abdominal pain, weight loss
  - Tumor location affects presenting signs and stage
    - **Head**: painless jaundice from compression of CBD
    - **Body/Tail**: pain (may radiate to back) and weight loss
- Treatment
  - Early stage — pancreaticoduodenectomy, followed by adjuvant chemo ± radiation
  - Advanced disease — palliative chemotherapy, supportive care

Pancreatic Neuroendocrine Tumors

- **Glucagonoma**: glucagon-secreting tumor that causes scaly, necrolytic migratory erythema, diarrhea, persistent hyperglycemia with plasma glucagon > 1,000 pg/dL
  - NME: eczematous or psoriasiform rash, often at skin flexures and orifices
- **Insulinoma**: insulin-secreting B-cell tumor
- **Gastrinoma (Zollinger-Ellison syndrome)**: covered in Gastroenterology presentation
- **VIPomas**
  - Tumors that secrete VIP (stimulates intestinal fluid/electrolytes)
  - Profuse secretory diarrhea
  - Dx: increased VIP level and low K^+

PEARLS — GI CANCERS

- Increasing rates of colorectal cancer in **young patients**: Take all symptoms seriously; do not assume bleeding is from hemorrhoids
- **CRC screening**
  - **Recall different risk groups**
- **Inherited CRC**
  - **Lynch syndrome** is a common hereditary syndrome: universal MSI testing on all CRC patients
  - **> 10 lifetime adenomas** — think polyposis syndrome!
- Endocarditis caused by *Strep bovis* or *Clostridium septicum* — think colorectal cancer
- Painless jaundice — think pancreatic cancer (head of pancreas)
- Esophageal cancer
  - Proximal 2/3 — squamous, from tobacco/EtOH
  - Distal 1/3 — adenocarcinoma, from GERD/Barrett's

LUNG CANCER

AR 7

A 67-year-old man with a 100-pack/year history of smoking (2 ppd for 50 years) is essentially dragged in by his wife, who says that he has withered away to nothing and has been acting very confused lately. He says he is fine but keeps calling you by his grandchild's name. You don't get much more information out of him.

PMH: HTN controlled on lisinopril; prostatectomy 5 years ago
ROS: 30-lb weight loss/6 months

Exam: oriented only to person
Chest: coarse scattered crackles; no focal findings
Abd: soft, benign

Laboratory: calcium = 11.5 mg/dL

CXR: central/hilar mass with area of cavitation

Based on your findings, which of the following types of lung cancer does this man most likely have?

A. Small cell
B. Adenocarcinoma
C. Squamous cell carcinoma
D. Bronchoalveolar carcinoma
E. Large cell

Answer:_____

Lung Cancer

- Risk factors
  - Smoking
  - Asbestos
  - Uranium, nickel, diesel exhaust, beryllium, silica, arsenic, heavy radon exposure
- Screening

Lung Cancer — Screening

- The USPSTF (revised 2021) recommends yearly lung cancer screening with low-dose CT scan for people who:
  1) Have a history of heavy smoking (≥ 20 pack years) **and**
  2) Smoke now or have quit within the past 15 years **and**
  3) Are between 50 and 80 years of age
- Radiation dose exposure is < 1/3 of a standard-dose diagnostic chest CT
- Informed consent and multidisciplinary evaluation critical
- When should screening stop?
  1) Turns 81 years old **or**
  2) Has not smoked in 15 years **or**
  3) Develops a health problem that makes him or her unwilling or unable to have surgery if lung cancer is found

Lung Cancer

- There are **2 major categories** of cancer:
  - **Non–small cell lung cancer (~ 85%)**
    - Adenocarcinoma
    - Squamous cell
    - Large cell
    - Others
  - **Small cell lung cancer (~ 15%)**

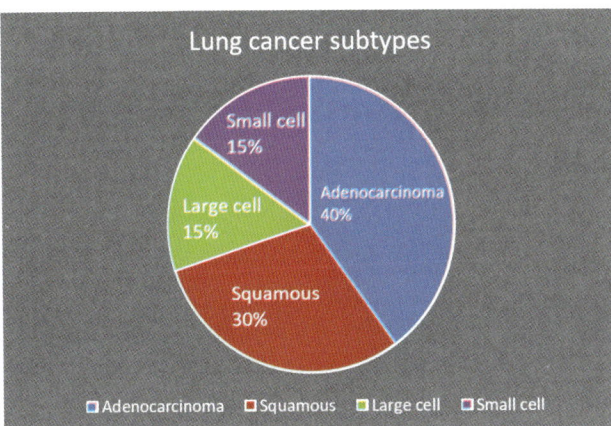

- **Squamous cell**
  - Usually starts near a central bronchus
  - Associated with **cavitary lesions**
  - Usually metastasizes by direct extension into the hilar node and mediastinum
  - Associated with **hypercalcemia**
    - From secretion of a parathyroid hormone-like substance
  - Histologic
    - **Keratin** production by tumor cells
    - Intercellular desmosomes "intercellular bridges"

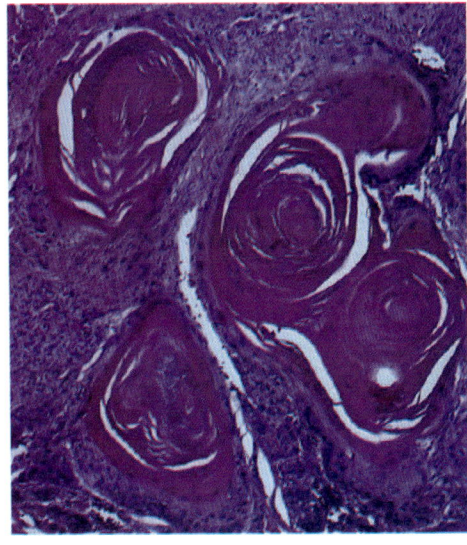

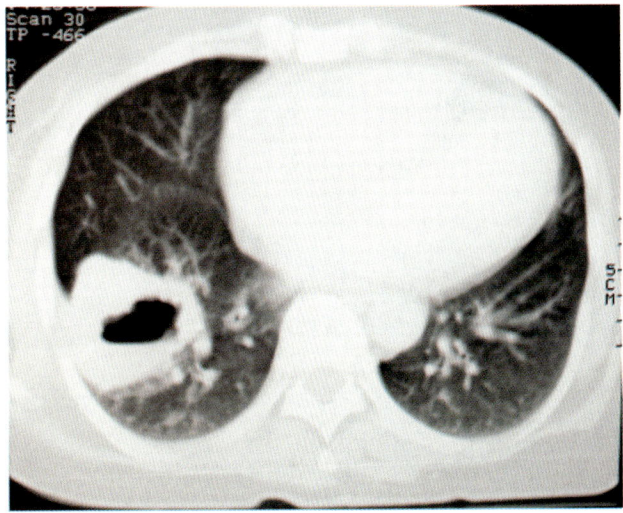

- **Adenocarcinoma**
  - **Most common lung cancer (~ 40% of all cases)**
  - **Higher incidence of driver mutations (i.e., EGFR)**
  - Pancoast tumor (superior sulcus tumor)
    - Named after the radiologist in 1924
    - Characteristic shoulder pain with weakness and numbness of the arm
    - Horner syndrome
      - Ptosis, miosis, anhidrosis

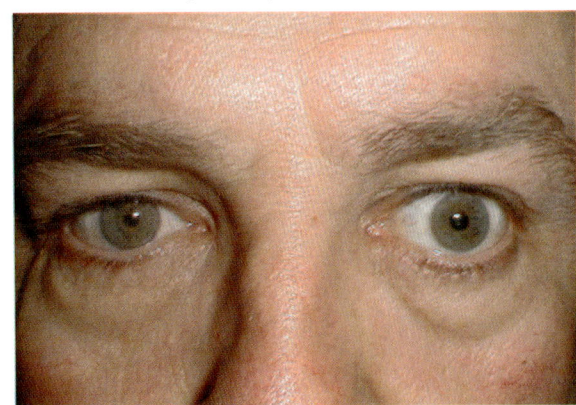

ONCOLOGY

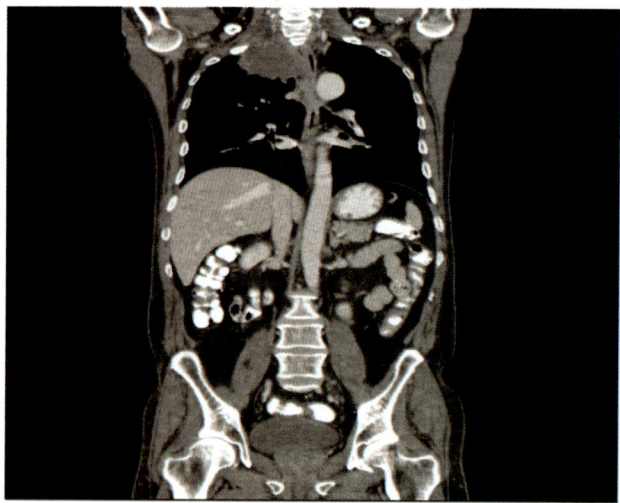

- **Adenocarcinoma in situ and minimally invasive adenocarcinoma**
  - **Formerly known as bronchoalveolar carcinoma**
  - Slow growing, indolent
  - Least association with smoking
  - Up to 50% arises in the setting of preexisting lung disease
  - Usually PET negative
    - Low-glucose metabolism

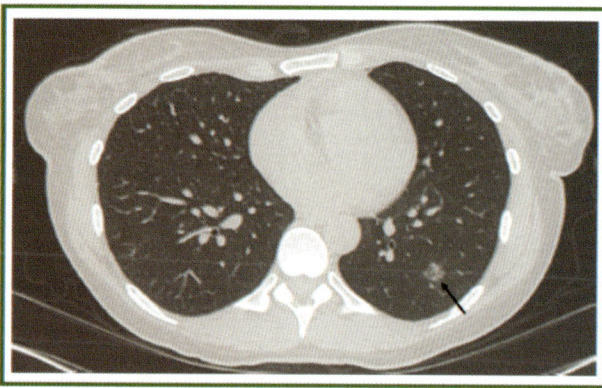

- **Small cell**
  - Previously called "oat cell"
  - The "oat cell" contains dense neurosecretory granules
    - Vesicles containing neuroendocrine hormones
  - Extremely aggressive
  - 80% of patients have metastases at the time of diagnosis
  - Paraneoplastic syndromes
    - SIADH
    - Ectopic ACTH production
    - Lambert-Eaton syndrome
    - Most common cause of SVC syndrome

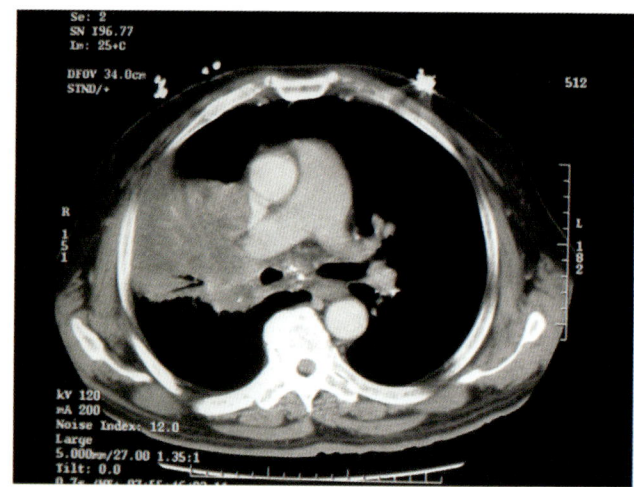

Lung Cancer — Management
- **Non–small cell**
  - Stage: I/II surgery ± adjuvant chemo
    - Lobectomy or pneumonectomy + MLND
    - Adjuvant cisplatin doublet × 4 cycles for high risk
  - Stage III: chemo-XRT
    - Concurrent chest XRT + platinum-chemo
    - Adjuvant immunotherapy × 1 year
  - Stage IV: palliative systemic therapy — tumor molecular testing is key (NGS for actionable mutations, PD-L1 testing)
    - Platinum-chemo
    - Targeted therapies (*EGFR, ALK, ROS1, BRAF* mutations)
    - Immunotherapy (checkpoint inhibitor)
- **Small cell**
  - Stage I/II/III: chemo-XRT
  - Stage IV: palliative chemoimmunotherapy
  - Prophylactic brain XRT responders
  - Surgery rarely indicated

Pearls — Lung Cancer
- Know screening guidelines
- Specific scenarios:
  - Lung mass and palpable neck nodes? — biopsy neck for diagnosis and staging
  - Lung mass and pleural effusion? — thoracentesis with cytology for diagnosis and staging
- Non–small cell
  - Adenocarcinoma — EGFR and other actionable mutations
  - Bronchoalveolar — less association with tobacco
  - Squamous cell — central, cavitates, hypercalcemia
  - Large cell — peripheral, "scar" carcinoma
  - Small cell — central
  - Paraneoplastic syndromes (SIADH, Cushing's, Lambert-Eaton's)

Solitary Pulmonary Nodule
- Most commonly found on CT chest
- Must assess risk of malignancy (1–35% in U.S.)
- Look at size, growth pattern/rate, and characteristics of nodule
- Management options include surveillance vs. PET/CT vs. biopsy
- Surveillance guided by Fleischner Society guidelines

HEAD AND NECK CANCER

- Risk factors
  - Tobacco and alcohol abuse
  - HPV-16/HPV-18 infections
  - EBV (nasopharyngeal carcinoma)
- Includes cancers of:
  - Oral cavity
  - Oropharynx
  - Nasopharynx
  - Hypopharynx
  - Larynx
- Histology
  - Squamous cell (95%)
- Clinical presentation
  - Depends on tumor site
  - Includes otalgia, hoarseness, oral ulcers
  - Cervical lymph node mass
- Diagnosis
  - Fiberoptic exam/scopes
  - CT/MRI imaging
  - FNA/biopsy
- If patient presents with cervical lymph node mass
  - Diagnose with FNA
  - If FNA positive for squamous cell cancer, then proceed with CT/MRI of head/neck and panendoscopy

Head and Neck Cancer — Management

- Early-stage disease
  - Surgical resection
  - Radiation
- Locally advanced disease — multimodality therapy
  - Surgery and postoperative radiation
  - Definitive combined chemoradiation with goal of organ preservation
- Metastatic disease
  - Platinum-based chemotherapy
  - PD-1 inhibitor immunotherapy
- Watch for increased risk of secondary malignancy (lung, esophageal) due to field defect

PRIMARY BRAIN CANCER

- Clinical presentation
  - Headache, seizures, N/V, focal neuro deficits
- Diagnosis: MRI brain with contrast
- Histology — astrocytoma most common
  - Anaplastic astrocytoma
  - Glioblastoma
  - Increasing use of molecular classification
    - IDH mutation status
- Management
  - Debulking surgery
  - Adjuvant radiation + temozolomide

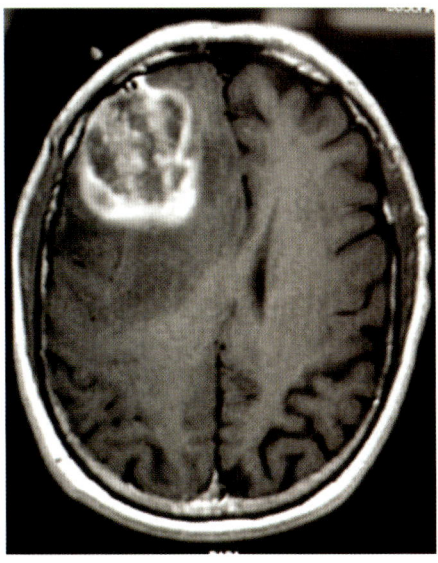

Carcinogens

- Tobacco — 30% of U.S. cancer-related deaths
- Alcohol — liver, head & neck, esophagus
- Asbestos — lung, mesothelioma
- Estrogens — breast, uterine, vaginal
- Nitrites — gastric
- Radiation (ionizing and UV) — leukemia, sarcoma, thyroid
- Viruses
  - *H. pylori* — gastric
  - Hepatitis B/C — liver
  - HPV — cervical, anal, oropharyngeal

PARANEOPLASTIC SYNDROMES

AR 8

A 62-year-old female undergoing treatment for metastatic breast cancer presents with confusion and a serum calcium of 12.5 mg/dL (normal is 8.5–10.3 mg/dL) with albumin of 2.5 mg/dL.

Which of the following should be done initially to manage her hypercalcemia?

A. Vigorous hydration with NS to maintain urine output 100–150 cc/hour followed by zoledronic acid
B. Zoledronic acid alone
C. Water restriction followed by zoledronic acid
D. Vigorous hydration with NS with HCTZ to maintain urine output at 100–150 cc/hour followed by zoledronic acid
E. Vigorous hydration with 1/4 NS with furosemide to maintain urine output at 100–150 cc/hour followed by zoledronic acid

Answer:_____

Paraneoplastic Syndromes

Clinical Syndrome	Underlying Cancer Type	Causal Mechanism
Hypercalcemia	Squamous cell lung Renal, breast, myeloma, T-cell leukemia/lymphoma	Bone metastasis PTH-rP Calcitriol/vit D
SIADH	Small cell lung Intracranial neoplasm	ADH (vasopressin)
Cushing syndrome	Small cell lung Pancreatic carcinoma Neural tumors	ACTH or ACTH-like substance
Carcinoid syndrome	Neuroendocrine tumors of GI tract	Serotonin Bradykinin
Polycythemia	Gastric and renal cancer Hepatocellular cancer	Erythropoietin

HYPERCALCEMIA OF MALIGNANCY

Hypercalcemia
- The most common paraneoplastic syndrome
- Malignancy is the most common cause of increased calcium in patients
- Most common associated cancers
  - Breast, renal, myeloma, squamous cell of lung, and head/neck
- Mechanisms
  - Increased osteolytic activity by bone metastasis
  - Ectopic PTHrP production
  - Vitamin D/Calcitriol overproduction
- Clinical presentation
  - Fatigue, constipation, polyuria/polydipsia, altered mental status
  - Elevated serum calcium
    - Correct for serum albumin
  - Cardiac dysrhythmias, renal dysfunction
  - Symptoms associated with severity and rate of development of hypercalcemia

Hypercalcemia — Management
- IV fluid hydration with normal saline
  - Most important initial step
- Diuretics
  - Use selectively only if volume overload develops
- Calcitonin
  - Useful in initial 48 hours, but watch for tachyphylaxis
- Osteoclast inhibitors
  - Mainstay of definitive therapy
  - Zoledronic acid preferred
  - Pamidronate preferred in renal dysfunction
  - Denosumab (RANKL inhibitor) in refractory cases
  - Watch for osteonecrosis of the jaw as rare toxicity
- Treat underlying tumor

Hypercalcemia — Summary of Acute Management
- Acute therapy — 3 things to give:
  1) Volume expansion with isotonic saline at initial rate of 200–300 mL/hour and then adjust to keep urine output 100–150 mL/hour
     - If fluid overload a problem, give furosemide (no longer standard for all)
  2) Calcitonin 4 IU/kg (if immediate reduction is needed — usually > 14 mg/dL and symptomatic), and then repeat q 6–12 hours if responsive
  3) Zoledronic acid 4 mg (dose adjust for renal dysfunction) IV over 15 minutes (becomes effective by day 2–4)

DIRECT TUMOR EFFECTS

- Superior vena cava syndrome
- Bone metastases
- Spinal cord compression
- Brain metastases
- Malignant pleural effusions
- Malignant pericardial effusions

SUPERIOR VENA CAVA (SVC) SYNDROME
- Results from occlusion of the superior vena cava, either by external compression or internal thrombus
- Most cases of external compression are secondary to malignancy
  - Lung cancer
  - Lymphoma
  - Mediastinal germ cell tumors
- Symptoms include:
  - Facial and neck swelling
  - Dyspnea
  - Headaches
  - Hoarseness (laryngeal edema)
  - Mental status changes (increased ICP)
- Physical findings include:
  - Facial plethora
  - Edema of the neck, upper extremities, and face
  - Neck vein distention
  - Collateral veins on the anterior chest
  - Mental obtundation

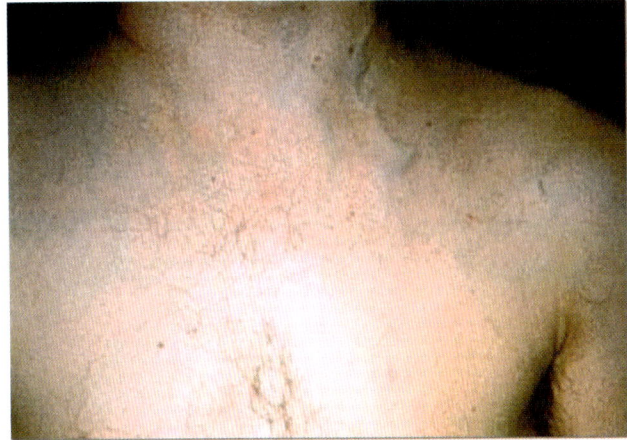

- Diagnosis
  - CT venogram of chest
  - Obtain tumor tissue diagnosis (if not known)
- Management
  - Supportive care
    - O_2, diuresis, steroids
  - Definitive therapy
    - Chemotherapy preferred for chemo-sensitive tumors
      - Small cell lung, lymphoma, germ cell
    - Radiation preferred for all others
      - Non–small cell lung
  - Other options
    - Anticoagulation, thrombolysis, stenting

BONE METASTASES
- Any malignancy may metastasize to the bone
- Most common would include:
  - Prostate
  - Breast
  - Lung
  - Renal cell
  - Myeloma
- Presenting symptoms include:
  - Pain
  - Pathologic fracture
- Common sites for bony involvement
  - Vertebral bodies
  - Femur
  - Ribs
  - Pelvis

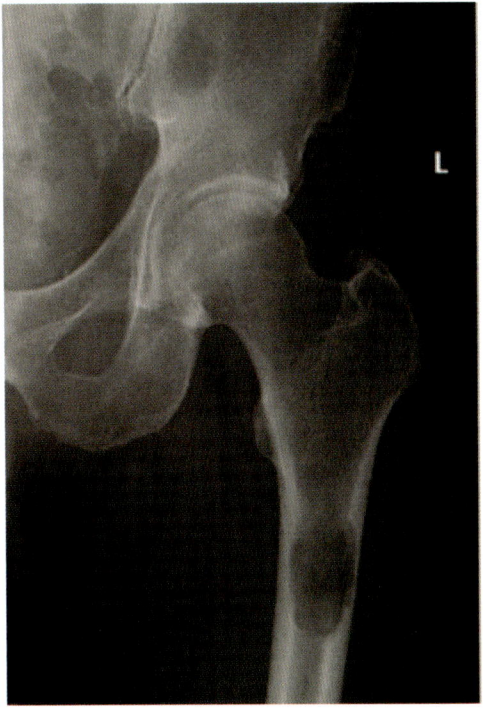

- Diagnosis should be made with:
  - Bone scan
  - Metastatic bone survey
    - Remember that purely lytic lesions will not appear on a bone scan
    - Should always confirm a "hot" bone scan with plain films
- Treatment should include:
  - Radiation therapy for pain control
  - Surgery in selected cases
    - Prophylactic rod
    - Vertebroplasty
  - Osteoclast inhibitors — reduce risk of skeletal-related events
    - Bisphosphonates
    - RANK ligand inhibitor — denosumab

AR 9

A 50-year-old man with a Hx of limited stage small cell lung cancer underwent chemoradiation 6 months ago, with complete response. The patient presents with bilateral leg weakness × 3 weeks, and mid-back pain × 3 days. Yesterday he soiled his clothes × 1. On exam, point tenderness is T10.

What is the best approach to diagnosis and the next step in management?

A. EMG followed by neurology consultation
B. Urgent MRI/CT brain with contrast, followed by IV steroids if Dx confirmed
C. Restaging scans for evaluation of relapsed disease and oncology consultation
D. Urgent MRI spine; if Dx confirmed, then IV dexamethasone and radiation oncology consultation

Answer:_____

Spinal Cord Compression
- An oncologic emergency
- Should <u>always</u> be suspected in a patient with a diagnosis of malignancy and a complaint of back pain
- Most common tumors are:
  - Lung
  - Breast
  - Prostate
  - Myeloma
- Clinical presentation
  - Back pain that worsens with activity
  - Localized tenderness in spine
  - Radicular pain
  - Loss of bowel and bladder control
  - Sensory changes typically precede motor loss
- Diagnosis
  - MRI is the gold standard for diagnosis
  - Image the entire spine
- Need tissue diagnosis to decide best treatment

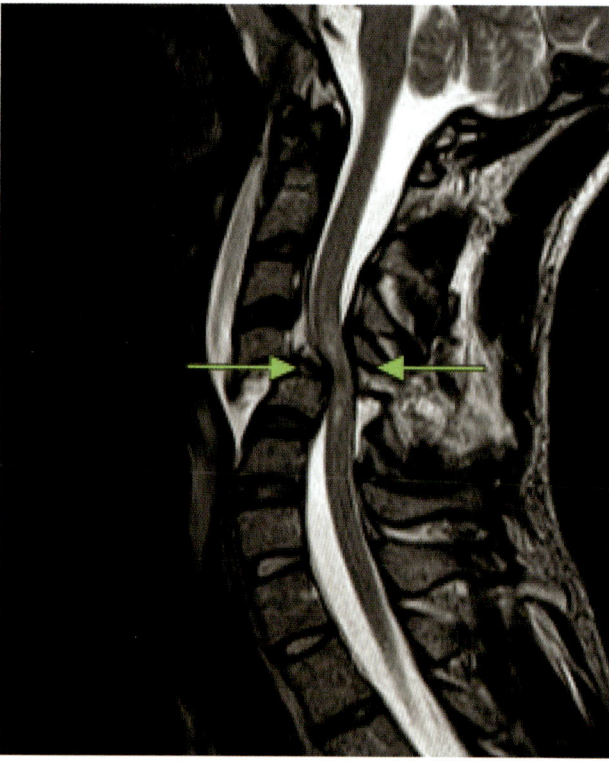

- Treatment best if done early
- If the patient is ambulatory at the initiation of therapy, then they are likely to remain so
- If they are already paraplegic, then only 10% recover the ability to walk
- Treatment options will depend upon patient's burden/type of disease, life expectancy, and values
  - Immediate steroids to reduce edema
  - Radiation often preferred therapy
  - Surgery (decompressive resection/stabilization) in selected cases
    - Unstable spine or progressive neurologic decline
    - Need tissue diagnosis
    - Unable to receive radiotherapy
  - Chemotherapy may be combined with radiation for sensitive tumors

BRAIN METASTASES
- Most common tumors associated are:
  - Lung
  - Breast
  - Melanoma
  - Renal cell carcinoma
- Symptoms include those of increased intracranial pressure
  - Headache
  - Nausea
  - Seizures
  - Progressive neurological changes
- Diagnosis: MRI is best

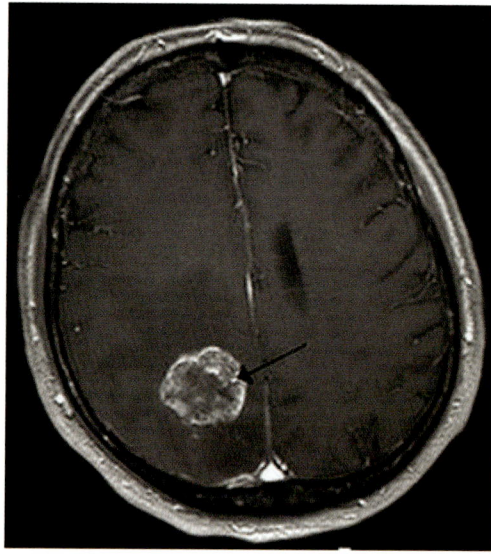

- Treatment includes:
  - Immediate large doses of steroids (usually IV dexamethasone)
  - For a solitary lesion with controlled systemic disease, consider **resection**
  - For multiple but limited disease, consider **stereotactic radiosurgery**
    - ≤ 3 lesions all ≤ 3 cm
  - For multiple or widespread lesions, and after any resection, **whole-brain radiation** therapy should be given

MALIGNANT EFFUSIONS

Malignant Pleural Effusions
- Occur either as an exudative reaction to a tumor or from lymphatic obstruction by the tumor
- Common tumors are those that metastasize to mediastinal nodes
  - Lung: **most common cause of exudative malignant effusion**
  - Breast
  - Lymphoma
- Diagnosis is by pleural fluid cytology
  - Exudative
- May require multiple samples and large volume for diagnosis
- Occasionally may need pleural biopsy or thoracoscopy for diagnosis
- Treatment involves:
  - Therapy directed to the primary tumor
  - Symptomatic management with thoracentesis
  - If recurrent, then needs definitive management
    - Pleurodesis
      - Talc, doxycycline, bleomycin
    - PleurX catheter

Malignant Pericardial Effusions
- Commonly occur in those tumors in the vicinity (direct extension)
  - Lung
  - Breast
- May occur via hematogenous spread
  - Leukemia
  - Lymphoma
- May cause tamponade
- Symptoms depend upon the rate of accumulation of the fluid
- Diagnose by echocardiogram
- Management
  - Pericardiocentesis
  - Pericardial window

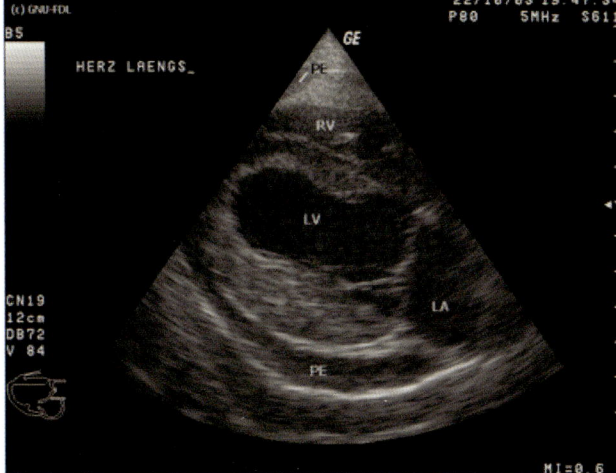

Systemic Cancer Therapy
- Cytotoxic chemotherapy — know key drug toxicities!
- Targeted therapy
  - Tyrosine kinase inhibitors
  - Monoclonal antibodies
- Endocrine therapy
- Immunotherapy

Chemotherapy — Side Effects to Be Aware Of
- General side effects would include count suppression, N/V, alopecia
- Some specific side effects include:
  - Cisplatin — renal, ototoxicity
  - Daunorubicin/Doxorubicin and trastuzumab — cardiac
  - Bleomycin — pulmonary fibrosis
  - Vincristine — neurotoxicity
  - EGFR inhibitors — skin rash
  - Alkylating agents — leukemogenic
  - Rituximab/monoclonal antibodies — infusion reactions

Immunotherapy — Checkpoint Inhibitors
- 2 major drug classes
  - PD-1 inhibitors (pembrolizumab, nivolumab, atezolizumab)
  - CTLA 4 inhibitors (ipilimumab)
- Work by immunomodulation of T cells; "release the brake" on the immune system to enhance its response to cancer cells
- Approved for use across wide variety of solid cancers, including:
  - Lung, renal, bladder, melanoma, gastric, liver, head and neck, breast, cervical, Hodgkin lymphoma

ONCOLOGY

**Immune-Related Adverse Events
(Autoimmune Toxicities)**
- Can affect virtually any organ
  - Colitis
  - Dermatitis
  - Hepatitis
  - Endocrinopathy
- Arise from general immunologic enhancement
- Caution in patients with preexisting autoimmune disease
- Can rarely lead to serious morbidity/mortality
  → prompt recognition and early intervention is key!
- Treat with immunosuppression
  - High-dose steroids

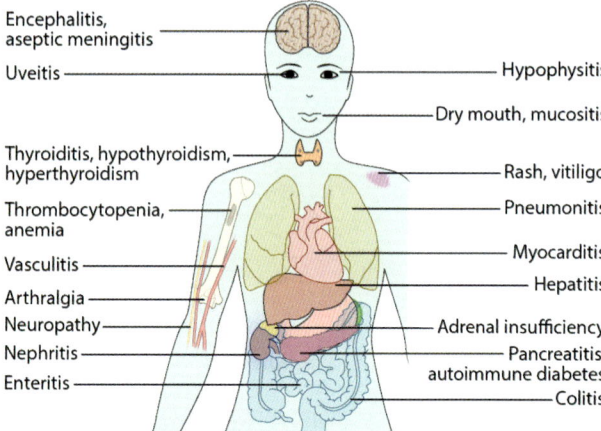

Molecularly Targeted Therapy
- Better understanding of oncogenic pathways and driver mutations
- Development of targeted agents with potential for greater efficacy and less toxicity vs. conventional chemotherapy
- Genomic tumor testing in search of "actionable" mutations
- Several recent FDA drug approvals based upon drug target, rather than tumor type
  - Tumor agnostic therapy (*NTRK* mutation, MSI, TMB)
- Key drug classes include:
  - Tyrosine kinase inhibitors
    - Imatinib for CML
    - Erlotinib for lung cancer
  - Monoclonal antibodies
    - Trastuzumab for breast cancer
    - Rituximab for lymphoma
    - Bevacizumab for colorectal, lung cancer

COMPLICATIONS OF CANCER THERAPY

Tumor Lysis Syndrome
- Rapid lysis of malignant cells leading to metabolic derangement
- Should be anticipated in rapidly growing tumors or those tumors that are sensitive to chemotherapy, such as Burkitt lymphoma or other non-Hodgkin lymphomas

AR 10

A 24-year-old male, HIV positive, presents with widespread peripheral lymphadenopathy. Biopsy confirms Burkitt lymphoma. Patient is admitted for staging and initiation of chemotherapy. On day 2 of treatment, nursing reports a marked decrease in urine output. Laboratory results:

	Admission	Current	Normal Value Range
Sodium	141 mEq/L	138 mEq/L	135–145 mEq/L
Potassium	4.5 mEq/L	6.4 mEq/L	3.5–5.0 mEq/L
Chloride	108 mEq/L	101 mEq/L	95–108 mEq/L
Bicarbonate	27 mEq/L	21 mEq/L	22–28 mEq/L
Calcium	8.9 mg/dL	7.1 mg/dL	8.5–10.3 mg/dL
Phosphate	3.6 mg/dL	8.2 mg/dL	3.0–4.5 mg/dL
Uric acid	7.6 mg/dL	12.2 mg/dL	2.5–8.0 mg/dL
BUN	14 mg/dL	42 mg/dL	7–30 mg/dL
Creatinine	1.1 mg/dL	1.9 mg/dL	0.7–1.2 mg/dL

Early treatment with which of the following may have prevented this condition?

A. Intravenous calcium
B. Intravenous furosemide
C. Intravenous rasburicase
D. Intravenous sodium bicarbonate
E. Intravenous steroids

Answer:_____

Tumor Lysis Syndrome
- Release of intracellular contents results in the development of:
  - Hyperuricemia
    - Uric acid nephropathy
  - Hyperkalemia
    - Cardiac arrhythmias
  - Hyperphosphatemia
    - Potentiates uric acid nephropathy and acute kidney injury
  - Hypocalcemia
    - Tetany or arrhythmias
- Prevention is the key
- Risk stratification to determine prophylaxis
- Management options
  - IVF hydration
  - Allopurinol — add for moderate-risk patients
    - Prevents new uric acid formation
  - Rasburicase — add for high-risk patients
    - Decreases existing uric acid
- Monitor electrolyte values closely after treatment

Febrile Neutropenia
- Potentially life-threatening complication of myelosuppressive cancer therapy
- Incidence has decreased with use of myeloid growth factor support
- Definition
  - A single temperature of ≥ 100.9°F (38.3°C) or ≥ 100.4°F (38.0°C) over 1 hour
- Perform thorough evaluation to identify source
  - H&P
  - Pan-cultures
  - LFTs, urine studies, chest imaging
- Rapid administration of empiric IV antibiotics
  - Cefepime or piperacillin/tazobactam
  - Add vancomycin if risk of gram-positive infection
  - Add antifungal later, if persistent fever

Cancer Survivorship
- Late effects of cancer or its treatment
  - Neuropathy
  - Infertility
  - Cardiovascular
- Monitoring for recurrence
  - Testing and follow-up
- Risk of second cancers
  - Behavioral modifications
- Psychosocial issues
  - Depression
- Financial burdens
  - Return to workplace

PEARLS — GENERAL ONCOLOGY

- Hypercalcemia — treatment for acute presentation
- Back pain in cancer patient or former cancer patient: MRI of entire spine
- Brain mets: IV steroids, resect, radiate
- Malignant pleural effusions: pleurodesis, if recurrent
- Tumor lysis syndrome — think prevention in high risk
  - Rasburicase, allopurinol
- Chemo drug toxicities — cisplatin, doxorubicin, bleomycin, vincristine
- Immunotherapy — recognize autoimmune toxicities
  - Treat with high-dose steroids

AUDIENCE RESPONSE ANSWERS

Audience Response 1
C. Adjuvant chemotherapy followed by radiation

AR 2
C. Bone density/DXA scan every 2 years

AR 3
C. Calculate her risk estimate for CIN-3, and then pursue colposcopy or excision if high risk.

AR 4
D. There is > 85% likelihood the mass is a germ cell tumor.

AR 5
C. Serum tumor markers and radical inguinal orchiectomy

AR 6
B. Transrectal ultrasound with multiple biopsies

AR 7
C. Squamous cell carcinoma

AR 8
A. Vigorous hydration with NS to maintain urine output 100–150 cc/hour followed by zoledronic acid

AR 9
D. Urgent MRI spine; if Dx confirmed, then IV dexamethasone and radiation oncology consultation

AR 10
C. Intravenous rasburicase

ONCOLOGY

ENDNOTES

[1]   Tessssa13 [CC BY-SA 4.0 (https://creativecommons.org/licenses/by-sa/4.0)]

[2]   UpToDate, 2019: Cancer Risks and management of BRCA carriers without cancer

[3]   http://www.dermnet.com/Acanthosis-Nigricans/picture/22985

[4]   Dr. Silke

MedStudy®

INTERNAL MEDICINE REVIEW

Psychiatry

Presented by

Y. Pritham Raj, MD

TABLE OF CONTENTS

Psychiatry Outline
- Psychiatric Conditions — an Overview
- Mood Disorders — Depression, Bipolar Disorder, Other Mood Disorders, Treatment[1]
- Suicide
- Anxiety Disorders
- Schizophrenia and Related Disorders
- Psychiatric Medications and Life-Threatening Side Effects
- Substance Use Disorders
- Personality Disorders
- Insomnia
- Other Topics in Psychiatry

Psychiatric Conditions
- General Pearls on Each Condition
  - Typical Age of Onset
  - Duration of Symptoms
  - Decline in Functionality
  - Pattern of Recurrence
  - Causative Agent (if applicable)

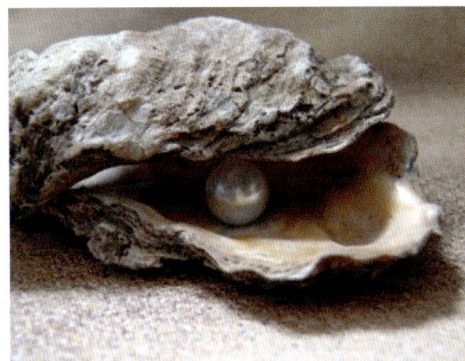

MAJOR DEPRESSIVE DISORDER (MDD)

- At least **2 weeks** of **depressed mood** and/or **anhedonia** with ≥ 5 **SIG E CAPS**:
  - **S**leep disturbance (insomnia or hypersomnia)
  - **I**nterest diminished
  - **G**uilt
  - **E**nergy loss or fatigue
  - **C**oncentration diminished
  - **A**ppetite changes
  - **P**sychomotor slowing (or agitation)
  - **S**uicidal thoughts
- General pearls
  - **Age of onset:** mean 32.5 years
  - **Duration of symptoms:** at least **2 weeks**
  - **Decline in functionality:** variable
  - **Prevalence:** more common in women; highest in transgender individuals (50%)
  - **Pattern of recurrence:** average of 5–9 episodes over a lifetime

- Lifetime prevalence of 20%
- 50% relapse after 1st episode
- 80% relapse after 3rd episode
- 80% of individuals can achieve a significant reduction in symptoms with proper treatment
- 50% of individuals may not respond to the initial treatment trial
- MDD is considered a relapsing, remitting illness

MDD — Assessment
- Medical, psychiatric, and social history
- **SIG E CAPS** captured in the Patient Health Questionnaire-9 (PHQ-9)
- **Suicidal and homicidal ideation**
- Substance use
- Physical exam/Laboratory assessment
- Medication reconciliation: β-blockers*****, corticosteroids, benzodiazepines, antiparkinsonian medications, hormones, stimulants, statins, antiseizure medications, proton pump inhibitors, and H_2 blockers, **interferons**

*The strongest association with β-blockers has been with low energy/fatigue, rather than MDD
- Laboratory assessment
  - Complete blood count (CBC)
  - Comprehensive metabolic panel (CMP)
  - Liver function tests (LFTs)
  - Urinalysis
  - Thyroid-stimulating hormone (TSH; free T_3, T_4 if TSH abnormal)
  - Vitamin B_{12}, vitamin B_1, folate
  - Pregnancy testing
  - Toxicology: drugs, heavy metal screen
  - Rapid plasma reagin (RPR)
  - Human immunodeficiency virus (HIV)

MDD — Treatment
- Psychotherapy and/or meds for 12 weeks
  - If no response to psychotherapy, start meds after 12 weeks

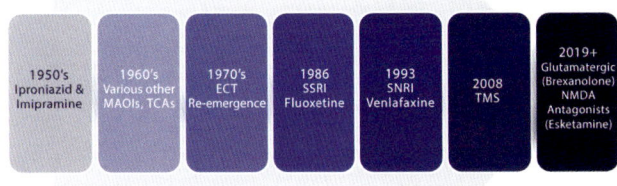

- After starting meds, monitor with **3 visits for mental healthcare during the first 12 weeks** per the National Committee for Quality Assurance
  - Increase dose if partial response in 4 weeks
  - Change to another medication if no response after 4–6 week trial at max dosing
  - Treatment-resistant depression (failure to respond to 1–2 antidepressants + psychotherapy) occurs in 30–45% of patients
- Consult a psychiatrist if there is treatment-resistant depression or a suspicion of hypomania, mania, or psychosis
- Seek emergent psychiatric assessment if suicidal or homicidal ideations present

MDD Treatment — SSRIs
- Selective serotonin reuptake inhibitors (SSRIs)
  - Fluoxetine, paroxetine, sertraline, citalopram, escitalopram, fluvoxamine
  - Also effective for anxiety disorders
  - May cause weight gain (+)
  - May cause GI side effects or headaches, usually resolve after 1–2 weeks
  - May cause decreased sexual function, dose dependence; consider adding or switching to **bupropion** or **mirtazapine**
  - If combined with aspirin or NSAIDs, mildly increased risk of gastrointestinal bleeding or abnormal uterine bleeding (AUB; formerly dysfunctional uterine bleeding)

Audience Response 1
A 65-year-old male presents with 4 weeks of depressed mood, poor sleep and appetite, and anhedonia. He denies any suicidal thoughts. He is diagnosed with MDD and agrees to start a trial of medication for his symptoms.

Which of the following medications is more likely to cause QT$_c$ prolongation in this patient?

A. Fluoxetine
B. Sertraline
C. Paroxetine
D. Citalopram
E. Escitalopram

Answer:_____

SSRI Pearls
- Longest half-life: **fluoxetine (4–14 days)**
- Shortest half-life: fluvoxamine, **paroxetine (21 hours without active metabolites)**
- Sedative: paroxetine
- Weight gain: paroxetine
- QT$_c$ prolongation: citalopram
- Least expressed in breast milk: sertraline

MDD Treatment — SNRIs
- Serotonin and norepinephrine reuptake inhibitors (SNRIs)
  - Venlafaxine, desvenlafaxine, duloxetine, levomilnacipran
  - Also effective for anxiety disorders
  - Also effective for neuropathic pain, fibromyalgia, and chronic musculoskeletal pain (duloxetine)
  - May cause weight gain (+)
  - May cause decreased sexual function
  - Dose-related BP effects

MDD Treatment — MAOIs
- Monoamine oxidase inhibitors (MAOIs)
  - Phenelzine, selegiline, isocarboxazid, tranylcypromine
  - Not 1st line treatment
  - May cause weight gain (+++)
  - May cause sexual dysfunction
  - Think **diet** and **tyramine → hypertensive crisis**
- Think serotonin
  - Give 2–4 weeks washout period
  - When switching to or from another serotonin med
  - **Serotonin syndrome**

MDD Treatment — TCAs
- Tricyclic antidepressants (TCAs)
  - Imipramine, amitriptyline, doxepin, desipramine, nortriptyline
  - Not 1st line treatment
  - Off-label use for migraine and chronic pain/fibromyalgia
  - May cause weight gain (+++)
  - May cause sexual dysfunction
  - Sedative (anticholinergic)
  - Consider checking serum levels
  - **Cardiotoxic (QT$_c$ prolongation and QRS widening)**

Recap — When Thinking Serotonin
- Good for depression and anxiety
- Also think:
  - Gastrointestinal
  - Platelets
  - Sexual dysfunction
  - **Sodium** (hyponatremia from syndrome of inappropriate antidiuretic hormone secretion [SIADH])
- Heart
  - Slight risk of QT$_c$ prolongation (citalopram)
  - Cardiotoxic (TCAs)

MDD Treatment — Bupropion
- Bupropion
  - Norepinephrine and dopamine reuptake inhibitor (NDRI)
  - Also used for smoking cessation
  - Off-label use for ADHD
  - May cause insomnia
  - May cause weight loss
  - No sexual dysfunction
  - Increased **seizure** risk in eating disorder and epilepsy patients

MDD Treatment — Mirtazapine

- Mirtazapine
  - Tetracyclic noradrenergic and specific serotonergic antidepressants (NaSSA)
  - Faster onset of action
  - May be used as augmenting agent in combination with other antidepressants for management of sleep, appetite, and sexual dysfunction
  - Sedative
  - Also an appetite inducer

MDD Treatment — Trazodone

- Trazodone
  - Sedative
    - Off-label use for sleep
- May increase appetite
- May cause priapism (rare)

AR 2

A 30-year-old woman presents with symptoms of depression. She has been treated successfully for depression in the past but gained 20 lb on pharmacotherapy and is reluctant to take medications due to fear of weight gain.

Which antidepressant would be the best option for her in regard to her concerns about weight gain?

A. Amitriptyline
B. Paroxetine
C. Mirtazapine
D. Bupropion
E. Fluoxetine

Answer:_____

Antidepressants and Weight Gain

- Least likely to most likely:
  - – Bupropion
  - + SSRIs (except paroxetine) and SNRIs
  - ++ Paroxetine, mirtazapine
  - +++ TCAs and MAOIs

Antidepressant Discontinuation Syndrome

- Withdrawal from antidepressants after sudden interruption of treatment
- Time course: 1–7 days after discontinuation
- Symptoms: dizziness, headaches, electric shock-like sensations, anxiety, irritability, insomnia, tremors
- More common with short half-life meds on higher doses
- Fluvoxamine, **paroxetine**, venlafaxine, sertraline
- Treatment
  - Use longer half-life medications
  - Slower taper off (5 half-lives)

BIPOLAR DISORDER

- Chronic and persistent mental illness consisting of alternating episodes of mania/hypomania and severe depression
- Lifetime prevalence of 1–4%
- Males and females are affected equally
- Onset usually before 25 years of age, 1st episode usually depressive
- 10-fold risk of bipolar disorder in 1st degree relatives
- 50% of individuals have psychotic symptoms at one point (bipolar disorder with psychosis)

Bipolar Disorder — Assessment

- Manic symptoms (**DIG FAST**)
  - **D**istractibility
  - **I**rritability/**I**ncreased goal-oriented activity
  - **G**randiosity (inflated self-esteem)
  - **F**light of ideas (racing thoughts)
  - **A**ctivity increase (e.g., social, sexual, occupational)
  - **S**leep decreased (e.g., feels rested after 3 hours)
  - **T**alkativeness (rapid vs. pressured)
- A manic episode requires at least one week of elevated or irritable mood plus **3** of the 7 symptoms described above
- Psychiatric and social history
- **DIG FAST** that is also captured in the Mood Disorders Questionnaire (MDQ)
- **Suicidal and homicidal ideation**
  - 50% of individuals with bipolar attempt suicide, and 20% complete it
- Substance use
- Physical exam/Laboratory assessment
- Medication reconciliation: corticosteroids, benzodiazepines, antiparkinsonian medications, antiseizure medications, hormones, stimulants, **antidepressants**
- Laboratory assessment
  - Complete blood count (CBC)
  - Comprehensive metabolic panel (CMP)
  - Liver function tests (LFTs)
  - Urinalysis
  - Thyroid-stimulating hormone (TSH; free T_3, T_4 if TSH abnormal)
  - Vitamin B_{12}, vitamin B_1, folate
  - Pregnancy testing
  - Toxicology: drugs, heavy metal screen
  - Rapid plasma reagin (RPR)
  - Human immunodeficiency virus (HIV)

Manic / Hypomanic Episode

- General pearls
  - **Age of onset:** usually prior to 25 years
  - **Duration of symptoms:**
    - **Manic episode (bipolar I): 7+ days***
    - **Hypomanic episode (bipolar II): 4+ days**
  - **Decline in functionality:**
    - Manic episode: significantly impaired
    - Hypomanic episode: none to mild
  - **Prevalence:** equal in women and men
  - **Pattern of recurrence:** 50% within 2 years of the initial episode

Bipolar Disorder — Treatment
- Treat bipolar spectrum disorder **with**:
  - Mood stabilizers
  - Antipsychotics
    - Most approved for acute manic episodes
    - Several approved for bipolar depression as well
  - No medications have approval for hypomania
- Lithium
  - Decrease risk of suicide (NNT 23)
  - Side effects **(LITHIUM)**:
    - **L**ethargy, leukocytosis (benign)
    - **I**ntention tremor
    - **T**eratogenicity
    - **H**ypothyroidism
    - **I**nsipidus (diabetes insipidus)
    - **U**rine (polyuria)
    - **M**etallic taste

AR 3

A 44-year-old woman presents having recently been prescribed lithium by her psychiatrist for bipolar mania. She is seeing you today for hypertension and joint pain.

Which medication combination would be the safest option for her 2 medical conditions when combined with lithium?

A. Chlorthalidone and acetaminophen
B. Amlodipine and acetaminophen
C. Spironolactone and ibuprofen
D. Olmesartan and ibuprofen
E. Lisinopril and aspirin

Answer:_____

Bipolar Disorder — Treatment
- **Valproic acid**
  - Monitor LFTs
  - Teratogenicity
- **Lamotrigine**
  - Increase dose gradually over weeks
  - **Stevens-Johnson syndrome**
- **Carbamazepine**
  - Strong CYP3A4 inducer
  - **SIADH**

CYCLOTHYMIC DISORDER
- For at least **2 years** numerous periods with hypomanic and depressive symptoms that do <u>not</u> meet full criteria for hypomanic episode and MDD
- Symptoms cause clinically significant distress or impairment in social, occupational, or other important areas of functioning

OTHER MOOD DISORDERS

SUBSTANCE-INDUCED MOOD DISORDER
- General pearls
  - **Causative agent: recreational substances, medications**
  - **Age of onset:** variable
  - **Duration of symptoms:** variable
  - **Decline in functionality:** variable
  - **Pattern of recurrence:** if reintroduced to causative agent

AR 4

A 65-year-old male with a history of Parkinson disease, on levodopa, has no known past psychiatric disorder. He currently lives at a nursing home and has been brought in by the nursing home staff for 10 days of increased energy, singing loudly at night, erotic behavior, and hypersexuality. He visited his neurologist 2 weeks ago, and his levodopa dose was increased for better management of his tremors.

What is the appropriate management for this patient?

A. Start a mood stabilizer.
B. He is depressed; start an antidepressant.
C. Refer the nursing home staff to therapy.
D. Decrease the levodopa dose.
E. Start an antipsychotic.

Answer:_____

MOOD DISORDER DUE TO ANOTHER MEDICAL CONDITION
- General pearls
  - **Causative agent: hypo-/hyperthyroidism, cancer, coronary heart disease, etc.**
  - **Age of onset:** variable
  - **Duration of symptoms:** variable
  - **Decline in functionality:** variable
  - **Pattern of recurrence:** if the causative condition returns

PREMENSTRUAL DYSPHORIC DISORDER
- General pearls
  - **Age of onset:** teens and 20s
  - **Duration of symptoms: luteal phase**
  - **Decline in functionality:** variable
  - **Pattern of recurrence:** with every menstrual cycle

AR 5

A 35-year-old G2P2 female with regular menstrual cycles presents with 10–12 days of mood swings and irritability. She lashes out verbally at her husband before every menstrual cycle. However, her symptoms resolve within a day of menstruation.

What is the appropriate 1st line treatment for her condition?

A. Continuous daily venlafaxine
B. Intermittent daily alprazolam for 2 weeks before menses
C. Cognitive behavioral therapy
D. Intermittent daily fluoxetine for 2 weeks before menses
E. Continuous daily spironolactone

Answer:_____

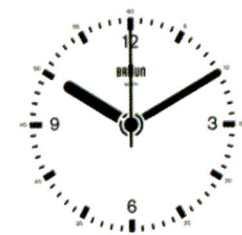

SUICIDE

Suicide Assessment
- Active suicidal thoughts vs. passive thoughts of death
- Acute vs. chronic
- Plan and intention
- Risk factors
  - Gender: male
  - Age: < 25 or > 60 years of age
  - Ethnicity: Caucasian
  - Psychiatric condition: bipolar > depression > psychosis
  - Previous attempts
  - Family history
  - Access to lethal means
  - Substance use
  - Lack of social support
  - Chronic medical illness/Chronic pain

Suicide and Medications
- FDA "black box warning": SSRIs may increase the risk of suicidal thinking and behavior in some children, adolescents, and young adults with MDD
- Lithium decreases suicidality in bipolar disorder
- Clozapine decreases suicidality in schizophrenia

ANXIETY DISORDERS

GENERALIZED ANXIETY DISORDER (GAD)
- Excessive anxiety and worry for **≥ 6 months**
- Difficulty controlling the worry
- Think **TICKES**[2]
- ≥ 3 of the following 6 symptoms for a majority of the past 6 months:
  - **T**ension in muscles
  - **I**rritability
  - **C**oncentration is poor
  - **K**eyed up/Restless
  - **E**asily fatigued
  - **S**leep disturbance

PANIC DISORDER
- Recurrent unexpected surge of intense fear or intense discomfort that reaches a peak within 10 minutes, with ≥ 4 of the following symptoms:
  - Feeling dizzy, lightheaded, or faint
  - Palpitations or pounding heart
  - Nausea or abdominal distress
  - Sweating
  - Trembling or shaking
  - Sensations of shortness of breath
  - Chest pain/discomfort
  - Chills or heat sensations
  - Paresthesia (numbness or tingling sensations)
  - Derealization (feelings of unreality)
  - Depersonalization (being detached from oneself)
  - Fear of losing control, going crazy, or dying

PHOBIAS
- **Agoraphobia:** individual fears and avoids situations when escape might be difficult or help might not be available in the event of developing panic-like symptoms or embarrassing events (e.g., falls, incontinence)
- **Social anxiety disorder (social phobia):** fear or anxiety about social situations
- **Specific phobias:** an irrational fear or anxiety due to the presence of a particular situation or object, resulting in avoidance of the situation or object

WORKUP AND MANAGEMENT

Anxiety Disorders — Workup and Management
- Female > male (2:1)
- Workup includes:
  - Toxicology for substance use
  - TSH for hyperthyroidism
  - ECG for arrhythmias
  - Pulmonary function test
- Management
  - **Cognitive behavioral therapy (CBT)**
  - SSRIs/SNRIs
  - Short course of benzodiazepines
    - Avoid long-term benzodiazepine therapy
  - Hydroxyzine or buspirone as alternatives to benzos
- Worsened by β-agonists

TRAUMA-RELATED STRESS DISORDERS
- Mood symptoms, irritability, sleep disturbances, "fight or flight" response; beginning after a traumatic event and lasting for:
  - 3–30 days — **acute stress disorder**
  - > 1 month — **posttraumatic stress disorder**

Posttraumatic Stress Disorder (PTSD)
- Can develop after an individual witnesses or experiences a serious threat of violence or death, resulting in disturbing thoughts, flashbacks, and nightmares related to the event
- Prevalence is about 3.5–9%
- Female > male
- Up to 75% of military veterans
- Rape is the most likely trigger of PTSD: 65% of men and 45.9% of women who are raped will develop PTSD
- Childhood sexual abuse is a strong predictor of lifetime likelihood for developing PTSD
- Symptoms
  - Mood and emotional symptoms
  - Irritability
  - Sleep-related symptoms and nightmares
  - Hyperarousal and hypervigilance
- Think "**RASH**"
  - **R**e-experiencing the traumatic event: images, thoughts, dreams, flashbacks (even when intoxicated), distress at exposure to cues (internal or external)
  - **A**voidance of **s**timuli
  - **H**yperarousal: difficulty falling asleep, irritability, poor concentration, hypervigilance, startles easily

PTSD — Treatment
- Psychotherapy
  - Cognitive behavioral therapy (CBT)
  - Exposure therapy
  - Eye movement desensitization and reprocessing (EMDR)
- Pharmaceutical
  - SSRIs and SNRIs for mood and irritability
  - **Prazosin** for nightmares
  - Benzodiazepines worsen the clinical course and should be avoided

Adjustment Disorder
- Emotional or behavioral symptoms in response to an identifiable stressor
- Causing significant impairment
- Symptoms improve after the stressor or its consequences have resolved
- **Acute: up to 6 months**
- **Persistent (chronic): > 6 months**
- Subtypes
  - With depressed mood
  - With anxiety
  - With disturbance of conduct
  - Mixed

SCHIZOPHRENIA AND RELATED DISORDERS

SCHIZOPHRENIA
- 1% of the population
- Male = Female
- Increased risk of suicide
- Very high prevalence of tobacco use (up to 80%)
- Age of onset
  - **Males: 15–25 years of age (mean age 19)**
  - **Females: 25–35 years of age (mean age 26)**
- Late-onset schizophrenia
  - ~ 45 years of age
  - Rare
  - Female > male
  - Mostly delusional

Schizophrenia Symptoms
- Positive symptoms
  - Auditory or visual hallucinations
  - Delusions
- Negative symptoms
  - Apathy
  - Lack of emotions
  - Poor social functioning
- Cognitive symptoms
  - Disorganized thoughts
  - Poor executive functioning
  - Poor attention
  - Impaired memory

Schizophrenia Assessment
- Psychiatric and social history
- **Suicidal and homicidal ideation**
- Substance use
- Physical exam/Laboratory assessment
- Medication reconciliation: **corticosteroids**, benzodiazepines, antiparkinsonian medications, hormones, stimulants, antidepressants
- Laboratory assessment
  - Complete blood count (CBC)
  - Comprehensive metabolic panel (CMP)
  - Liver function tests (LFTs)
  - Urinalysis
  - Thyroid-stimulating hormone (TSH; free T_3, T_4 if TSH abnormal)
  - Vitamin B_{12}, vitamin B_1, folate
  - Pregnancy testing
  - Toxicology: drugs, heavy metal screen
  - Rapid plasma reagin (RPR)
  - Human immunodeficiency virus (HIV)

SUBSTANCE-INDUCED PSYCHOSIS
- *Cannabis*/cannabinoids use in susceptible individuals increases psychosis by 2–3 times
- Psychostimulant (cocaine, methamphetamines, hallucinogens) use increases the odds 10-fold

PSYCHOSIS DUE TO ANOTHER MEDICAL CONDITION

- Causative Agent: **major neurocognitive disorder, hyperthyroidism, cancer, lupus, etc.**
- Age of Onset: variable
- Duration of Symptoms: variable
- Decline in functionality: variable
- Pattern of Recurrence: if the causative condition returns

DELUSIONAL DISORDER

- Isolated delusion for ≥ 1 month with no other psychotic symptoms present
- **Daily functioning is preserved**
- Somatic type
  - Delusional about bodily functions or parasites

ANTIPSYCHOTIC DRUGS

- **First generation (typical)**
  - Chlorpromazine, fluphenazine, haloperidol, perphenazine
  - Side effects
    - Extrapyramidal symptoms
    - Neuroleptic malignant syndrome
    - Tardive dyskinesia
    - Hyperprolactinemia
- **Second generation (atypical)**
  - Risperidone, olanzapine, clozapine, quetiapine, aripiprazole, ziprasidone, lurasidone, paliperidone, asenapine, brexpiprazole, cariprazine, lumateperone
  - Side effects
    - Less extrapyramidal symptoms
    - Higher risk of **metabolic syndrome**
    - Weight gain
    - Neuroleptic malignant syndrome
    - Less hyperprolactinemia
      - <u>Except</u> **risperidone** (higher risk)

Antipsychotic Drugs — Pearls

- Most antipsychotics may cause hyperprolactinemia
  - Except aripiprazole (most sparing)
- Most antipsychotics may cause extrapyramidal side effects
  - Except clozapine
- Most antipsychotics may cause QT_C prolongation
  - Except lurasidone

Clozapine

- In addition to positive symptoms, also effective for managing negative and cognitive symptoms
- Decrease suicide risk in schizophrenia patient
- Continue monitoring for **agranulocytosis**

COMPLICATIONS OF PSYCHOTROPIC DRUG THERAPY

Life-Threatening Psychiatric Medication Side Effects

- Lithium toxicity
- Serotonin syndrome
- Neuroleptic malignant syndrome

AR 6

A 36-year-old woman presents with agitation and confusion. She reports feeling well until developing a cough and a cold yesterday. She was seen at an urgent care clinic and given a medication but doesn't know what it was.

PMH: depression

Meds: citalopram, bupropion

Exam: T 102.8°F (39.3°C), BP 160/100 mmHg, P 120 bpm; anxious, tremulous, hyperreflexic

Which medication is likely contributing to her condition?

A. Acetaminophen
B. Amoxicillin
C. Dextromethorphan
D. Ibuprofen
E. Azithromycin

Answer:_____

Life-Threatening Psychiatric Medication Side Effects

- Course
  - Patient is on some therapeutic psych medication
  - Something happened that caused a major shift
    - Intentional or unintentional overdose
    - Another med was added
      - Same effect on the same neurotransmitter
      - Med-med interaction
    - Organ failure (e.g., acute kidney injury)

LITHIUM TOXICITY

- Thiazide diuretics > loop diuretics, angiotensin-converting enzyme (ACE) inhibitors, angiotensin receptor blockers (ARBs), and **nonsteroidal antiinflammatory drugs (NSAIDs)** may increase lithium levels
- Symptoms
  - Cardiac: prolonged QT_C, arrhythmias
  - GI: nausea, vomiting, diarrhea
  - CNS: ataxia, confusion, tremors, myoclonic jerks, seizures
  - Renal: deteriorating renal function
- Management
  - Stop the agent
  - ABCs and supportive care
  - Fluids
  - Gastrointestinal decontamination
    - Polyethylene glycol
    - Activated charcoal <u>not</u> effective
  - Hemodialysis
    - Lithium levels > 5 mEq/L (4 mEq/L in patients with renal impairment)

SEROTONIN SYNDROME

- "Too much CNS and peripheral serotonin"
- Antidepressants, **dextromethorphan**, amphetamines, cocaine, ecstasy, LSD , lithium, levodopa, **linezolid**, tramadol, ritonavir, buspirone, **St. John's wort**, ginseng, fentanyl, sumatriptan, ondansetron are associated with serotonin syndrome
- Clinical diagnosis, no confirming diagnostic labs; symptoms may range from mild tremor to life-threatening shock
- **Hunter** criteria — patient is on a serotonergic agent and has 1 of the following features or groups of features:
  - Spontaneous **clonus**
  - Inducible **clonus plus** agitation or diaphoresis
  - **Ocular clonus plus** agitation or diaphoresis
  - Tremor **plus hyperreflexia**
  - Hypertonia **plus** temperature > 100.4°F (38.0°C) **plus** ocular clonus or inducible clonus

Serotonin Syndrome — Treatment

- Stop precipitating agent(s)
- Sedate using **benzodiazepines** in order to target:
  - Agitation
  - Tremor, clonus
  - Heart rate and blood pressure
- Oxygen to keep sat ≥ 94%
- Fluids
- Cardiac monitoring: Vital signs fluctuate widely and rapidly
- Cyproheptadine if benzodiazepines fail
- Severe hyperthermia (> 105.9°F [> 41.1°C]): sedate, paralyze, intubate
  - Avoid antipyretics such as acetaminophen

NEUROLEPTIC MALIGNANT SYNDROME

- "Too little dopamine" or "too much dopamine blockage"
- Antipsychotics (1st generation > 2nd generation) and antiemetic drugs (e.g., metoclopramide)
- Discontinuation of antiparkinsonian medications
- Risk factors
  - Organic brain abnormalities
  - Antipsychotic-naïve patients
  - Low serum iron levels
  - Dehydration
  - Lithium
  - Simultaneous use of multiple antipsychotics
- Symptoms
  - Mental status changes
  - **Muscular rigidity ("lead pipe")**
  - Fever
  - Autonomic instability: tachycardia, hypertension, tachypnea, diaphoresis
- Diagnostics
  - Elevated serum **creatine kinase** (CK)
  - Leukocytosis
  - Electrolyte abnormalities and metabolic acidosis are common

Neuroleptic Malignant Syndrome — Treatment

- Stop precipitating agent (or reinstitute the stopped medication)
- Supportive care
- Fluids, fluids, fluids
- Benzodiazepines
- Off label: dantrolene, bromocriptine, amantadine
- Electroconvulsive therapy if available, in severe cases

Overlapping Features of Serotonin Syndrome and Neuroleptic Malignant Syndrome

- Vitals: tachycardia, tachypnea, hypertension, hyperthermia
- Mucosa: hypersalivation (dry in anticholinergic poisoning)
- Diaphoresis (dry in anticholinergic poisoning)
- Altered mental status
- Increased muscle tone, "lead pipe" rigidity in neuroleptic malignant syndrome

Features to Distinguish Neuroleptic Malignant from Serotonin Syndrome

	Serotonin Syndrome	Neuroleptic Malignant Syndrome
Medication History	Serotonergic agent	Dopaminergic agent
Time until Onset	< 12 hours	1–3 days
Reflexes	Hyperreflexia	Hyporeflexia
Pupils	Dilated	Normal
Bowel Sounds	Hyperactive	Normal to decreased

AR 7

A 68-year-old man is brought to the ED by his wife for evaluation of fever and confusion.

PMH: Parkinson's, HTN

Meds: omeprazole, lorazepam, enalapril; he stopped taking levodopa-carbidopa 1 week ago

Exam: T 104.2°F (40.1°C), BP 185/110 mmHg, P 135 bpm, diaphoretic; Ext: marked muscle rigidity with hypoactive reflexes

Labs: Hgb 13, WBC 13,000, Ca^{2+} 8.7, CK 605

What is the most likely diagnosis?

A. Parkinson disease
B. Meningitis
C. Depression
D. Neuroleptic malignant syndrome
E. Serotonin syndrome

Answer:_____

SUBSTANCE USE DISORDERS

Stages of Change
- Precontemplation (not ready to quit)
- Contemplation (considering a quit attempt)
- Preparation (actively planning a quit attempt)
- Action (actively involved in a quit attempt)
- Maintenance (achieved cessation)

NICOTINE
- 10% of population are active smokers
- 80% of schizophrenia patients
- Increased tobacco use among mental health patients
- Address mood, anxiety, habits, and stress management
- Nicotine is a potent parasympathomimetic stimulant

Smoking Cessation Medications
- Nicotine replacement therapy
  - Patch (baseline)
  - Gum or lozenge (short-acting form)
- Varenicline: partial nicotine agonist
  - **Side effect: depression and mood symptoms**
- Bupropion: dopamine/norepinephrine reuptake inhibitor

ALCOHOL
- Psychotherapy
  - Alcoholics Anonymous
  - Cognitive behavioral therapy
- Medications
  - Naltrexone: opioid antagonist
    - **Contraindicated in patients on opioids**
  - Acamprosate: GABA agonist/glutamate antagonist
  - Aldehyde dehydrogenase inhibitor

Alcohol Withdrawal
- Withdrawal seizures: 12–48 hours
- Alcoholic hallucinosis: 12–24 hours of abstinence and typically resolves within 24–48 hours
- Delirium tremens
  - 5% of patients who undergo withdrawal
  - Hallucinations, disorientation, tachycardia, hypertension, hyperthermia, agitation, and diaphoresis
  - Begins 48–96 hours after the last drink and lasts 1–5 days

Alcohol Withdrawal — Treatment
- Supportive
- Long half-life benzodiazepines (e.g., chlordiazepoxide)
- Delirium tremens is treated more aggressively with IV lorazepam in the intensive care unit (ICU)
- Alternatives to benzos: antiseizure medications
- Folic acid, vitamin B_{12}, thiamine

OPIATES
- Psychotherapy
  - Narcotics Anonymous
  - Cognitive behavioral therapy
- Medications
  - Methadone: opiate replacement therapy
    - Decrease craving
    - **QT_c prolongation**
  - Buprenorphine/Naloxone: reduce euphoria/cravings
- Supportive care with symptom management for withdrawal

OTHER SUBSTANCES

Cocaine
- Intoxication: agitation, paranoia, tachycardia, tachypnea, hypertension, diaphoresis, **mydriasis**
- Complications: **myocardial ischemia or infarction**, stroke, pulmonary edema, and **rhabdomyolysis**, substance-induced mood disorder, substance-induced psychosis, "coke nose"

Amphetamines
- Intoxication: tachycardia, hypertension, anorexia, insomnia, **scratches and tactile hallucinations**, mood disorder, psychosis
- Complications: substance-induced mood disorder, substance-induced psychosis, tooth decay, "meth mouth"

Cannabis
- Intoxication: clinically significant, problematic behavioral or psychological changes (e.g., impaired motor coordination, euphoria, anxiety, sensation of slowed time, impaired judgment, social withdrawal), conjunctival infection, increased appetite, dry mouth, tachycardia
- No current evidence in use of *cannabis* in management of mood or anxiety; may worsen anxiety over time
- Complications: substance-induced anxiety, psychosis, and mood disorder with acute use; psychosis with chronic use; hastens the onset of schizophrenia in predisposed individuals

PERSONALITY DISORDERS (PDs)

- Cluster A
  - Paranoid personality disorder
  - Schizoid personality disorder
  - Schizotypal personality disorder
- Cluster B
  - Antisocial personality disorder
  - **Borderline personality disorder**
  - Narcissistic personality disorder
  - Histrionic personality disorder
- Cluster C
  - Dependent personality disorder
  - Avoidant personality disorder
  - **Obsessive-compulsive personality disorder (OCPD)**
- An enduring pattern of inner experience and behavior that differs markedly from the expectations of the individual's culture, is pervasive and inflexible, has an onset in adolescence or early adulthood, is stable over time, and leads to distress or impairment
- Cluster B with elevated risk of:
  - Substance use
  - Depression
  - Poor impulse control and aggression
    - Borderline personality disorder
    - **Black or white thinking and splitting**
    - Therapy: **dialectical behavior therapy**

AR 8

A 28-year-old female presents to the clinic for changes in her mood. She reports she experiences multiple mood swings, sometimes up to 5–6 times a day. She sometimes feels high on energy, feeling great, motivated, wants to dance all day. Her mood, however, can change to very depressed and low energy within an hour, with urges to cut herself. She reports she hates her previous doctor because he made her wait every time she visited his office. She can tell by now that you are the best doctor ever and that you will be taking great care of her.

What is the most likely etiology of her mood swings?

A. Depression
B. Cyclothymia
C. Bipolar disorder
D. Borderline personality disorder
E. Delusional disorder

Answer:_____

OBSESSIVE DISORDERS

- Obsessive-compulsive personality disorder (OCPD)
  - "Perfectionist" personality
  - Provides rational explanations for their obsessions
  - Bothersome to others
- Obsessive-compulsive disorder (OCD)
  - Aware their obsessions are not rational
  - Bothersome to patient and others

Obsessive-Compulsive Disorder
- OCD is characterized by distressing, intrusive, obsessive thoughts and/or repetitive compulsive physical or mental acts
  - Obsessions: recurrent and persistent thoughts, urges, or images that are intrusive and inappropriate and cause marked anxiety and distress
  - Compulsions: repetitive behaviors or mental acts performed in response to an obsession or according to rules that must be applied rigidly
- Treatment
  - Therapy
    - Cognitive behavioral therapy
    - Exposure and response prevention therapy
  - Medication
    - High-dose SSRIs

INSOMNIA

- Repeated difficulty with sleep initiation, maintenance, consolidation, or quality that occurs despite adequate time and opportunity for sleep, resulting in daytime impairment
- Difficulty initiating sleep
- Difficulty maintaining sleep (most common)
- Early-morning awakening with inability to return to sleep
- Slightly more common among women
- Individuals suffering from insomnia are 10× and 17× more likely to suffer from depression and anxiety, respectively
- Associated with increased suicidal thoughts
- Medical comorbidities
  - Diabetes
  - Coronary heart disease
  - COPD
  - Pain
  - Nocturia
  - Restless leg syndrome
  - Menopause
  - Substance use
- Management
  - Address **predisposing conditions** and **medication reconciliation**
  - **Sleep hygiene**
    - Cognitive behavioral therapy
    - Establish bedtime and wake time
    - Reduce time in bed
    - Encourage bed use only for sleep and sex
    - Avoid daytime naps
    - Avoid substances that interfere with sleep
    - Breathing and relaxation techniques
    - Address expectations about sleep
    - Management of anxious and catastrophic thoughts

- Medications
  - Benzodiazepines: triazolam, estazolam, lorazepam, temazepam, flurazepam, and quazepam
  - Nonbenzodiazepine hypnotics: zaleplon, zolpidem, eszopiclone
  - Melatonin agonists: ramelteon
  - Orexin receptor antagonists: suvorexant
  - Antidepressants: doxepin; (off-label use: trazodone and amitriptyline)
  - Diphenhydramine
  - Antipsychotics
  - Barbiturates
  - Herbal over the counters and melatonin
- Medications by duration of effect
  - Short-acting: zaleplon, zolpidem, triazolam, lorazepam, **ramelteon**
  - Longer-acting: zolpidem (extended release), eszopiclone, temazepam, estazolam, **doxepin**, **suvorexant**

Insomnia — Bottom Line
- Address underlying medical, psychiatric, and/or social conditions
- **Behavioral approaches and CBT first**
- Medication reconciliation and avoid stimulants
- Avoid hypnotics in patients with alcohol use disorder
- Avoid anticholinergics in older adults
- Acute (< 1 month) insomnia: stress management, education, reassurance
- Chronic (> 1 month) insomnia
  - **Onset insomnia: short-acting meds**
  - **Maintenance insomnia: longer-acting meds**
- Follow-up

EATING DISORDERS

ANOREXIA NERVOSA (AN)
- Epidemiology: onset usually in adolescent girls
- Female > male
- Clinical features
  - Weight loss of 15% under ideal, **low BMI**
  - Preoccupation with food, intense fear of becoming fat, and distorted self-image
  - Bradycardia, hypotension, anemia, electrolyte abnormalities
  - Absence of ≥ 3 consecutive menstrual cycles
- May require inpatient aggressive nutrition
- Elevated risk for:
  - Refeeding syndrome
  - Arrhythmias and QT_c prolongation

BULIMIA NERVOSA (BN)
- Binge eating + purging (vomiting or laxatives)
- Epidemiology: usually women 20–30 years of age (older than anorexia patients)
- **Normal or elevated BMI**
- Clinical clues
  - **Erosion of dental enamel**
  - Erosive skin lesions on fingers
  - Young patient with Mallory-Weiss tears or severe GERD
- Lab abnormalities
  - **Hypokalemic** and **hypochloremic alkalosis**

SOMATIC SYMPTOM AND RELATED DISORDERS

SOMATIC SYMPTOM DISORDER
- Somatic symptom disorder is characterized by thoughts, feelings, or behaviors related to somatic symptoms
- Involvement of multiple organ systems
- History of extensive workup with unremarkable physical examination and laboratory findings
- Absence of psychiatric disorders
- Schedule regular appointments
- One symptom to focus on during each appointment
- Set limits for workups and diagnostics

CONVERSION DISORDER
- Symptoms or deficits affecting voluntary **motor or sensory function**, suggesting a **neurologic** or general medical condition
- After a thorough evaluation, no neurologic explanation exists, or the examination findings are inconsistent with the complaint

FACTITIOUS DISORDER
- **Falsification** of medical or psychological signs and symptoms in oneself or others for the principal purpose of assuming the sick role (imposed on self)
- Factitious disorder (formerly Munchausen syndrome)
- Factitious disorder imposed on another (formerly Munchausen syndrome by proxy) primarily victimizes others
- No known secondary gain

MALINGERING
- Malingering is the fabricating of symptoms of mental or physical disorders for **secondary gain** such as financial compensation, avoiding school, work or military service, obtaining drugs, or as a mitigating factor for sentencing in criminal cases

AUDIENCE RESPONSE ANSWERS

Audience Response 1
D. Citalopram

AR 2
D. Bupropion

AR 3
B. Amlodipine and acetaminophen

AR 4
D. Decrease the levodopa dose.

AR 5
D. Intermittent daily fluoxetine for 2 weeks before menses

AR 6
C. Dextromethorphan

AR 7
D. Neuroleptic malignant syndrome

AR 8
D. Borderline personality disorder

ENDNOTES

[1]   Raj YP, Christensen JF, Feldman MD. Mental & Behavioral Disorders: Depression in *Behavioral Medicine*, 5th Edition, McGraw-Hill Professional, New York, NY; 2020.
Raj YP, Parker J, Safani D, Nam K. Psychiatric Disorders: Bipolar and Related

Disorders in *Primary Care Psychiatry*, 2nd Edition, Wolters Kluwer, Philadelphia, PA; 2019.

[2]   Raj YP. The Patient with Depressive Symptoms. In: Jiang W, Gagliardi JP, Krishnan KR, eds. Clinician's Guide to Psychiatric Care. New York, NY: Oxford University Press; 2009. P 51.

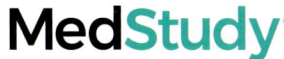

MedStudy

INTERNAL MEDICINE REVIEW

Pulmonary Medicine

Presented by

Raj Dasgupta, MD

TABLE OF CONTENTS

Why Some Topic Names Are Not Printed in This Section

At MedStudy, we do all we can to optimize your self-testing and learning.

In this section, the speaker has chosen to introduce topics with an Audience Response question to help you learn. In the syllabus, we've intentionally "hidden" some topic names that would give away the answers—so you can self-test more effectively. Where we've done this, instead of the topic name, you'll see an empty teal band or some extra space, but you can still find the topic on the page using the Table of Contents.

Why We Moved Some Slide Information to the Audience Response Answers Page

At MedStudy, we do all we can to optimize your self-testing and learning.

In this presentation, the speaker will give some extra information after their AR questions to help explain the correct and incorrect answers. To keep from interfering with your self-testing, we've moved that explanatory text to the Audience Response Answers page(s) at the end of the section.

Be assured, all the content on the slides is in your syllabus—so you can focus on the teaching instead of taking detailed notes.

Pulmonary Medicine Outline
- **Pulmonary Medicine**
  - PFTs
  - Asthma
  - COPD
  - Interstitial Lung Diseases
  - Pulmonary Nodules and Lung Cancer
  - Pleural Effusions
  - Latent and Active Tuberculosis
  - Pulmonary Embolism and DVT
- **Sleep Medicine**
  - Obstructive and Central Sleep Apnea
- **Critical Care Medicine**
  - ARDS and Ventilator Management
  - Evaluation of Shock and Defining Sepsis

Pulmonary Medicine

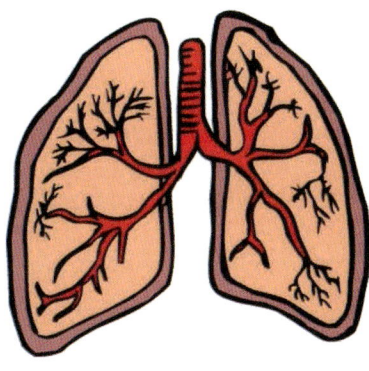

PULMONARY FUNCTION TESTS (PFTs)

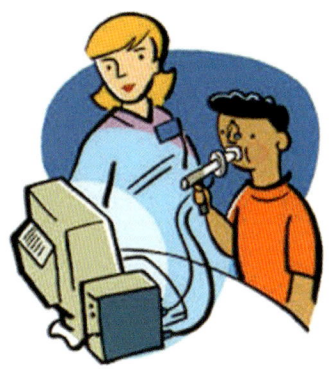

- **Consist of 3 tests:**
  1) **Airflow**
     - Dynamic compliance
       - FEV_1, FVC, FEV_1/FVC, FEF 25–75%
  2) **Static lung compartments**
     - Measured by lung volumes
       - TLC, RV
  3) **Alveolar membrane permeability**
     - DLCO

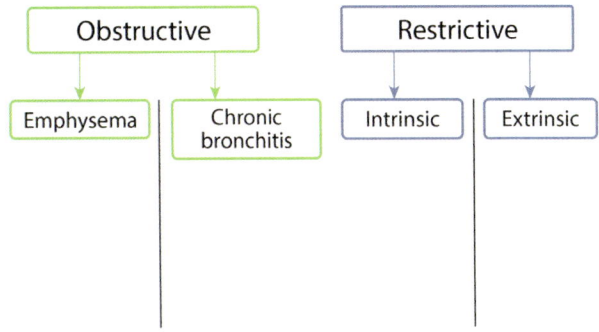

- **In your office**
  - With spirometry you can determine most of the:
    - Lung volumes and capacities
    - Flow-volume loops
    - Bronchodilator response
- **Pulmonary function lab**
  - Total lung capacity
    - Helium dilution
    - Nitrogen wash-out
    - Plethysmography
  - DLCO
    - Corrected for alveolar volume and Hgb
  - Methacholine challenge

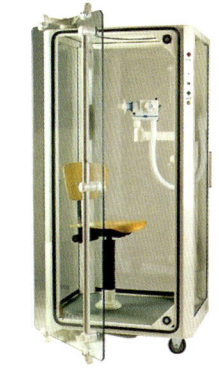

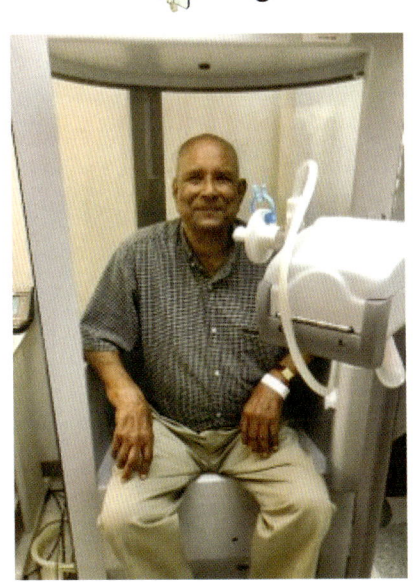

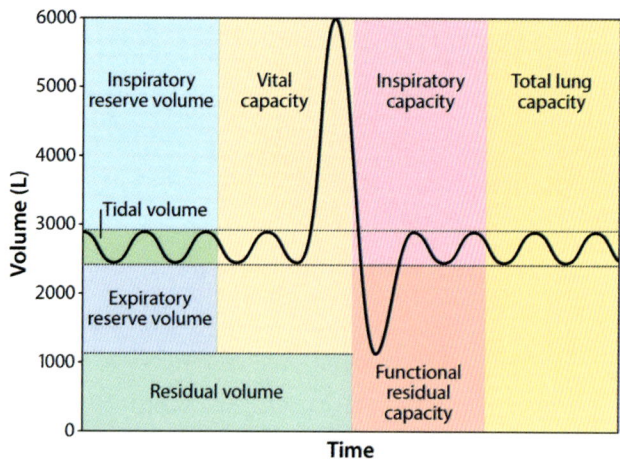

Forced Expiratory Volumes

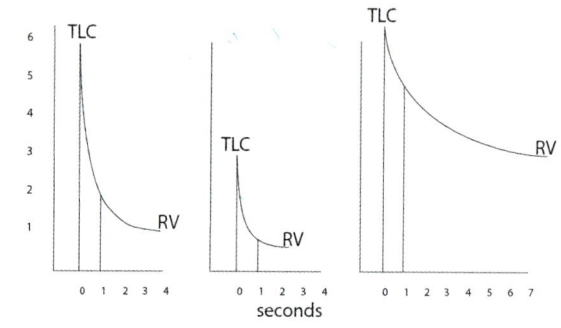

	Normal	Restrictive	Obstructive
FEV$_1$/FVC =	0.8	0.9	0.4

Carbon Monoxide Diffusing Capacity (DLCO)

- Decreased by anything that interrupts **gas-blood** oxygen exchange
  1) Alveoli
  2) Interstitium
  3) Capillary
- Decreased DLCO is seen in anemia and reduced blood volume in pulmonary circulation
  - Correct for hemoglobin

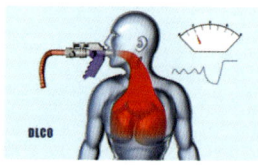

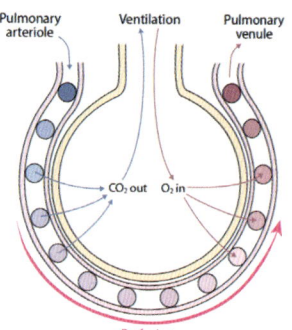

Pulmonary Function Tests

- **Bottom-line point**
  - **TLC** to assess restrictive lung disease
    - < 80% of predicted is abnormal
  - **FEV$_1$/FVC** to assess obstructive lung disease
    - < 70% of predictive is abnormal
  - **DLCO** determines how much oxygen travels from the alveoli of the lungs to the blood stream

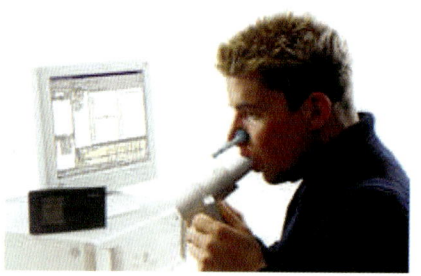

Audience Response 1

A 60-year-old woman is evaluated for a 4-month history of progressive fatigue and dyspnea on exertion. She does not smoke cigarettes and denies chest pain, palpitations, dizziness, or syncope. She has a 12-year history of limited cutaneous systemic sclerosis.

A screening cardiopulmonary evaluation 3 years ago was normal. She also has GERD and Raynaud phenomenon and intermittently develops ulcers on the fingertips.

Current medications are amlodipine, omeprazole, and nitroglycerin ointment.

On physical exam: Temp 98.6°F (37°C), BP 120/80, HR 86, RR 16. Cardiac examination reveals a loud S$_2$ with fixed splitting. The lungs are CTA.

The abdominal examination is unremarkable. Sclerodactyly is present, and pitting scars are visible over several fingertips. There is no peripheral edema.

CBC and ESR are normal. ECG shows evidence of right ventricular hypertrophy.

Chest radiograph shows no infiltrates.

Pulmonary function studies:

FEV$_1$: 84% of predicted and FVC: 82% of predicted

FEV$_1$/FVC: 80% of predicted

TLC: 85% of predicted

DLCO: 44% of predicted

Which of the following is the most likely diagnosis?

A. Atrial septal defect
B. Interstitial lung disease
C. Left ventricular failure
D. Pulmonary arterial hypertension

Answer:_____

PFT Summary of Common Disorders

	Asthma	COPD: Chronic Bronchitis	COPD: Emphysema	Pulmonary Fibrosis	PAH
FEV$_1$/FVC	nl or ↓	↓	↓	↑	nl
TLC	nl	nl	↑	↓	nl
DLCO	nl	nl	↓	↓	↓

FLOW-VOLUME LOOPS

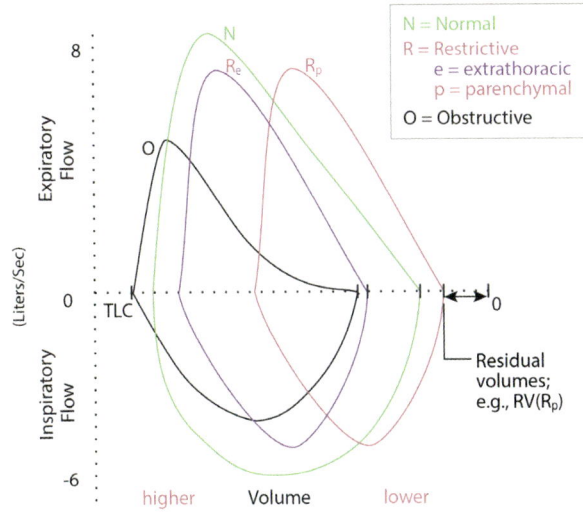

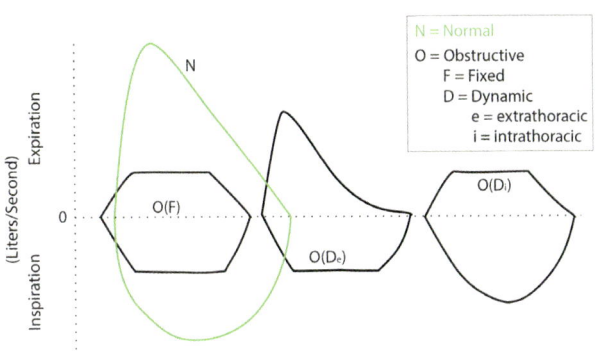

Common way of expressing **airflow** in the different lung diseases
- Derived from spirometry data, are plotted on:
  - A *y*-axis (flow rate)
  - An *x*-axis (volume in liters)
- We get most of our information by the **shape** of the loop

Flow-Volume Loops for Upper Airway Obstruction
- **Fixed**
  - Tracheal stenosis
  - Extrinsic compressive tumor
- **Dynamic**
  - Extrathoracic
    - Flattening of the **inspiratory loop** — vocal cord dysfunction
    - Flattening of the **expiratory loop** — tracheomalacia
      - Flaccidity of the tracheal **support cartilage**, which leads to tracheal collapse
      - Trachea normally dilates slightly during inspiration and narrows slightly during expiration
      - These processes are exaggerated in tracheomalacia, leading to airway collapse on expiration

AR 2
A 65-year-old male presents with chronic cough and dyspnea on exertion.

	Pre-BD			Post-BD	
Test	**Actual**	**Pred**	**% Pred**	**Actual**	**% Chg**
FVC (L)	3.17	4.22	75	3.98	25
FEV$_1$ (L)	2.16	3.39	63	2.86	30
FEV$_1$/FVC (%)	68	80		72	

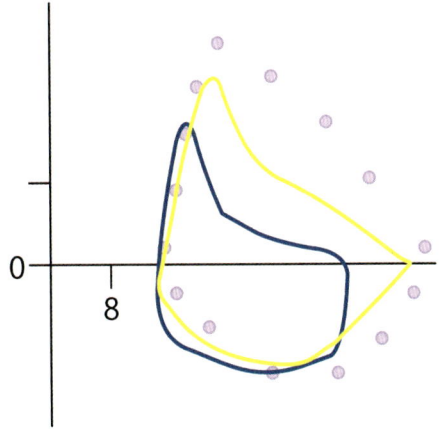

Which of the following is the patient's most likely diagnosis?

A. Variable extrathoracic obstruction
B. Mild lower airway obstruction with reversibility
C. Severe lower airway obstruction without reversibility
D. Variable intrathoracic obstruction
E. Fixed obstruction

Answer:_____

AR 3

A 30-year-old female tax accountant with a German shepherd and a cockatiel develops progressive dyspnea on exertion.

Test	Pre-BD Actual	Pre-BD Pred	Pre-BD % Pred	Post-BD Actual	Post-BD % Chg
FVC (L)	1.70	4.38	39	1.76	4
FEV$_1$ (L)	1.55	3.62	43	1.54	0
FEV$_1$/FVC(%)	91	83		88	− 3
RV (L)	1.03	1.98	52		
TLC (L)	2.66	6.10	44		
DLCO	5.00	31.98	16		

Which of the following flow-volume loops would be expected for this patient?

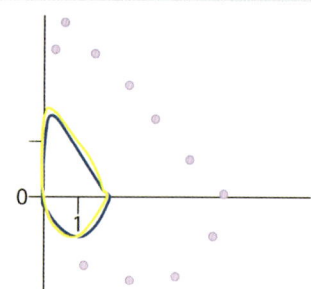

A.

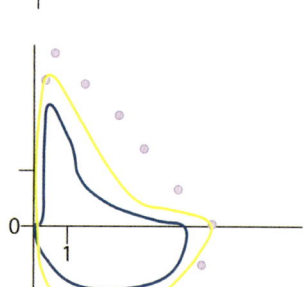

B.

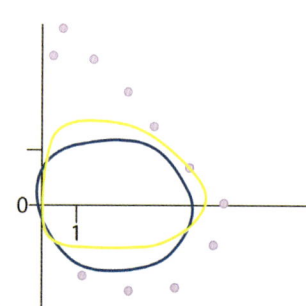

C.

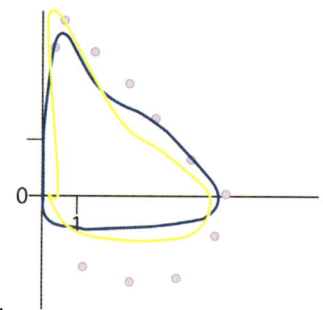

D.

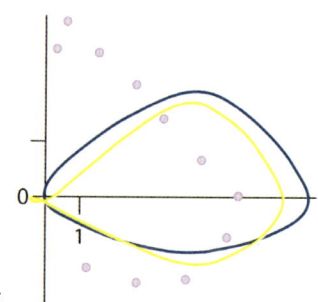

E.

Answer:_____

OBSTRUCTIVE LUNG DISEASES

ASTHMA

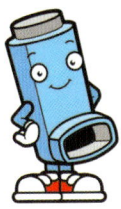

2 Main Types of Asthma

- Allergic
  - Atopic
  - Extrinsic
  - The most common form
  - Triggered by inhaled antigens
    - Dust mites
    - Pollen
    - Pet dander
    - Mold
  - Biologics
  - Review your immunology!!!
- Nonallergic
  - Nonatopic
  - Intrinsic
  - About 10% of asthmatics
  - Triggered by factors not related to allergies
    - Exercise
    - Cold and dry air
    - Smoke
    - Viruses
    - Stress and anxiety
    - Perfumes and fumes
    - Medications: β-blockers
  - Bronchial thermoplasty

AR 4

What is the main antigen-presenting cell in the lung for asthmatics?

A. Mast cell
B. Eosinophil
C. Macrophages
D. Neutrophil

Answer:_____

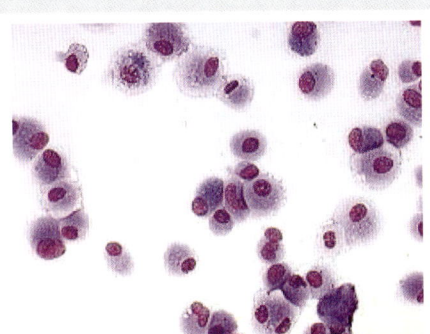

BAL showing an abundant amount of macrophages

AR 5

What is the main inflammatory cell in the airways of asthmatics?

A. Mast cell
B. Eosinophil
C. Neutrophil
D. Basophil

Answer:_____

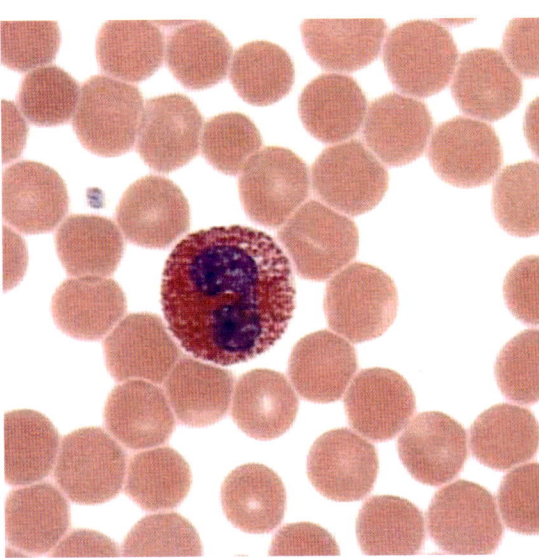

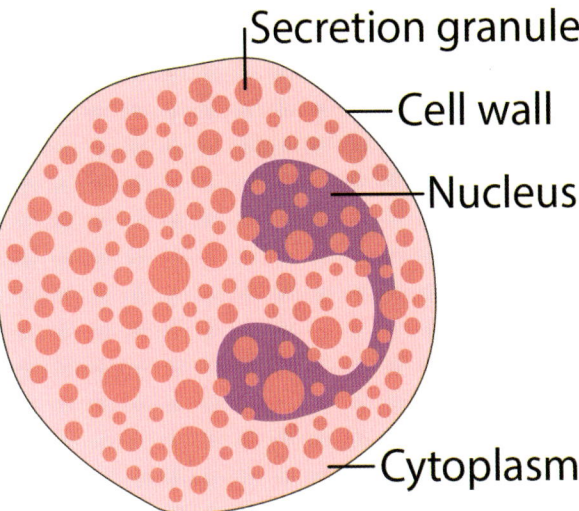

Secretion granule
Cell wall
Nucleus
Cytoplasm

Asthma Definition and Diagnosis

- Definition
  - **Chronic** inflammatory disease of the respiratory tree to various **sensitizing** stimuli, resulting in **reversible** airway obstruction
  - Characterized by:
    1) **Bronchial hyperresponsiveness** (BHR)
       - Role for challenge testing
    2) Abnormalities in airway **smooth muscle** function
       - Role for bronchial thermoplasty

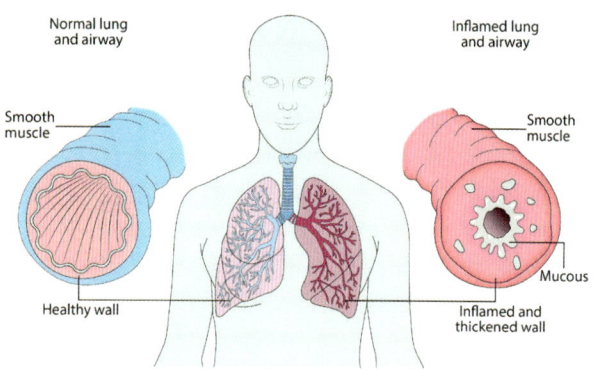

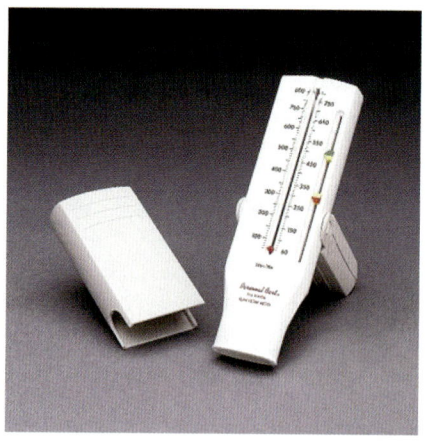

Asthma Diagnosis

- **Traditional**
  - Pattern of symptoms and response to therapy
  - Spirometry and/or PFTs + BD response
    - FEV_1/FVC, FEV_1, PEF
    - TLC, DLCO
  - Challenge testing
    - Exercise-induced bronchoconstriction and chronic cough
      - Exercise, cold air, methacholine
- **Other considerations**
  - Fraction of exhaled NO (FENO)
    - Eosinophilic inflammation in the airways stimulates airway epithelial cells to produce NO

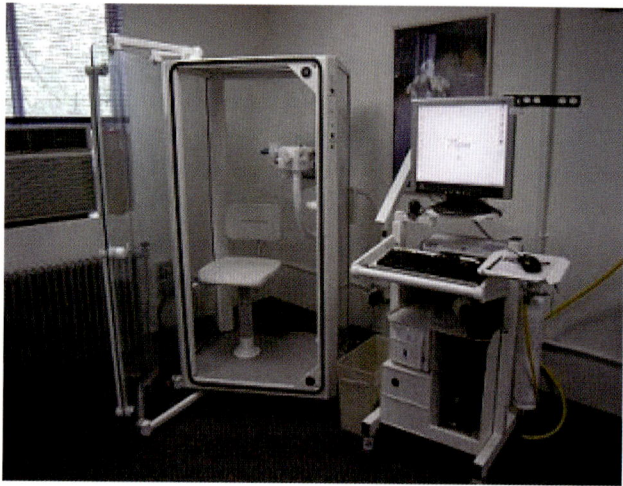

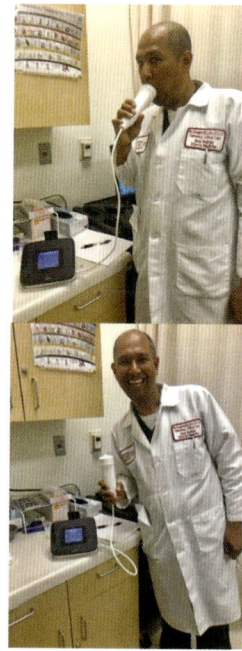

- The **classic** signs and symptoms of asthma are:
  - Intermittent dyspnea
  - Cough
  - Wheezing
- Clinically classified according to:
  - Frequency of symptoms
  - Forced expiratory volume in 1 second (FEV_1)

Pharmacologic Asthma Treatment

- **Antiinflammatory medicines**
  - **Corticosteroids**
    - Route: oral, inhaled, IV, and intramuscular
- **Direct bronchodilators** (short- and long-acting)
  - **β_2-Agonists** (increases cAMP)
    - Salbutamol, albuterol, levalbuterol
  - **Anticholinergics** (M3 receptor in smooth muscle)
    - Helpful and recommended in the acute setting
    - Ipratropium bromide
  - **Methylxanthines** (relaxes bronchial smooth muscle)
    - Theophylline
    - Aminophylline (short-acting)
  - **Adrenergic agonists** (inhaled epinephrine)
    - FDA reapproves Primatene Mist OTC (Nov. 2018)
- **Mast-cell stabilizers**
  - Cromolyn sodium
    - Not for adults or asthma attack
    - 2 puffs QID
    - 4 weeks to get optimal effect
- **Leukotriene inhibitors**
  - Zileuton
    - Leukotriene synthesis inhibitor
  - Montelukast
    - Leukotriene receptor antagonist

AR 6

A 47-year-old man is evaluated for worsening of asthma symptoms characterized by frequent daytime wheezing and cough, as well as nocturnal awakening related to asthma 2–3 times per week.

He has been using his inhalers regularly without adequate relief. He has not had recent URI infection, sinusitis, postnasal drip, or new exposures. He is taking an inhaled corticosteroid and inhaled albuterol.

On exam, temp 98.6°F (37.0°C), BP 135/80, HR 80, and RR 18. Lung exam reveals scattered **bilateral wheezing**. Spirometry shows an FEV_1 of **70%** of predicted. Following an inhaled bronchodilator, FEV_1 improves to **90%** of predicted.

Which of the following is the most appropriate next step in management?

A. Add a leukotriene receptor antagonist.
B. Add prednisone.
C. Observe the patient using his inhalers.
D. Obtain a 2-week symptom and peak flow diary.

Answer:_____

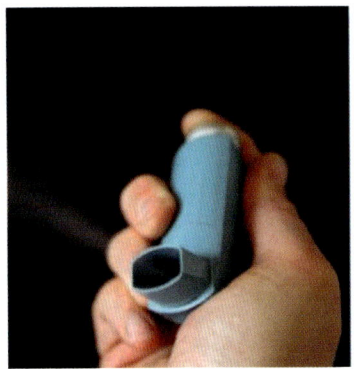

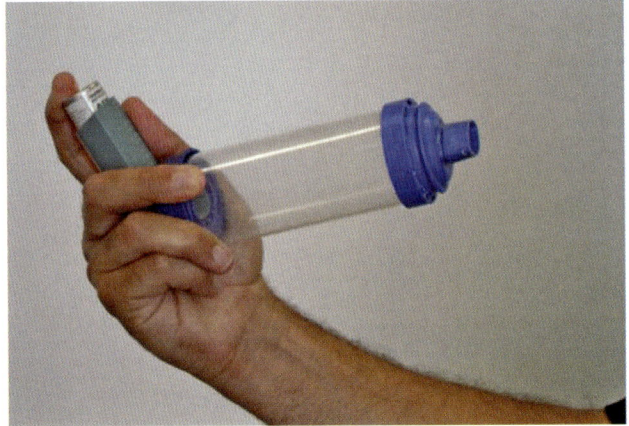

Th2 Pathway and Allergic Asthma

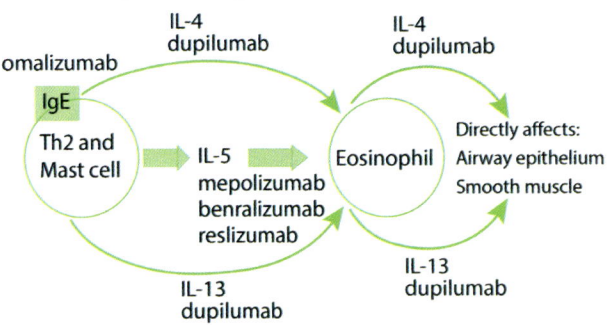

Asthma Immunologic Therapy[1]

- **Omalizumab**
  - Subcutaneous injection
  - Moderate-to-severe persistent allergic asthma
  - Dosed on **IgE levels** and weight
  - Epinephrine auto-injector

Asthma risk vs. Serum IgE concentration

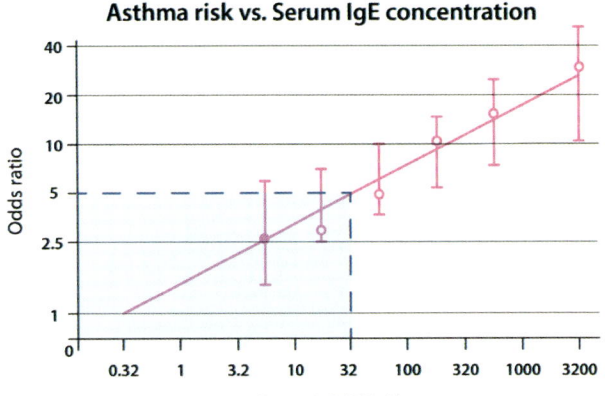

AR 7

Should you follow IgE levels after starting omalizumab?

A. Yes
B. No
C. Please tell me.

Answer:_____

IL-5 — "Nucala," "Fasenra," and "Cinqair"

- FDA has recommended mepolizumab, benralizumab, and reslizumab (IV) for add-on maintenance treatment in patients 18 years of age and older with severe eosinophilic (peripheral) asthma
- Monoclonal antibody that binds to and inactivates interleukin-5

Mepolizumab (Nucala)

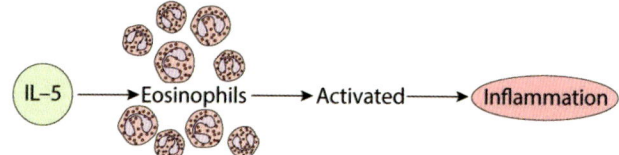

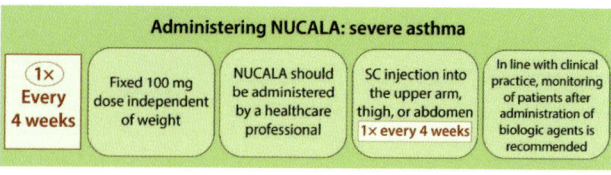

Administering NUCALA: severe asthma

| 1× Every 4 weeks | Fixed 100 mg dose independent of weight | NUCALA should be administered by a healthcare professional | SC injection into the upper arm, thigh, or abdomen 1× every 4 weeks | In line with clinical practice, monitoring of patients after administration of biologic agents is recommended |

Opportunistic Infections: Herpes Zoster
In controlled clinical trials, 2 serious adverse reactions of herpes zoster occurred with NUCALA compared to none with placebo. Consider vaccination if medically appropriate.

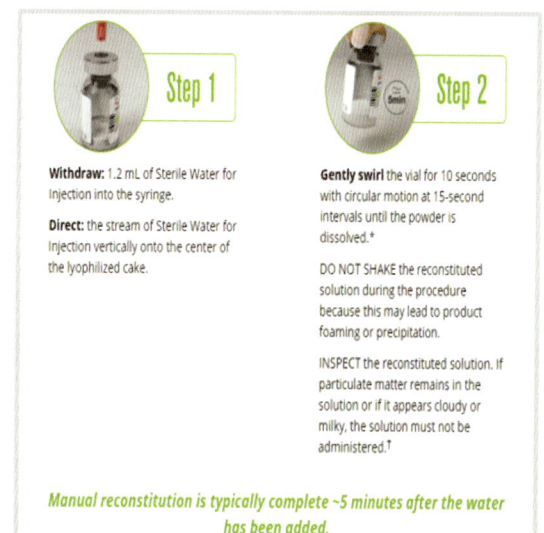

Step 1

Withdraw: 1.2 mL of Sterile Water for Injection into the syringe.

Direct: the stream of Sterile Water for Injection vertically onto the center of the lyophilized cake.

Step 2

Gently swirl the vial for 10 seconds with circular motion at 15-second intervals until the powder is dissolved.*

DO NOT SHAKE the reconstituted solution during the procedure because this may lead to product foaming or precipitation.

INSPECT the reconstituted solution. If particulate matter remains in the solution or if it appears cloudy or milky, the solution must not be administered.†

Manual reconstitution is typically complete ~5 minutes after the water has been added.

Benralizumab (Fasenra)

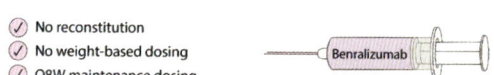

✓ No reconstitution
✓ No weight-based dosing
✓ Q8W maintenance dosing

	Benralizumab (Fasenra)	Omalizumab (Xolair)	Mepolizumab (Nucala)	Reslizumab (Cinqair)
Number of Doses in Year 1	8	13–26	13	13
Maintenance Dosing	Every 8 weeks	Every 2–4 weeks	Every 4 weeks	Every 4 weeks
Prefilled Syringe (No Reconstitution)	✓	X	X	X
Fixed Dose (No Weight-Based Dosing)	✓	X	✓	X
Subcutaneous Injection	✓	✓	✓	X

The recommended dose of benralizumab is 30 mg administered once every 4 weeks for the first 3 doses, and then once every 8 weeks thereafter by subcutaneous injection into the upper arm, thigh, or abdomen.

Reslizumab (Cinqair)

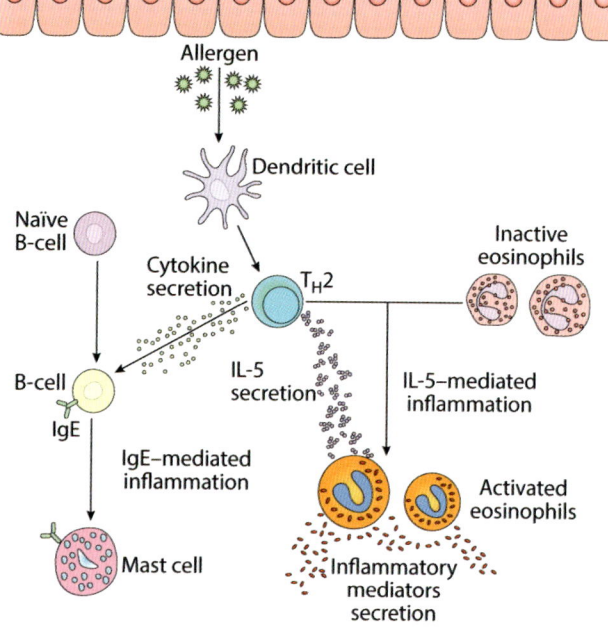

- Only intravenous therapy approved for patients with severe asthma and an eosinophilic phenotype
- Individualized, weight-based IV infusion; 3 mg/kg doses every 4 weeks
- Administration time of 20–50 minutes
- Anaphylaxis observed in 0.3% of patients

Dupilumab (Dupixent)
- Inhibits **IL-4** and **IL-13** signaling
- At home **self-injection** given subcutaneous
- The approved group is 12 years of age and older with either an eosinophilic phenotype or with an oral corticosteroid-dependent asthma

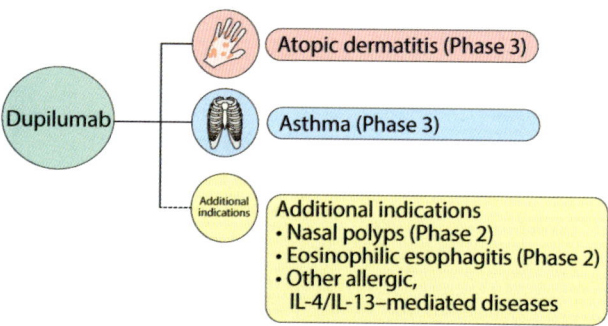

Dupilumab

- Atopic dermatitis (Phase 3)
- Asthma (Phase 3)
- Additional indications
  - **Additional indications**
    - Nasal polyps (Phase 2)
    - Eosinophilic esophagitis (Phase 2)
    - Other allergic, IL-4/IL-13–mediated diseases

Bronchial Thermoplasty
- FDA approved in 2010
- Nonpharmacologic therapy for severe asthma in patients 18 years of age and older not well controlled with currently available medical therapies
- Targets airway remodeling by reducing airway smooth muscle mass that is responsible for:
  - Bronchoconstriction
  - Mucus production
  - Airway hyperresponsiveness

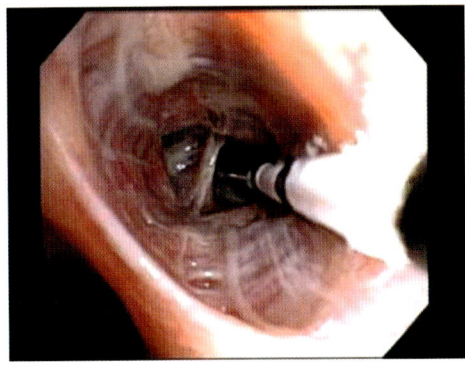

A

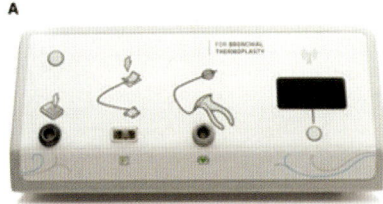

B

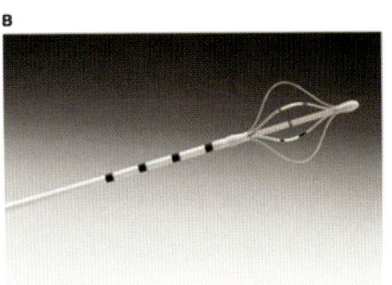

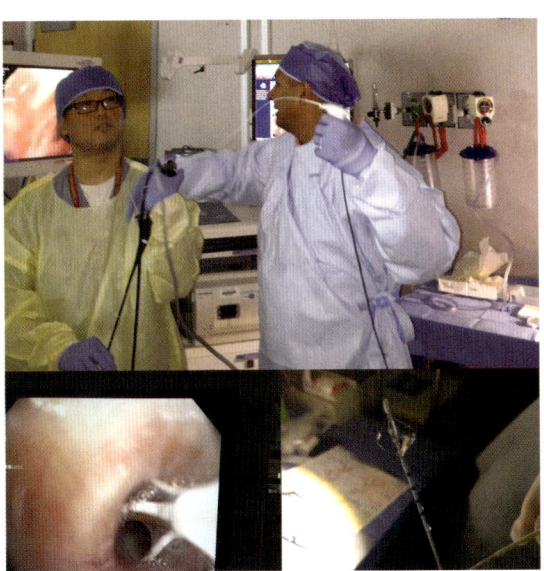

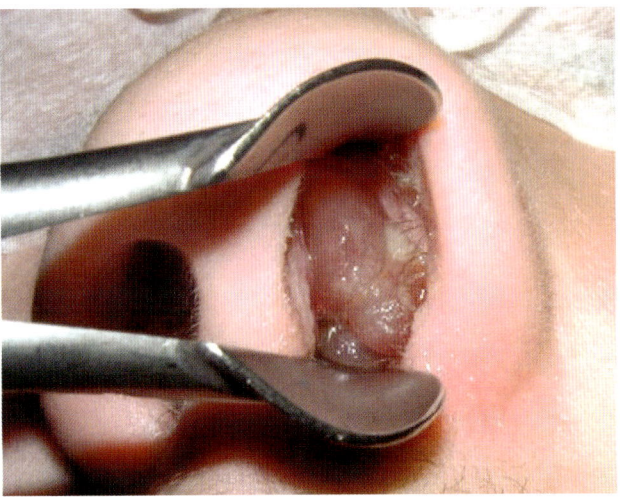

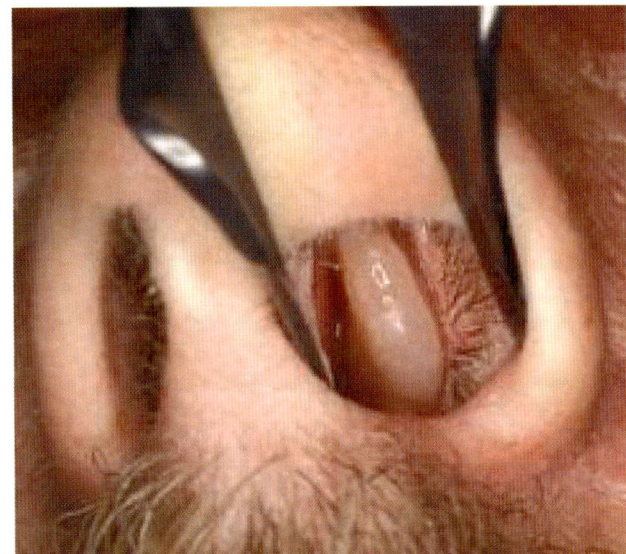

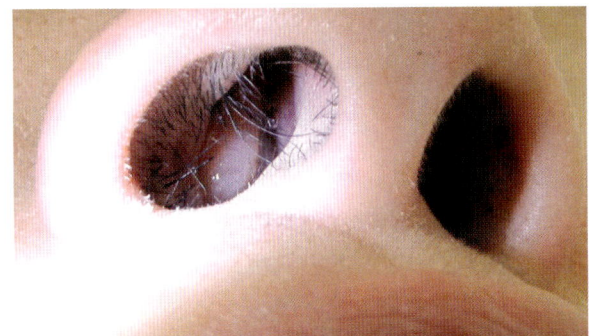

Drugs to Be Careful with in Patients with Asthma
- Aspirin and NSAIDs
  - Samter triad
    1) Nasal polyps
    2) Asthma
    3) Aspirin intolerance
- Nonselective β-blockers
- ACE inhibitors

Asthma-Related Diseases
Allergic bronchopulmonary aspergillosis (ABPA)
- Major features
  - History of asthma
  - Immediate skin test reactivity to *Aspergillus* antigens
  - Elevated serum total IgE
  - Peripheral blood eosinophilia
  - Central bronchiectasis on chest CT
  - Elevated specific serum IgE and IgG to *A. fumigatus*

Eosinophilic granulomatosis with polyangiitis (EGPA)
- ACR has 6 criteria:
  1) Asthma
  2) Greater than 10% peripheral eosinophils on the differential
  3) Mononeuropathy or polyneuropathy
  4) Migratory or transient pulmonary opacities detected radiographically
  5) Paranasal sinus abnormality
  6) Biopsy containing a blood vessel showing the accumulation of eosinophils in extravascular areas

CHRONIC OBSTRUCTIVE PULMONARY DISEASE (COPD)

COPD Definition
- The Global Initiative for Chronic Obstructive Lung Disease (**GOLD**)
  - **Preventable** and treatable disease
  - Pulmonary component is characterized by airflow limitation that **is reversible**
  - Associated with an abnormal inflammatory response of the lungs to **noxious** particles or gases

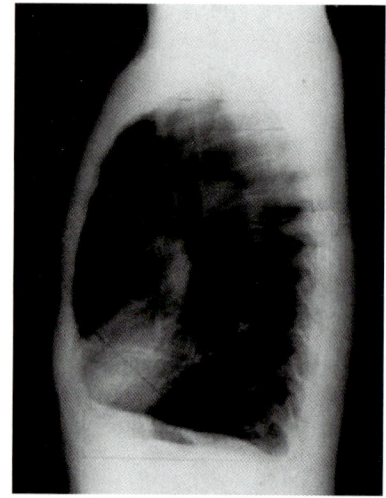

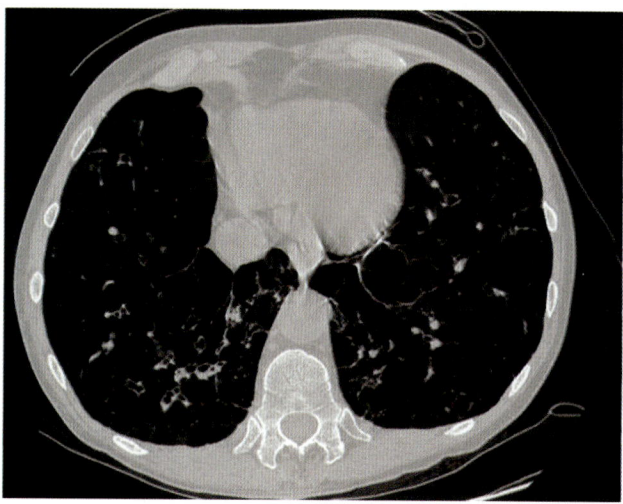

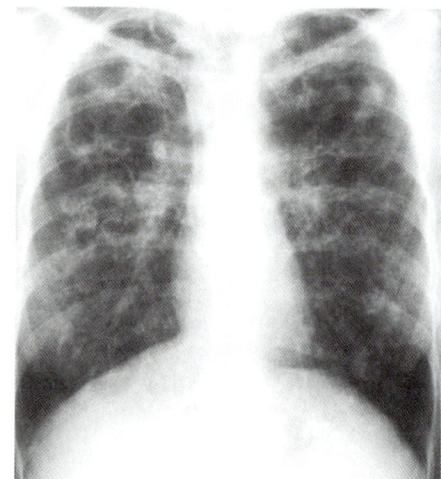

COPD
- COPD is a mixture of:
  - **Emphysema** (pink-puffer)
    - Anatomic/histologic diagnosis
  - **Chronic bronchitis** (blue bloater)
    - Epidemiologic diagnosis
      - Cough and sputum > 3 months for 2 years
  - **Asthma and COPD overlap syndrome** (ACOS)
- Most patients have characteristics of both with a predominance of one

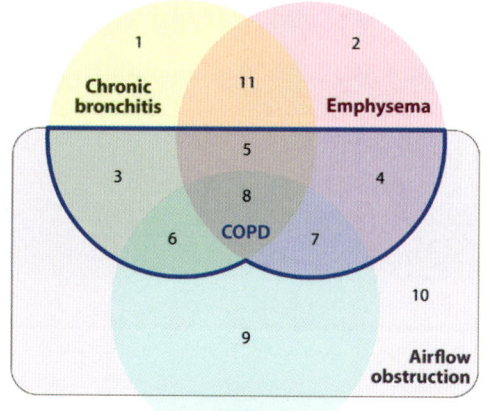

GOLD Classification of Severity Based on Airflow Limitation

I. Mild
- $FEV_1/FVC < 0.70$
- $FEV_1 \geq 80\%$ predicted

II. Moderate
- $FEV_1/FVC < 0.70$
- $50\% \leq FEV_1 \geq 80\%$ predicted

III. Severe
- $FEV_1/FVC < 0.70$
- $30\% \leq FEV_1 < 50\%$ predicted

IV. Very severe
- $FEV_1/FVC < 0.70$
- $FEV_1 < 30\%$ predicted or $FEV_1 < 50\%$ predicted plus chronic respiratory failure

Active reduction of risk factor(s): influenza vaccination
Add short-acting bronchodilator (when needed)

Add regular treatment with one or more long-acting bronchodilators (when needed)
Add pulmonary rehabilitation

Add inhaled glucocorticosteroids if repeated exacerbations

Add long-term oxygen if chronic respiratory failure
Consider surgical treatments

GOLD Combined Assessment (Spirometry and Symptom Score)

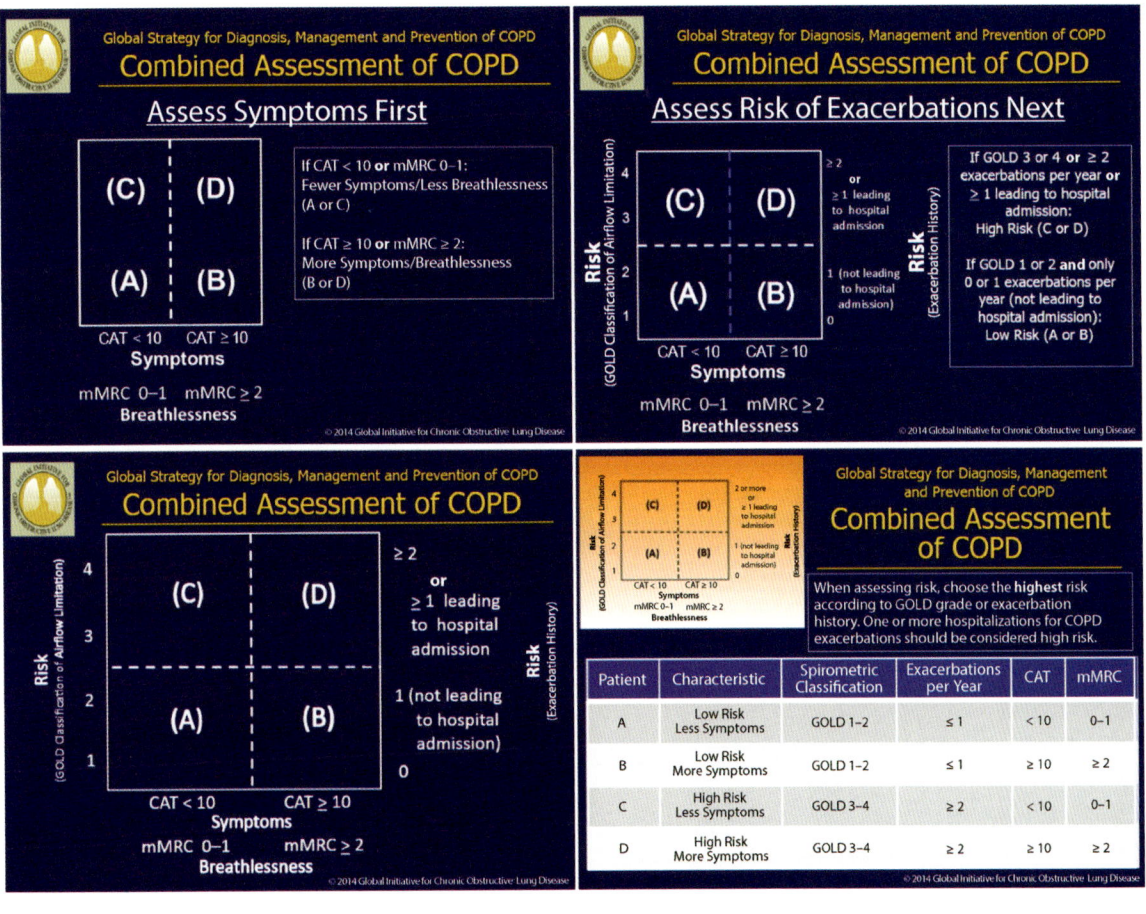

PULMONARY MEDICINE

MMRC Questionnaire for Assessing Severity of Breathlessness		
Severity	**Score**	**Level of Breathlessness**
None	0	Not troubled with breathlessness except with strenuous exercise
Mild	1	Troubled by shortness of breath when hurrying or walking up a slight hill
Moderate	2	Walks slower than people of the same age due to breathlessness or has to stop for breath when walking at own pace on the level
Severe	3	Stops for breath after walking approximately 100 meters or after a few minutes on the level
Very Severe	4	Too breathless to leave the house or breathless when dressing or undressing

Treatment Categories and Options
- **Smoking cessation**
  - Varenicline titrating up to 2 mg daily for 12 weeks
  - Bupropion titrating up to 300 mg daily
  - Nicotine replacement
  - CBT
- **Bronchodilator therapy**
  - β_2-Agonist
  - Anticholinergic
  - Methylxanthines
  - LABA and LAMA combinations
- **Corticosteroids**
  - Inhaled (controversial)
  - Systemic
- **Supplemental oxygen therapy**
  - OSA and the "overlap syndrome"
- **Drugs for reducing exacerbations**
  - Azithromycin
  - Roflumilast
- **Pulmonary rehabilitation**
- **Surgical therapy**
  - Lung volume reduction surgery (LVRS)
  - Lung transplant

Bronchodilator Treatment
1) **Anticholinergic agents**
   - Short-acting (GOLD Stage I)
     - Ipratropium bromide
   - Long-acting
     - Tiotropium — **UPLIFT** trial, reduced exacerbations
2) **β_2-Agonists**
   - Short-acting (GOLD Stage I)
     - Albuterol, levalbuterol
   - Long-acting
     - Combination therapy reduced exacerbations
     - **SUN**, **TORCH**, and **SHINE**
3) **Methylxanthines**
   - Theophylline
     - 200 mg extended release PO daily

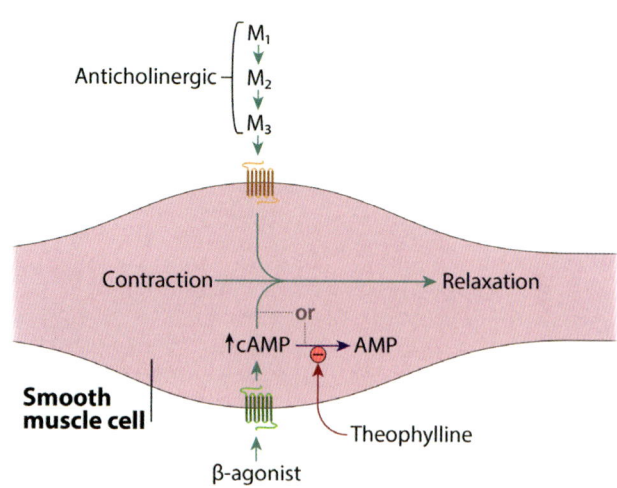

Oxygen Therapy for COPD
- Criteria for starting home oxygen (**mortality reduction**)
  1) Resting $P_aO_2 < 55$ or
  2) O_2 sat (S_aO_2) < 88% or
  3) $P_aO_2 < 59$ mmHg (O_2 sat > 89%) with evidence of:
     - Cor pulmonale
     - Erythrocytosis
       - Hematocrit > 55%
- Decreases morbidity and mortality in severe **chronic** COPD
  - Keep these patients on supplemental oxygen 24 hours/day
    - Long-term continuous oxygen treatment in COPD: Nocturnal Oxygen Treatment Trial (NOTT)

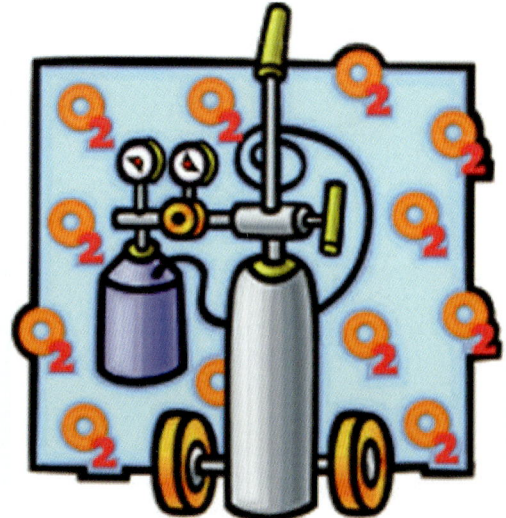

Lung Volume Reduction Therapy[2]

- **Lung volume reduction surgery**
  - The idea is that removing ruined areas of the lung
    - Reduces dead space
    - Improves chest wall and diaphragm dynamics
  - There was no overall survival advantage in the LVRS group, **except** for mainly upper-lobe emphysema + poor exercise capacity
- **Endobronchial valves**
  - Permit exhalation and drainage of secretions but no air entry during inspiration
  - First valve therapy was FDA approved in 2018

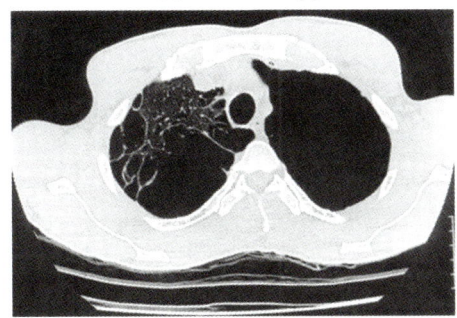

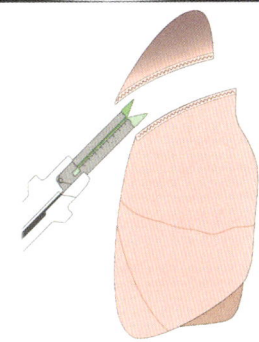

Lung Transplant

- Substantial improvement in exercise tolerance and quality of life
- Transplantation (over the past few years) **has convincingly** been shown to prolong survival from this disease
- Transplant recipients face
  - Infection secondary to immunosuppression
  - Toxic effects of immunosuppressant drugs
  - Acute and chronic rejection of lung allograft
- Can get **single** and double lung transplant

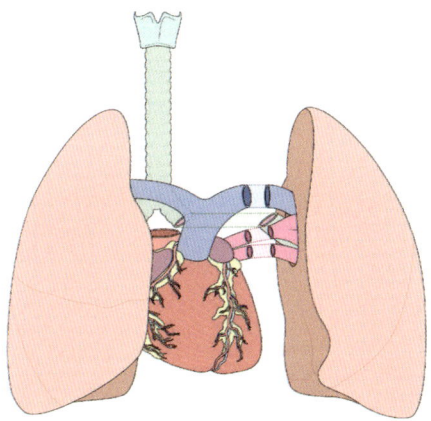

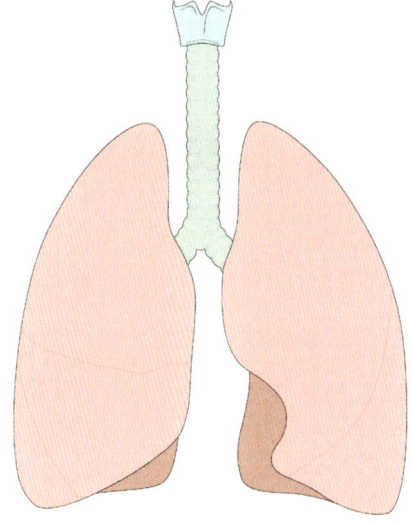

AR 8

A 59-year-old man who has a long-standing history of COPD with **chronic bronchitis** is evaluated in follow-up of his most recent exacerbation 6 weeks ago, which necessitated a visit to the ED. At that time, he was treated with a 7-day outpatient course of oral prednisone and azithromycin. His symptoms are now at baseline, but still has a productive morning cough which is "minimal."

The patient reports that he has dyspnea climbing stairs, but he is able to work as an accountant without difficulty. He smoked 2 packs of cigarettes daily for 20 years, before quitting at age 50. He has had **2 COPD exacerbations** in the past year. His current therapeutic regimen is tiotropium, 18 mcg daily, and salmeterol/fluticasone propionate, 50/250 mcg twice daily.

On exam, temp 98.6°F (37.0°C), HR 78 bpm, RR 12 bpm, and BP 130/80 mmHg. Spirometry reveals FEV_1 45%, FVC 58%, and FEV_1/FVC 61%. Oxygen saturation 93% at rest on RA. Serum α_1-antitrypsin levels are normal.

Which of the following should you recommend to reduce the frequency of this patient's exacerbations?

A. Add prednisone, 5 mg daily.
B. Add roflumilast, 500 mcg daily.
C. Change salmeterol/fluticasone to 50/500 mcg twice daily.
D. Discontinue salmeterol/fluticasone, and add roflumilast, 500 mcg daily.

Answer:_____

AMERICAN JOURNAL OF

Respiratory and Critical Care Medicine

Effect of Roflumilast and Inhaled Corticosteroid/Long-Acting β_2-Agonist on Chronic Obstructive Pulmonary Disease Exacerbations (RE^{2}SPOND)
A Randomized Clinical Trial

American Journal of Respiratory and Critical Care Medicine Volume 194 Number 5 | September 1 2016

Conclusions: Roflumilast failed to statistically significantly reduce moderate and/or severe exacerbations in the overall population. Roflumilast improved lung function and reduced exacerbations in participants with frequent exacerbations and/or hospitalization history. The safety profile of roflumilast was consistent with that of previous studies.

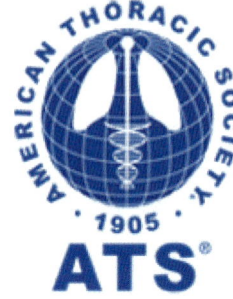

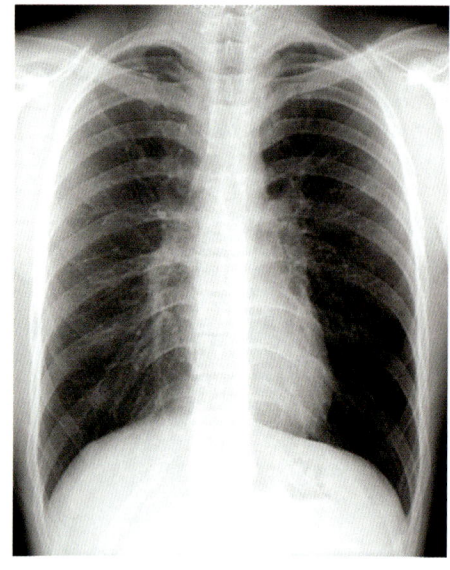

AR 9

A 68-year-old man with a history of COPD (FEV_1 and P_aCO_2 measured under **stable conditions** of 550 mL and 58 mmHg respectively) is admitted with a 3-day history of increasing cough, purulent sputum, and dyspnea.

His only medications are an inhaled β_2-agonist and an inhaled anticholinergic agent.

The patient weighs 65 kg.

Temp 100.9°F (38.3°C); RR 28; irregular HR 120; and BP 100/65.

He is using his accessory muscles of respiration and appears anxious. Heart sounds are diminished, and breath sounds are decreased bilaterally.

CXR shows hyperinflation but no evidence of PNA, HF, PNX, or rib fracture

ABG drawn on 5 L/min of nasal oxygen shows a pH of 7.22, P_aCO_2 74, and P_aO_2 92

ECG shows MAT

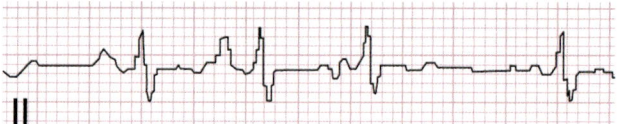

II

AR 9

In the management of the previous patient, which of the following reduces mortality in severe acute exacerbations of COPD?

A. Oxygen
B. Smoking cessation
C. Corticosteroids
D. A and B
E. Other

Answer:_____

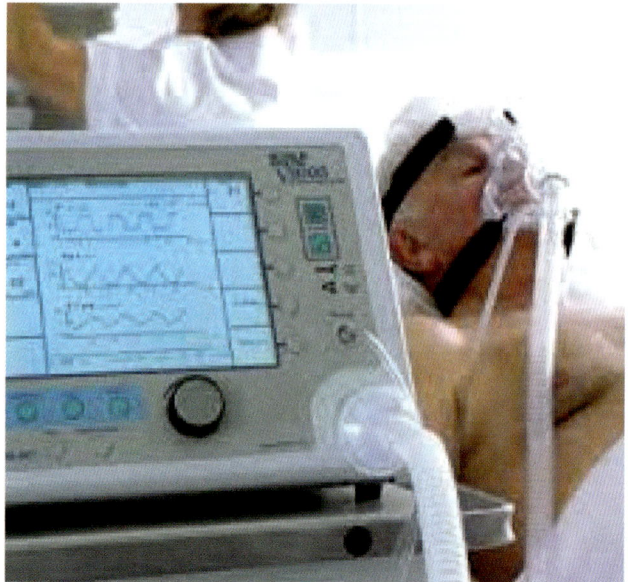

Noninvasive bilevel positive pressure ventilation

AR 10

A 62-year-old woman is evaluated in the ED for a 2-day history of increased dyspnea. She has advanced COPD with an FEV$_1$ of 35% of predicted. She has a 75-pack-year smoking history and continues to smoke. Her current medications are tiotropium bromide and albuterol.

Exam: She is difficult to arouse. Temp 98.6°F (37.0°C); BP 145/90, HR 95, RR 25; and BMI 30. Lung exam discloses prolonged expiration and wheezing. Bilateral pitting leg edema is noted. Oxygen saturation by pulse oximetry is 93%.

Which of the following is the most appropriate diagnostic test to perform next?

A. Arterial blood gas studies
B. Chest CT scan
C. Complete blood count
D. Echocardiography

Answer:_____

AR 11

A 63-year-old woman who has had COPD for 10 years is evaluated because of **easy bruising** that is making her increasingly **self-conscious**. Three years ago, the patient had 1 hospitalization related to an exacerbation. One year ago, she had an exacerbation that was treated with oral medications at **home**. She has had no exacerbations since.

The patient **quit smoking** 3 years ago, and she does not have cough and sputum. She is **physically active** and able to do her own shopping and housework. Her current medications are fluticasone/salmeterol 250/50 mcg bid and tiotropium 18 mcg daily. This regimen has been **unchanged** since her hospitalization 3 years ago.

On physical examination, temperature is 98.6°F (37.0°C). Pulse is 78 bpm, respirations are 14 breaths/min, and blood pressure is 110/70 mmHg. FEV$_1$ is 1.4 L (45% of predicted), unchanged during the past 3 years. S$_a$O$_2$ is 92% on ambient air.

Which of the following is the most appropriate recommendation?

A. Make no changes in medications.
B. Taper and discontinue fluticasone/salmeterol.
C. Taper and discontinue fluticasone/salmeterol and add formoterol/budesonide.
D. Taper and discontinue fluticasone/salmeterol and add indacaterol.

Answer:_____

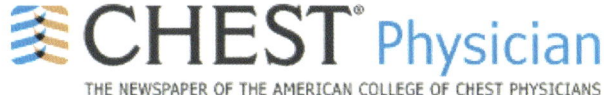

LAMA/LABA may allow withdrawal of inhaled steroids

An option in severe but stable COPD.

BY SHARON WORCESTER
Frontline Medical News

AT CHEST 2014

AUSTIN, TEX. – Inhaled corticosteroids can be successfully withdrawn without increasing the risk of exacerbations in patients who have chronic obstructive pulmonary disease and are receiving dual bronchodilator therapy with a long-acting muscarinic antagonist and a long-acting beta$_2$-agonist, according to findings from the WISDOM study.

However, inhaled corticosteroid (ICS) withdrawal should be conducted with caution, as a small but statistically significantly greater decrease in lung function occurred in patients who withdrew completely, compared with those who did not during the 12-month, double-blind, parallel-group study, Dr. Helgo Magnussen reported at the annual meeting of the American College of Chest Physicians.

"In patients with severe but stable COPD who are receiving combination therapy with tiotropium, salmeterol and ICS, a stepwise withdrawal of ICS was noninferior to continuation of ICS with respect to the risk of moderate or severe

See **COPD** · page 5

[3]

INTERSTITIAL LUNG DISEASES (ILDs)

- **Overview**
  - Diffuse parenchymal lung disease (DPLD)
  - Diverse (> 100) group of disorders that affect the **interstitium**, a potential space between the capillaries and the alveoli
  - Partly a **misnomer**, because there is often bronchial and alveolar involvement

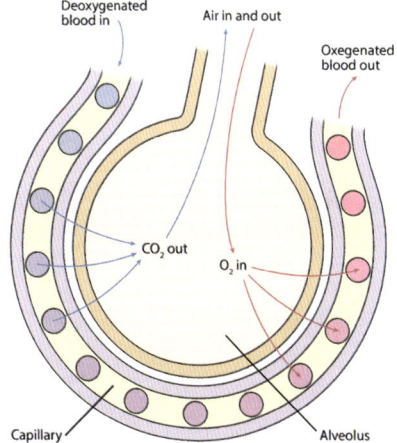

Interstitial Lung Diseases
- **Diagnosis**
    1) Bronchoscopy
        - BAL
        - TBB
        - EBUS
    2) Surgical biopsy
        - VATS
        - Thoracotomy
- **Common factors in their clinical presentation**
    1) Diffuse disease on chest imaging
        - Reticulonodular disease on CXR
        - Ground-glass on CT scan
    2) Restrictive intrinsic PFTs
    3) Elevated A-a gradient
    4) Dyspnea on exertion

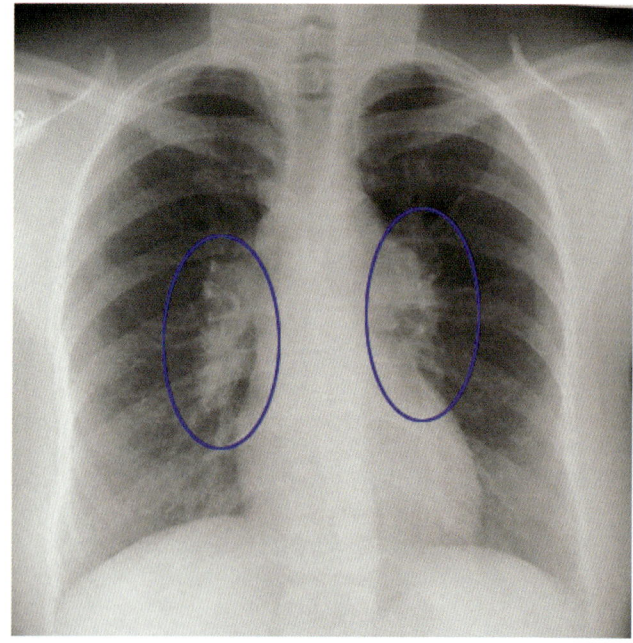

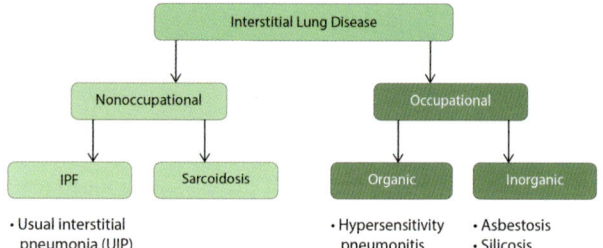

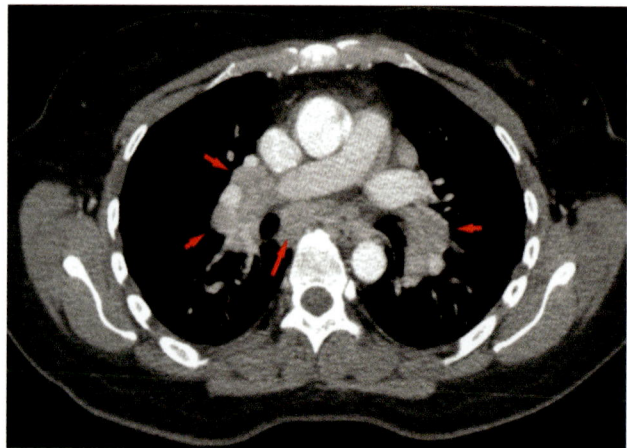

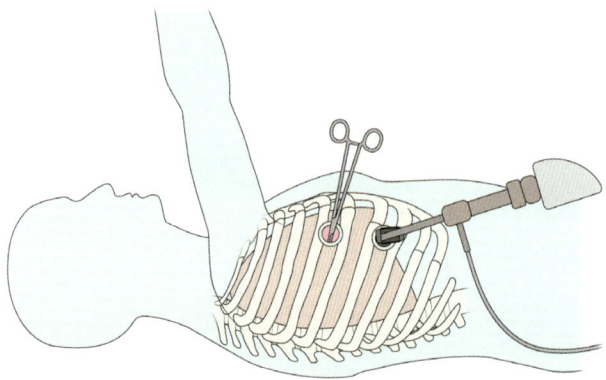

- Usual interstitial pneumonia (UIP)
- Hypersensitivity pneumonitis
- Asbestosis
- Silicosis
- Berylliosis
- Coal worker's pneumoconiosis

Two Distinct Syndromes
- **Löfgren Syndrome**
    - Acute
    - Erythema nodosum
    - Arthritis
    - Hilar adenopathy

SARCOIDOSIS
- **Definition**
    - A systemic disease of unknown etiology
    - Characterized by the presence of noncaseating granulomas
- **Clinical manifestations**
    - Can involve almost any organ system
        - Ocular, skin, myocardial, rheumatologic, GI, and CNS
    - Pulmonary involvement is most common

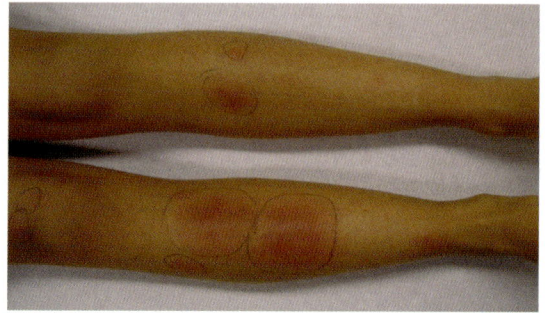

- **Heerfordt-Waldenström**
  - Subacute to chronic
  - Fever
  - Parotid enlargement
  - Uveitis
  - Facial palsy

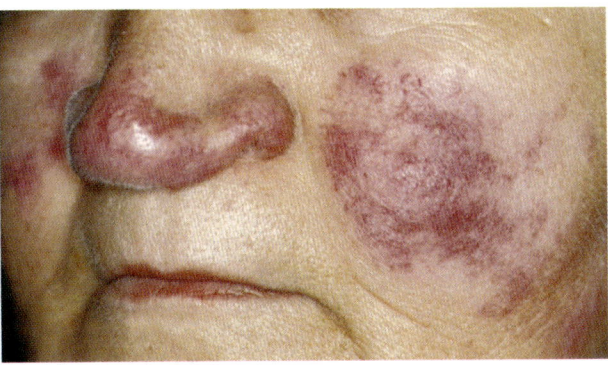

Sarcoid Diagnosis
- **Exclude the other granulomatous diseases**
  - Hypersensitivity pneumonitis
  - Berylliosis
  - Infectious diseases caused by mycobacteria and fungi
- **Biopsy most easily accessible tissue**
  - Noncaseating granulomas
- **If lung involvement, usually start with bronchoscopy with TBB ± EBUS**

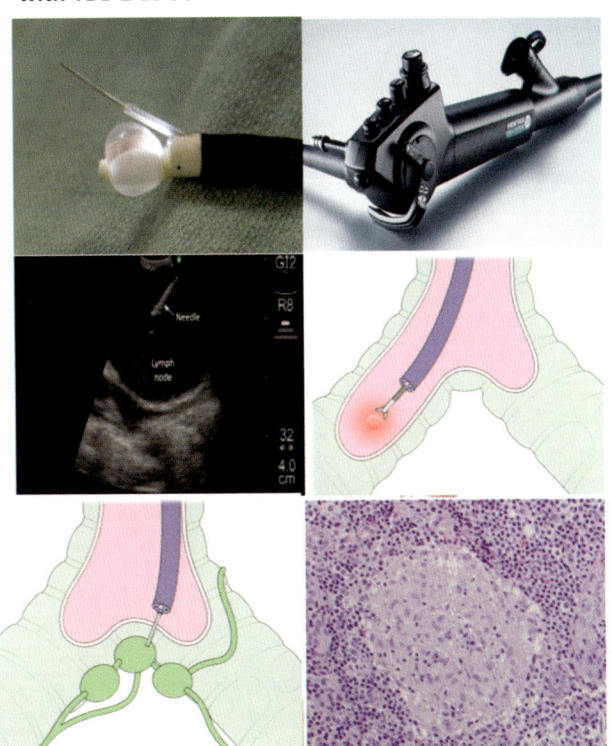

Sarcoid Treatment
- Majority of patients do not require treatment
- Treat acute symptomatic disease with corticosteroids
- Corticosteroids
  - Do not induce remission or alter the course of disease
  - Decrease symptoms
  - Improve PFTs
  - Numerous side effects
- **Indications** for systemic corticosteroids
  - Eyes
  - Heart
  - CNS
  - Symptomatic pulmonary involvement
  - Symptomatic hypercalcemia

Sarcoid Steroid-Sparing Agents
- The evidence in support of individual 2nd line cytotoxic agents is largely **observational**
- The agents that appear to have the greatest likelihood of benefit with an acceptable side effect profile are:
  - Methotrexate
  - Azathioprine
  - Leflunomide
  - Antimalarial
  - TNF-inhibitors
  - Mycophenolate mofetil
  - Corticotropin injection

Methotrexate (MTX)
- Most commonly used steroid-sparing agent
- For lungs, skin, eyes, and CNS
- Oral or intramuscularly
- Begin PO **7.5 mg weekly** with folic acid daily
- Dose is gradually increased by 2.5 mg q 2 weeks until a dose of **15–20 mg** per week
- Intramuscular MTX for refractory nausea

Azathioprine
- Weight-based dosing
- 2–3 mg/kg start at 50 mg and increase slowly every 2–3 weeks to reduce GI side effects
- Toxicity is largely related to its metabolites, which are broken down by the enzyme thiopurine-S-methyltransferase (**TPMT**)
- TPMT enzyme activity can be genotyped or measured

Leflunomide
- Start at **10 mg** and increase to 20 mg daily
- Nausea, diarrhea, abdominal pain, hepatotoxicity
- Reasonable alternative if patient cannot tolerate the side effects of MTX

Antimalarials
- Chloroquine and hydroxychloroquine have immunomodulating properties
- For **cutaneous** sarcoidosis, but several reports have described its use in pulmonary disease
- Glucose-6-phosphate dehydrogenase (**G6PD**) levels must be determined prior to initiating therapy
- Used for hypercalcemia because it decreases 1,25 dihydroxyvitamin D
- Side effects irreversible retinopathy and blindness require exam at baseline and q 6–12 months

TNF Inhibitors

- The two main TNF agents used in the treatment of sarcoidosis are:
  - Infliximab (Remicade)
  - Adalimumab (Humira)

Mycophenolate Mofetil (MMF)

- Inhibitor of lymphocyte proliferation and activity, has been used to treat a variety of ILDs associated with rheumatic disease
- Data regarding the use of MMF in sarcoidosis is **limited**
- Start at 500 mg PO bid up to 2 g daily
- Nausea and diarrhea may be dose limiting

Corticotropin Injection (Acthar Gel)

- **FDA approved** for sarcoidosis after steroids and cytotoxic agents are used
- Work on **melanocortin** receptors
- 40–80 units SubQ 2–3 times per week

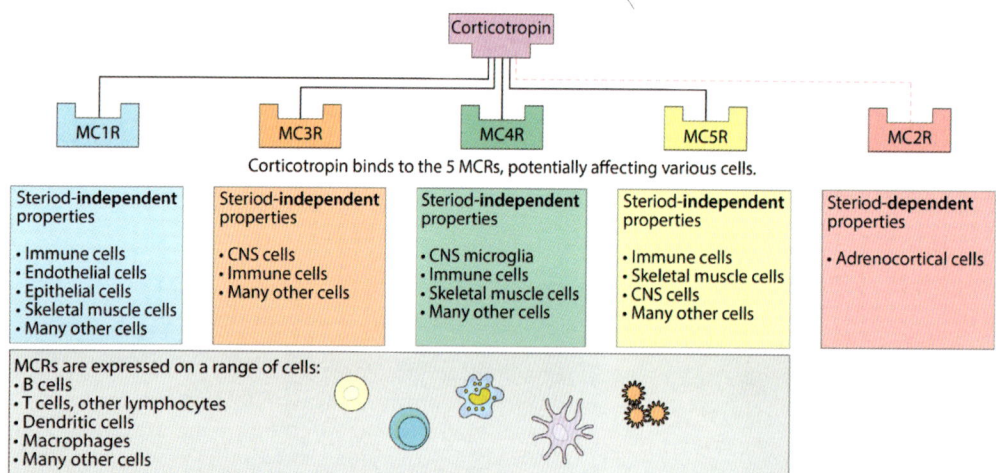

Corticotropin binds to the 5 MCRs, potentially affecting various cells.

Steroids have been demonstrated not to bind to any of the 5 MCRs.

AR 12

A **65-year-old** female is evaluated for a 10-month history of cough and dyspnea. She reports no other symptoms or medical problems and takes no medications. She is a **former smoker** with a 20-pack-year history. She has **no pets**.

On exam, BP 120/70 mmHg, HR 80 beats/minute, and RR 24 breaths/minute. Oxygen saturation is 87% on RA. There is **no JVD**. Cardiac examination is normal. Lung exam — bilateral **inspiratory crackles** at the lung bases. Digital **clubbing** is present.

PFT: Decreased TLC, decreased FEV_1, decreased FVC, normal FEV_1/FVC, and a decreased DLCO.

A CT scan is done.

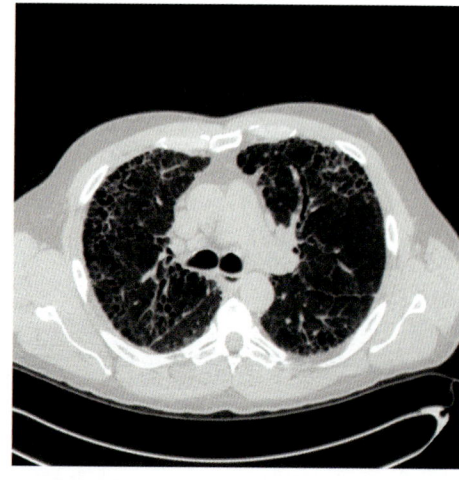

Which of the following is the most likely diagnosis?

A. Emphysema
B. Heart failure
C. Hypersensitivity pneumonitis
D. Idiopathic pulmonary fibrosis

Answer:_____

- Etiology is unknown
- Diagnosis of exclusion
  - Occupation and exposures
  - Drugs
    - Bleomycin, amiodarone, MTX
  - Rheumatologic symptoms
- Physical exam
  - Velcro rales and clubbing
- Diagnostic workup includes:
  - High resolution CT chest
    - Fleischner Society
  - PFTs
    - Intrinsic restrictive pattern
  - ABG
    - A-a gradient
  - Histologic tissue diagnosis if necessary based on ILD board recommendation
    - TBB
    - Wedge resection

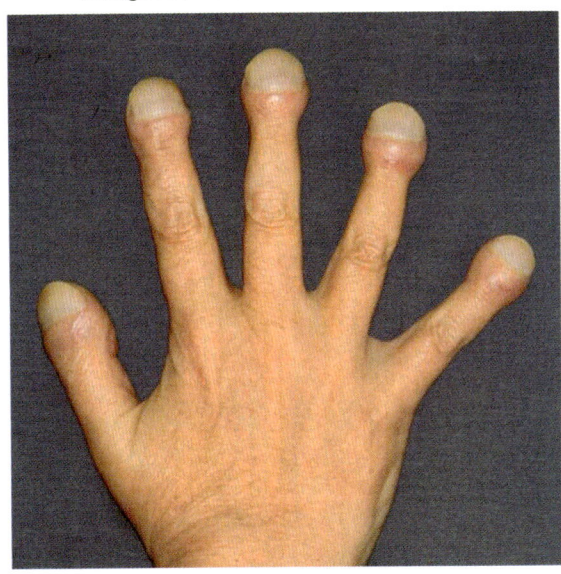

Idiopathic Pulmonary Fibrosis

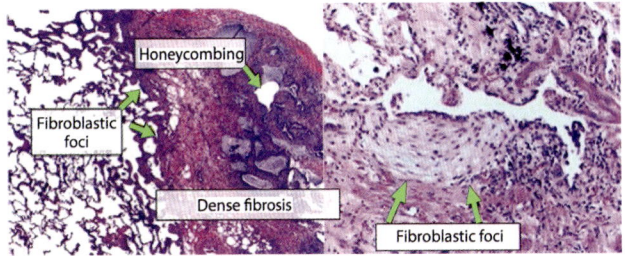

The histologic hallmark and chief diagnostic criterion is a heterogeneous appearance with alternating areas of normal lung, interstitial inflammation, fibroblast foci, and honeycomb change.

GERD and Chronic Microaspiration[5]
- Up to **90%** of patients with IPF have GERD
- GERD is an important risk factor for the **progression** of IPF
- In a review, 67–76% of patients with IPF assessed with **ambulatory pH** probe had GERD
- Classic symptoms of GERD were **poor predictors** of increased esophageal acid exposure among patients with moderate-to-severe IPF

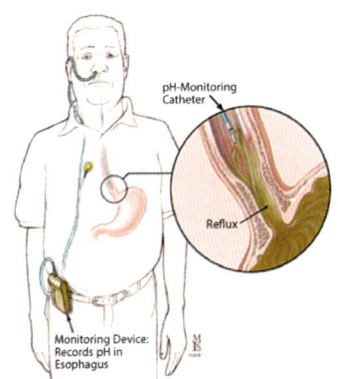

The Role of CT is Expanded to Permit Diagnosis of IPF Without Surgical Lung Biopsy in Select Cases[4]

	Typical UIP CT Pattern	Probably UIP CT Pattern	CT Pattern Indeterminate for UIP	CT Features Most Consistent with non-IPF Diagnosis
Distribution	Basal predominant (occasionally diffuse), and subpleural predominant; distribution is often heterogeneous	Basal and subpleural predominant; distribution is often heterogeneous	Variable or diffuse	Upper-lung or mid-lung predominant fibrosis; peribronchovascular predominance with subpleural sparing
Features	Honeycombing; reticular pattern with peripheral traction bronchiectasis or bronchiolectasis; absence of features to suggest an alternative diagnosis	Reticular pattern with peripheral traction bronchiectasis or bronchiolectasis; honeycombing is absent; absence of features to suggest an alternative diagnosis	Evidence of fibrosis with some inconspicuous features suggestive of nonUIP pattern	Any of the following: predominant consolidation, extensive pure ground glass opacity (without acute exacerbation), extensive mosaic attenuation with extensive sharply defined locular air trapping on expiration, diffuse nodules or cysts

AR 13

Which of the following is the most common side effect of nintedanib in the treatment of idiopathic pulmonary fibrosis (IPF)?

A. Diarrhea
B. Headache
C. Hypertension
D. Liver enzyme elevation

Answer:_____

- Nintedanib (Ofev)
  - Tyrosine kinase inhibitor
  - Slows rate of disease progression in IPF
  - 150 mg PO twice daily
  - Side effects
    - Diarrhea 62%
    - Nausea 24%
    - Vomiting 12%
    - Elevation in LFTs 14%
- Pirfenidone (Esbriet)
  - Antifibrotic agent
  - Slows rate of disease progression in IPF
  - Start 267 mg (1 capsule) PO TID
    - After 1st week increased to 534 mg PO TID
    - After 2nd week increased to 801 mg PO TID
  - Side effects
    - Rash 30%
    - Photosensitivity 9%
    - Nausea 36%
    - Diarrhea 26%
    - Abdominal discomfort 24%

Treatment

- **Supportive care**
  - Supplemental oxygen
  - Pulmonary rehabilitation
  - Vaccinations
  - Information regarding participation in randomized trials
- **For patients who desire active therapy rather than supportive care and are not interested in participating in a clinical trial**
  1) Pirfenidone; the dose ranges up to 40 mg/kg per day in 3 divided doses
  2) Nintedanib
- **Do <u>not</u> use for chronic therapy**
  1) Glucocorticoid monotherapy
  2) Combination therapy with azathioprine, prednisone, and N-acetylcysteine
- **Early referral for lung transplantation evaluation**
- **In patients with an acute exacerbation of IPF can consider:**
  - Broad-spectrum antibiotics
  - High-dose glucocorticoids in combination with a cytotoxic agent, such as azathioprine

AR 14

A **77-year-old** man is evaluated in the hospital for idiopathic **pulmonary fibrosis**. He was diagnosed 3 years ago and has gradually worsened despite therapy with prednisone, azathioprine, and N-acetylcysteine.

All therapy has been discontinued over the past 6 months because of failure to respond and side effects. He has been **homebound** on high-flow oxygen and has been hospitalized 3 times in the past year. He just finished 7 days of levofloxacin. He has indicated that he **does not want** additional aggressive therapy.

On exam, patient is in severe respiratory distress; BP 144/80 mmHg, HR 118 bpm, RR 28 bpm, and afebrile. Oxygen saturation is 88% with the patient breathing 100% oxygen by nonrebreather. Patient with neck retraction and accessory muscles use. Bilateral crackles are noted posteriorly.

WBC is 5,000 cells/mm^3 with a normal differential count. CXR and CT chest are shown.

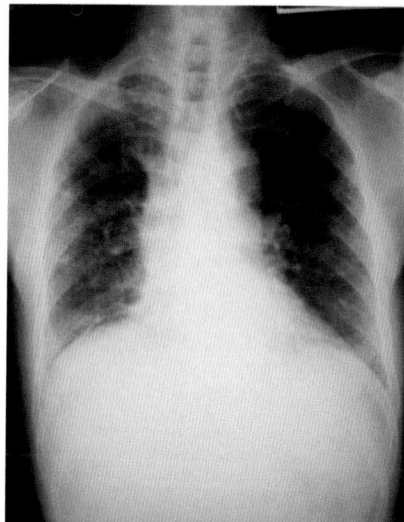

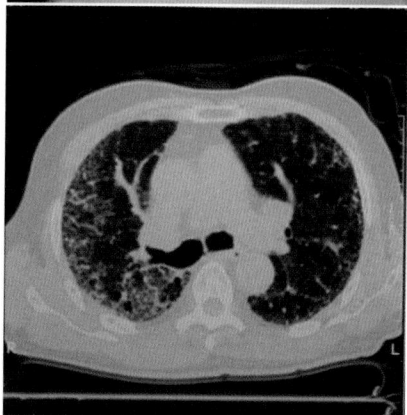

Which of the following is the most appropriate recommendation?

A. Intravenous methylprednisolone 120 mg IV q 6 hours
B. Mechanical ventilation with pressure control mode
C. BiPAP with initial settings of 10/5 cm H_2O
D. Palliative care consult

Answer:_____

PULMONARY NODULES

SOLITARY PULMONARY NODULE

- **Differential diagnosis**
  1) **Malignancy**
     - Bronchogenic carcinoma
     - Pulmonary metastases
  2) **Benign disease**
     - Granulomas
     - Benign tumors (hamartomas)
     - Resolving infarction
     - Rheumatoid and vasculitic nodules
     - AV malformations
     - Pulmonary sequestration
     - Rounded atelectasis
     - Rounded pneumonia

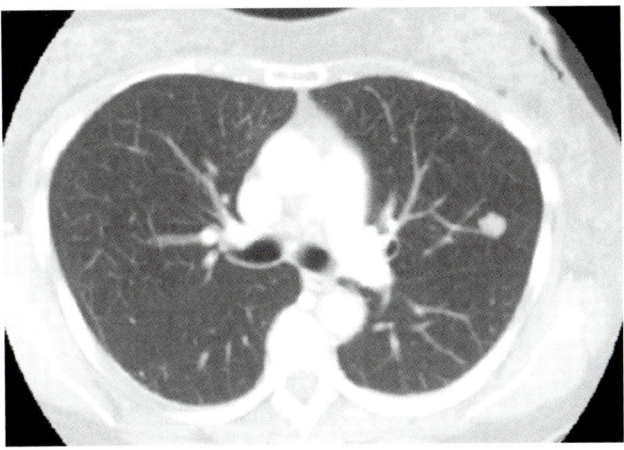

Granuloma

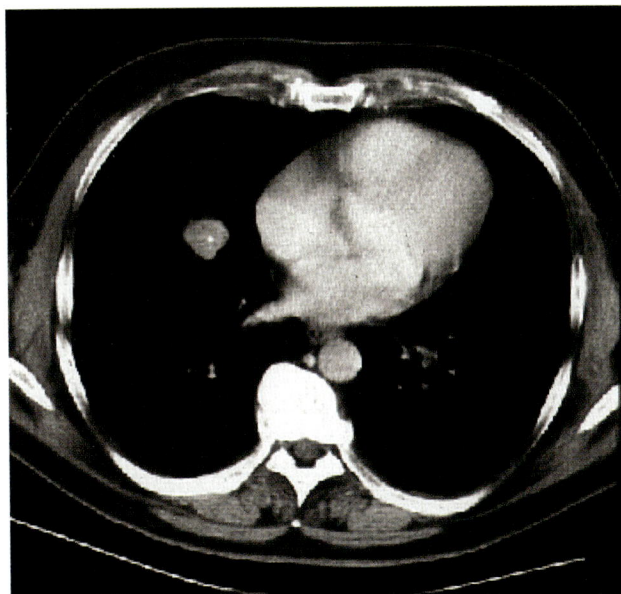

Target-like calcification in the right lower lobe granuloma

Pulmonary Hamartoma

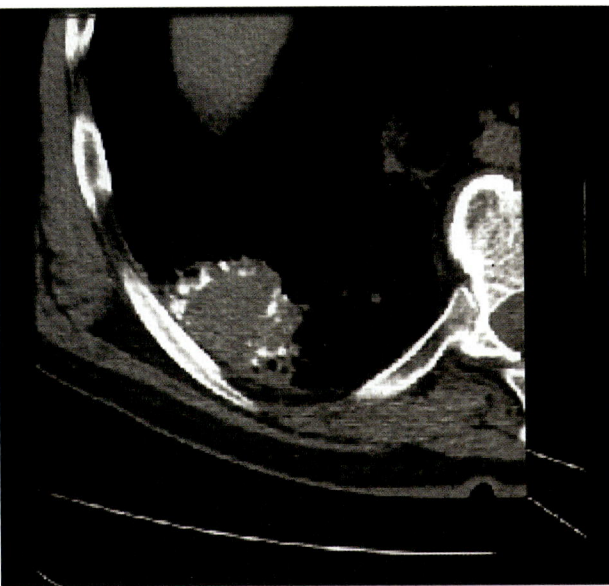

Characteristic popcorn configuration suggestive of a hamartoma

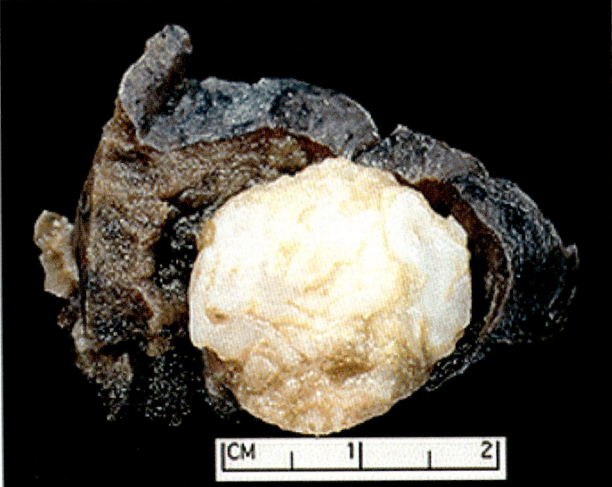

Well-circumscribed mass with a variegated yellow and white appearance, which corresponds to fat and cartilage

Pulmonary AVM

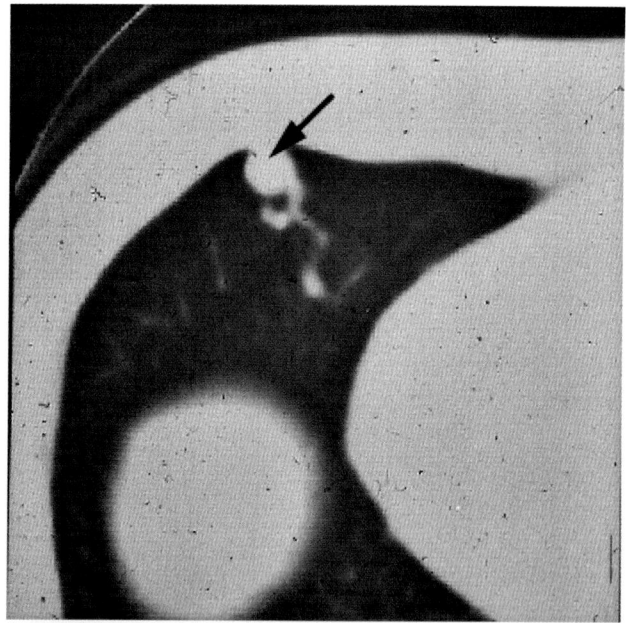

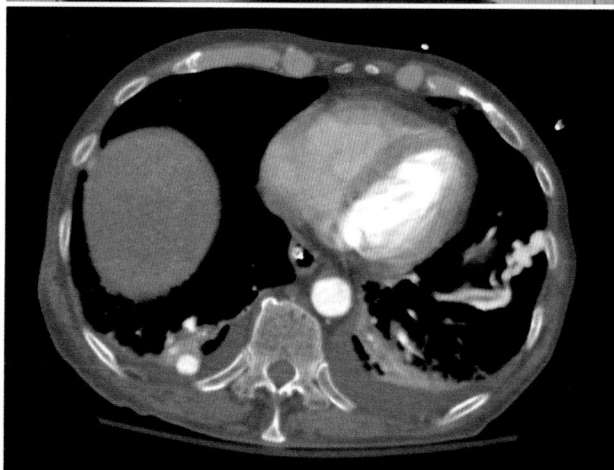

Hereditary hemorrhagic telangiectasia

Pulmonary Sequestration

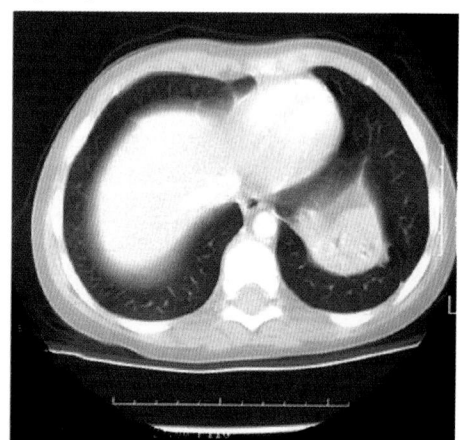

3.5 × 3 × 2.5-cm soft tissue mass located immediately above the diaphragm on the left side of the chest; a large artery from the descending aorta was identified

Rounded Atelectasis

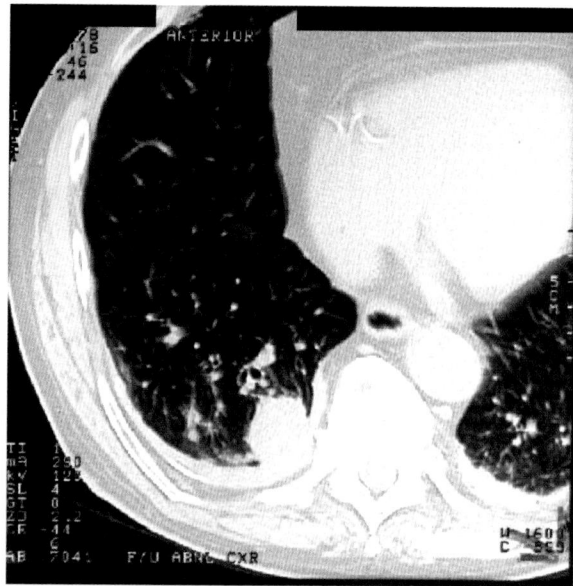

Seen in asbestosis and TB

Pulmonary Tuberculoma

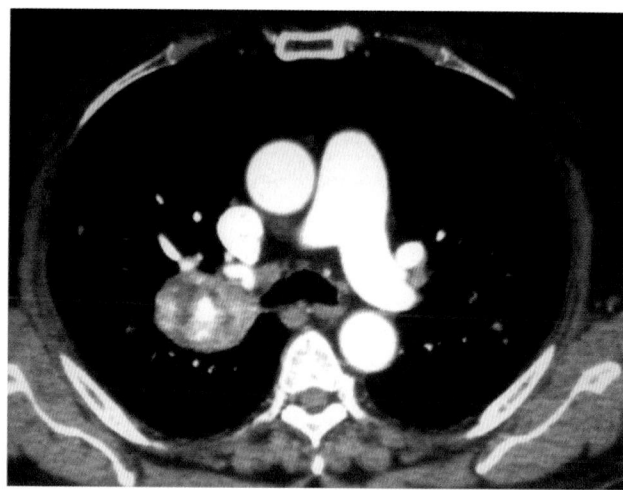

Pulmonary Nodule Evaluation
- **2 key elements:**
  1) **History**
     - Smoking
     - Age > 30 years
     - Previous malignancy
  2) **Appearance of the nodule**
     - CT scan
     - Calcifications
- **Low risk**
  - Follow-up imaging
  - Fleischner Society recommendations
- **High risk**
  - Fine-needle aspiration
  - Bronchoscopy/EBUS
  - Open-lung biopsy
- **Intermediate risk**
  - If nodules are > 0.8-cm diameter, 5-fluorodeoxyglucose + PET

Thoracic Positron Emission Tomography

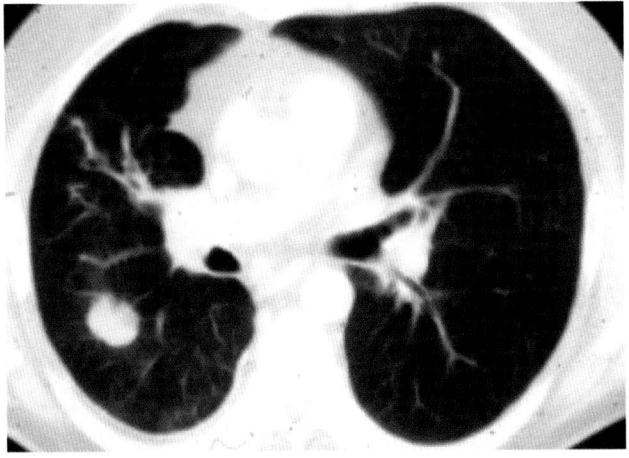

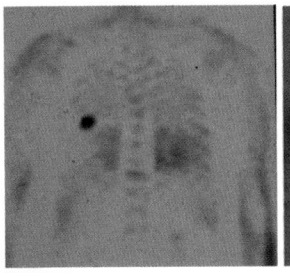 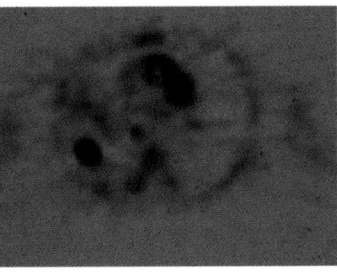

AR 16

A **57-year-old man** is evaluated after a **CXR** taken in a **preoperative assessment** for a knee replacement shows a **1-cm nodule** in the right lower lobe of the lung. The patient lives in Montana and has not traveled recently. He does not recall ever having been exposed to tuberculosis or having been tested for the disease.

His most recent chest radiograph was 10 years ago. The result was normal, and the radiograph is no longer available. About 6 months ago, he had abdominal pain that was evaluated with an **abdominal CT scan**, and the pain has since resolved. The patient has a 20-pack-year history of cigarette smoking but quit 10 years ago. He is otherwise healthy.

On exam, VS are normal, lungs are clear, and there is no lymphadenopathy.

Which of the following is the most appropriate next step in the management of this patient?

A. Fluorodeoxyglucose and positron emission tomography (FDG-PET) scan
B. MRI of the chest
C. Repeat CT scan in 3 months
D. Review of lung images from CT scan of the abdomen
E. Thin-section CT scan of the chest

Answer:_____

AR 15

In which of the following circumstances would a PET scan give the most useful clinical information in order to make a decision about proceeding to surgical resection?

A. A 45-year-old woman from Ohio, who has never smoked, who has a history of histoplasmosis, and is now found to have a 2.5-cm pulmonary nodule on chest CT; no prior radiographs are available
B. A 55-year-old man with a history of smoking who has a 2-cm left lower lobe nodule on chest CT with normal-sized mediastinal nodes
C. A 58-year-old woman with a 3.5-cm right lower lobe adenocarcinoma with new neurologic findings
D. A 46-year-old woman with a new 0.7-cm left lower lobe nodule with a history of adenocarcinoma in situ resected 1 year ago
E. A 52-year-old man with poorly controlled DM with HbA1c of 10.2 and a 60-pack-year smoking history with an undiagnosed 3-cm right lower lobe nodule

Answer:_____

Management of Nodules Smaller than 8 mm

Type	Size			Follow-Up	
Solid	< 6 mm (< 100 mm³)	Single	Low risk	No routine follow-up	
			High risk	Optional CT at 12 months	
		Multiple	Low risk	No routine follow-up	
			High risk	Optional CT at 12 months	
	6–8 mm (100–250 mm³)	Single	Low risk	CT at 6–12 mos, then consider CT at 18–24	
			High risk	CT at 6–12 mos, then CT at 18–24	
		Multiple	Low risk	CT at 3–6 mos, then consider CT at 18–24	
			High risk	CT at 3–6 mos, then CT at 18–24	
	> 8 mm (> 250 mm³)	Single	All	Consider CT at 3 mos, PET/CT or biopsy	
		Multiple	Low risk	CT at 3–6 mos, then consider CT at 18–24	
			High risk	CT at 3–6 mos, then CT at 18–24	

Nodules Detected Incidentally at Nonscreening CT Based on 2017 Fleischner Society Guidelines

Subsolid	Size	Follow-Up
Ground-Glass	< 6 mm	No follow-up indicated
	≥ 6 mm	CT at 6–12 months to confirm persistence, then CT at 3 and 5 years
Part-Solid	< 6 mm	No follow-up indicated
	≥ 6 mm	CT at 3–6 months to confirm persistence, then annual CT for 5 years
Multiple	< 6 mm	CT at 3–6 months; If stable CT at 2 and 4 years
	≥ 6 mm	CT at 3–6 months; Subsequent management based on most suspicious nodule

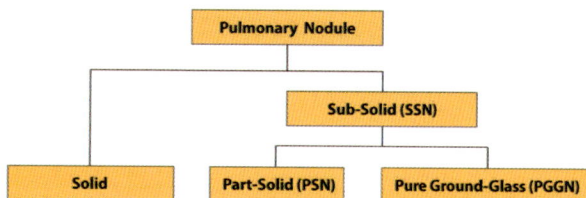

Nonsolid (ground-glass) or partly solid nodules may require longer follow-up to exclude indolent adenocarcinoma.

PLEURAL EFFUSIONS

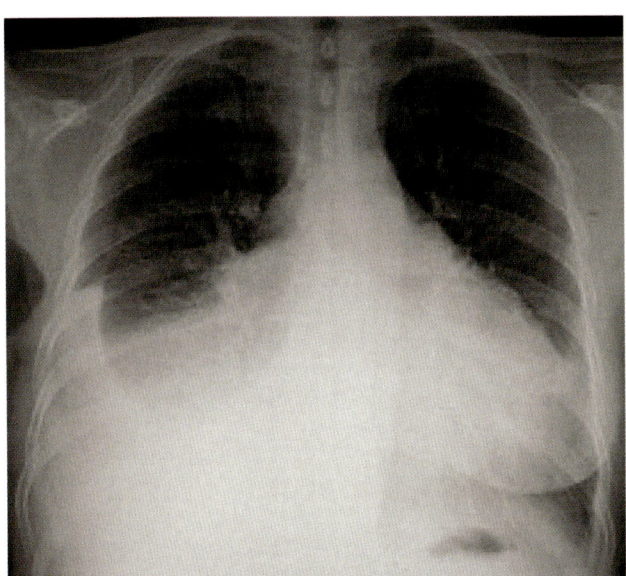

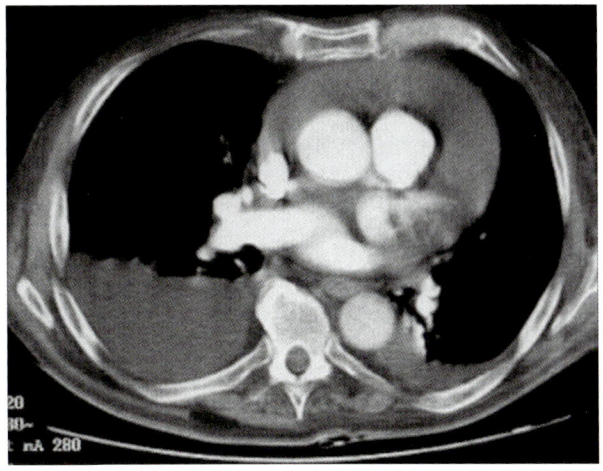

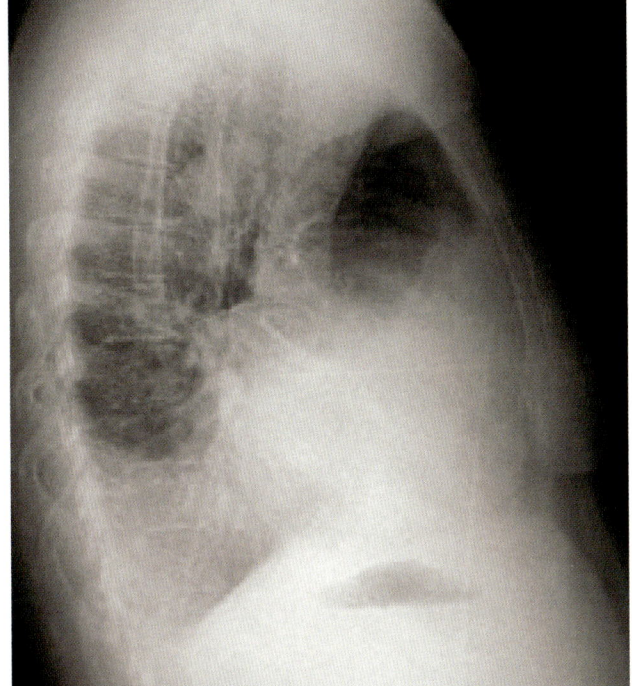

Light Criteria

If any **one** of the following criteria is met, the fluid is an **exudate**:

- Pleural LDH > 2/3 upper limit of normal for serum LDH
- Pleural LDH/serum LDH > 0.6
- Pleural protein/serum protein > 0.5

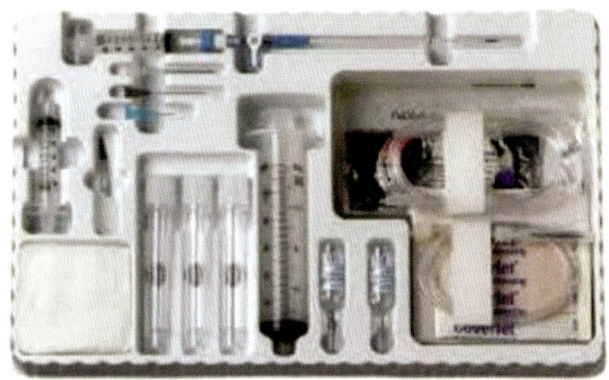

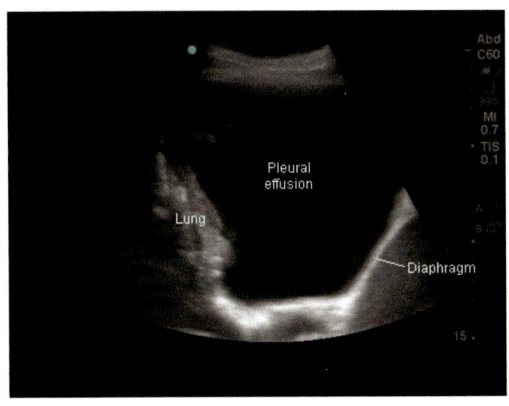

Pleural effusion

Lung

Diaphragm

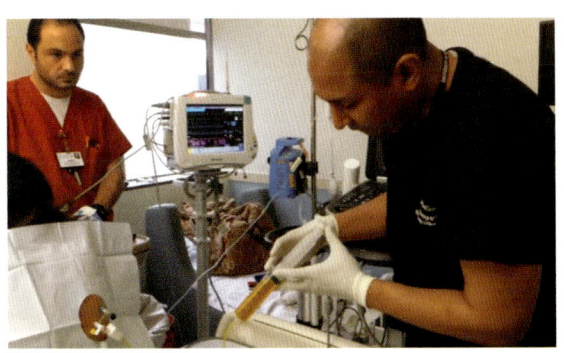

PULMONARY MEDICINE

EXUDATIVE vs. TRANSUDATIVE

Pleural Effusions
- **Transudative effusions**
  - HF (LV failure)
    - Increased hydrostatic pressure
  - Hypoalbuminemia (decreased oncotic pressure)
    - Cirrhosis
    - Nephrotic syndrome
  - Atelectasis
  - Pulmonary embolism
- **Exudative effusions**
  - Pneumonia and malignancy
    - 80% of all exudates
  - Pulmonary embolism
  - Tuberculosis
  - Chylothorax
  - Dressler syndrome
  - Pancreatitis
  - Rheumatologic disease
- **Indications for a chest tube**
  1) Pus in pleural space
  2) Positive culture on pleural space fluid
  3) Complicated parapneumonic effusion

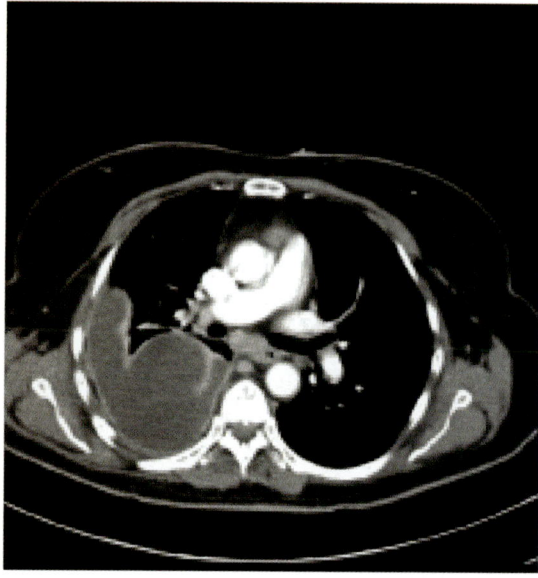

- **Mesothelial cells**
  - Normally line the cavity
  - No mesothelial cells — think tuberculous effusion
- **Eosinophils**
  - Drug reaction, parasites
- **Lymphocytes**
  - TB (pleural biopsy)
  - Malignancy (cytology)
- **Neutrophils**
  - Pneumonia
- **Glucose**
  - Low in RA and empyema
- **Amylase**
  - Pancreatitis (fistula)
  - Esophageal rupture
  - Tumor
- **pH**
  - pH < 7.20 suggests complicated effusion and **possible need for chest tube** or seen in RA
- **ANA**
  - Drug-induced SLE and native SLE
- **Triglycerides**
  - Chylous effusions
    - Associated with leakage of thoracic duct
    - Trauma, lymphoma, LAM

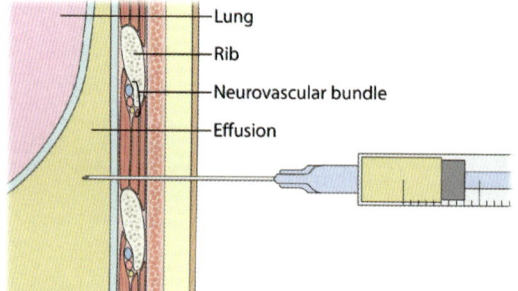

AR 17

A **62-year-old** male complains of a nonproductive **cough** and **weight loss** of 20 lb over the last 3–4 months. He has also noted a hoarse voice for the last month. He has a 45- to 50-pack-year smoking history but quit recently.

On exam, vitals are WNL; BMI is 19 kg/m²; auscultation reveals decreased breath sounds with dullness to percussion on the right along with (+) egophony and decreased tactile fremitus prolonged expiration. The remainder of the exam is unremarkable.

Chest CT shows a **pleural effusion** on the right and a **right upper lobe mass.**

Diagnostic thoracentesis is performed, and 100 mL of fluid is removed that reveals a lymphocytic exudate.

Cytology is negative for malignancy.

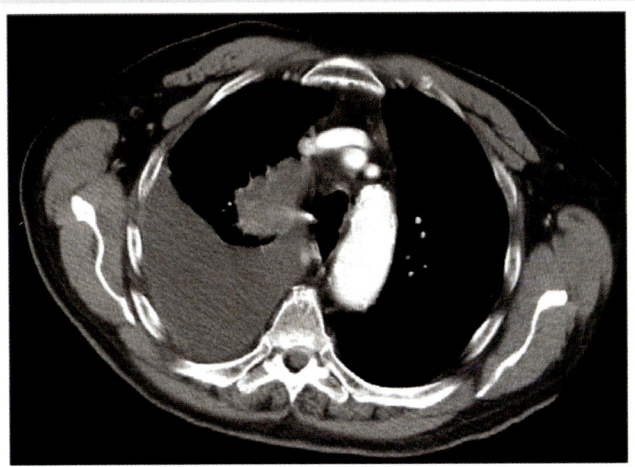

Which of the following is the most appropriate next step in the evaluation of this patient?

A. Bronchoscopy ± EBUS
B. Closed pleural biopsy
C. PET scan
D. Repeat thoracentesis and pleural fluid cytology.

Answer:_____

Indwelling Pleural Catheter (PleurX Catheter)
- For symptomatic reaccumulating malignant and nonmalignant pleural effusions
- Can combine with chemical pleurodesis

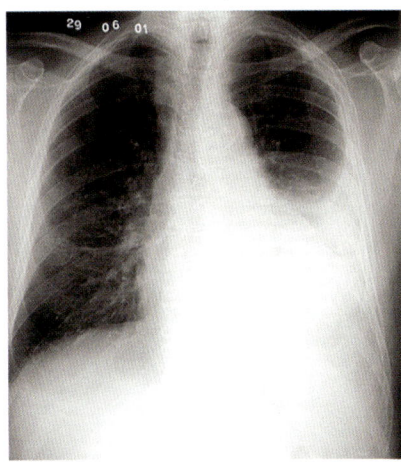

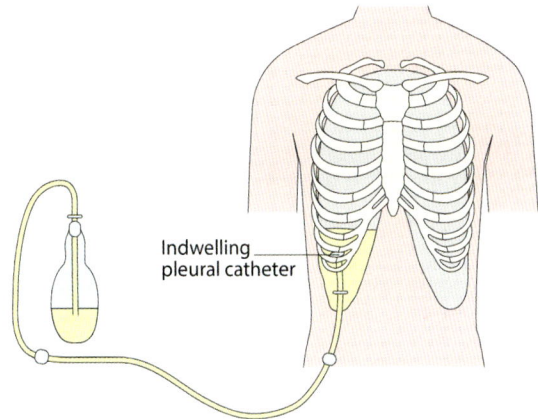

Indwelling pleural catheter

FDA Clears BD's PleurX Catheter System for Specific Non-Malignant Recurrent Pleural Effusions

MYCOBACTERIAL INFECTIONS

TUBERCULOSIS (TB)

Latent and Active Tuberculosis

What is Tuberculosis?
- Tuberculosis (TB) is an infectious disease caused by *Mycobacterium tuberculosis* bacteria and is transmitted person to person via droplets in the **air**
- Although TB can affect multiple organs, it primarily affects the lungs (a.k.a. **primary or pulmonary TB**)
- There are 2 TB-related conditions:
  1) Latent TB — no symptoms
  2) Active TB — bacteria defeat the immune system defenses and begin multiplying, causing symptoms

What is Latent TB?
- Infected with *M. tuberculosis*, but bacteria are inactive in the body
- No symptoms
- Not contagious
- Causes positive tuberculin skin test or TB blood test

Screening for Latent TB Infection
- The Mantoux test
  - 0.1 mL of purified protein derivative (PPD) injected intradermally in forearm to form a wheal
  - Test is time sensitive and must be read 48–72 hours after being placed
  - Diameter of the induration (**not the red area**) is measured **perpendicularly** to the long axis of the arm

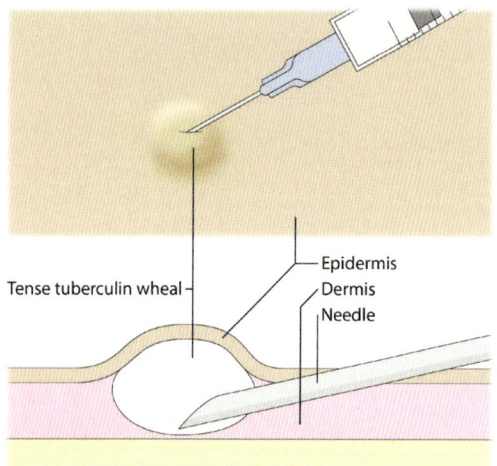

Tense tuberculin wheal — Epidermis / Dermis / Needle

- **CDC** criteria determines positive test and takes into consideration the **clinical suspicion** of LTBI
- PPD is used for asymptomatic patients, not acutely ill patients

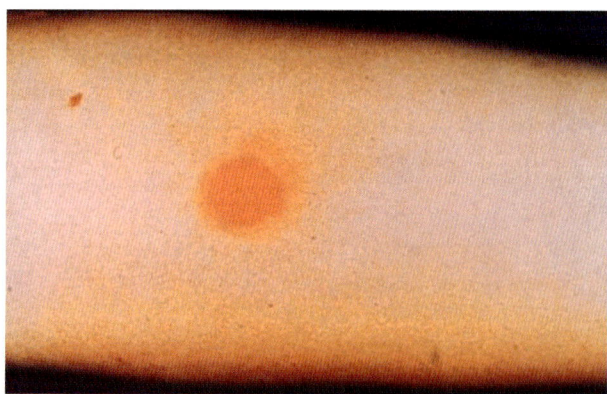

- 5 mm
  - Is positive for those in the high-risk group
    - **HIV** or major cell-mediated dysfunction
    - Fibrotic changes on CXR consistent with prior TB
    - Close contact with a documented case
    - Patients with organ transplant and other immunosuppressed patients
      - Receiving the equivalent of > 15 mg/day of prednisone for 1 month or more
- 15 mm
  - Is positive for the low-risk group
    - No known risk factors
- 10 mm
  - Is positive for those in the moderate-risk group
    - Homeless persons
    - Recent immigrants
      - Within 5 years from high-prevalence countries
    - IV drug users who are HIV negative
    - Incarcerated individuals
    - Health care workers
    - Nursing home patients and staff
    - Chronic kidney disease
    - Hematologic malignancy
    - Immunosuppressive therapy
      - < 15 mg/day prednisone

- Summary
  - Who should be tested in general?
    - Asymptomatic patients who are at risk
  - What is a positive test?
    - > 5 mm
      - HIV, CXR (+), close contacts, severely immunocompromised
    - > 15 mm
      - No risk factors
    - > 10 mm
      - All the rest
- "New converter" and "booster effect"
  - Are terms to discuss patients who are monitored with yearly PPD
- Booster effect
  - Stimulating T cells with bad memory
  - Significant induration on the 2nd test but not the 1st
  - Effect can **persist for several months**, so it becomes difficult to diagnose a "new converter"
- 2-step TB skin test
  - For patients with annual screening on the **1st screening**
  - Help diagnose "new converter" by getting a "**baseline**" with the 2nd step if the 1st is nonreactive
  - The risk of TB reactivation is highest in the first 2 years of a new converter
- What is treatment for a positive test?
  - 9 months of isoniazid (**4 options per CDC**)
- Who should be treated?
  - Everyone (**controversial**)
- What is the risk of developing TB with a positive test?
  - 10% lifetime risk (**5% in the 1st two years**)
  - HIV (+) the risk is 10% per year
  - After INH treatment, the lifetime risk is 1–2%
- What is the effect of previous BCG vaccination on these recommendations?
  - Means nothing (**use γ release assay**)
- When is anergy testing the answer?
  - Never

Anergy Skin Testing
- Persons who do not mount a delayed-type hypersensitivity response are considered to be **anergic**, such as HIV
- The **1991** guidelines recommended the use of companion or "control" antigens in conjunction with PPD testing to provide additional information about a person's ability to mount a DTH response
- If the PPD is (–), and at least 1 antigen from the anergy panel is reactive, this individual's immune system is considered **healthy** enough to mount an immune response

Screening for Latent TB
- 2 IGRAs are approved by the U.S. Food and Drug Administration (FDA) and are available in the U.S.
  1) QuantiFERON-TB Gold In-Tube (QFT-GIT) test
  2) T-SPOT.*TB* (T-SPOT) test

QuantiFERON-TB Gold

- Approved by the FDA in **2005** as a means of diagnosing tuberculosis
- The CDC considers the test to be an alternative to skin testing
- Incubating the patient's blood for 16–24 hours with synthetic peptides representing 2 TB-specific antigens
  - These antigens will stimulate interferon-γ release from the patient's white blood cells, which is then measured by ELISA
  - Results are reported as positive, negative, or **indeterminate**

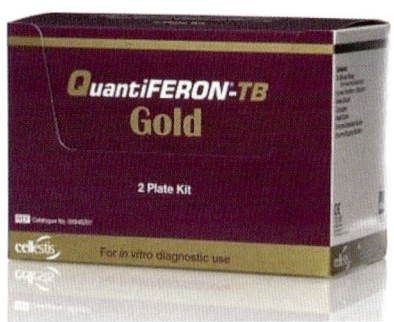

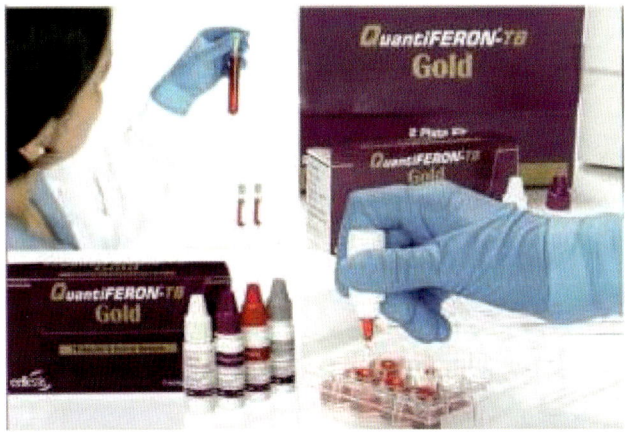

T-SPOT

- FDA approved in **2008**
- The T-SPOT is a unique, single-visit blood test for tuberculosis (TB) screening, also known as an interferon-γ release assay (IGRA)
- The T-SPOT is the only blood test for latent TB that has demonstrated both sensitivity and specificity exceeding **95%**

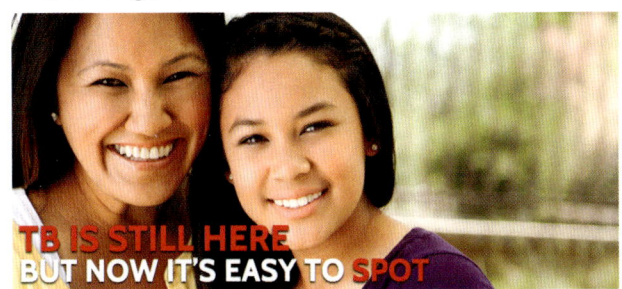

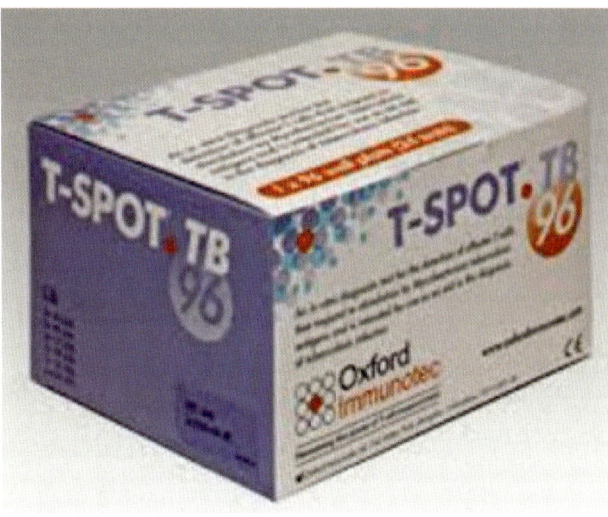

Principles of the TSPOT Assay System

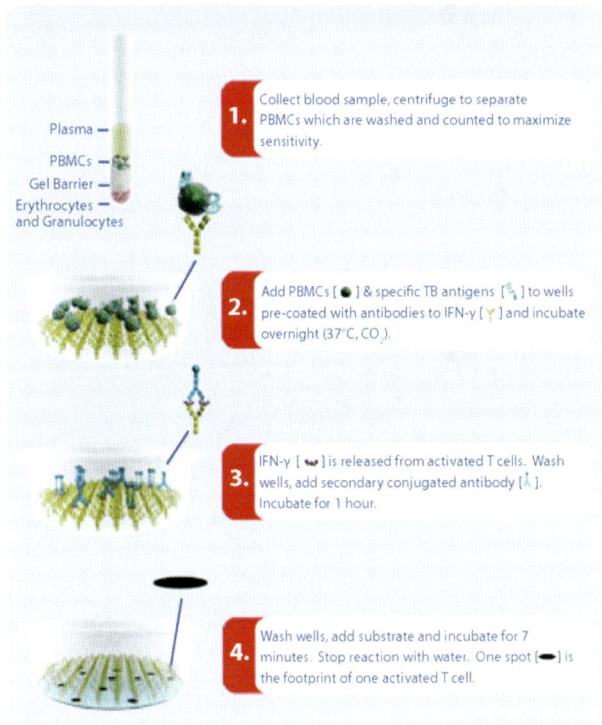

Plasma
PBMCs
Gel Barrier
Erythrocytes and Granulocytes

1. Collect blood sample, centrifuge to separate PBMCs which are washed and counted to maximize sensitivity.

2. Add PBMCs [●] & specific TB antigens [ ] to wells pre-coated with antibodies to IFN-γ [γ] and incubate overnight (37°C, CO_2).

3. IFN-γ [ ] is released from activated T cells. Wash wells, add secondary conjugated antibody [ ]. Incubate for 1 hour.

4. Wash wells, add substrate and incubate for 7 minutes. Stop reaction with water. One spot [ ] is the footprint of one activated T cell.

- Positive > 8 spots
- Negative < 4 spots
- Borderline 5, 6, or 7 spots

Advantages of QuantiFERON-TB Gold and T-SPOT

- The patient does not need to return for a reading
- Results are available within 24 hours
- There is no booster phenomenon
- There is no reader bias (as can affect skin test interpretation)
- The result is not affected by prior BCG vaccination
- Not affected by HIV (anergy)

Latent TB Treatment

- It is essential to rule out **active TB**
- Latent TB treatment to someone with active TB presents a serious risk of developing **drug-resistant** strains of TB
- There are 4 (CDC 2014) treatment regimens:
  1) 9 months of isoniazid is the gold standard (93% effective)
  2) 6 months of isoniazid based on cost effectiveness, patient compliance, and drug toxicity
  3) 4 months of rifampin for those who are unable to take INH or had exposure to INH-resistant TB
  4) 3-month (12-dose) regimen of weekly rifapentine and isoniazid

Latent TB Facts

- It isn't easy to catch TB; you need consistent exposure to the contagious person for a long time; for that reason, you're more likely to catch TB from a relative than a stranger
- It is assumed by most medical doctors that latent tuberculosis is the normal or regular strain of tuberculosis
- There are 3 other types of tuberculosis recognized in the world today:
  1) Multidrug-resistant tuberculosis (**MDR TB**)
     - Resistant to at least INH and rifampin
  2) Extensively drug-resistant tuberculosis (**XDR TB**)
     - INH and rifampin, plus any fluoroquinolone and at least 1 of 3 injectable 2nd line drugs
  3) Totally drug-resistant tuberculosis (**TDR TB**)

Case — History and Physical Exam

- 39-year-old **homeless** man comes to the clinic with a several-month history of a productive cough
- He also reported nightly fevers to **103.1°F (39.5°C)** associated with chills; during the past 6 months, he has had a **20-lb weight loss**
- He is a nonsmoker, and his medical history is significant for a hospitalization 4 months ago; he was lost to follow-up after discharge
- Temp 101.1°F (38.4°C), BP 105/60 mmHg, HR 88 bpm, and RR 20 bpm
- He is thin and unkempt appearing, in no acute distress; He has bitemporal wasting, poor dentition, and multiple **1- to 2-cm mobile cervical lymph nodes**
- Cardiac and pulmonary examinations are normal; examination of his abdomen is benign, and extremities are normal
- **Differential diagnosis**
  - Active TB
  - Lung abscess
  - Bronchiectasis
  - Lung cancer
  - Pneumonia
- **Initial diagnostic plan**
  - Respiratory isolation
  - Sputum for AFB culture, smear, and PCR
    - Induced
    - Bronch with BAL ± TBB
  - CXR/CT
- **Results**
  - Cavitary lesion in the right upper lobe
  - Acid-fast bacilli on smear
  - MTB PCR (+)

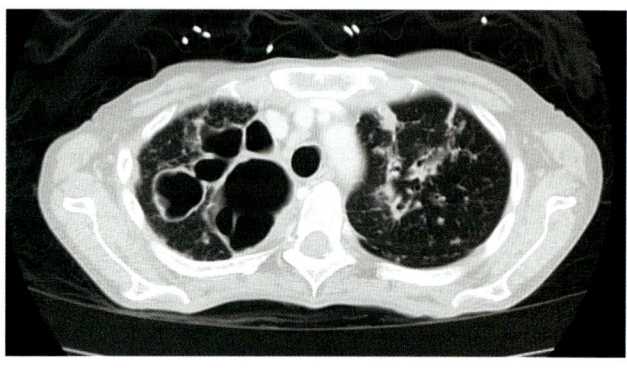

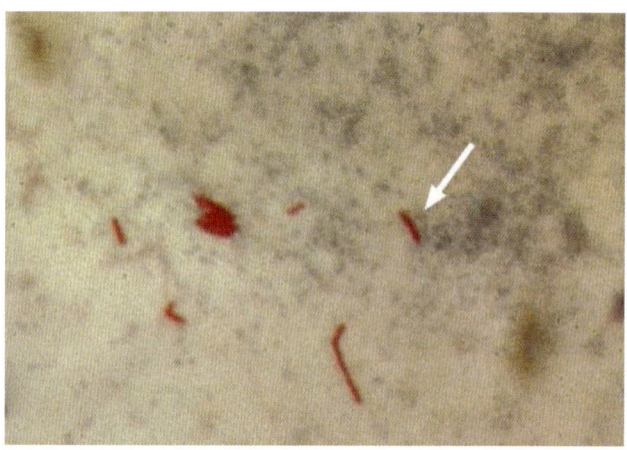

Case — Treatment

- **Suspect the diagnosis**
  - High-risk group
  - Worrisome chest x-ray
  - Consistent symptoms
- **Isolate early**
  - Airborne precautions
    - Negative pressure ventilation room
    - N95 respirator
- **Treatment plan**
  1) Isoniazid (INH) with vitamin B_6
  2) Rifampin
  3) Pyrazinamide
  4) Ethambutol
- Used for the first 2 months; after that, isoniazid and rifampin are continued for 4 months, making it 6-months total

Active Tuberculosis

- **Epidemiology**
  - TB is still a leading cause of death in the world
  - World Health Organization (WHO) estimates that about 1/3 of the world's population is infected
  - The global incidence of active TB is increasing
    - Mainly due to TB associated with HIV infections
- **Sites of TB disease**
  - Lungs (**80–85%**)
  - Pleura
  - CNS
  - Lymphatic system
  - Genitourinary system
  - Bones and joints
  - Peritoneum

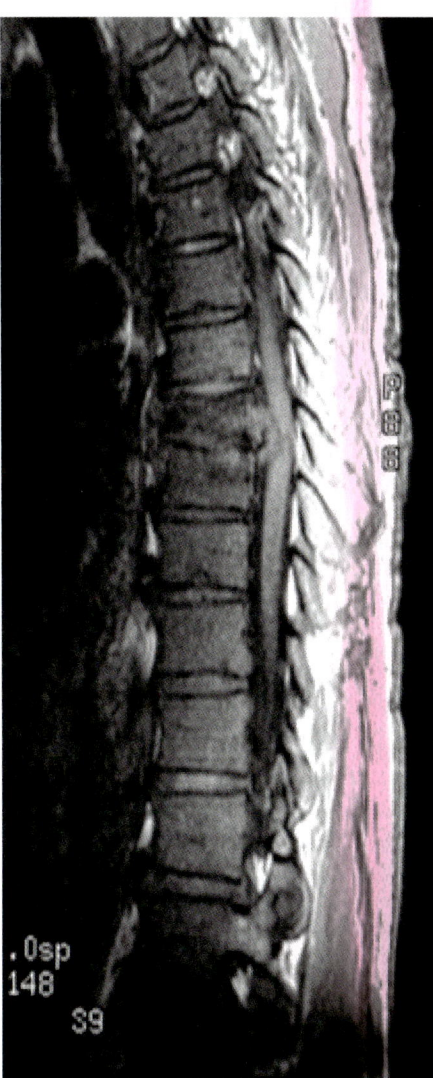

ATS / IDSA Criteria for Diagnosing NTM

Clinical

Pulmonary symptoms, nodular or cavitary opacities on chest radiograph, or a high-resolution computed tomography scan that shows multifocal bronchiectasis with multiple small nodules	+	Appropriate exclusion of other DX

Microbiologic

Positive culture results from at least 2 separate expectorated sputum samples	OR	Positive culture results from at least 1 BAL	OR	Typical biopsy + tissue culture or typical biopsy + positive sputum AFB culture

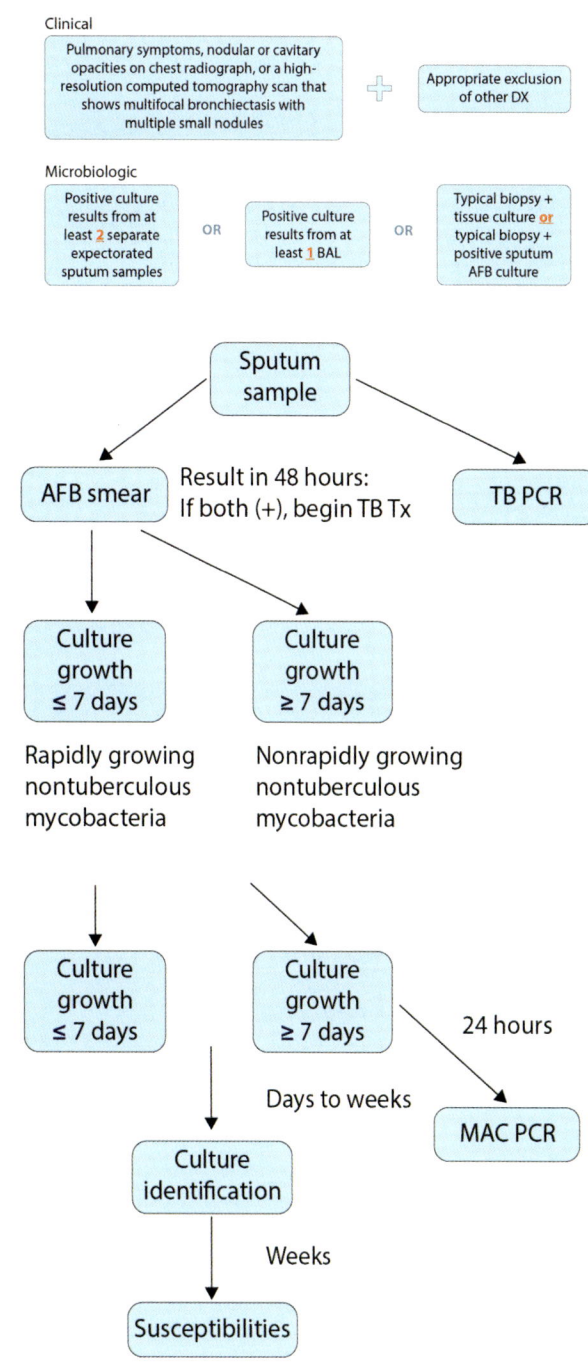

Sputum sample

AFB smear → Result in 48 hours: If both (+), begin TB Tx

TB PCR

Culture growth ≤ 7 days → Rapidly growing nontuberculous mycobacteria

Culture growth ≥ 7 days → Nonrapidly growing nontuberculous mycobacteria

Culture growth ≤ 7 days

Culture growth ≥ 7 days → 24 hours → MAC PCR

Days to weeks

Culture identification

Weeks

Susceptibilities

- **Pulmonary complications of TB include:**
  - Hemoptysis
  - Pneumothorax
  - Bronchiectasis
  - Extensive pulmonary destruction
  - Malignancy
  - Chronic pulmonary aspergillosis

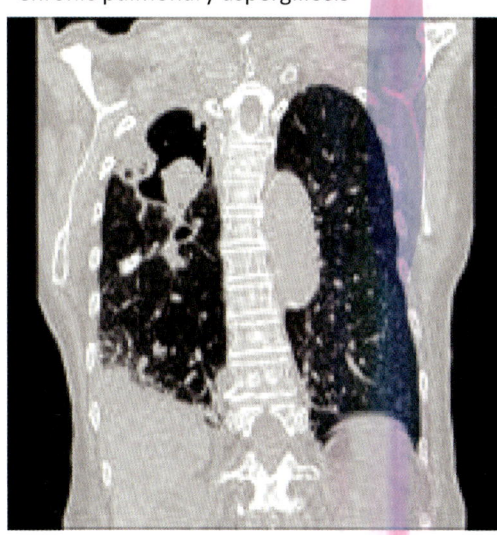

NONTUBERCULOUS MYCOBACTERIA (NTM)
- **Rapidly growing**
  - *M. abscessus*
  - M. chelonae
  - M. fortuitum
- **Nonrapidly growing**
  - **MAC**
  - *M. kansasii*
  - M. malmoense
  - M. xenopi
  - M. szulgai
  - M. simiae

NTM as a pulmonary pathogen in the U.S.
- **Most common**
- **2nd most common**
- **3rd most common**

Why is This Important?
- **Rapidly growing AFB culture**
  - Resistant to antituberculous therapy
  - Mortality up to 20% for severe infections
- **Nonrapidly growing AFB culture**
  - Resistant to conventional antibiotics
  - Many regimens include rifampin or rifabutin

VENOUS THROMBOEMBOLIC DISEASE

Overview of Pulmonary Embolism and DVT
- Most pulmonary emboli are self-limited and resolve quickly
- PE is still the **3rd** most common cardiovascular cause of death
- The incidence has **not** declined
  - Inadequate prophylaxis of hospitalized patients

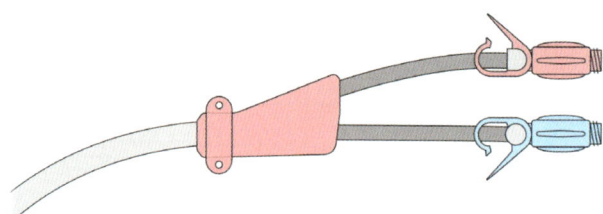

- The majority of emboli are from the lower extremities
  - Virtually all from above the knee
- Newer data demonstrates the significance of **upper extremity** DVT being a more frequent cause of PE than previously expected
  - Internal jugular vein
  - Subclavian vein

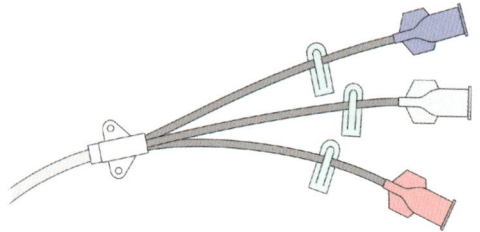

Risk Factors for PE and DVT
- Pregnancy
- Smoking
- Birth control
- Nephrotic syndrome
- Paroxysmal nocturnal hemoglobinuria
- Perioperative
- Virchow triad
  1) Alternations in blood flow
  2) Injury to the vascular endothelium
  3) Hypercoagulability
- Diabetes mellitus
- Age (> 60 years)
- Obesity
- Prolonged immobility
- HF
- IBD
- Rheumatoid arthritis
- COPD
- **Occult cancer**
  - 8% of idiopathic DVT develop cancer in 2 years
  - 17% of recurrent idiopathic DVT associated with malignancy
    - Especially lung and GI
  - Routine screening and exam recommend
    - Not extensive cancer search
- **Coagulation abnormalities**
  - Factor 5 Leiden gene mutation
    - **Not** deficiency
    - Most common inherited hypercoagulable disorder
    - Resistance to activated protein C
  - Protein C and S deficiency
  - Antithrombin (AT) deficiency
  - *G20210A* prothrombin mutation
  - Elevated homocysteine levels
  - Antiphospholipid antibodies
    - Lupus anticoagulant
    - Anticardiolipin
    - β_2-Microglobulin

Overuse of the Hypercoagulable Workup
- **Controversy**
  - Not for 1st episode of unprovoked VTE
  - If thrombophilia is detected in a patient with no history of VTE, anticoagulation is usually not necessary
  - Conversely, patients with recurrent VTE should be anticoagulated even if their workup is negative
- **Indications**
  - Recurrent thromboembolic episodes
  - Thromboembolism at a young age (< 40 years)
  - Family history for thromboembolism
  - Thrombosis in an unusual site

Specific Recommendations for a Hypercoagulable Workup
- Hepatic or portal vein thrombosis should be evaluated for:
  - *JAK2* mutations
  - Paroxysmal nocturnal hemoglobinuria (CD 55 and CD 59)
- Patients with VTE who have a history of warfarin-induced skin necrosis test for **protein C deficiency**
- For arterial thrombosis test for **antiphospholipid syndrome**
- Most of the hypercoagulable tests should be performed **2 weeks** following the discontinuation of anticoagulation

DVT Diagnosis
- **Venography**
  - Nonpractical gold standard
- **D-dimer**
  - Elevated D-dimer nonspecific in chronically ill and hospitalized
  - If pretest probability of DVT is low, DVT can be safely excluded in patients with a normal D-dimer
  - 2 main assays
    1) Latex agglutination (no value)
    2) ELISA

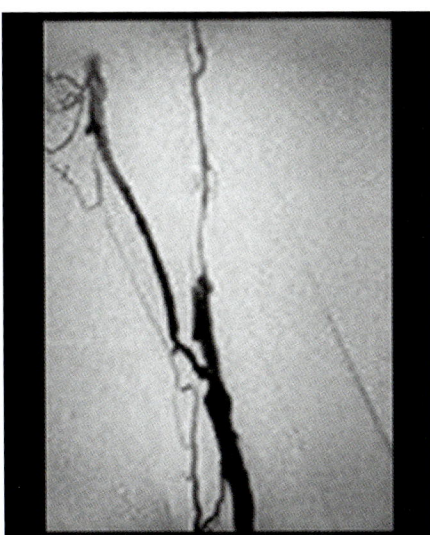

DVT Diagnosis
- **Compression ultrasonography**
  - Has become the procedure of choice
- **MRI**
  - Possible advantage for renal, iliac, and pelvic veins

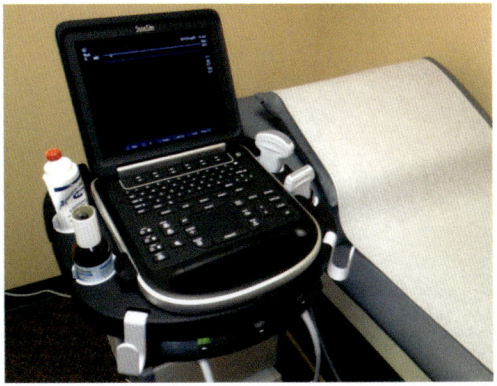

Clinical Question
- Are DVTs more common in the left or right lower extremity?

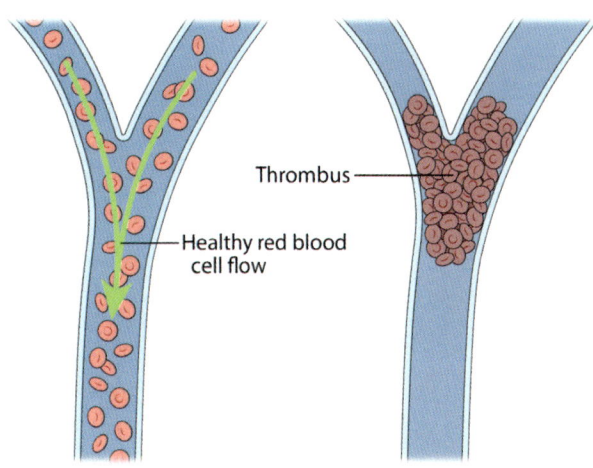

Thrombus

Healthy red blood cell flow

Answer
- **Left**
  - **May-Thurner syndrome**
    - In contrast to the right common iliac vein, which ascends almost vertically to the IVC
    - The left common iliac vein takes a more transverse course
      - Along this course, it underlies the right common iliac artery, which may compress it against the lumbar spine

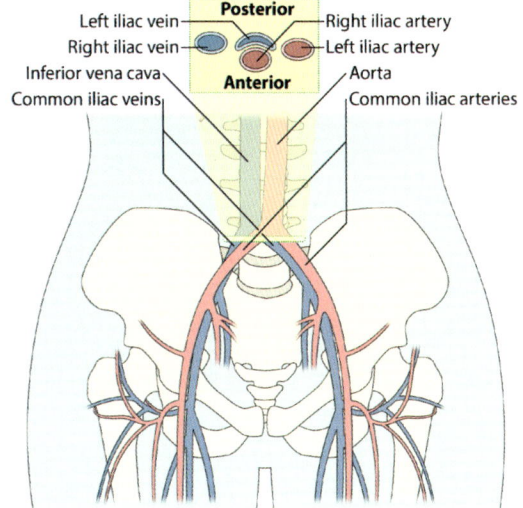

Left iliac vein — **Posterior** — Right iliac artery
Right iliac vein — Left iliac artery
Inferior vena cava — **Anterior** — Aorta
Common iliac veins — Common iliac arteries

Pulmonary Embolism

- There are 10 techniques used in the evaluation of possible PE
  1) ABG
  2) CXR
  3) ECG
  4) V/Q scan
  5) Venous studies
     - Venography
       – Invasive
       – Noninvasive
     - Ultrasonography
  6) D-dimer
  7) Pulmonary angiography
  8) CT angiogram
  9) MRI/MRA
  10) Echocardiography

10

- **ABG**
  – Indicate hypoxia
  – Necessitating further inquiry
  – A-a gradient

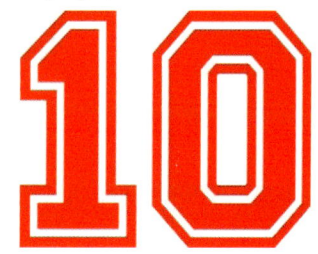

- **Chest x-ray**
  – Helps rule out other causes in the differential
  – "**Hampton hump**"
    - Pleural-based, wedge-shaped defect from infarction just above the diaphragm
  – "**Westermark sign**"
    - It is a lack of vascular markings in the area downstream of the embolus
  – "**Fleischner lines**"
    - Atelectasis
  – Pleural effusions
  – The most common CXR finding in PE
    - Normal (controversial)

Hampton Hump

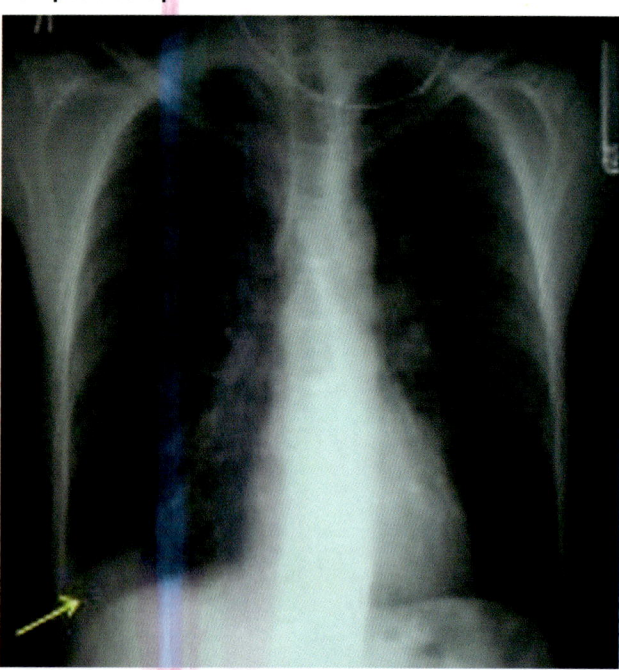

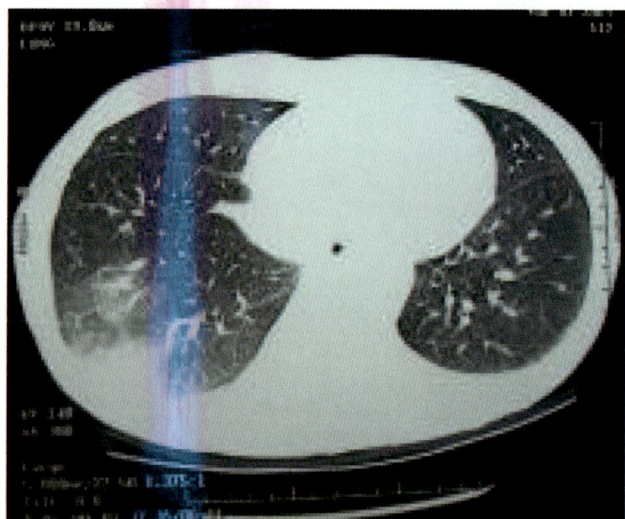

Westermark Sign

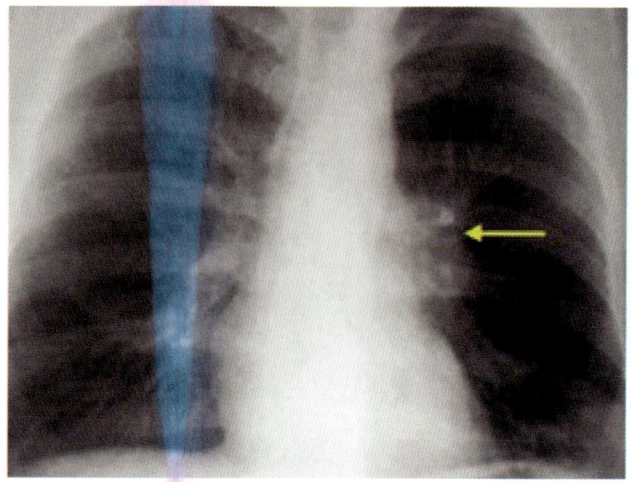

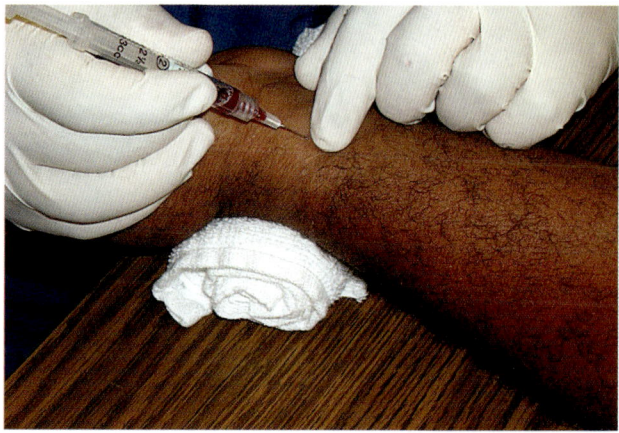

© 2022 MedStudy Internal Medicine Review – Pulmonary Medicine

Pulmonary Embolism

- **ECG**
  - Right-axis deviation
  - S_1, Q_3, T_3
    - Deep S in lead I
    - Q wave in lead III
    - Inverted T wave in lead III
  - Sinus tachycardia is the most common ECG change

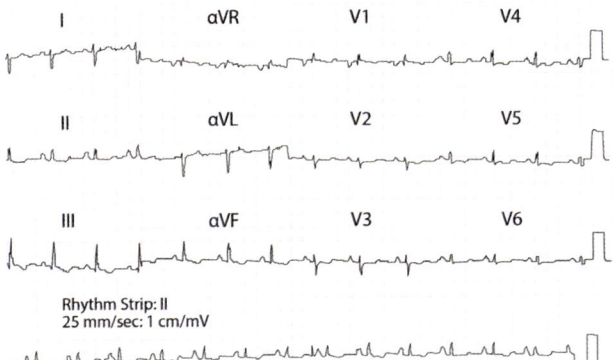

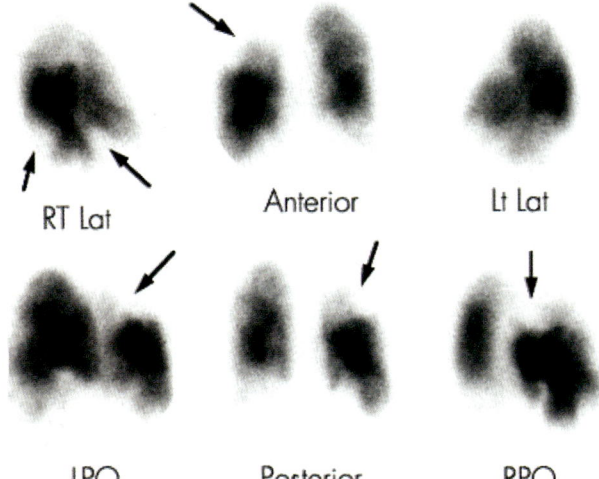

Ventilation/Perfusion Scan

RT Lat   Anterior   Lt Lat

LPO   Posterior   RPO

- **Ventilation/Perfusion lung scan**
  - 2 parts to the V/Q scan
    1) Tagged albumin is injected into the pulmonary circulation
    2) Patient inhales a tagged gas that is distributed into the airways
  - Results
    - Normal
    - Low probability
    - Moderate probability
    - High probability
- **Venous studies**
  - PE and DVT are 2 manifestations of the same disease process
    - Venography
      - Invasive
      - Noninvasive
    - Ultrasonography

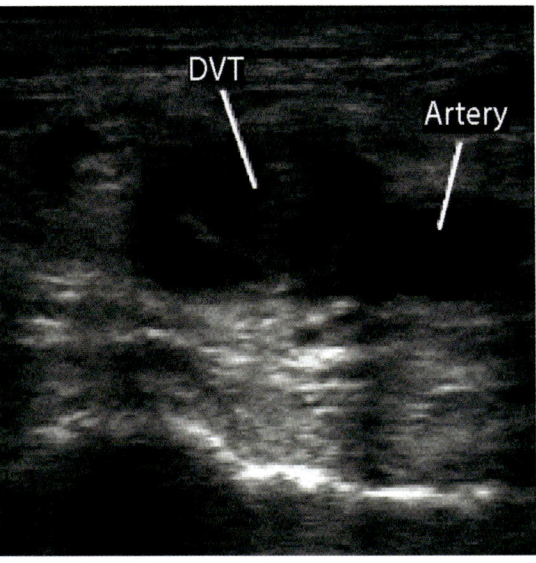

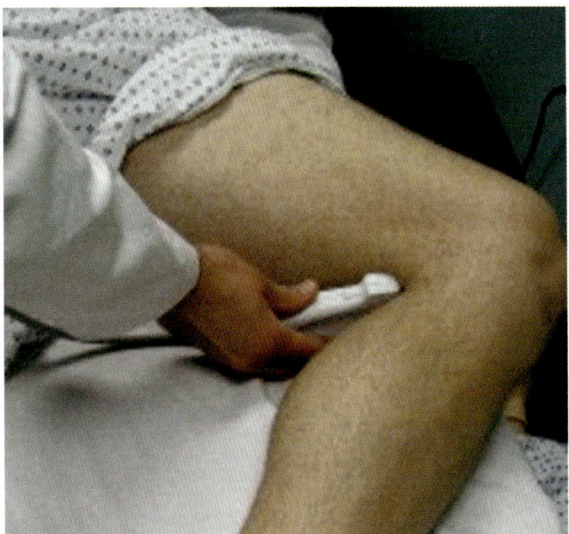

- **CT angiogram**
  - Limited to 4th order vessels
  - Requires contrast
  - Requires a 10- to 20-second breath hold
    - May lead to motion artifact
  - Is almost always used in place of a V/Q scan
- **Question**
  - What study answered the question that a CT scan and **clinical suspicion** are the best combination to diagnose PE?

PIOPED II
- "The Prospective Investigation of Pulmonary Embolism Diagnosis"[6]
  - Patients with suspected PE (n = 773)
  - All got
    - CT scan
    - Lower-extremity ultrasound
    - V/Q
    - Angiogram when diagnosis not made by U/S or V/Q scan
  - CT sensitivity 83%, specificity 96%

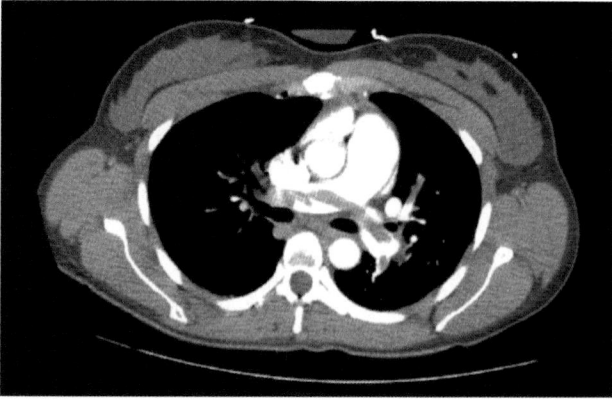

AR 18

Majority of patients with PE identified by CT have negative leg ultrasound.

A. True
B. False

Answer:_____

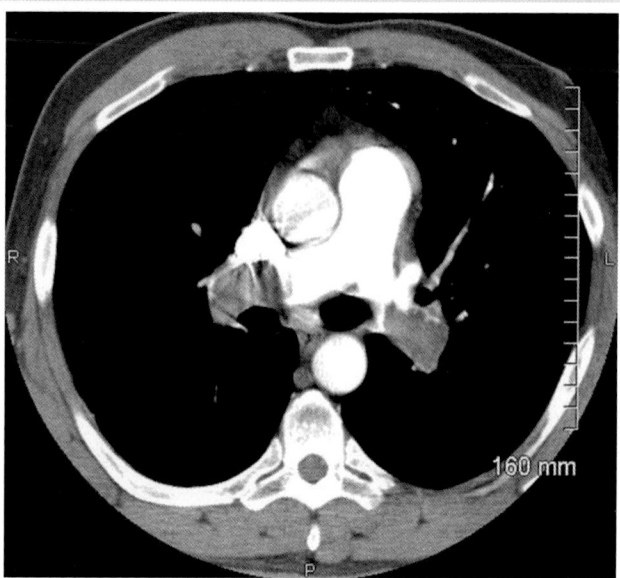

Pulmonary Embolism
- **TTE/TEE**
  - Not indicated for the diagnosis of PE
  - Useful for determining right ventricular strain
  - Evaluate other etiologies for the patient's symptoms

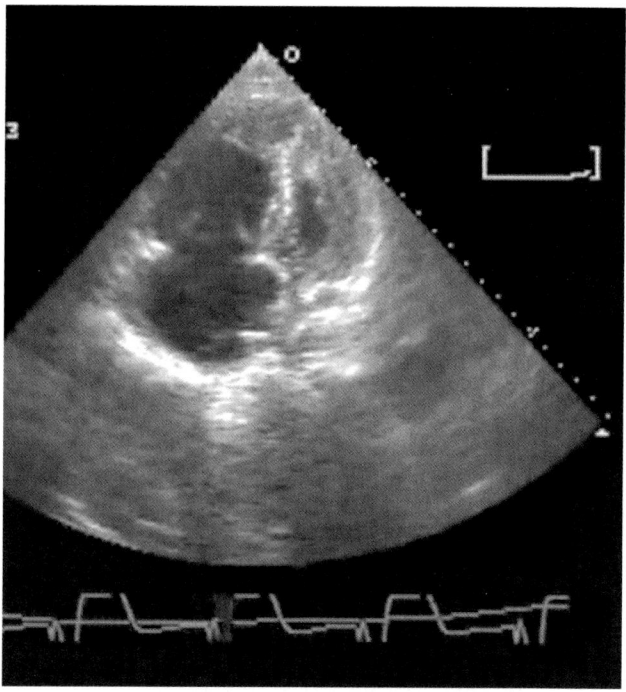

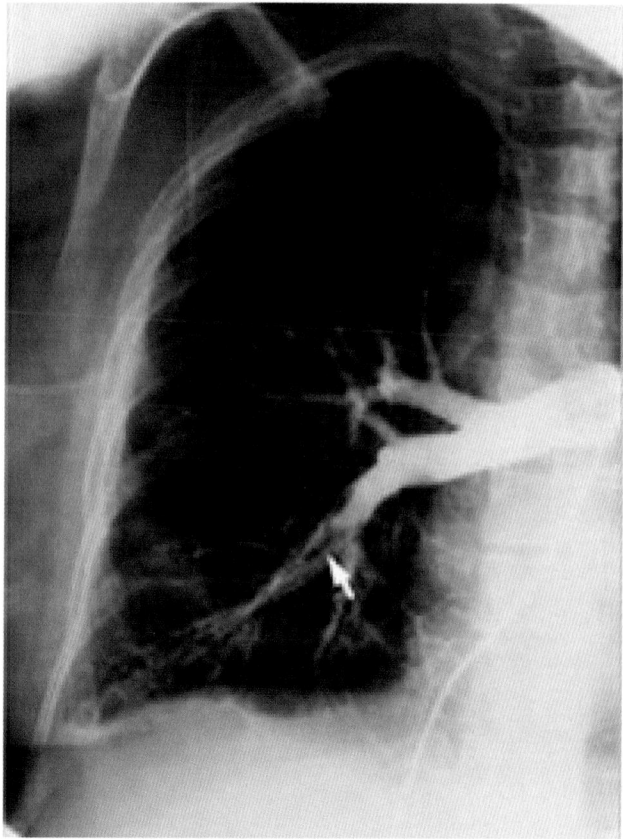

- **Pulmonary angiogram**
  - An invasive test
  - Consider for patients with:
    - High probability of PE but negative workup
    - Chronic thromboembolic pulmonary hypertension

Clinical Question
- Can you treat pulmonary embolism as an outpatient?

Answer: Yes
- **Pulmonary Embolism Severity Index (PESI)**
  - 11 variables
    1) Age
    2) Sex
    3) Cancer
    4) HF
    5) Chronic lung disease
    6) HR > 110 beats/minute
    7) SBP < 100 mmHg
    8) RR > 30 breaths/minute
    9) Temp < 96.8°F (36.0°C)
    10) Altered mental status
    11) S_aO_2 < 90%

AR 19
A 26-year-old man is evaluated in the ED for a 24-hour history of swelling of the left leg and calf. Medical history is unremarkable, but he reports his uncle had a DVT. He takes no meds.

On exam, temp 98.0°F (36.7°C), BP 120/75 mmHg, HR 85 bpm, RR 14 breaths/min. Swelling of the left lower extremity is noted, and dorsiflexion of the foot elicits pain. Doppler ultrasonography confirms acute left lower extremity **DVT** of the **popliteal vein**.

Based on updated American College of Chest Physicians guidelines, which of the following is the most appropriate initial management?

A. Compression stockings
B. Rivaroxaban
C. Tissue plasminogen activator
D. Warfarin

Answer:_____

AR 20
A 28-year-old man is evaluated in the ED for a 24-hour history of swelling of the left lower extremity. Medical history is noncontributory, and he takes no meds.

On exam, temp 97.0°F (36.1°C), BP 120/75 mmHg, HR 80 bpm, and RR 14 bpm. Pulses are intact. He has a swollen left calf that is slightly tender to palpation.

Labs show an activated partial thromboplastin time of 32 seconds, platelet count of 256,000 cells/mm³, and INR of 1.0. Doppler ultrasonography of the left leg shows an acute **DVT** in the left popliteal vein extending to the iliac vein.

The patient expresses significant concern about anticoagulant therapy. An uncle died of a **cerebral hemorrhage** while being treated for acute coronary syndrome.

According to several trials on treatment of venous thromboembolism, which of the following is the most appropriate treatment for this patient?

A. Apixaban
B. Aspirin
C. Clopidogrel
D. LMWH followed by warfarin

Answer:_____

Introduction — Importance of Initial Anticoagulation[7]
- Venous thromboembolism (**VTE**) is comprised of 2 entities: DVT and PE
- VTE has significant morbidity and **mortality** for both the inpatient and outpatient population
- The risk of recurrent thrombosis and embolization is highest in the **1st few days and weeks** following diagnosis
- Thus, initial anticoagulation during the 1st few days (**0–10 days**) is critical in the prevention of recurrence and VTE-related death

Indications for Anticoagulation
- Patients with ultrasound-proven **proximal** DVT
  - Popliteal, femoral, or iliac vein
- Most cases of symptomatic **distal** DVT
  - Below the knee and in the calf veins
- Pulmonary embolism
- For each patient, the decision to anticoagulate must weigh the risk of morbidity and mortality without anticoagulation against the risk of **bleeding** on anticoagulation

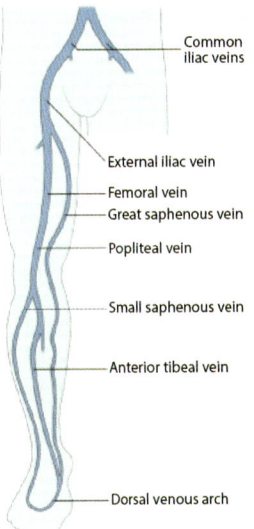

Traditional Treatment of DVT / PE
- **UF heparin** (IV and SubQ) nomogram ± bolus
  - Adjusted by aPTT to 1.5–2 times control
  - HIT
- **LMWH** 1 mg/kg bid or 1.5 mg/kg daily
  - Renal adjustment
    - GFR < 30
  - Studies have shown that patients on LMWH for VTE after **2 weeks** have almost total resolution showing the importance of immediate therapeutic anticoagulation
- **Warfarin**
  - Begin on day 1
  - Overlap by 5 days and INR 2–3
    - Takes 5 days to suppress the activity of the intrinsic pathway
    - Factor **7** shortest half-life

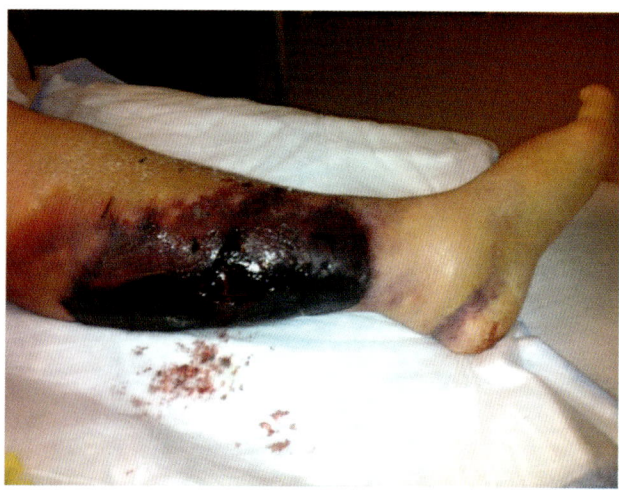

Options for Initial Anticoagulation Include the Following:
1) Unfractionated heparin (UFH)
2) Low-molecular-weight (LMW) heparin
3) Fondaparinux
4) Oral Factor 10a inhibitors

Bleeding Risk
- Tools are available for estimating the risk of bleeding in anticoagulated individuals (**HAS-BLED score**)
- However, none of these tools have been validated in patients anticoagulated for **VTE**
- Many clinicians use a **gestalt** estimate for assessing bleeding risk

HAS-BLED		
Letter	**Clinical Characteristic**	**Points**
H	Hypertension	1
A	Abnormal liver or renal function	1 or 2
S	Stroke	1
B	Bleeding	1
L	Labile INR	1
E	Older patients (age > 65)	1
D	Drugs or alcohol	1 or 2
Maximum Score		9

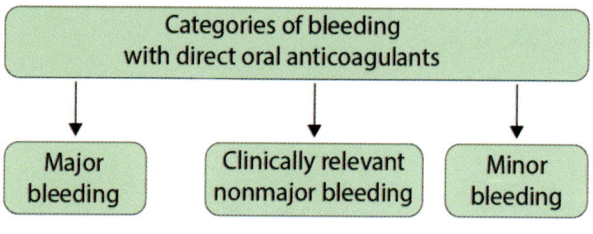

Categories of bleeding with direct oral anticoagulants

Major bleeding
- Hgb drop > 2 g/dL
- Blood transfusion
- Bleeding into a vital organ such as CNS & GI

Clinically relevant nonmajor bleeding
- Does not meet definition of major or minor bleeding

Minor bleeding
- Reported by the patient such as bruising and menorrhagia

Bleeding Risk with Direct Oral Anticoagulant (DOAC) Therapy
- **Intracranial Hemorrhage**
  - All DOACs have decreased risk compared to warfarin
  - Studies are predominantly in atrial fibrillation patients

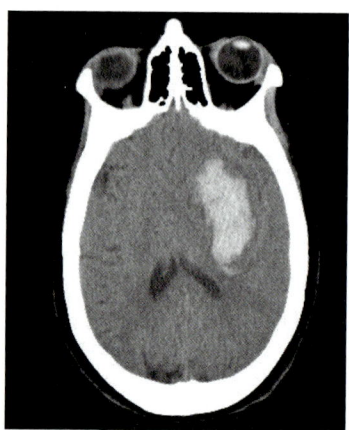

- **GI Bleeding**
  - All DOACs have increased risk compared to warfarin except apixaban
  - Apixaban had the same risk as warfarin
  - Dabigatran has the highest risk of GI bleed

Special Populations — For Initial Anticoagulation
- **Kidney disease**
  - IV UFH is preferred anticoagulant in those with severe renal failure (CrCl < 30 mL/min)
- **Hemodynamic instability and extensive clot burden**
  - IV UFH for extensive DVT or those with massive or submassive PE based upon an anticipated need for a procedural or surgical intervention
  - Direct oral anticoagulants and LMWH have not been adequately tested in this population
- **Anticipated need for discontinuation or reversal**
  - IV UFH has a short half-life and a known reversibility agent (protamine sulfate)
- **Obesity or poor subcutaneous absorption**
  - No preferred agent in patients who are obese or have massive edema; however, therapeutic anticoagulation can be assured with IV UFH
- **Malignancy**
  - LMWH
  - Apixaban
- **Pregnancy**
  - LMWH has a more favorable safety profile, especially when compared with warfarin

IVC Filter for DVT / PE
- IVC filter
  - If anticoagulation contraindicated
  - If recurrence despite adequate anticoagulation
  - Bleeding requires discontinuation of anticoagulation
- There currently is **insufficient data** to compare the safety and efficacy of specific types of IVC filters (retrievable vs. permanent)

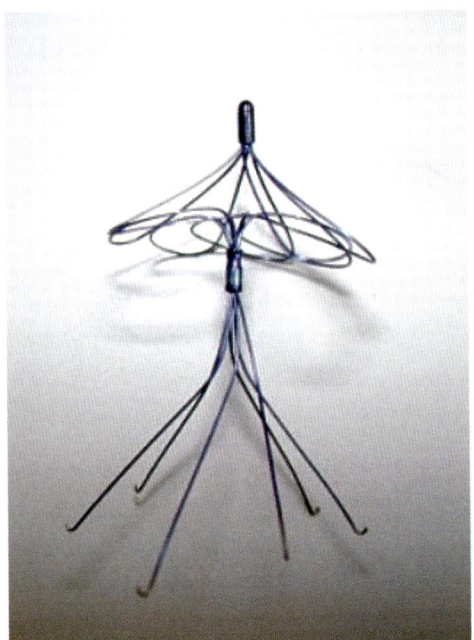

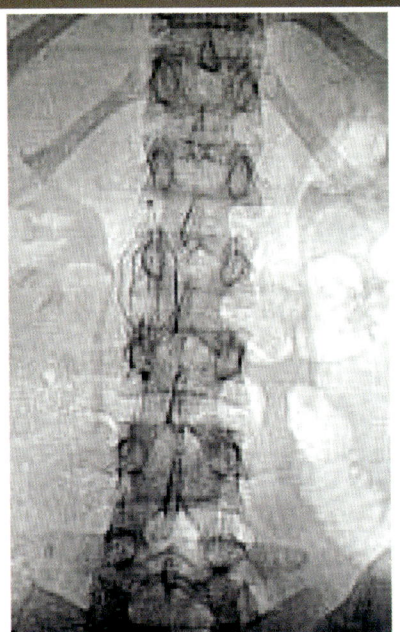

Thrombolytic Therapy for PE

- **Systemic** and **direct catheter**
  - 2 indications (FDA approved)
    1) Persistent hypotension
    2) Persistent severe hypoxemia despite maximization of oxygen therapy
  - tPA (FDA approved)
    - 100 mg as a continuous IV infusion administered over 2 hours
      - Can give a 40 mg bolus
  - Used to treat DVT (direct catheter)
    - Prevent postphlebitis syndrome

Thrombectomy for PE

- **Mechanical thrombectomy**
  - Qualifies for thrombolytic therapy but has contraindications
  - Fails thrombolytic therapy
  - Associated with a high operative mortality rate

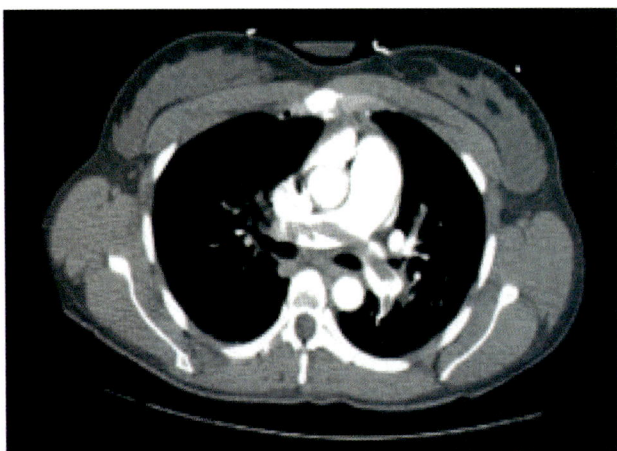

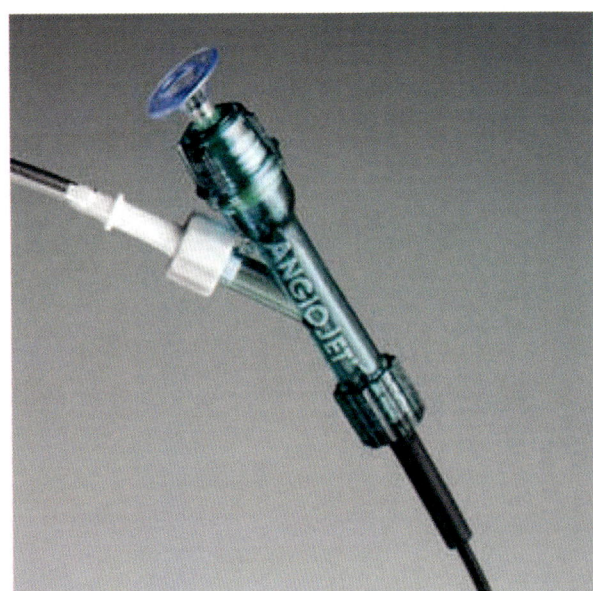

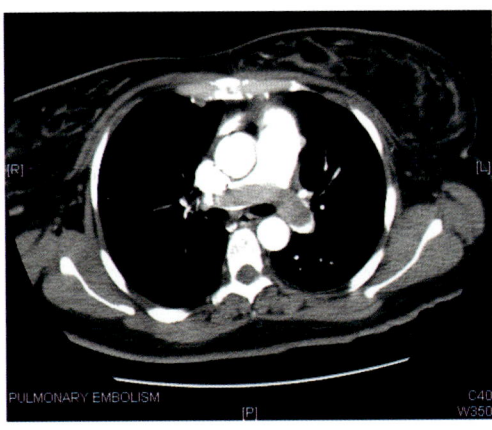

Systemic Thrombolysis of a Massive Pulmonary Embolism

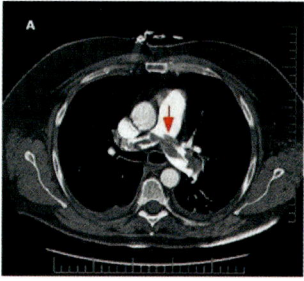 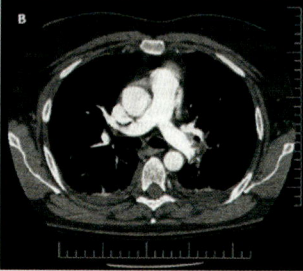

AR 21

Radiology calls you to say the CT scan reveals emboli in the right lower and middle segmental arteries. You begin LMWH and warfarin. The patient asks how long they need to take the warfarin.

You tell the patient ...

A. 3 months
B. 6 months
C. 12 months
D. Indefinitely
E. Not enough information to determine this

Answer:_____

AR 22

A 44-year-old man is evaluated in follow-up for an episode of **unprovoked** left proximal leg DVT 3 months ago. Following initial anticoagulation with LMW heparin, he began treatment with warfarin.

INR testing done every 3 to 4 weeks has shown a stable therapeutic INR. He has mild left leg discomfort after a long day of standing, but it does not limit his activity level.

He tolerates warfarin well. Family history is unremarkable, and he takes no other medications.

On physical exam, VS are normal. He has mild edema of the left leg below the knee, with postthrombotic pigmentation. The remainder of the examination is unremarkable.

Which of the following is the most appropriate management?

A. Continue anticoagulation indefinitely.
B. Discontinue warfarin in another 3 months.
C. Discontinue warfarin now.
D. Discontinue warfarin and perform thrombophilia testing.

Answer:_____

Clinical Question

Does aspirin prevent the recurrence of venous thromboembolism?

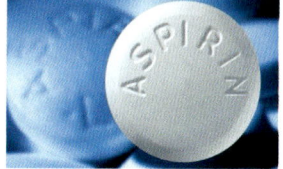

Answer: Yes

- "Aspirin for Preventing the Recurrence of Venous Thromboembolism" *NEJM*, May 30, 2012
  - The risk of recurrence of venous thromboembolism persists for many years after anticoagulant treatment is withdrawn
  - This risk is particularly high among patients with **unprovoked** venous thromboembolism, about **20% of whom have a recurrence within 2 years** after treatment with vitamin K antagonists has been discontinued
  - Extending treatment with these agents reduces the risk of recurrence but is associated with an increased risk of bleeding, as well as the inconvenience and expense of laboratory monitoring and dose adjustments

Prospectively planned combined analysis of the WARFASA and ASPIRE trials reported that aspirin, as compared with placebo, significantly reduced the rate of VTE reoccurrence by 32% with no excess risk of bleeding.

Clinical Question

- Does D-dimer predict the recurrence of an unprovoked venous thromboembolism?

Answer: Yes

- Verhovsek M, et al. Systematic review: D-dimer to predict recurrent disease after stopping anticoagulant therapy for unprovoked venous thromboembolism. *Ann Intern Med*. 2008 Oct 7; 149(7):481–90, W94
- D-dimer is a **fibrin degradation product** (FDP), a small protein fragment present in the blood after a blood clot is degraded by fibrinolysis (the main enzyme is plasmin).

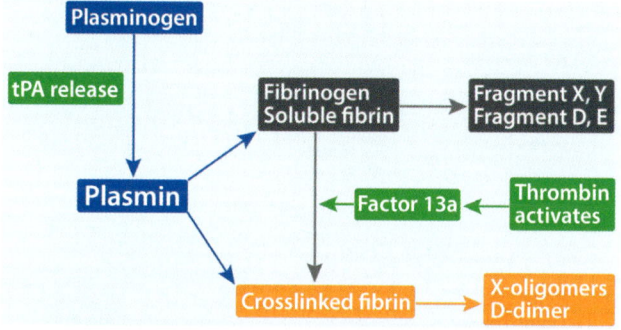

Clinical Question

- Is gender a risk factor for recurrence of an unprovoked venous thromboembolism (VTE)?

Answer: Yes[8]

- The risk for recurrence in patients with a first unprovoked VTE who have **negative D-dimer** results is not low enough to justify stopping anticoagulant therapy in **men** but may be low enough to justify stopping therapy in women
- The risk of recurrent venous thromboembolism is higher among men than women
- Why the women had a low risk of recurrent venous thrombosis is **unknown**

Common Clinical and Exam Questions

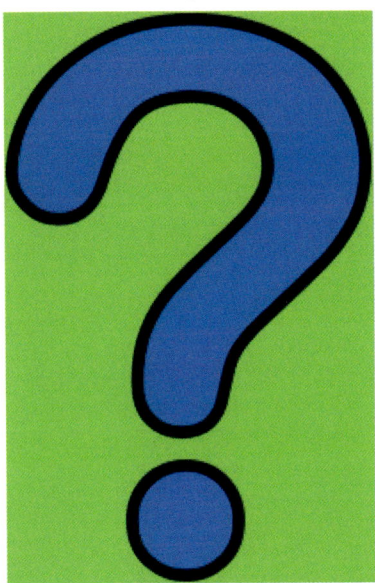

"What about IV Direct Thrombin Inhibitors for DVT and PE?"
- IV direct thrombin inhibitors include:
  - Bivalirudin (Angiomax)
  - Argatroban
- These agents have very short half-lives and specific clinical indications such as:
  - Percutaneous coronary intervention (**PCI**)
  - Heparin-induced thrombocytopenia (**HIT**)

"What Labs Should I Check Before Starting the New Oral Anticoagulants?"
- DOACs are generally administered at fixed doses without lab monitoring
- Lab testing prior to administration of these agents should include:
  - Prothrombin time (**PT**) and activated partial thromboplastin time (**aPTT**), to assess and document coagulation status before anticoagulation
  - Measurement of serum **creatinine**

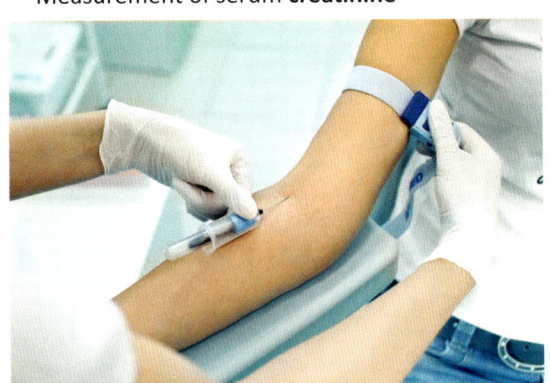

"How Do I Transition to the DOAC?"
- **LMWH**
  - Stop LMWH and wait until **next dose** to start DOAC
- **Warfarin**
  - Stop warfarin and wait until **INR < 2.0**, then start DOAC

Sleep Medicine

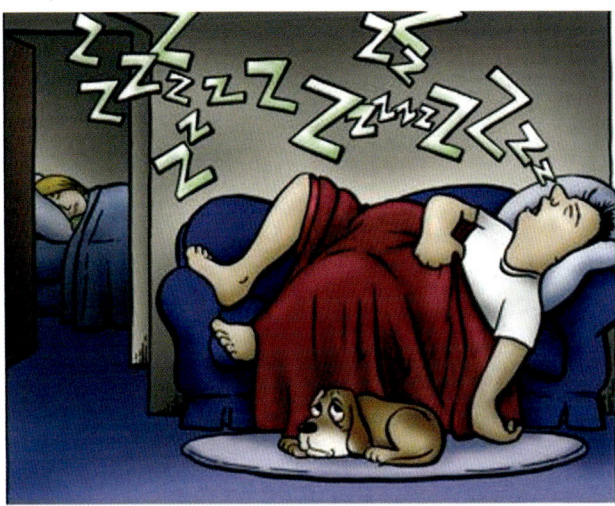

OBSTRUCTIVE SLEEP APNEA-HYPOPNEA SYNDROME (OSAHS)

Sleep Apnea Scoring
- **Obstructive apnea criteria**
  - Cessation of airflow > 90% in the thermal sensor and 10 seconds duration; oxygen desaturation is **not** part of the definition
- **Obstructive hypopnea has 2 main criteria:**
  - 1A scoring (AASM)
    - Cessation of airflow > 30%, 3% decrease in oxygenation from baseline or arousal and lasting 10 seconds
  - 1B scoring (Medicare)
    - Cessation of airflow > 30%, 4% decrease in oxygenation from baseline and lasting 10 seconds
- **RERA (respiratory effort-related arousals)**
  - Last for 10 seconds; the event is not an apnea or hypopnea

Obstructive Sleep Apnea

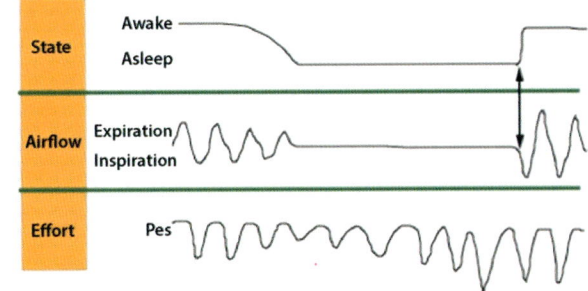

Continuing respiratory effort, as shown by esophageal pressure ("Pes") at the time of cessation of airflow

PULMONARY MEDICINE

Sleep Apnea

- **Previously the best initial test**
  - Overnight pulse oximetry desaturation study
    - Good to evaluate **hypoxemia in patients using PAP**
- **Confirmation test**
  - Polysomnography (gold standard) vs. home sleep study
    - ECG, EEG, EMG, oximeter, tidal CO_2 recorder
    - Split study
    - Differentiates obstructive and central sleep apnea
      - Presence or absence of inspiratory effort during the apneic episodes
    - The frequency of hypoxic apneic episodes determines the severity of the disease
      - Normal < 5/hour
      - Mild 5–15/hour
      - Moderate 15–30/hour
      - Severe > 30/hour
- **Obstructive sleep apnea (OSA)**
  - Is sleep apnea occurring despite continuing ventilatory effort
  - Frequently associated with:
    - Abnormal airway
      - **Neck circumference**
        - » Seems to be the most important determinant of OSA in both men and women
      - Tonsillar hypertrophy or lymphoma
      - Micrognathia
      - Acromegaly
      - Goiter
      - TMJ disease
    - Obesity
      - Not a necessary feature
- **Obesity-hypoventilation syndrome (OHS)**
  - **Not all patients** with OHS have OSA
  - Pickwickian syndrome
    - These patients not only have extreme daytime sleepiness but also have hypoventilation (**high pCO_2**) while awake

Sleep Apnea Treatment

- **Lifestyle modifications**
  - Weight loss
  - Avoiding
    - Alcohol
    - Sedatives
    - Hypnotics
  - Not sleeping in the supine position

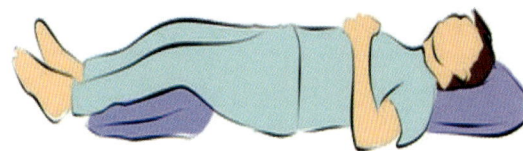

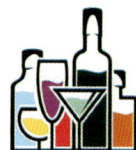

Mainstay Therapy

- **PAP ventilation**
  - **CPAP**
    - Continuous positive airway pressure
  - **BiPAP**
    - Bilevel positive airway pressure

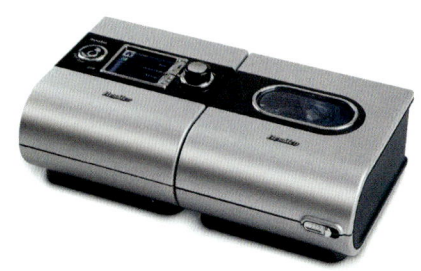

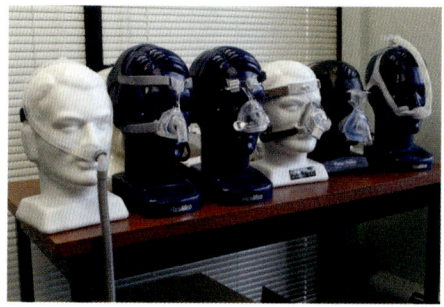

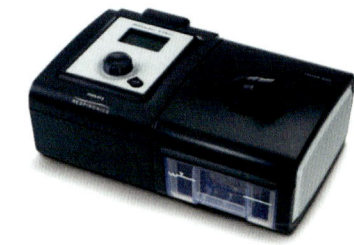

Unfortunately, Not Everyone Tolerates PAP Therapy

- Dental devices
- Provent
- Surgery
- Tracheostomy
- Inspire

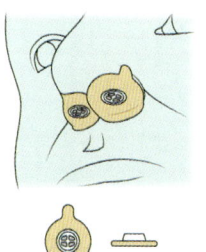
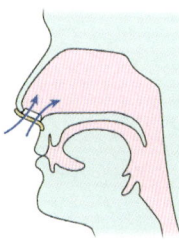
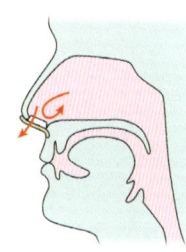

Inspiration   Expiration

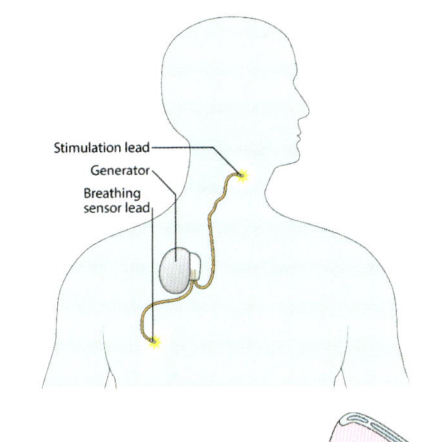

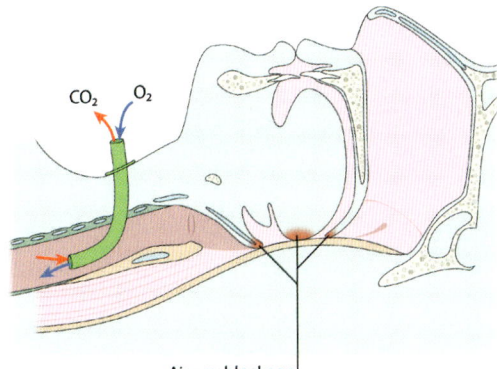

CO$_2$ O$_2$

Airway blockage

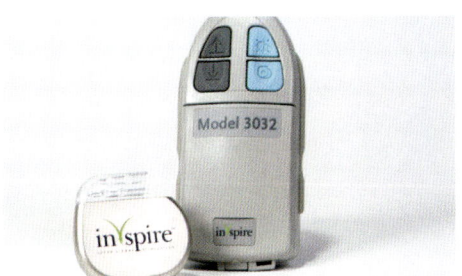

Model 3032

in·spire   in·spire

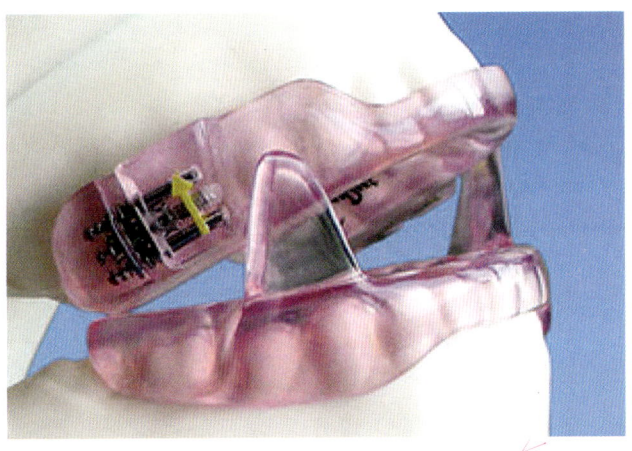

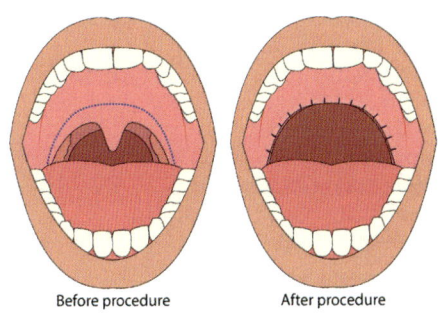

Before procedure   After procedure

CENTRAL SLEEP APNEA SYNDROME (CSAS)

Central Sleep Apnea

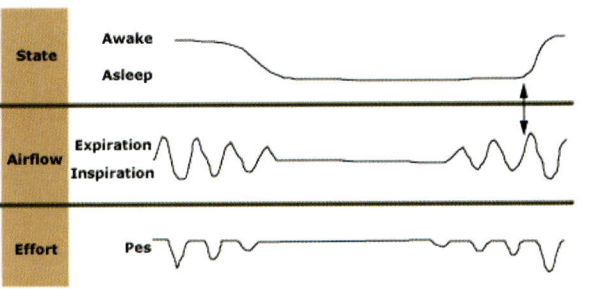

No respiratory effort, as shown by absence of changes in esophageal pressure ("Pes"), at the time of cessation of airflow

Central Sleep Apnea Classification — Hypercapnic
- High **sleep** and **waking** P$_a$CO$_2$
- **Decreased** ventilatory response to hypercapnia
- Causes
  - Neuromuscular disorders
    - ALS, myasthenia gravis, Guillain-Barré, muscular dystrophy
  - Chronic use of long-acting opioids
    - Biot respiration

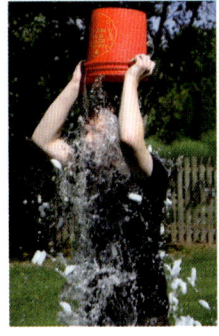

[9]

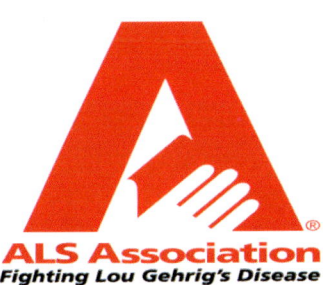

ALS Association
Fighting Lou Gehrig's Disease

Central Sleep Apnea Classification — Nonhypercapnic
- Normal or **low** waking P_aCO_2
- **Increased** ventilator response to hypercapnia
- Causes
  - Primary or idiopathic CSA
  - Sleep-onset CSA
  - Cheyne-Stokes respiration
  - High-altitude periodic breathing
  - Complex sleep apnea

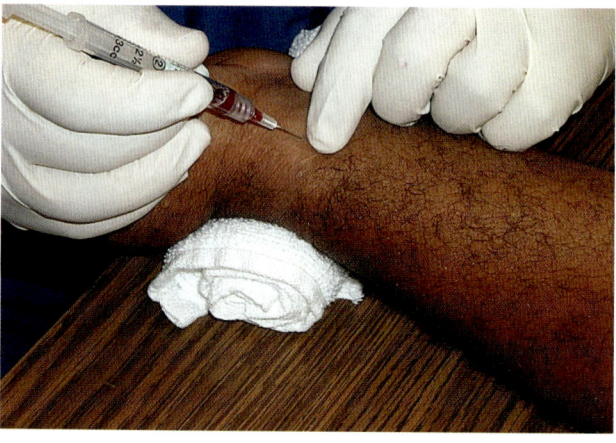

Central Sleep Apnea Treatment[10]
- Treatment is not standardized
- Try different therapies
  - Lifestyle modifications
    - Weight loss
    - Avoid alcohol
  - Supplemental oxygen
    - CPAP for remaining obstructive apneas
    - BiPAP with back up rate
    - Avoid ASV in HF (EF <40%)
  - Medications
    - Acetazolamide (causes a metabolic acidosis)

The Respicardia remedē System is a pacemaker-like implantable device designed to improve cardiovascular health by restoring natural breathing during sleep in patients with central sleep apnea.

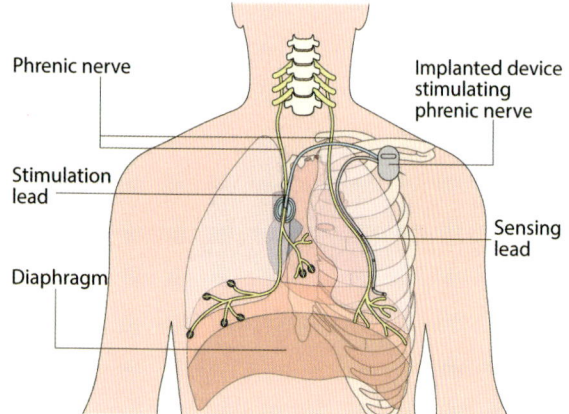

Phrenic nerve

Implanted device stimulating phrenic nerve

Stimulation lead

Sensing lead

Diaphragm

Central Sleep Apnea
- Congenital central alveolar hypoventilation syndrome (Ondine curse)
  - Failure of autonomic control of breathing
  - Diminished responsiveness to O_2 and CO_2
  - Onset in infancy
  - Many cases involve mutations in **PHOX2B** gene

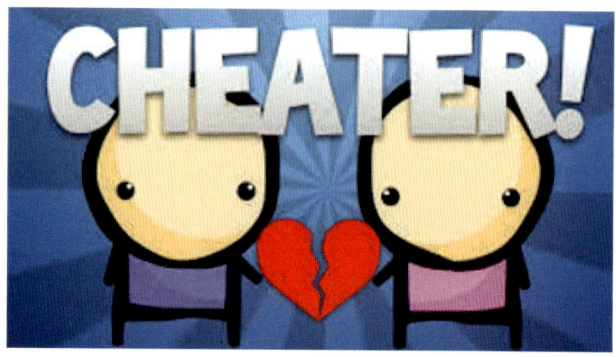

CRITICAL CARE

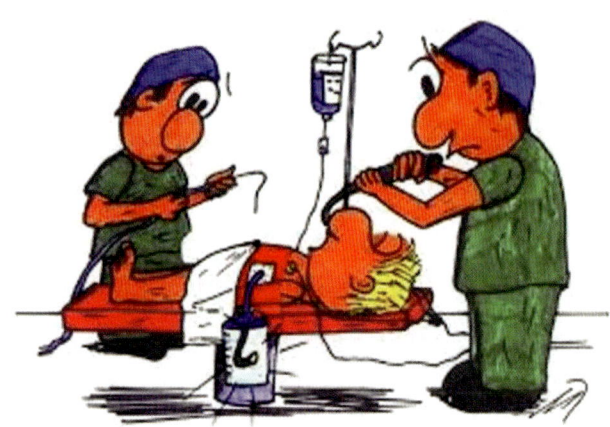

ACUTE RESPIRATORY DISTRESS SYNDROME (ARDS)
- **Classic definition (American-European Consensus Conference's definition 1994)**
  1) Ratio of $P_aO_2/F_iO_2 < 200$
  2) Acute bilateral pulmonary infiltrates
  3) PCWP < 18 mmHg
     - Measured by Swan-Ganz catheter or no clinical evidence of left-heart failure

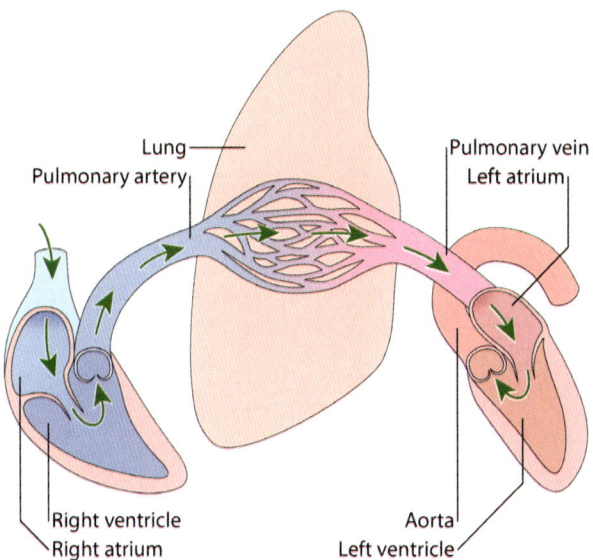

- **Direct causes**
  - Aspiration
  - Pneumonia
  - Inhalation injuries
- **Indirect causes**
  - Sepsis
  - Pancreatitis
  - TRALI
  - Trauma
- **Grouped together under the term ARDS due to similarities of**:
  - Clinical
  - Physiological
  - Pathological
  - Management

Berlin Definition of ARDS 2012

- The Berlin Definition of ARDS requires that **all of the following** criteria be present to diagnose ARDS:
  - Symptoms must have begun within 1 week of a known clinical insult
  - Bilateral opacities consistent with pulmonary edema must be present on CXR or CT
  - Respiratory failure must not be explained by cardiac failure or fluid overload
- The severity of the hypoxemia defines the severity of the ARDS
  - **Mild ARDS**
    - P_aO_2/F_iO_2 is > 200 mmHg, but ≤ 300 mmHg, on ventilator settings that include PEEP ≥ 5
  - **Moderate ARDS**
    - P_aO_2/F_iO_2 is > 100 mmHg, but ≤ 200 mmHg, on ventilator settings that include PEEP ≥ 5
  - **Severe ARDS**
    - P_aO_2/F_iO_2 is ≤ 100 mmHg on ventilator settings that include PEEP ≥ 5

ARDS

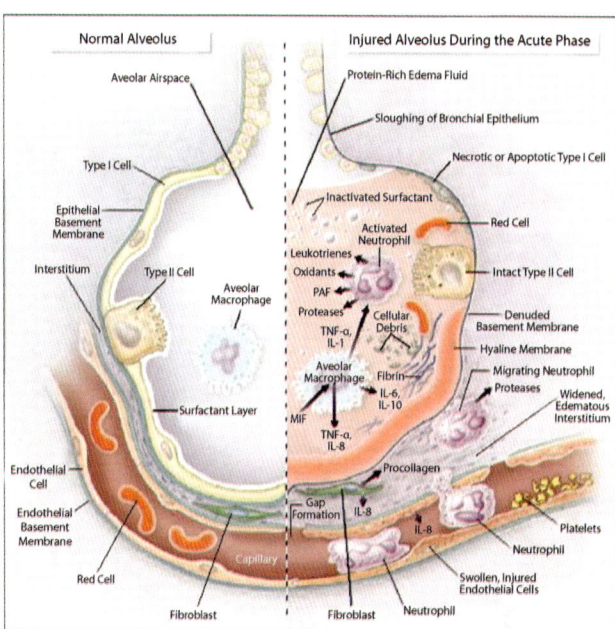

- **Overview**
  - ARDS is characterized by increased permeability of the alveolar-capillary membrane
    - Causes pulmonary edema
    - Leads to severe hypoxemia
    - Decreases pulmonary compliance
  - It is unknown what factors cause the leaky lungs
  - There is a 24- to 72-hour lag time between injury and ARDS
  - There is no prophylactic treatment for ARDS

ARDS Physiology

- Healthy lungs regulate the movement of fluid to maintain a small amount of interstitial fluid and dry alveoli
- This is interrupted by lung injury, causing excess fluid in both the **interstitium** and **alveoli**
- Consequences include impaired gas exchange, decreased compliance, and increased pulmonary arterial pressure

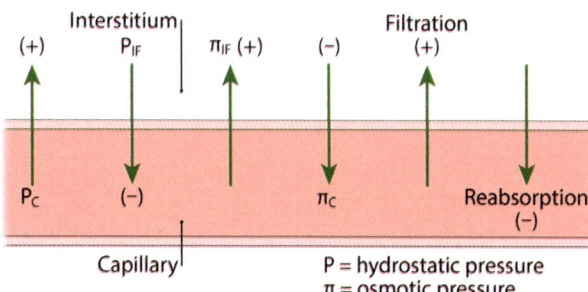

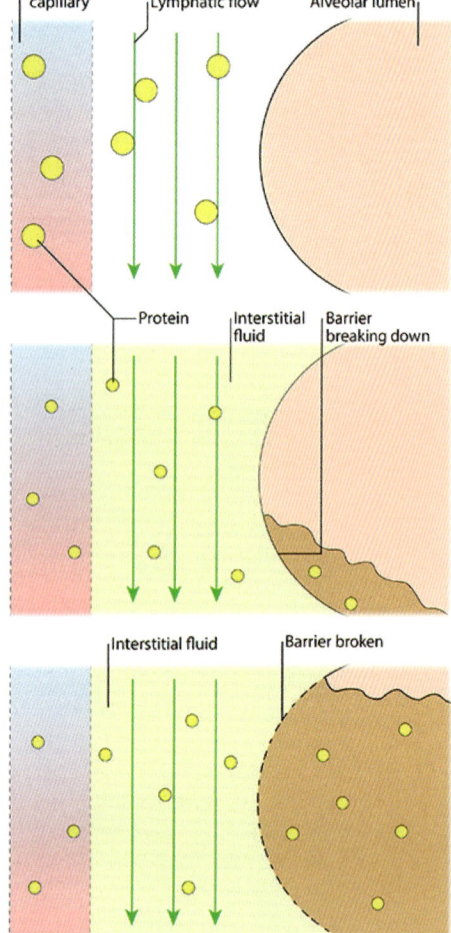

ARDS Treatment

- Treat the causative condition
  - If a patient has an abscess, push surgeons to remove it or IR to drain it
  - Give empiric antibiotics if **sepsis** is thought to be the cause
- Optimize cardiopulmonary support
  - Maintain adequate cardiac output
  - Prevent worsening lactic acidosis
- Nutrition
  - Should be enteral rather than parenteral
- Medications
  - Glucocorticoids
    - Trials are ongoing

Efficacy and Safety of Corticosteroids for Persistent ARDS[11]

- **Conclusions**
  - These results do not support the routine use of methylprednisolone for persistent ARDS despite the improvement in cardiopulmonary physiology
  - In addition, starting methylprednisolone therapy more than **2 weeks after** the onset of ARDS may increase the risk of death

Methylprednisolone Infusion in Early Severe ARDS[12]

- **Objective**
  - To determine the effects of low-dose prolonged methylprednisolone infusion on lung function in patients with **early** severe ARDS
  - Methylprednisolone infusion (1 mg/kg/day) vs. placebo
- **Conclusion**
  - Reduction in duration of mechanical ventilation and ICU length of stay

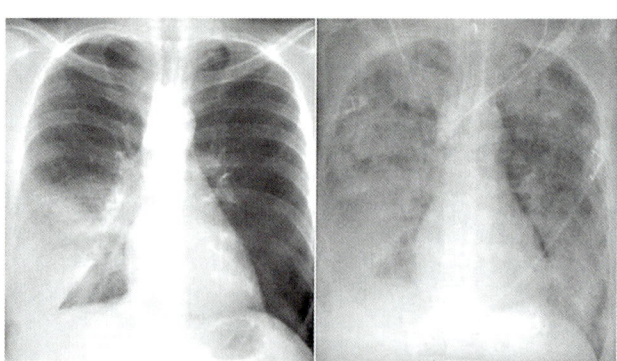

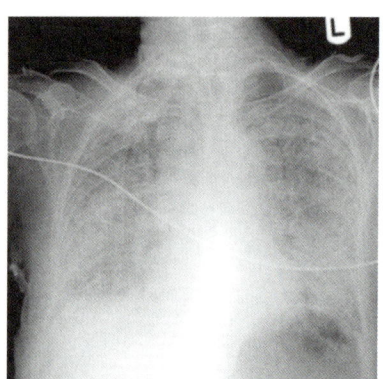

ARDS Stages

1	Exudative Stage: Characterized by accumulation in the alveoli of excessive fluid, protein, and inflammatory cells that have entered the air spaces from the alveolar capillaries. The exudative phase unfolds over the first 2–4 days after onset of lung injury.
2	Fibroproliferative (or Proliferative) Stage: Connective tissue and other structural elements in the lungs proliferate in response to the initial injury. Under a microscope, lung tissue appears densely cellular. Also at this stage, there is a danger of pneumonia sepsis and rupture of the lungs causing leakage of air into surrounding areas.
3	Resolution and Recovery: During this stage, the lung reorganizes and recovers. Lung function may continue to improve for as long as 6–12 months and sometimes longer, depending on the precipitating condition and severity of the injury. It is important to remember that there may be (and often are) different levels of pulmonary recovery among individuals who suffer from ARDS.

Patients with ARDS tend to progress through 3 relatively discrete pathologic stages: the **exudative** stage, the **proliferative** stage, and the **fibrotic** stage.

ARDS Ventilator Management
- **ARDS is that it has shunt physiology**
  - The only way to improve oxygenation is to recruit, or "pop open" some of the fluid-filled alveoli
  - To "pop open" alveolar unit use PEEP
- **Low tidal volumes**
  - 6–8 mL/kg is considered optimal
- **Permissive hypercapnia**
  - Low tidal volumes result in an elevated P_aCO_2
- **Positioning**
  - Lateral decubitus position is usually tried first

AR 23

A 63-year-old woman is admitted to the hospital for septic shock secondary to CAP. After antibiotics, fluids, and vasopressors, her condition stabilizes. However, she subsequently develops ARDS and is intubated. Her O_2 requirement increases until she is receiving 100% O_2. Vent settings are in the volume-controlled continuous mandatory ventilation mode with RR **22 breaths/min**, TV **330 mL** (6 mL/kg of ideal body weight), F_iO_2 **100%**, and PEEP **5**. Peak pressure of 25 cm H_2O, and a plateau pressure of 22 cm H_2O and a plateau pressure of 22 cm H_2O.

On exam, Temp 100.4°F (38.0°C), BP 115/60 mmHg, HR 105 beats/min, and RR 22 breaths/min. The skin is cool. There is no JVD. Heart sounds are rapid and regular but otherwise unremarkable. Diffuse crackles are heard on pulmonary exam. There is no edema. The remainder of the physical exam is noncontributory.

ABG show a pH **7.31**, P_aCO_2 **50 mmHg**, and P_aO_2 of **54 mmHg**. CXR shows extensive patchy areas of opacification of the lung fields.

Which of the following is the most appropriate management?

A. Decrease the TV.
B. Implement a prone positioning maneuver.
C. Start inhaled NO.
D. Decrease the RR.
E. Increase the PEEP.

Answer:_____

AR 24

A patient with ARDS is on the ventilator with the settings of 12 mL/kg for the patient's tidal volume. This was switched appropriately to ARDSNet protocol of 6 mL/kg to improve survival.

What physiologic changes would you expect?

A. Increased compliance and oxygenation
B. Decreased compliance and oxygenation
C. No change in compliance and oxygenation
D. Decreased compliance and increased oxygenation
E. Increased compliance and decreased oxygenation

Answer:_____

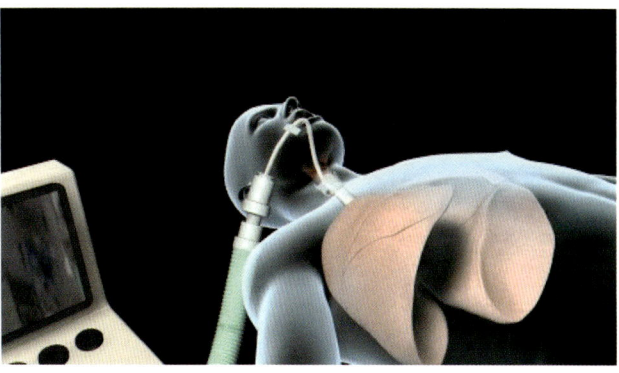

Advanced ARDS Management
- **ECMO (extracorporeal membrane oxygenation)**
  - VV or VA (for hemodynamic support)
- **High-frequency ventilation**
  - Combines a very high respiratory rate, very low tidal volumes (smaller than anatomical dead space) and high mean airway pressure (PEEP)
  - May increase in-hospital mortality
- **APRV** (airway pressure release ventilation)
- **Prone position**
- **Paralytics: careful of critical illness neuropathy/myopathy**

Paralytics in ARDS
- In patients with severe ARDS, early administration of a neuromuscular blocking agent improved the adjusted **90-day survival** and increased the time off the ventilator without increasing muscle weakness
  - However, follow up studies from 2019 show no benefit

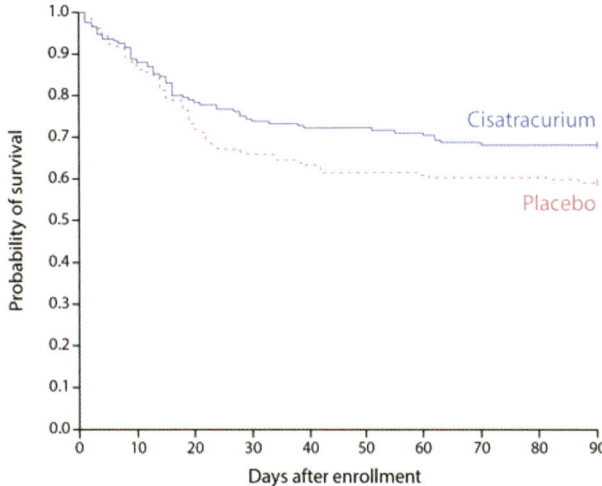

Probability of survival through day 90, according to study group.

[13]

Question

- Does prone position ventilation decrease mortality in ARDS?

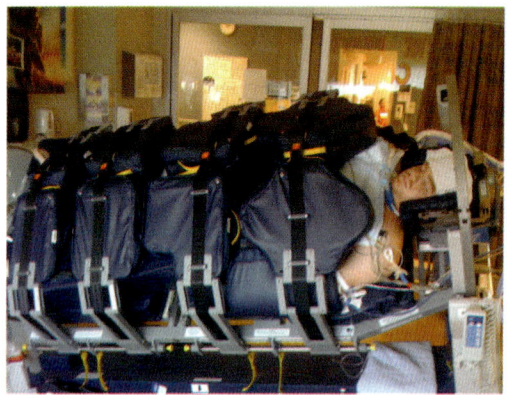

Answer

- **Yes**
  - "Prone Positioning in Severe Acute Respiratory Distress Syndrome" (*NEJM*, May 20, 2013)
    - Prospective, multicenter, randomized, controlled trial to explore
    - Showed that patients with ARDS and severe hypoxemia (as confirmed by a P_aO_2:F_iO_2 ratio of < 150 mmHg, with an F_iO_2 of ≥ 0.6 and a PEEP of ≥ 5 cm of water) can benefit from prone treatment when it is used early and in relatively long sessions

ARDS Ventilator Settings

- No ventilator mode has **proven better** than another for ARDS
- Commonly recommend initial setting
  - Assist-control, volume-cycled
  - F_iO_2 = 100%
    - Lower to < 60% ASAP
  - Tidal volume = 6–8 mL/kg
  - Inspiratory flow = 60 L/min
  - PEEP = start at 5 cm H_2O
    - Usually goes up to 10–20 cm H_2O
    - Titrate to **plateau pressure** ≤ 30 cm H_2O

Peak and Plateau Pressures

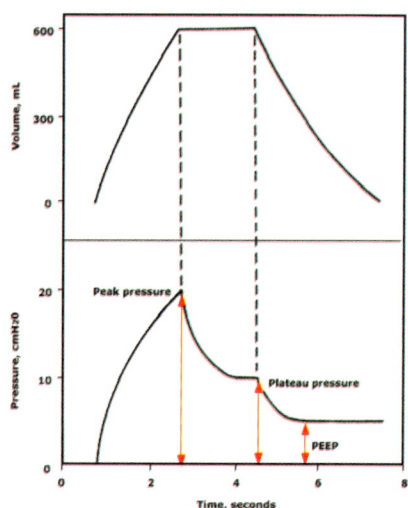

If peak pressures are increasing:

- Check plateau pressures by allowing for an **inspiratory pause**
- If peak pressures are high and plateau pressures are low, then you have an **obstruction**
- If both peak pressures and plateau pressures are high, then you have a lung **compliance** issue

High Peak Pressures Low Plateau Pressures	High Peak Pressures High Plateau Pressures
Mucus plug	ARDS
Bronchospasm	Pulmonary edema
ET tube blockage	Pneumothorax
Biting	ET tube migration to a single bronchus
	Effusion

SHOCK STATES

Evaluation of Shock in the MICU

What Tubes and Lines are Seen in this CXR?

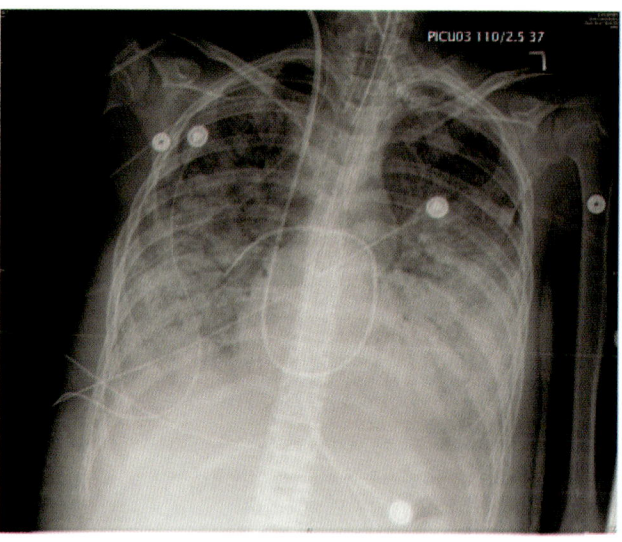

Basics of Shock Evaluation

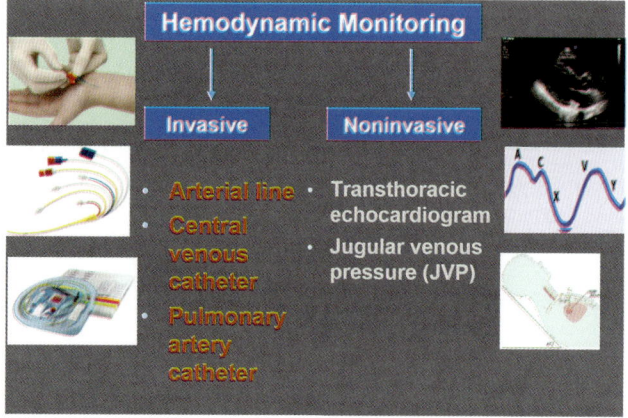

- The goal of hemodynamic monitoring is to maintain adequate **tissue perfusion ($S_{cv}O_2$)**
  1) Oxygen delivery: CO + Hgb
  2) Oxygen consumption

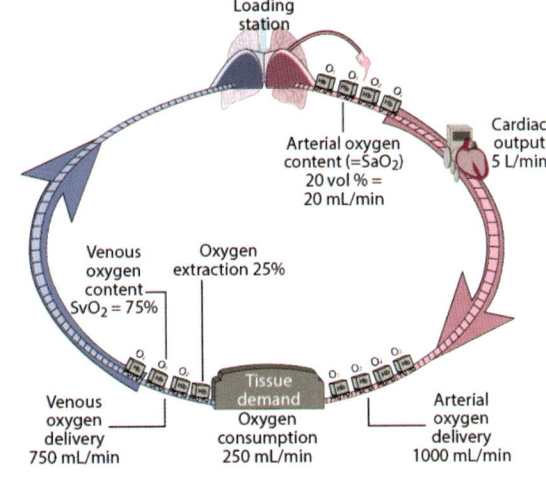

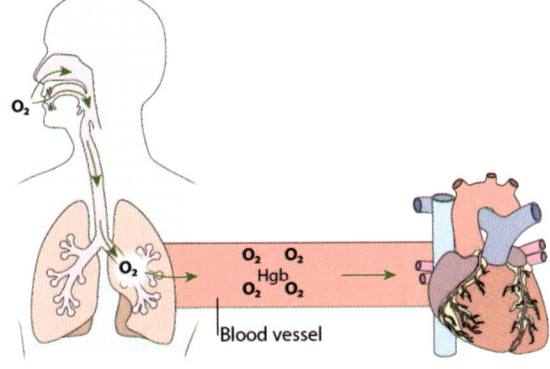

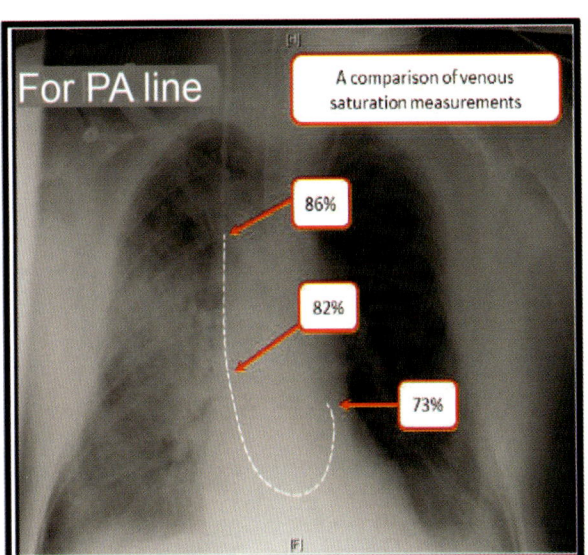

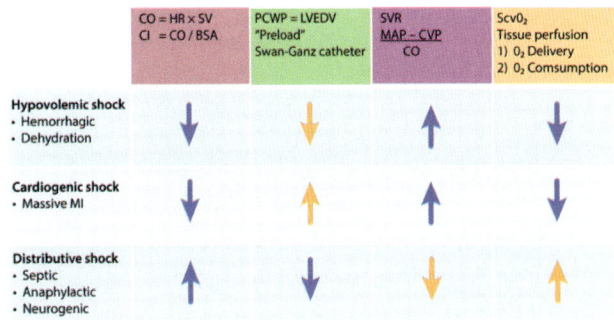

CO = HR × SV\nCI = CO / BSA	PCWP = LVEDV\n"Preload"\nSwan-Ganz catheter	SVR\nMAP – CVP\nCO	ScvO$_2$\nTissue perfusion\n1) O$_2$ Delivery\n2) O$_2$ Comsumption
Hypovolemic shock\n• Hemorrhagic\n• Dehydration	↓	↓	↑	↓
Cardiogenic shock\n• Massive MI	↓	↑	↑	↓
Distributive shock\n• Septic\n• Anaphylactic\n• Neurogenic	↑	↓	↓	↑

Practice Questions

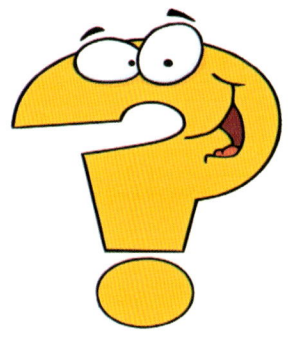

AR 25
What is the diagnosis of a patient with the following hemodynamic profile on Swan-Ganz monitoring?

CO: 3.4 L/min (normal 5–6)

PCWP: 6 mmHg (normal 8–12)

SVR: 2,500 dynes (normal 700–1,600)

A. Distributive shock, secondary to anaphylaxis
B. Hypovolemic shock
C. Cardiogenic shock

Answer:_____

AR 26
A 68-year-old male presents to the hospital with increasing shortness of breath, orthopnea, PND, and palpitations. He has a long history of recurrent HF.

Physical exam reveals bi-basilar rales, and he is hypotensive with BP 70/40 mmHg.

Swan-Ganz reveals the following:

Cardiac index 1.4 (normal 2.6–4.2)

PCWP 34 mmHg (normal 8–12)

SVR 2,400 dynes (normal 700–1,600)

AR 26A
What is the diagnosis?

A. Cardiogenic shock from left heart failure
B. Hypovolemic shock from blood loss
C. Distributive shock secondary to sepsis

Answer:_____

AR 26B

In the previous patient, what is the preferred drug of choice for this type of shock?

A. Norepinephrine
B. Dopamine
C. Dobutamine
D. Phenylephrine
E. Vasopressin

Answer:_____

AR 26C

In the same patient, what is the expected mixed venous O$_2$ saturation (S$_v$O$_2$)?

A. Low (< 60%)
B. Normal (60–75%)
C. High (> 75%)

Answer:_____

AR 27

A 71-year-old male is admitted with hypotension, tachypnea, and tachycardia. His HR is 122 reg, BP 83/48, and RR 28.

A Swan-Ganz PA catheter is inserted:

CO 9.3 L/min (normal 5–6)

PCWP 8 mmHg (normal 8–12)

SVR 550 dynes (normal 700–1,600)

What is the hemodynamic picture consistent with?

A. Hypovolemic shock
B. Distributive shock secondary to sepsis
C. Cardiogenic shock from left heart failure

Answer:_____

3rd International Consensus Definition for Sepsis & Septic Shock

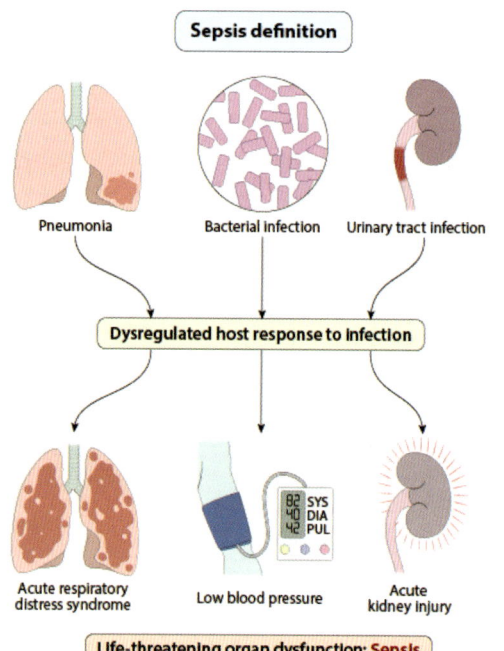

Sepsis clinical criteria

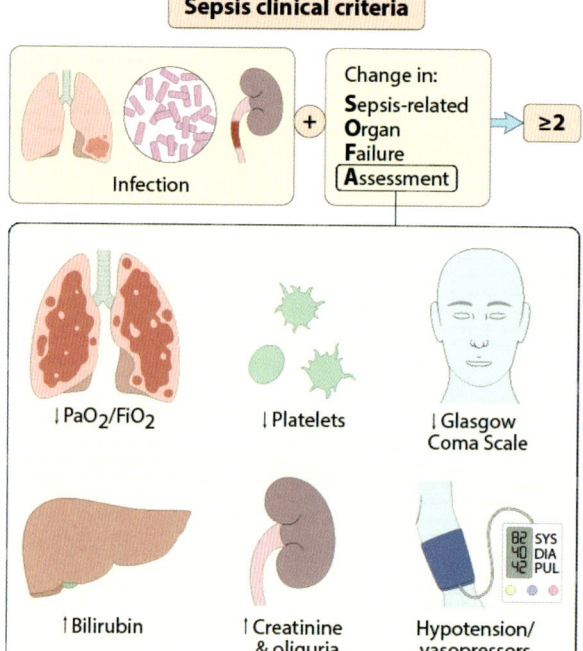

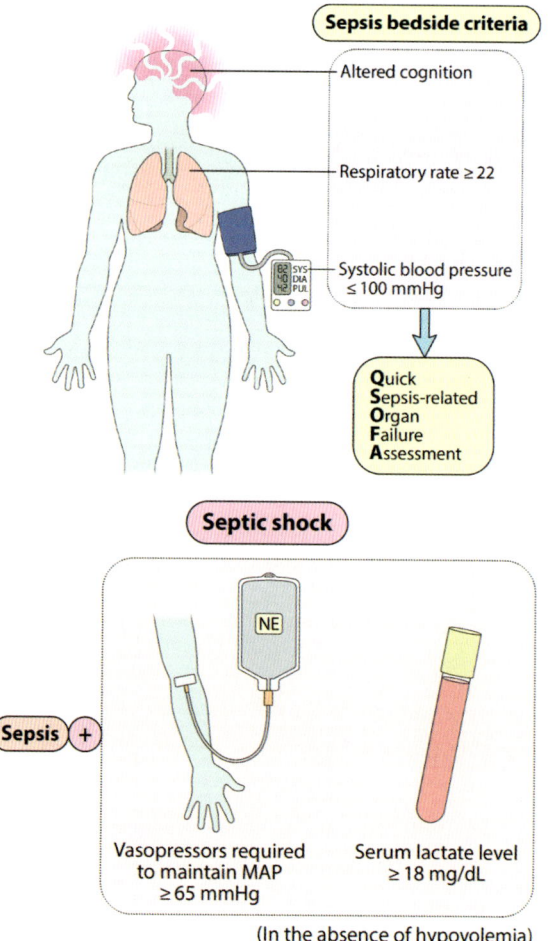

AR 28
Which of the following approaches to treatment of sepsis has been demonstrated to improve outcomes?

A. Blood transfusion at hemoglobin levels of 7 g/dL compared with 9 g/dL
B. Early administration of appropriate antimicrobials
C. Early goal-directed therapy
D. Protocol-based therapy
E. Target resuscitation to achieve a mean arterial blood pressure of 80–85 mmHg compared with 65–70 mmHg with angiotensin II acetate (Giapreza)

Answer:_____

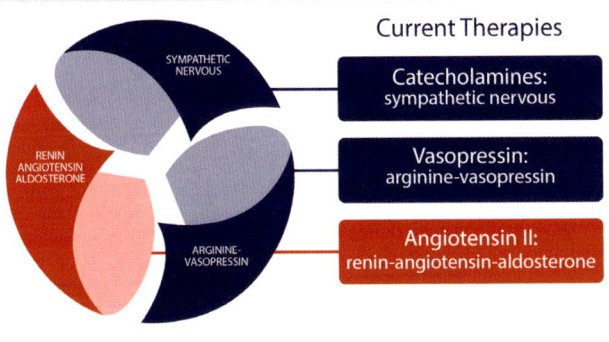

Current Therapies
Catecholamines: sympathetic nervous
Vasopressin: arginine-vasopressin
Angiotensin II: renin-angiotensin-aldosterone

[14]

Thank You
Website: beyondthepearls.net

AUDIENCE RESPONSE ANSWERS AND EXPLANATORY INFORMATION

Audience Response 1
D. Pulmonary arterial hypertension
- This patient most likely has pulmonary arterial hypertension (PAH) associated with collagen vascular disease related to systemic sclerosis particularly in those with limited cutaneous disease
- PFTs with PAH usually reveal an isolated decreased DLCO in the setting of normal airflow and lung volumes (excluding restrictive lung disease)

AR 2
B. Mild lower airway obstruction with reversibility

AR 3
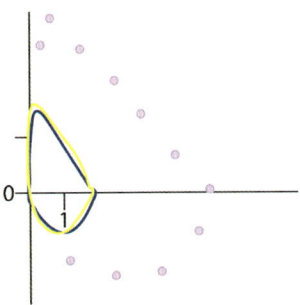
A.

AR 4
C. Macrophages

AR 5
B. Eosinophil

AR 6
C. Observe the patient using his inhalers.
Poor inhaler technique is a common cause of lack of response to asthma therapy; inhaler technique should be evaluated before therapy is adjusted.

AR 7
B. No
- Total IgE levels are elevated during treatment above the patient's baseline
- Retesting of IgE levels during omalizumab treatment is unnecessary and cannot be used as a guide for dose determination

AR 8
B. Add roflumilast, 500 mcg daily.

AR 9
E. Other

AR 10
A. Arterial blood gas studies
With the presence of somnolence, there is a high chance that she has arterial hypoxemia and alveolar hypoventilation with carbon dioxide retention; both are best evaluated by obtaining ABG.

AR 11
D. Taper and discontinue fluticasone/salmeterol and add indacaterol.

AR 12
D. Idiopathic pulmonary fibrosis
Idiopathic pulmonary fibrosis has the classic CT findings of basal and peripheral disease with evidence of honeycomb changes.

AR 13
A. Diarrhea

AR 14
D. Palliative care consult
End-of-life care should be discussed with all patients with idiopathic pulmonary fibrosis, ideally in the outpatient setting with family present and when there is no urgency to intervene.

AR 15
B. A 55-year-old man with a history of smoking who has a 2-cm left lower lobe nodule on chest CT with normal-sized mediastinal nodes

AR 16
D. Review of lung images from CT scan of the abdomen
Evaluation of a pulmonary nodule should always begin by review of any previous images.

AR 17
D. Repeat thoracentesis and pleural fluid cytology.
*   Imaging demonstrates a unilateral pleural effusion with an ipsilateral **lung mass** suspicious for bronchogenic carcinoma with pleural metastasis
*   Initial evaluation is with thoracentesis, because positive cytology for non–small cell carcinoma will effectively establish a diagnosis and simultaneously establish the malignancy as **Stage IV**
*   The overall sensitivity of pleural fluid cytology averages 60%, with 65% of positive results obtained on the initial sampling; an additional **27%** are identified on the 2nd sampling, and **5%** on the 3rd

AR 18
A. True
True
Which is why excluding the diagnosis of PE based on negative LE ultrasound makes no sense.

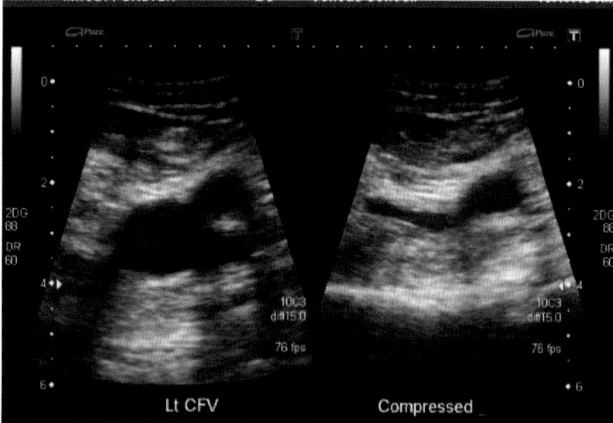

AR 19
B. Rivaroxaban
According to guidelines from the American College of Chest Physicians, the use of a target-specific anticoagulant (apixaban, rivaroxaban) alone is recommended over warfarin in patients with proximal deep venous thrombosis.

AR 20
A. Apixaban
A metaanalysis of numerous studies shows that target-specific oral anticoagulants, such as apixaban, were associated with a lower odds ratio of fatal bleeding, case fatality due to bleeding, and a higher likelihood of survival following a major bleed compared with LMW heparin and warfarin.

AR 21
E. Not enough information to determine this

AR 22
A. Continue anticoagulation indefinitely.
Long-term anticoagulation therapy is recommended for patients with unprovoked proximal leg deep venous thrombosis or pulmonary embolism who have low or moderate bleeding risk.

AR 23
E. Increase the PEEP.
In patients with severe acute respiratory distress syndrome, current recommendations are to use a positive end-expiratory pressure level that achieves adequate oxygenation with an FiO_2 of < 0.6 and does not cause hypotension.

AR 24
B. Decreased compliance and oxygenation

AR 25
B. Hypovolemic shock

AR 26A
A. Cardiogenic shock from left heart failure

AR 26B
C. Dobutamine

AR 26C
A. Low (< 60%)

AR 27
B. Distributive shock secondary to sepsis

AR 28
B. Early administration of appropriate antimicrobials

ENDNOTES

[1]   Burrows B, et al. Association of asthma with serum IgE levels and skin-test reactivity to allergens. N Engl J Med. 1989;320:272–277.

[2]   N Engl J Med. 2003;348(21):2059.

[3]   Magnussun H, et al. Withdrawal of Inhaled Glucocorticoids and Exacerbations of COPD. N Engl J Med 2014; 371: 1285-1294.

[4]   https://www.thelancet.com/journals/lanres/article/PIIS2213-2600(17)30433-2/fulltext

[5]   Am J Respir Crit Care Med. 1998;158:1804.

Eur Respir J. 2006;27:136.

Ann Thorac Surg. 2006;82:1570; author reply 1570.

[6]   Stein, P, et al. Multidetector Computed Tomography for Acute Pulmonary Embolism. N Engl J Med 2006; 354:2317-2327.

[7]   Barritt DW, Jordan SC. Anticoagulant drugs in the treatment of pulmonary embolism: A controlled trial. Lancet. 1960; 1(7138):1309.

[8]   Keron C, et al. D-Dimer Testing to Select Patient with a First Unprovoked Venous Thromboembolism who can Stop Anticoagulant Therapy: A Cohort Study. Ann Intern Med 2015; 162: 27-34.
Kylre P, et al. The Risk of Recurrent Venous Thromboembolism in Men and Women. N Engl J Med 2004; 350:2558-2563.

[9]   slgckgc [CC BY 2.0 (https://creativecommons.org/licenses/by/2.0)], via Wikimedia Commons

[10]   Cowie M, et al. Adaptive Servo-Ventilation for Central Sleep Apnea in Systolic Heart Failure. N Engl J Med 2015; 373:1095-1105.

[11]   The National Heart, Lung, and Blood Institute Acute Respiratory Distress Syndrome (ARDS) Clinical Trials Network. New Engl J Med. 2006; 354(16);1671–1684.

[12]   Meduri, et al. Chest. 2007; 131:954–963.

[13]   Papazian L, et al. Neuromuscular Blockers in Early Acute Respiratory Distress Syndrome. N Engl J Med 2010; 365.

[14]   Holst L, et al. Lower versus Higher Hemoglobin Threshold for Transfusion in Septic Shock. N Engl J Med 2014; 371:1381-1391.
ProCESS Investigators. A Randomized Trial of Protocol-Based Care for Early Septic Shock. N Engl J Med 2014; 370:1683-1693.
Khanna, A, et al. Angiotensin II for the Treatment of Vasodilatory Shock. N Engl J Med 2017; 377:419-430.
Delaney A, et al. Goal-Directed Resuscitation for Patients with Early Septic Shock. N Engl J Med. 2014 Oct 16;371(16):1496-506.
Asfar P, et al. High versus Low Blood-Pressure Target in Patients with Septic Shock. N Engl J Med 2014; 370:1583-1593.

MedStudy

INTERNAL MEDICINE REVIEW

Rheumatology

Presented by

R. Michelle Koolaee, DO

TABLE OF CONTENTS

Rheumatology Outline

- Interpreting Rheumatology Labs
- Patterns of Arthritis
- Synovial Fluid Analysis
- Rheumatoid Arthritis (RA)
- Seronegative Spondyloarthritis
- Osteoarthritis (OA)
- Crystalline Arthritis
- Systemic Lupus Erythematosus (SLE)
- Other Connective Tissue Diseases
  - Systemic Sclerosis, Sjögren's, Inflammatory Myositis
- Vasculitis
- Office Orthopedics

- HLA-B27: seronegative spondyloarthritis
- HLA-B51: Behçet disease
- HLA-B*58:01: allopurinol hypersensitivity syndrome

Audience Response 1
Which of the following labs has _not_ been commonly associated with the disease?

A. Anti–CCP antibody and rheumatoid arthritis
B. Anti-RNA polymerase III and limited sclerosis
C. Anti-dsDNA and systemic lupus erythematosus
D. HLA-B*58:01 and allopurinol hypersensitivity syndrome

Answer:_____

INTERPRETING RHEUMATOLOGY LABS

- Rule 1: Labs can be helpful to support the diagnosis
- Rule 2: Don't rely on labs alone to make the diagnosis!

Common (a.k.a. Board-Testable) Rheumatology Labs

- ANA: okay for screening but nonspecific; significant if > 1:80; patterns are not generally helpful
- dsDNA and anti-Smith (Sm) antibodies: specific for SLE
- RNP: mixed connective tissue disease; also seen in SLE
- Antihistone: drug-induced lupus
- SSA/SSB: Sjögren syndrome
- C3, C4: low in SLE (may correlate with disease activity)
- Antiphospholipid markers:
  - DRVVT (lupus anticoagulant)
  - Anticardiolipin IgG/IgM
  - β_2-Glycoprotein-1 IgG/IgM

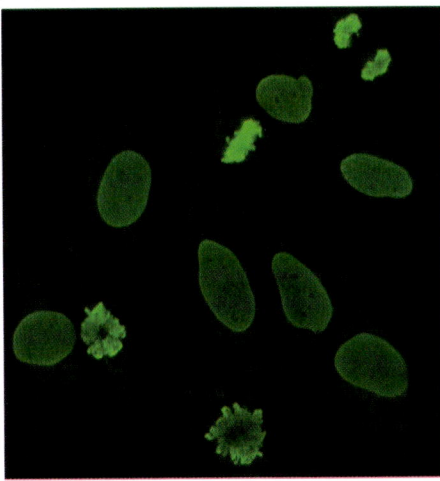

- RF: RA, vasculitis, chronic lung disease/infections, Sjögren's*
- CCP: more specific in RA, poor prognosis*
- Anticentromere Ab/anti-Scl-70: systemic sclerosis limited/diffuse
- Anti-RNA polymerase III: scleroderma renal crisis
- Antisynthetase antibodies (anti-Jo-1, PL-7, PL-12, OJ, and EJ)
- HMGCR antibody: statin-induced necrotizing myopathy
- ANCA: c-ANCA (PR3) = GPA; p-ANCA (MPO) = nonspecific
- ESR, CRP, ferritin: acute phase reactants
- ACE: sarcoidosis
* Hint: 20% of patients who have RA will be seronegative

PATTERNS OF ARTHRITIS

Categorizing Arthropathies

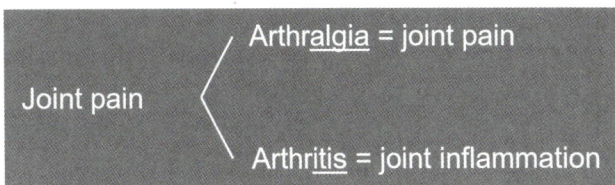

Joint pain
Arthralgia = joint pain
Arthritis = joint inflammation

- **Cardinal signs of inflammation**
  - Erythema (rubor)
  - Swelling (tumor)
  - Heat (calor)
  - Pain (dolor)

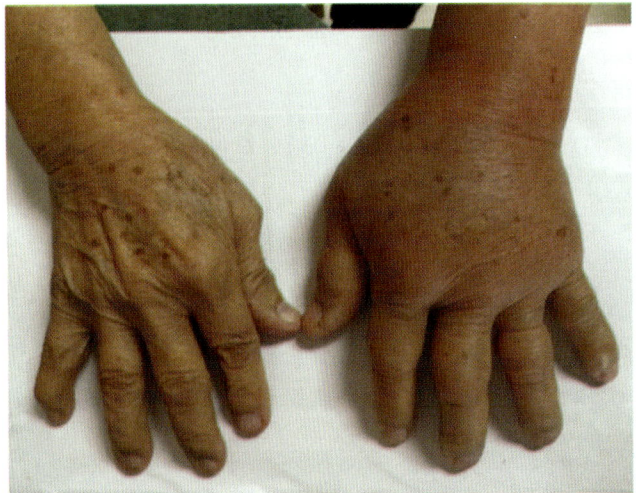

[1]

Common Forms of Arthritis
- **Inflammatory**
  - Rheumatoid arthritis
  - Crystal-induced arthritis
    - Gout
    - Pseudogout
    - Hydroxyapatite
  - Seronegative spondyloarthropathies
    - Ankylosing spondylitis
    - Reactive arthritis
    - Psoriatic arthritis
    - IBD-associated arthritis
- **Noninflammatory**
  - Osteoarthritis

Hint: Look for patterns to help make the diagnosis

High Yield — Distinguishing Inflammatory vs. Noninflammatory Pain

History	Noninflammatory Pain	Inflammatory Pain
Morning Stiffness	< 30 minutes	> 60 minutes
Activity	Worse with activity; improves with rest	Better with activity
Exam	No synovitis; bony hypertrophy in OA	Synovitis (swelling/heat)
Synovial Fluid	Noninflammatory	**Inflammatory (WBC count > 2,000 cells/mm³ [2 × 10⁹/L])**
Labs	Normal ESR/CRP	Elevated ESR/CRP, anemia of chronic disease, thrombocytosis
Imaging	No erosions	Juxtaarticular osteopenia, erosions, deformities

Joint Swelling vs. Bony Enlargement

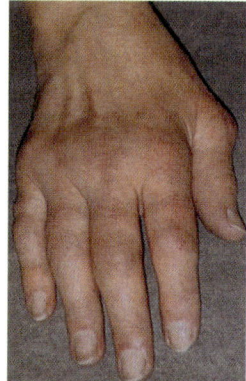

- MCPs + PIPs
- Spongy/Boggy/Painful
- DIPs spared
- Wrist swelling
= **Inflammatory arthritis (like RA)**

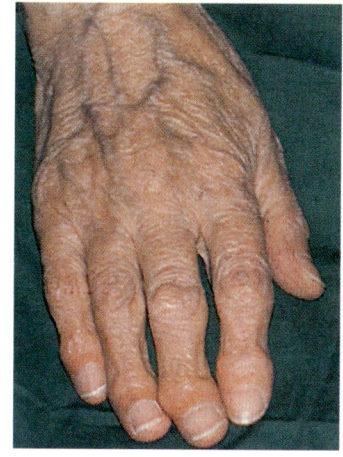

- DIPs + PIPs
- Bony/Firm
- MCPs spared
- Wrist spared
= **OA**

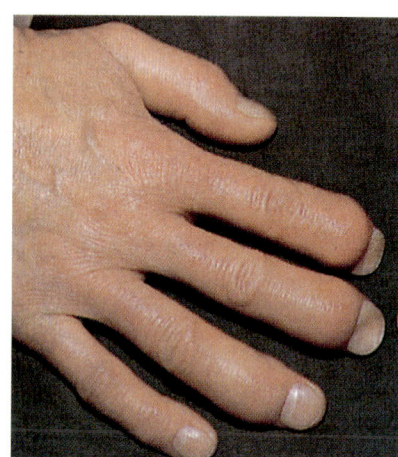

- DIPs
- Nail pitting
= **Psoriatic arthritis**

X-rays of Common Arthritides

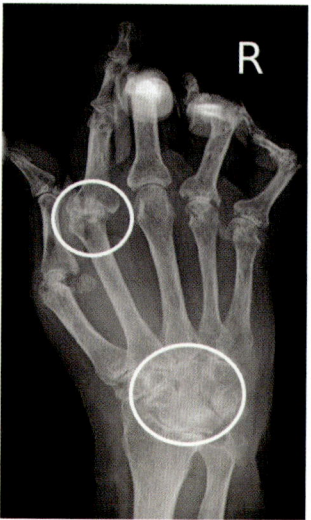

Rheumatoid arthritis

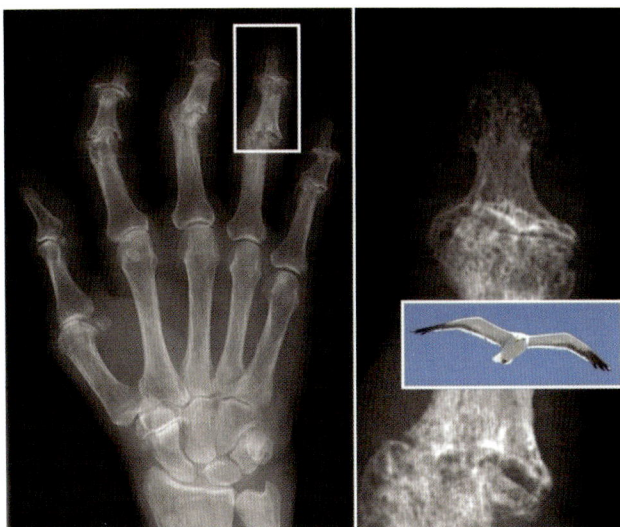

Hand OA; erosive OA

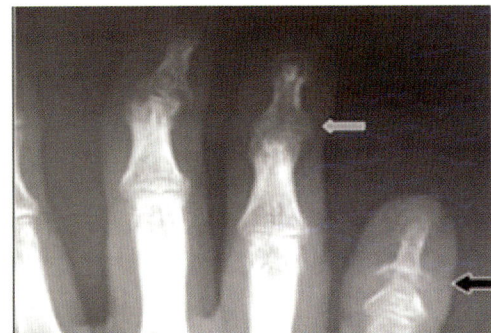

Psoriatic arthritis

Synovial Fluid Analysis

Type of Fluid	Color	WBC/mm³
Normal	Clear (colorless)	< 200 (< 25% PMN)
Noninflammatory	Clear yellow	200–2,000 (< 25% PMN)
Inflammatory	Cloudy yellow	2,000–100,000 (> 50% PMN)
Septic	Purulent	> 50,000 (> 75% PMN)

- Order on synovial fluid: cell count with differential, crystal analysis, and Gram stain with culture and sensitivity
- Protein, glucose, LDH not important

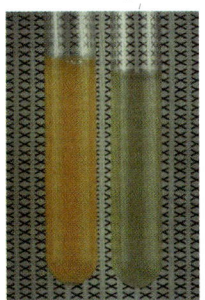

- Synovial fluid analysis is the only way to definitively diagnose gout or pseudogout
- "Birefringent" crystals = 2 colors
  - Uric acid = negatively birefringent (**yellow** when **parallel** to direction of red compensator), needle shaped
  - Calcium **p**yrophosphate = **p**ositively birefringent (**b**lue), rhomboid

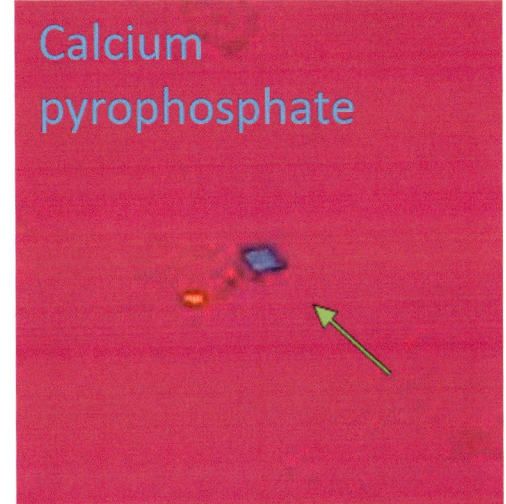

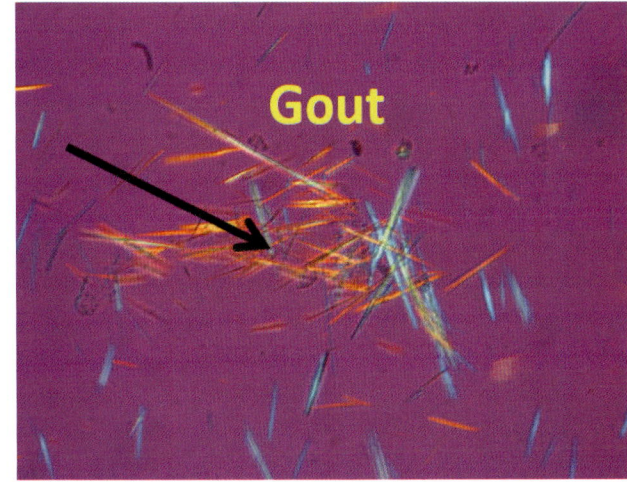

RHEUMATOLOGY

AR 2

A 34-year-old Hispanic female presents with 12 weeks of pain in both hands and wrists. Morning stiffness lasting 2 hours. She denies rashes, fever, diarrhea, weight loss, Raynaud's, photosensitivity, oral ulcers, sicca symptoms, sick contacts, or family history of autoimmune diseases. Her hands are shown.

Labs: RF negative, CCP negative, ANA positive at 1:80 speckled pattern, ESR 48 mm/hour, CRP 1.31 mg/dL, Hgb 11.7 mg/dL

X-rays of her hands show juxtaarticular osteopenia of her MCPs and PIPs.

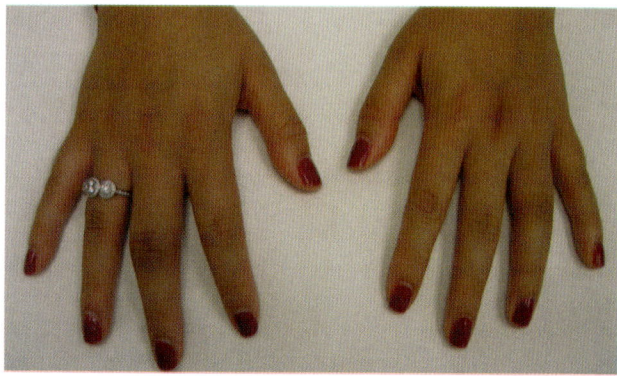

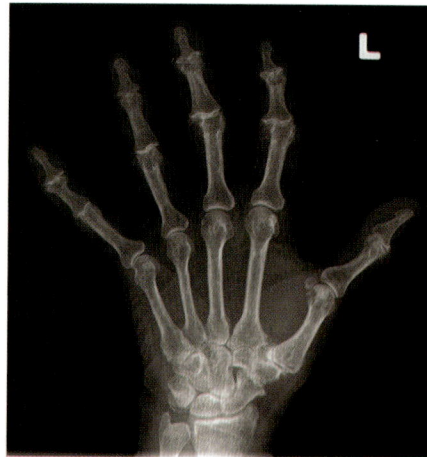

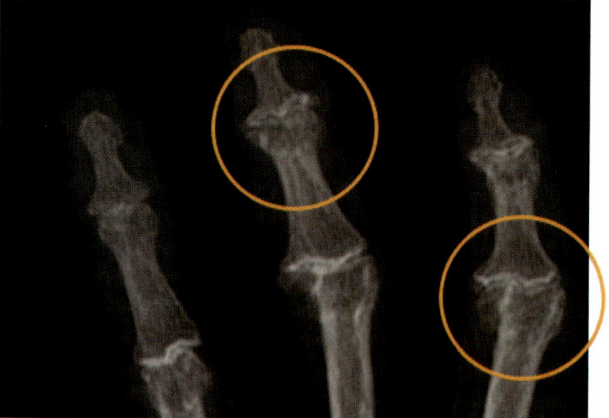

What is the most likely diagnosis?

A. Systemic lupus erythematosus
B. Seronegative rheumatoid arthritis (RA)
C. Calcium pyrophosphate deposition arthropathy
D. Osteoarthritis
E. Parvovirus infection

Answer:_____

AR 3

A 60-year-old female presents with 5 years of pain in the PIPs/DIPs of both hands; rings no longer fit.

20 minutes of morning stiffness

Intermittent erythema and swelling in DIPs/PIPs

PE: firmness with bony enlargement of the DIPs/PIPs with tenderness; no swelling noted

Labs: Hgb 13.1 g/dL, ESR 11 mm/hour, RF/CCP negative

X-rays: DIPs/PIPs with severe joint space narrowing, central erosions; DIPs with gull wing deformities; no marginal erosions or periarticular osteopenia

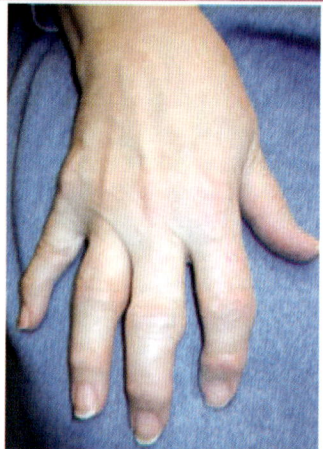

Which of the following is the most likely diagnosis?

A. Erosive osteoarthritis
B. Rheumatoid arthritis
C. Fibromyalgia
D. Seronegative spondyloarthritis
E. Lupus

Answer:_____

INFLAMMATORY ARTHRITIDES

RHEUMATOID ARTHRITIS

Rheumatoid Arthritis (RA)
- Immune-mediated inflammatory arthritis
- Chronic (≥ 6 weeks), symmetric, polyarticular
- Prolonged morning stiffness > 1 hour
- Joints involved: TMJs, PIPs, MCPs, wrists, elbows, shoulders, hips, knees, ankles, tarsus, MTPs; **spares DIPs, T- and L-spine, and SI joints**
- +RF and/or CCP antibodies in 80%, seronegative in 20%
- ↑ ESR or CRP

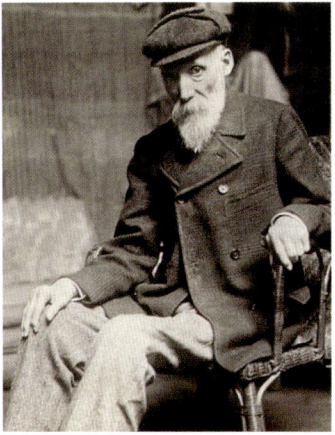
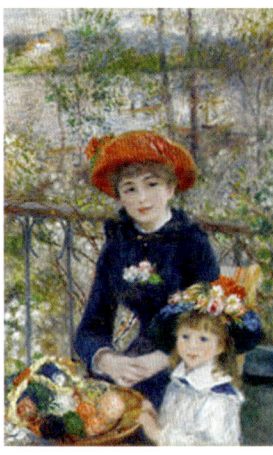

Pierre-Auguste Renoir
(February 25, 1841–December 3, 1919)

- RF ± CCP positive, worse prognosis
  - Joint erosions
  - Deformities
  - Cervical spine atlantoaxial (C1–C2) subluxation
  - Extraarticular manifestations
  - Lymphoma

Diagnosis of RA
- Differential diagnoses
  - SLE
  - Sjögren's
  - Psoriatic arthritis
  - Sarcoidosis
  - ***High yield*: viral arthritis, especially parvovirus**

Clinical Findings of RA
- Demineralization, joint erosions/destruction in bilateral wrists with carpal bone fusion (patients will have limited wrist extension on physical exam)

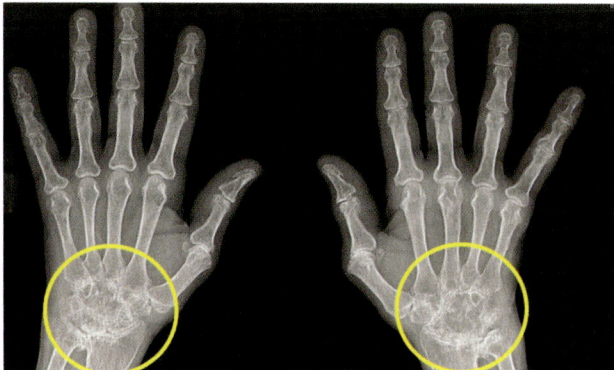

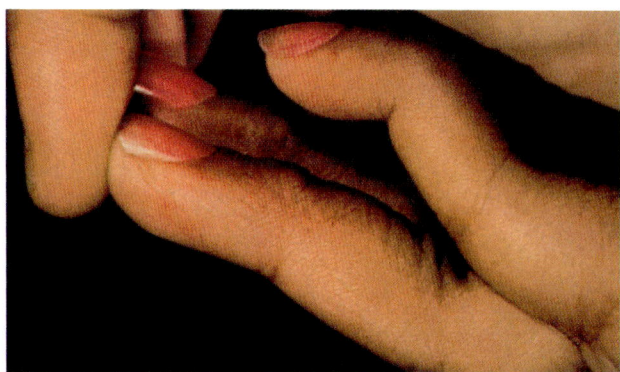

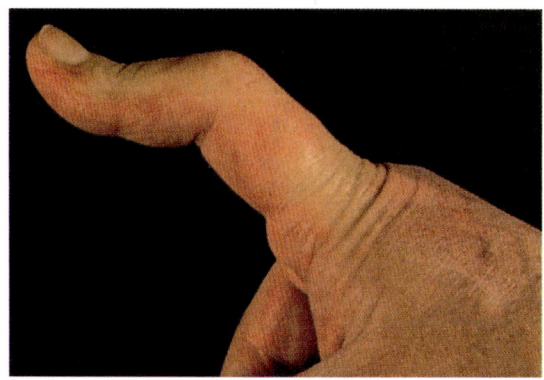

Swan-neck deformity and Boutonnière deformity

Extraarticular Manifestations of RA

- Pulmonary
- Skin
- Cardiac
- Muscular
- Ocular
- Neurologic

RA — Pulmonary Disease

- Pleuritis
- **Exudative** pleural effusion with low glucose, low pH, high LDH
- Pulmonary rheumatoid nodule
- Organizing pneumonia
- Interstitial lung disease/fibrosis (NSIP and UIP are the most common types of ILD in RA)

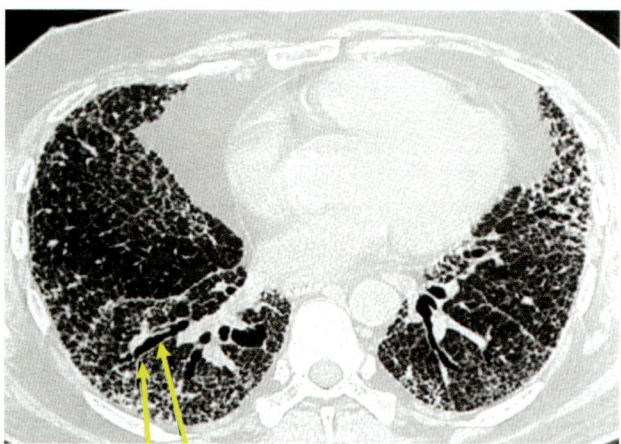

RA — Skin Disease

- Subcutaneous nodules — 25%
- Vasculitis
  - Nailfold infarcts
  - Palpable purpura
  - Ulcers
- Drug-induced (steroid) bruising

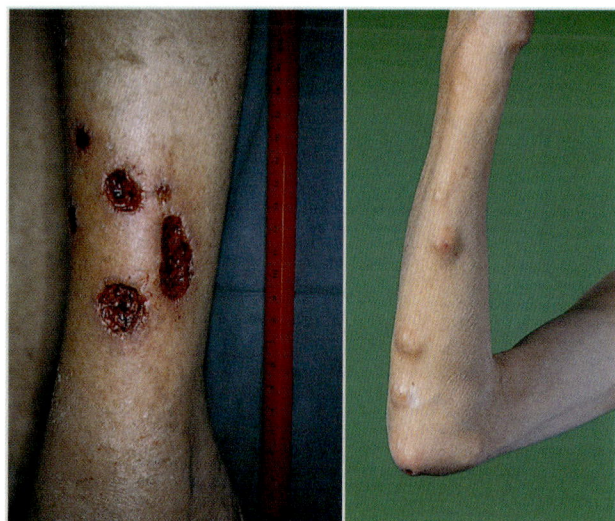

Ulcers   Nodules

RA — Cardiac, Neurologic, and Ocular Disease

- Cardiac
  - ****Pericarditis = Most common cardiac manifestation of RA****
  - Myocarditis
  - Valvular nodules
  - ***Atherosclerosis (3× ↑ CV risk)**
- Neurologic
  - Mononeuritis multiplex
  - Carpal tunnel syndrome
  - Atlantoaxial subluxation
- Ocular
  - Sicca
  - Episcleritis
  - Scleritis
  - Scleromalacia perforans

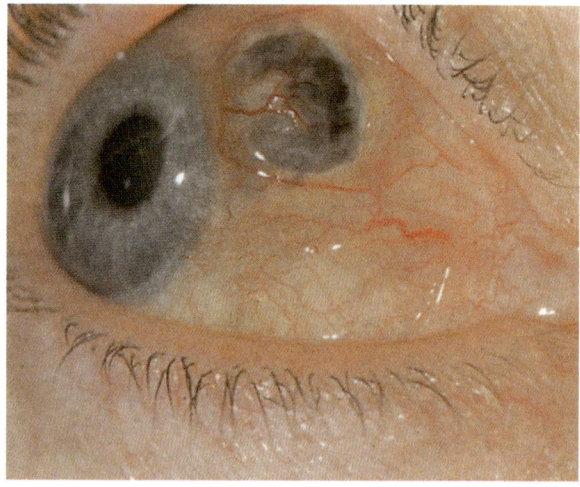

Scleromalacia perforans

Treatment of RA

- Analgesics
- NSAIDs   } **Immediate Pain Relief**
- Glucocorticoids

- **D**isease-**m**odifying **a**nti**r**heumatic **d**rugs **(DMARDs)**
  - Nonbiologics: methotrexate, leflunomide, hydroxychloroquine, sulfasalazine, tofacitinib, baricitinib, upadacitinib
  - Biologics: TNF inhibitors, non-TNF inhibitors
- **NSAIDs**
  - Provide pain relief but do not change the disease course!
  - Side effects: GI (gastritis/ulcers/hepatotoxicity), CV (HF exacerbation, MI, HTN), renal (interstitial nephritis), hematologic (platelet dysfunction)
- **Glucocorticoids**
  - Used as bridging agents, do modify the disease
  - Side effects: weight gain, adrenal insufficiency, Cushing's, diabetes, bruising, skin fragility, HTN, hyperlipidemia, osteoporosis, mood changes, acne

Nonbiologic DMARDs
- **High-yield facts**
  - **Methotrexate** = #1 DMARD prescribed in U.S.
    - **Dihydrofolate reductase inhibitor, antidote folate**
    - Side effects: marrow suppression, hepatotoxicity, pneumonitis
    - Contraindicated in pregnancy and EtOH abuse
    - High drug interaction with sulfamethoxazole-trimethoprim
  - **Hydroxychloroquine:** retinal toxicity; okay in pregnancy
  - **Sulfasalazine**
    - Okay in pregnancy
  - **Leflunomide** similar to MTX (fewer pulmonary risks)
- **Small-molecule inhibitors (JAK inhibitors)**
  - Tofacitinib
  - Baricitinib
  - Upadacitinib
  - Advantages: effective, short half-lives, orally administered
  - High risk for shingles, much higher than TNF inhibitors
  - TB, fungal, opportunistic infections are similar to biologics
  - Possibly increased risk for thrombosis

Biologic DMARDs
- <u>Tumor necrosis factor inhibitor (TNFi) agents</u>
  - Etanercept
  - Adalimumab
  - Infliximab
  - Golimumab
  - Certolizumab
- <u>Non-TNF agents</u>
  - Tocilizumab and sarilumab (anti-IL6)
  - Abatacept (CTLA-4 Ig)
  - Rituximab (inhibits B cells)
  - Anakinra (IL-1 inhibitor)
- **Pearls:**
  - Increased risk for nonserious and serious infections, opportunistic infections (check for latent TB, HBV, HCV)
  - Avoid live vaccines: MMR, varicella, nasal flu, oral polio, Zostavax (Shingrix is **not** a live vaccine)
  - Avoid TNFi in HF Class III/IV

AR 4

A 55-year-old patient with seropositive rheumatoid arthritis, on methotrexate, presents to you with a urinary tract infection.

Which of the following antibiotics would you avoid prescribing due to high risk for drug interaction?

A. Nitrofurantoin
B. Ciprofloxacin
C. Cefuroxime
D. Sulfamethoxazole-trimethoprim

Answer:_____

SERONEGATIVE SPONDYLOARTHRITIS

Seronegative Spondyloarthritis — The Spectrum
- Ankylosing spondylitis
- Reactive arthritis
- Psoriatic arthritis
- Arthritis associated with inflammatory bowel disease

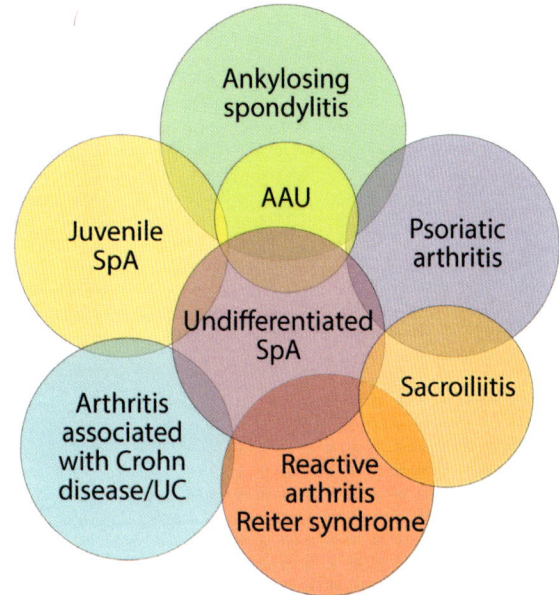

Clinical Findings of Seronegative Spondyloarthritis
- Common clinical features
  - **RF negative**
  - **Axial arthritis** (spine, SI joints)
  - **Peripheral arthritis**
    - Asymmetric: knees and ankles
    - Dactylitis "sausage digits"
    - Enthesitis: achilles
  - **Ocular** involvement: conjunctivitis, uveitis
  - HLA-B27: high association with axial disease
  - Colitis
  - Psoriasis/skin

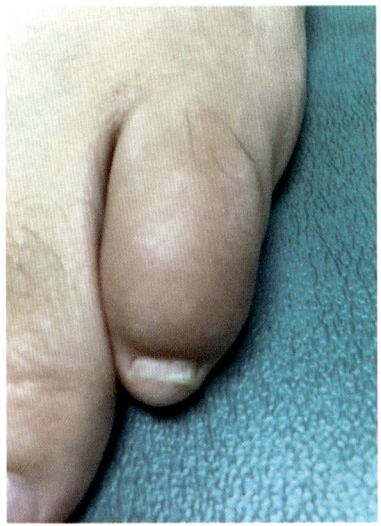

Dactylitis "sausage digits"

Ankylosing Spondylitis

- Onset 20–30 years of age, mostly male
- Diagnosis = symmetrical, symptomatic sacroiliitis with no bowel disease or psoriasis
- Pain is decreased with exercise and wakes patient from sleep
- HLA-B27 > 90% in AS, low specificity
- Uveitis
- Aortitis
- Apical fibrosis of lungs (upper lobe)

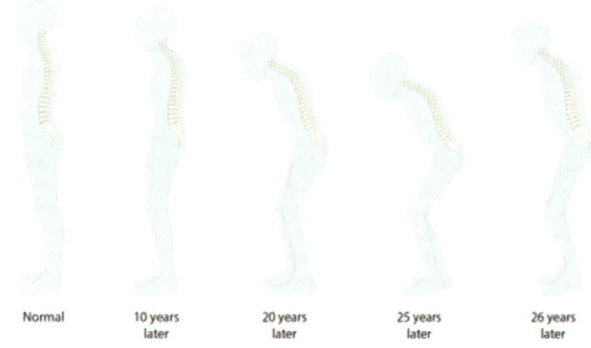

| Normal | 10 years later | 20 years later | 25 years later | 26 years later |

"Bamboo Spine" in Ankylosing Spondylitis

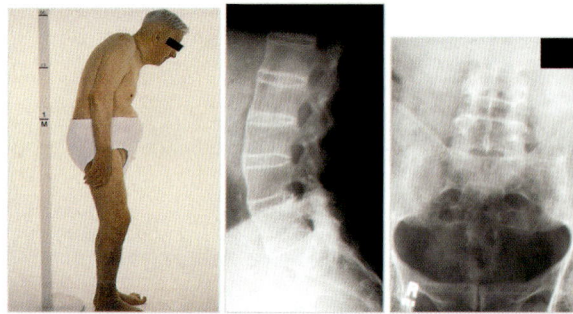

- **Hallmarks of disease**
  - "Flowing syndesmophytes"
  - Bilateral sacroiliitis

Treatment of Ankylosing Spondylitis

- Exercise
- NSAIDs
- DMARDs: for peripheral arthritis, skin/GI disease
  - SSZ, MTX
- Biologics: for axial and peripheral arthritis, enthesitis, skin/GI/GU/eye disease
  - TNF inhibitors
  - Secukinumab: IL-17 inhibitor
  - Ixekizumab: IL-17A inhibitor

Reactive Arthritis

- Peripheral or axial inflammatory arthritis 2–4 weeks after infection (typically following GI or GU infection)
- Etiologies
  - GU
    - *Chlamydia trachomatis*
  - GI
    - *Salmonella*, *Shigella*, *Yersinia*
    - *Campylobacter*, *Clostridioides* (formerly *Clostridium*) *difficile*
- Classic triad: Look for it!
  1) Ocular involvement
     - Conjunctivitis
     - Uveitis
  2) Urethritis
  3) Arthritis
     - Dactylitis
     - Enthesitis
     - Asymmetric oligoarthritis

"Can't see, can't pee, can't climb a tree."

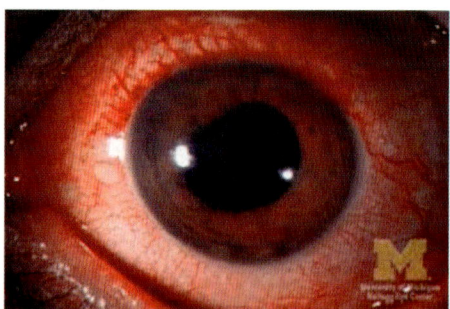

[2]

Uveitis

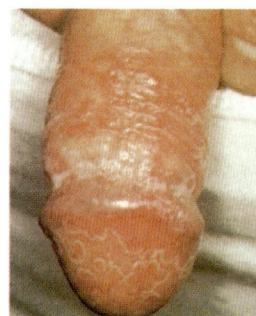

Circinate balanitis

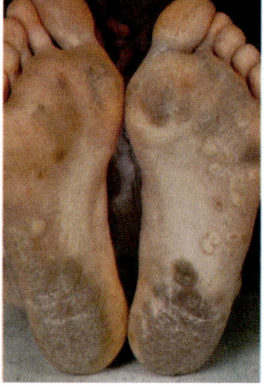

Keratoderma blennorrhagicum

- Bacteria frequently undetectable during arthritis → presumed infection = look at the history!
- Disease is usually self-limited and resolves within 6 months without erosive damage; 25% can have persistent disease
- Treatment
  - NSAIDs
  - Intraarticular ± systemic steroids
  - Antibiotics: controversial
  - MTX, sulfasalazine, TNF inhibitors for refractory disease

Psoriatic Arthritis

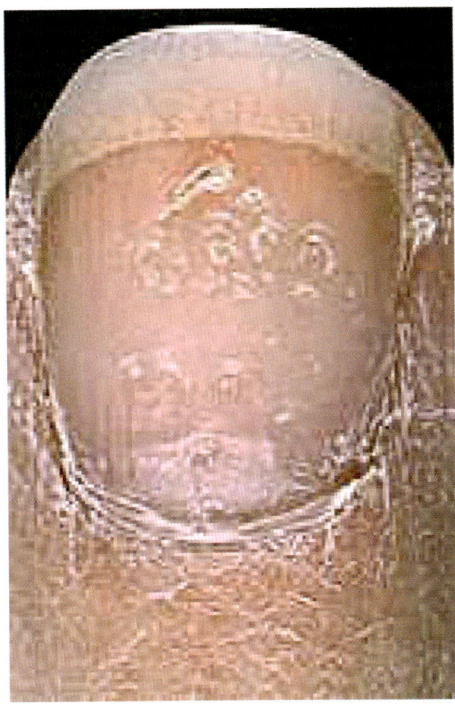

Dystrophic nail beds with pitting

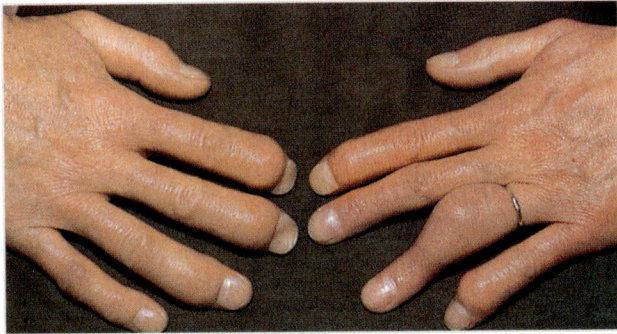

Asymmetrical arthritis with DIP and PIP involvement

Treatment of Psoriatic Arthritis
- Exercise
- NSAIDs
- DMARDs: for peripheral arthritis, skin disease
  - SSZ, MTX
  - Apremilast, tofacitinib
- Biologics: for axial and peripheral arthritis, enthesitis, skin/GI/GU/eye disease
  - TNF inhibitors
  - Secukinumab, ixekizumab, IL-17 inhibitor
  - Ustekinumab: anti-IL-12/23
  - Abatacept: CTLA4-Ig

AR 5

A 28-year-old man with 3 months of L foot pain and swelling and pain in the posterior area of the heels.

Meds: ibuprofen with little improvement

Synovial fluid analysis L knee: WBC 4,500 cells/mm³, 85% neutrophils; no crystals

Exam: as shown below

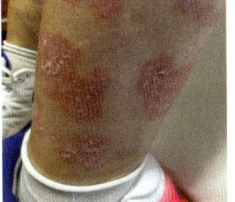 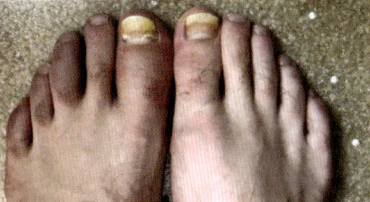

Which of the following has been commonly associated with his disease?

A. Interstitial lung disease
B. Sjögren syndrome
C. Glomerulonephritis
D. Uveitis
E. Raynaud phenomenon

Answer:_____

OSTEOARTHRITIS

Degenerative Joint Disease — Osteoarthritis (OA)

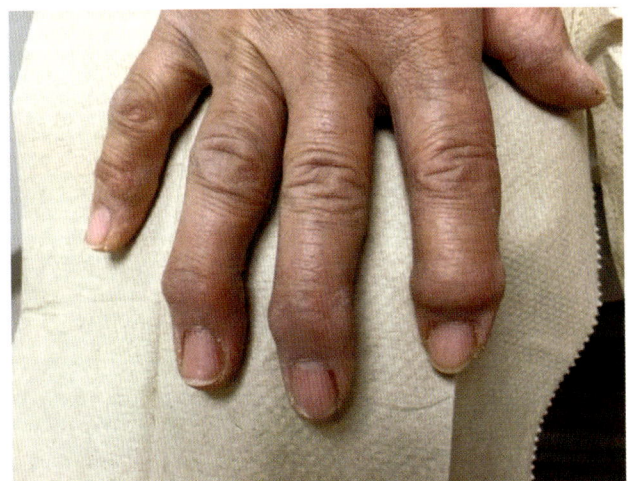

- <u>Primary OA</u>: asymmetric, DIPs, PIPs, knees, hips, cervical and lumbar spine
  – Less commonly shoulders and ankles
- Pain is exertional, weight bearing
- Morning stiffness < 30 minutes
- Fluid WBC < 2,000 cells/mm³
- Asymmetric joint space narrowing with new bone formation (osteophytes)
- Usually not erosive (except for erosive OA affects DIPs)
- <u>Secondary OA</u>: MCPs, shoulder, elbow, wrist, ankle, **or** erosions **should make you think something else**
- Diagnosis is clinical
- Treatment = education + physical therapy
  – Oral analgesics
    • Acetaminophen
    • NSAID or COX-2 selective NSAID
    • Glucosamine/chondroitin **does not** work
    • Tramadol/opiates for severe pain
  – Topical NSAIDs and/or capsaicin (when intolerant of oral NSAIDs)
  – Intraarticular steroids (when 1–2 joints affected)
  – Intraarticular hyaluronic acid
  – Surgery for joint replacement

Osteoarthritis vs. Rheumatoid Arthritis

	OA	RA
Joint Distribution	Asymmetric monoarticular, oligoarticular, polyarticular	Symmetric polyarticular
Synovitis	No, only bony enlargement	Yes
Target Joint	DIP, PIP, CMC, hips, knees, spine, feet, toes	PIP, MCP, wrists, elbows, knees, hips, ankles, toes, shoulders; never the spine!
A.M. Stiffness	< 30 minutes knees, < 60 minutes hips	> 1 hour
Labs	Noninflammatory	Inflammatory: elevated plt, anemia of chronic disease, elevated ESR
Bone Changes	Bony enlargement with new bone formation (osteophytes), subchondral cysts	Bone loss: periarticular osteopenia, marginal erosions

What Do You See?

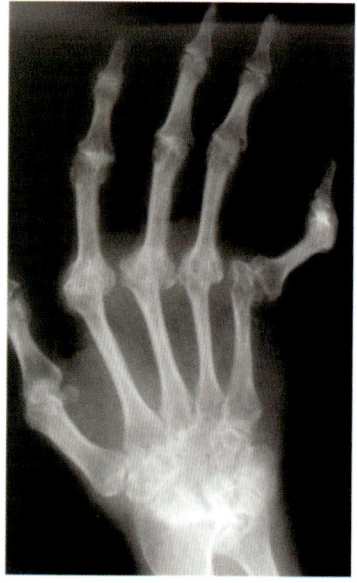

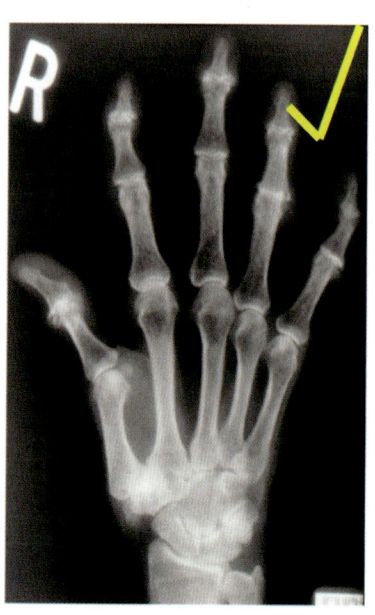

CRYSTALLINE ARTHRITIS

OVERVIEW

Crystalline Arthropathies
- Gout: uric acid
- Pseudogout: calcium pyrophosphate deposition (CPPD)
- Hydroxyapatite: basic calcium phosphate

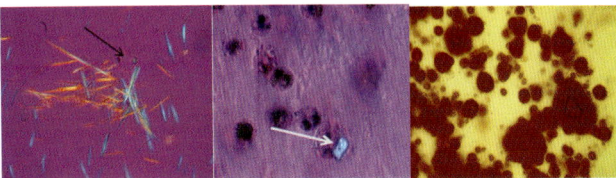

GOUT
"The king of diseases and the disease of kings"

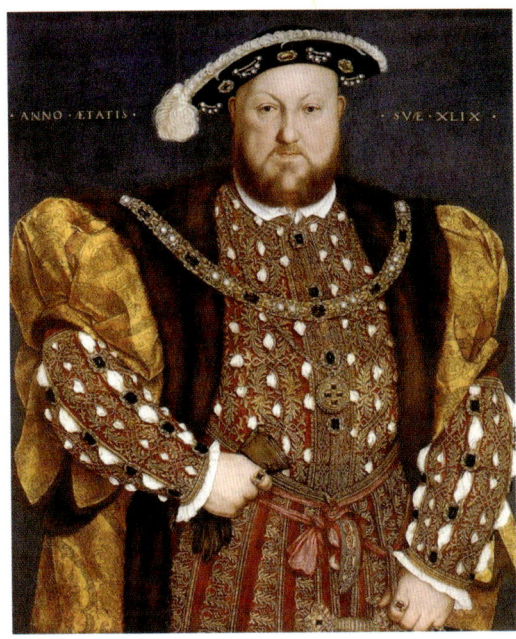

King Henry VIII of England 16th Century

- Acute peripheral inflammatory arthritis after years of hyperuricemia
- Risks
  - Trauma, surgery, starvation, dehydration
  - Chronic kidney disease
  - Diet: purine-rich meat, seafood, high-fructose corn syrup/processed sugars, ethanol
  - Medications: diuretics, low-dose aspirin, cyclosporine
- Definitive Dx: needle-shaped, negatively birefringent uric acid crystals
- Hyperuricemia alone does not diagnose gout

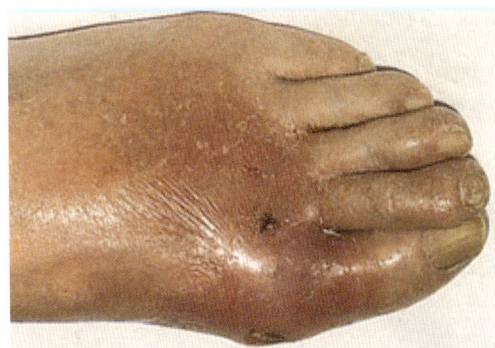

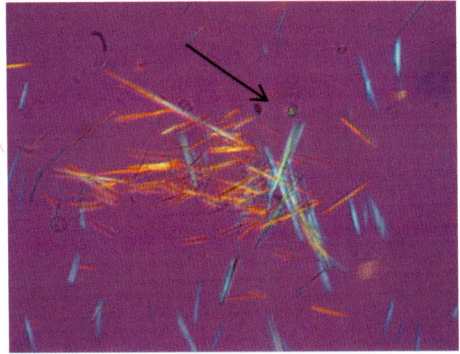

Gout — Acute Treatment
- NSAIDs
- Oral or intraarticular glucocorticoids
- Oral colchicine
- Any shifts in uric acid (↑ or ↓) can worsen flare; as such:
  - Do not first start allopurinol during a flare
  - If their home meds include allopurinol, do <u>not</u> stop it during a flare

Gout — Chronic Treatment
- **Know: goal uric acid for nontophaceous gout < 6 mg/dL**
- Lifestyle modifications: diet, avoid aggravating factors (diuretics)
- Xanthine oxidase inhibitors: 1st line
  1) Allopurinol: **Check *HLA-B58:01* in Asians and African Americans to avoid allopurinol hypersensitivity syndrome**
  2) Febuxostat (Uloric): Monitor LFTs, okay for use if GFR < 30 mL/min — choose this if patient cannot use allopurinol
- Uricosuric (inhibits URAT1)
  - Probenecid: **requires normal GFR; has GI side effects**
- Pegloticase (Krystexxa, Puricase)
  - Approved for refractory **tophaceous** gout
  - Expensive
  - 20% infusion reaction, 6% anaphylaxis
  - Monitor uric acid prior to each infusion

RHEUMATOLOGY

Gout — Prophylaxis during Urate-Lowering Therapy
- Why prophylaxis? Prevents flares while lowering uric acid to goal
- **Use colchicine, NSAIDs, or low-dose prednisone**
- Duration of prophylaxis (whichever is longer)
  - 6 months after the last gout flare
  - 3 months after reaching target urate level in patients without tophi
  - 6 months after target urate level reached in patients with tophi

CALCIUM PYROPHOSPHATE DEPOSITION DISEASE

Calcium Pyrophosphate Deposition (CPPD) Disease
- Think about CPPD when:
  - Acute onset of inflammatory arthritis
  - Risk factors
    - Surgery/trauma
    - Older age (frequently ≥ 75 years of age)
    - Diuretics (in setting of dehydration)
    - Hyperparathyroidism
- Chondrocalcinosis on radiograph is tip-off
- Polarized light microscopy is definitive diagnosis
  - **CP**PD = **P**ositively birefringent crystals = **B**lue

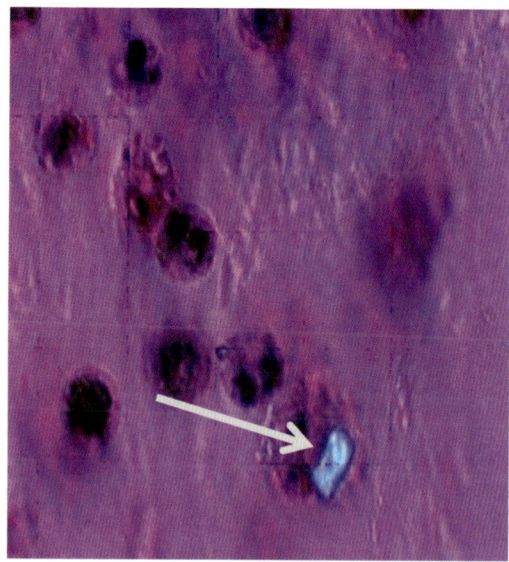

CPPD Management
- NSAIDs
- Oral steroid taper
- Steroid injection
- Colchicine
- **Test for associated diseases**
  - Hemochromatosis: iron studies, *HFE* gene
  - Thyroid disease: thyroid function tests
  - Hyperparathyroidism: intact PTH, ionized calcium
  - CKD: calcium, Mg, phos

Chondrocalcinosis

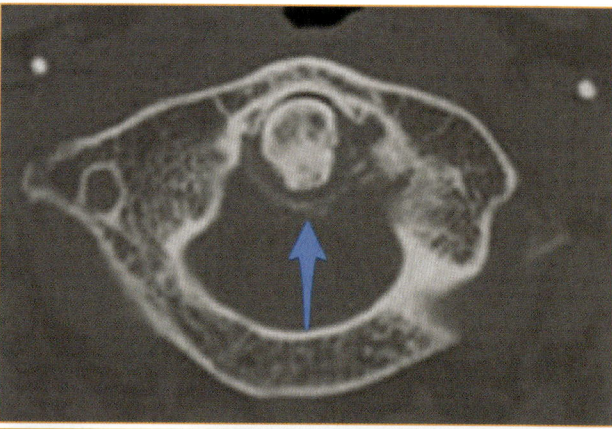

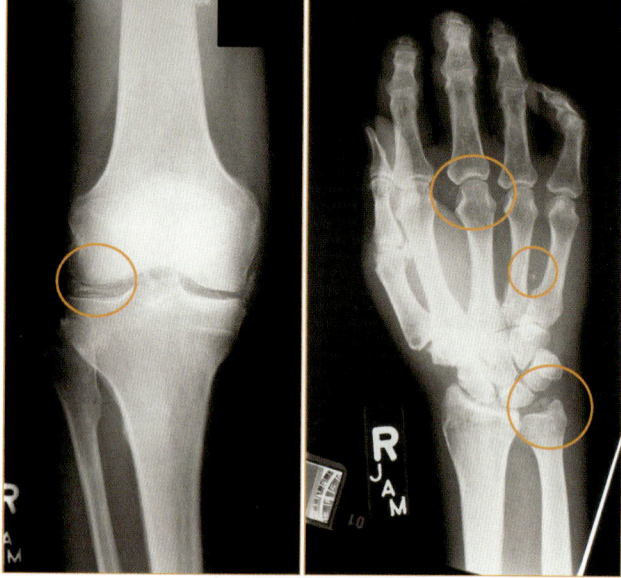

- **Pearls: Look for calcifications**
  - Neck pain, meningitis-like symptoms → think crowned dens syndrome
  - Hooked osteophytes at 2nd and 3rd MCP with chondrocalcinosis → think hemochromatosis

HYDROXYAPATITE ARTHROPATHY (HAA)
- Also known as **basic calcium phosphate (BCP)** arthropathy or calcium apatite deposition disease
- Associated with aging and:
  1) Acute synovitis (rare)
  2) Destructive arthropathy (Milwaukee shoulder — hemorrhagic shoulder effusion in older women)
  3) Calcific tendinitis/bursitis — more common
  4) Tumoral calcinosis/Heterotrophic calcification
- Only visualized by electron microscopy or alizarin red stain

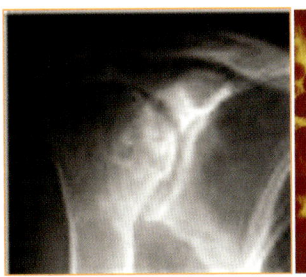
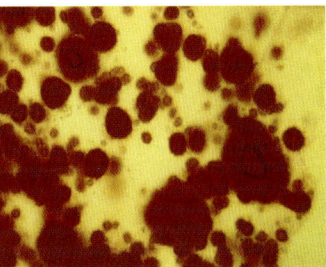

AR 6

A 53-year-old man with a 15-year history of gout presents for evaluation. He has had 4–5 flares/year, usually L big toe and ankles. Episodes last about 5–7 days, but the last one, 2 months ago, lasted for more than 2 weeks. He is currently asymptomatic but noted a firm nodule on his R elbow that is not painful, but he can squeeze out chalky white material.

Exam: BP 140/80 mmHg, HR 75 bpm

Uric acid 8.7 mg/dL, serum creatinine 1.5 mg/dL

X-ray of his L foot is shown

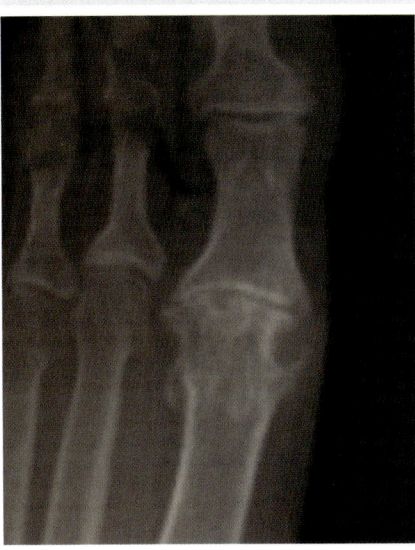

Which of the following is the most appropriate next step in management?

A. Start allopurinol and target uric acid to goal < 6.0 mg/dL.
B. Start febuxostat and target uric acid to goal < 6.0 mg/dL.
C. Start allopurinol and colchicine; target to uric acid goal < 5.0 mg/dL.
D. Start indomethacin 75 mg PO bid.
E. Start colchicine 0.6 mg PO bid.

Answer:_____

SYSTEMIC LUPUS ERYTHEMATOSUS (SLE)

DIAGNOSIS OF SLE

2019 Classification Criteria for SLE[3]

Clinical Domains	Points
Constitutional Domain Fever	2
Cutaneous Domain Nonscarring alopecia Oral ulcers Subacute cutaneous or discoid lupus Acute cutaneous lupus	2 2 4 6
Arthritis Domain Synovitis in at least 2 joints or tenderness in at least 2 joints, and at least 30 minutes of morning stiffness	6
Neurologic Domain Delirium Psychosis Seizure	2 3 5
Serositis Domain Pleural or pericardial effusion Acute pericarditis	5 6
Hematologic Domain Leukopenia Thrombocytopenia Autoimmune hemolysis	3 4 4
Renal Domain Proteinuria > 0.5 g/24 hour Class II or V lupus nephritis Class III or IV lupus nephritis	4 8 10
Immunologic Domains	**Points**
Antiphospholipid Antibody Domain Anticardiolipin IgG > 40 GPL or anti-β_2GP1 IgG > 40 units or lupus anticoagulant	2
Complement Proteins Domain Low C3 or low C4 Low C3 and low C4	3 4
Highly Specific Antibodies Domain Anti-dsDNA antibody Anti-Smith antibody	6 6

ANA ≥ 1:80 (HEp-2 IF)

10 points

Must have 1 clinical

In each domain, highest score counts

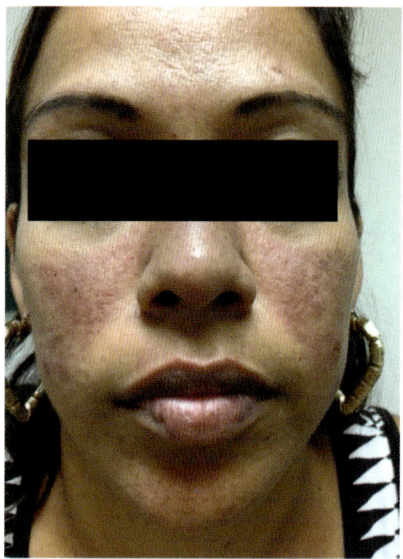

SLE Labs
- ANA: > 95% are ANA positive (if ANA is negative, it's not likely lupus)
- Anti-dsDNA: specific for SLE, associated with renal involvement if present and trends with disease activity, good biomarker
- Hypocomplementemia: C3, C4, if can trend — can use as a biomarker
- Anti-Smith: specific for SLE
- Anti-RNP: MCTD
- Ro/SSA and La/SSB = Sjögren's, SCLE, neonatal lupus
- Antiribosomal P antibody: neuropsychiatric lupus
- Leukopenia/lymphopenia, ITP, hemolytic anemia

TREATMENT OF SLE

SLE Therapy[4]
- SLE therapy is based on the most severe manifestation
- Death is typically from SLE disease (renal/CNS), infection, or CV mortality
- Benefits of hydroxychloroquine
  - Decreases mortality
  - Decreases severity/number of flares
  - Improves pregnancy outcomes
  - Decreases thrombosis
  - Improves glucose tolerance

DRUG-INDUCED LUPUS

High Yield — Drug-Induced Lupus (DIL)
- **Procainamide, hydralazine, INH, phenothiazines, β-blockers, TNF inhibitors**
- Fever, rash, joint aches/arthritis, pleuritis
- Usually no kidney or CNS involvement
- ANA positive
- **> 95% antihistone antibodies (if on exam, think DIL)**
- Seldom have anti-dsDNA or anti-Smith
  - Exception is TNF inhibitors
- Treatment: Discontinue the offending drug

AR 7
A 22-year-old African American female with a 1-year history of inflammatory arthritis, alopecia, fatigue with sun exposure, +ANA, +RNP, WBC 3.1. U/A noted RBC casts and 3+ proteinuria.

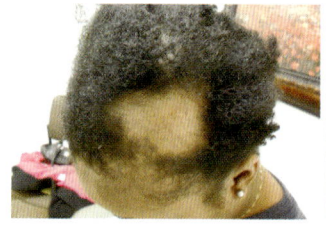
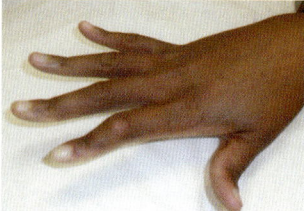

[5]

Which of the following increases her risk for morbidity/mortality?

A. +ANA
B. +RNP
C. Lupus nephritis
D. Inflammatory arthritis
E. Leukopenia

Answer:_____

RAYNAUD PHENOMENON

- Primary: benign
  - Up to 10% of the general population
  - May occur in up to **20–30% of young, healthy women, especially thin runners**
  - Normal nailfold capillaries (abnormal nailfold capillaries are a predictor for developing future connective tissue disease [CTD])
- Secondary: associated with CTD
  - Abnormal nailfold capillaries (demonstrates dilatation and dropout) — SLE, dermatomyositis, SSc
  - Due to vasospasm, microvascular injury
  - Ulcers, gangrene

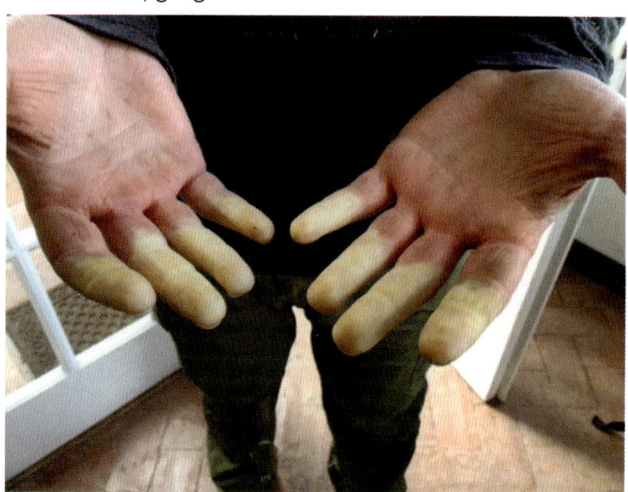

Treatment of Raynaud's
- Avoid cold exposure
- **Calcium channel blockers — best 1st option**
- Antiplatelet agents
- Topical nitrates
- Advanced disease consider phosphodiesterase-5 inhibitors (sildenafil, tadalafil), endothelin receptor antagonists
- For impending gangrene, aggressive inpatient management with prostacyclin analogues, sympathetic nerve blocks

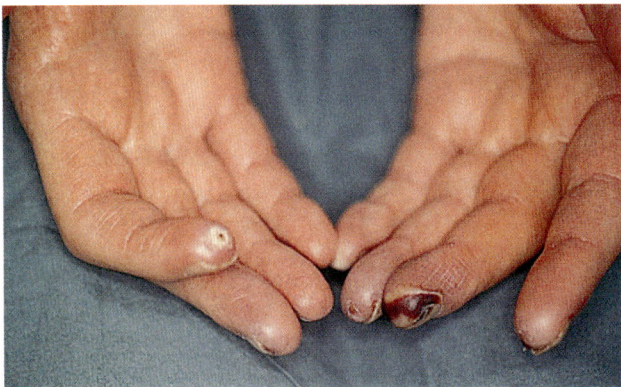

SYSTEMIC SCLEROSIS (SSc)

- Diffuse cutaneous SSc
  - Raynaud's, nailfold capillary changes
  - **Skin involvement above flexure of elbows and knees**
  - GI: dysphagia, GERD, esophageal dysmotility
  - Interstitial lung disease >> pulmonary HTN
  - **Scleroderma renal crisis (10–20%)**
    - **Associated with RNA Polymerase III**
    - **Prednisone > 15 mg daily can trigger**
    - **Rx: ACE inhibitor**

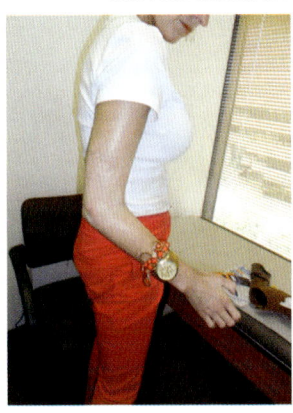
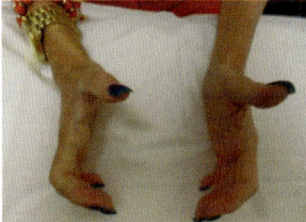

- Limited SSc
  - Raynaud's
  - Nailfold capillary changes
  - **Skin: Face and distal extremities and does not progress beyond flexure of elbows or knees, calcinosis, telangiectasias**
  - GI: Dysphagia, GERD, esophageal dysmotility
  - Interstitial lung disease
  - **Pulmonary HTN in 10–40%, especially if anticentromere Ab+**

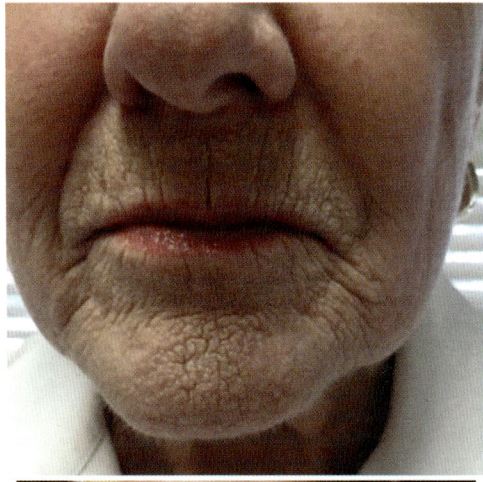

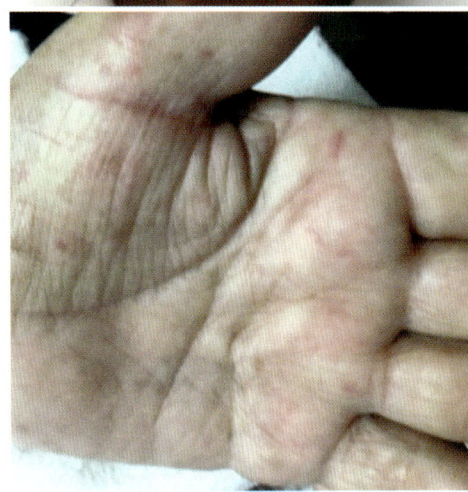

Management of SSc
- No therapies exist for overall disease modification
- Monitor BP regularly, renal function
- No proven benefit of prophylactic ACE — for scleroderma renal crisis
- Aggressive use of proton pump inhibitors for GERD
- Annual PFTs (ILD) and echocardiogram
  - High-resolution CT chest if concern for ILD
  - Do R heart cath if pulmonary hypertension is present on echo
- Interstitial lung disease
  - Mycophenolate mofetil
  - New: recent FDA approval of tocilizumab for SSc-related ILD
  - Azathioprine
  - Cyclophosphamide

SSc Autoantibodies for Exams
- Antitopoisomerase I (anti-Scl-70) = diffuse SSc, ILD, reduced survival
- Anticentromere = limited SSc, pulmonary HTN
- Anti-RNA polymerase III = scleroderma renal crisis, in diffuse SSc
- ANA = > 95% are ANA positive

SJÖGREN SYNDROME

Primary Sjögren Syndrome
- Sicca syndrome: dry eyes, dry mouth, dry skin
  - Usually annoying
  - < 20% complications: salivary gland enlargement, Type 1 distal RTA, ILD, neurologic manifestations, lymphoma
- Autoantibodies: anti-SSA/SSB antibodies (not all patients with Sjögren syndrome have these antibodies), ANA, RF
- Diagnosis: clinical features + salivary gland biopsy + serology
- **Pearl**: Many Sjögren's patients will have fibromyalgia

Systemic Manifestations of Sjögren's
- Musculoskeletal: arthralgias, myalgias
- Cutaneous: dry skin, hyperglobulinemia purpura, vasculitis
- Pulmonary: interstitial lung disease
- GI: esophageal dysmotility, pancreatitis, hepatitis
- Renal: RTA, interstitial nephritis
- Neurologic: peripheral neuropathy, cranial neuropathy, CNS
- Hematologic: leukopenia, anemia, lymphoma

Risk of Malignancy in Sjögren's
- 1° Sjögren's = ~ 20–40× increased risk of developing non-Hodgkin lymphoma; **typically a B-cell lymphoma or MALToma — this point is high yield for boards**
- Heralded by the development of:
  - A monoclonal protein
  - New-onset leukopenia
  - New-onset anemia
  - New lymphadenopathy

MYOSITIS AND MYOPATHIES

- Polymyositis
- Dermatomyositis
- Inclusion body myositis
- Drug-induced myopathy
  - Glucocorticoids (not inflammatory!)
  - Colchicine
  - Statins
  - Cocaine
  - Alcohol

POLYMYOSITIS AND DERMATOMYOSITIS
- 40–50 years of age; females > males (2:1)
- Clinical features
  - Insidious-onset **proximal** muscle weakness
  - Dysphagia (esophageal dysmotility or oropharyngeal involvement), SOB (ILD, diaphragm weakness)
  - Dermato: Gottron papules, heliotrope rash, shawl sign, holster sign
  - Malignancy is associated and occurs before, with, or after myositis diagnosis (± 2 years)
    - 9% in polymyositis
    - 15% in dermatomyositis

Gottron Papules

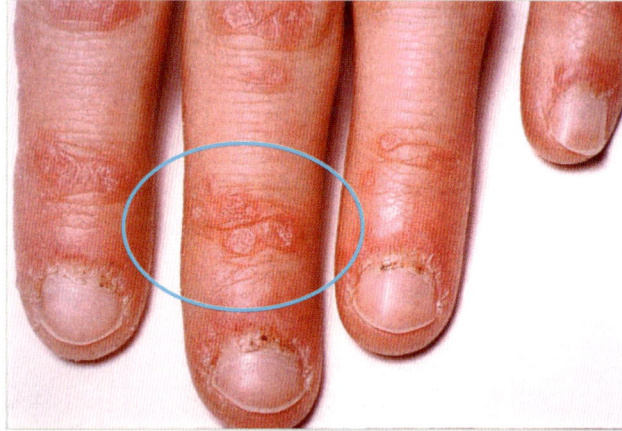

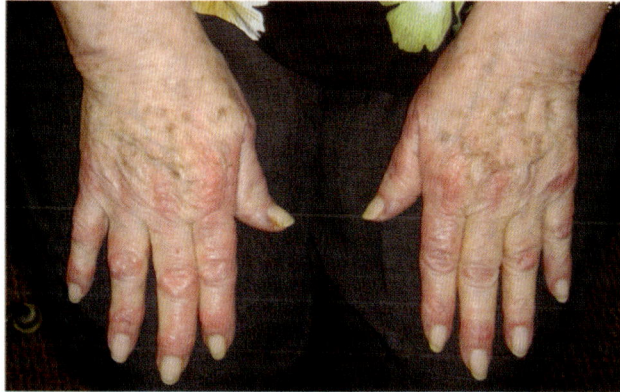

- Diagnosis
  - ↑ CPK, aldolase, AST, and ALT
  - Abnormal EMG/MRI
  - Definitive test: muscle biopsy
- Autoantibodies (antisynthetase syndrome)
  - Anti-SRP antibodies in aggressive polymyositis
  - Anti-tRNA synthetase antibodies (e.g., anti-Jo-1) = increased risk of ILD
  - Anti-Mi-2: Classic DM with V sign and shawl sign
- Pathologic features
  - Polymyositis (PM): inflammation in muscle fascicle, cytotoxic CD8-positive T lymphocytes
  - Dermatomyositis: Inflammation is perifascicular, with vasculopathy, B cells and CD4-positive T cells

Treatment of Myositis

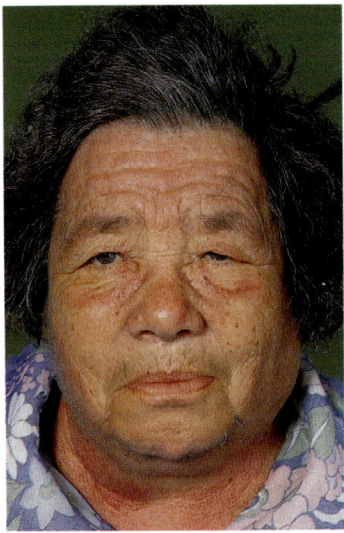

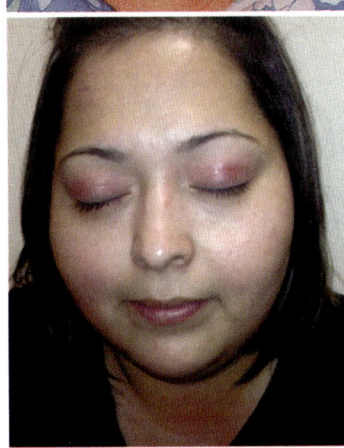

Treatment of inflammatory myositis:
glucocorticoids ± immunomodulators

Heliotrope and shawl rash — photosensitive rashes

INCLUSION BODY MYOSITIS
- More common in males and > 50 years of age
- Slow onset of asymmetrical weakness (years)
- **Both proximal and distal muscle weakness**
- CK usually normal or just mildly increased
- Associated with NT5C1A antibody
- EMG/MRI similar to PM/DM
- Muscle biopsy for diagnosis
- Poor response to steroids and immune modulation

GLUCOCORTICOID MYOPATHY
- Risk proportional to dose
- Diagnosis
  - Normal muscle enzymes
  - Normal EMG
  - Biopsy: no inflammation; atrophy
  - Test: dose reduction → improvement
- Treatment: dose reduction

Statin Myopathy / Statin Myositis
- Present with myalgias, rhabdomyolysis, asymptomatic elevated CK
- Highest offending agents are most lipophilic (simvastatin, atorvastatin, lovastatin)
  - Least likely: pravastatin, rosuvastatin, and fluvastatin
- Stopping statin will improve symptoms and CK
- **High yield: If symptoms and high CK persist, consider immune-mediated necrotizing myopathy; patients test + for HMGCR Ab or anti-SRP antibodies → treat with DMARDs**

AR 8
A 53-year-old female with COPD and hyperlipidemia presents with progressive weakness for 4 months and itchy rash on her arms, face, scalp. Her arms tire when combing her hair. She is unable to climb one flight of stairs without stopping for rest.

She denies fever and pain or swelling of any joints or muscles.

Noted weight loss 20 lb in 3 months

Meds: salmeterol, prednisone 3 mg/day, rosuvastatin 10 mg/day

Exam: violaceous rash on her eyelids and knuckles; R axillary 3-cm firm, fixed mass; motor 4/5 upper and lower extremity; normal reflexes

This patient is most likely to have:

A. Polymyositis
B. Malignancy-associated dermatomyositis
C. Statin-induced myopathy
D. Steroid-induced myopathy
E. Inclusion body myositis

Answer:_____

AR 9
A 45-year-old female presents with fatigue, severe myalgias, and weakness after starting simvastatin 6 months ago.

Which of the following is the most appropriate next step?

A. Check creatine kinase (CK) and thyroid function tests.
B. Stop the statin and see if her symptoms improve.
C. Check for illicit drug use.
D. Prescribe coenzyme Q10.
E. Reduce the dose of simvastatin.

Answer:_____

VASCULITIS

OVERVIEW

Vasculitis Classification
- **Large vessel vasculitis**
  - Giant cell arteritis (temporal arteritis)
  - Takayasu arteritis
- **Medium vessel vasculitis**
  - Polyarteritis nodosa (PAN)
  - Kawasaki's (pediatric patients)
- **Small vessel vasculitis**
  - Granulomatosis with polyangiitis (GPA)
  - Microscopic polyangiitis (MPA)
  - Eosinophilic granulomatosis with polyangiitis (EGPA)
  - IgA vasculitis
  - Cryoglobulinemic vasculitis, hypersensitivity vasculitis, hypocomplementemic urticarial vasculitis

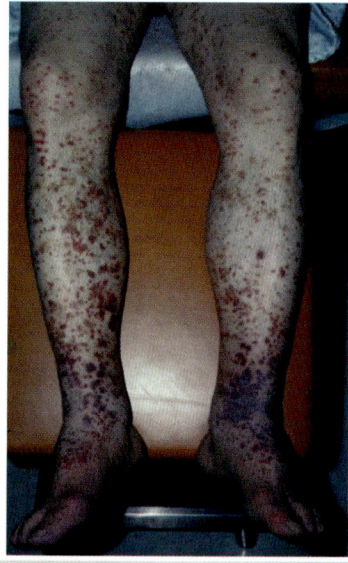

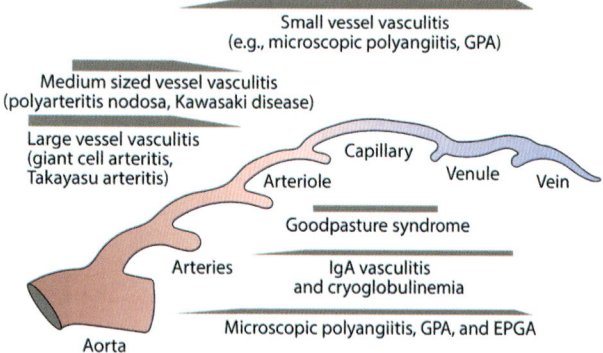

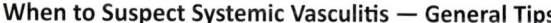

When to Suspect Systemic Vasculitis — General Tips
- **Multiorgan involvement**
- Constitutional: fevers (DDx in FWS*), weight loss, fatigue
- Acute kidney injury ± glomerulonephritis (if RBC casts or dysmorphic RBCs in the urine sediment, think small vessel vasculitis)
- Respiratory failure ± diffuse alveolar hemorrhage (DAH)
- Rashes: palpable purpura, skin necrosis
- Neurologic symptoms: foot drop, peripheral neuropathy
- Inflammatory arthritis
- Elevated ESR/CRP
- +ANCA

*FWS = fever without a source

Palpable Purpura
- Raised, nonblanching
- Due to small vessel damage (postcapillary venules)
- Favors dependent areas

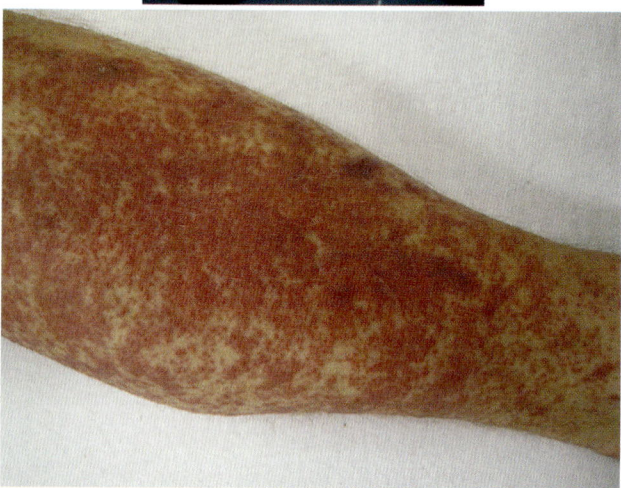

Hypersensitivity Vasculitis
- **Palpable purpura**
- Skin biopsy reveals leukocytoclastic vasculitis
  - Neutrophilic infiltrate surrounding and disrupting small vessels; fibrin deposits and nuclear debris
- Causes: infection, meds (antibiotics, thiazide diuretics, allopurinol), systemic vasculitis

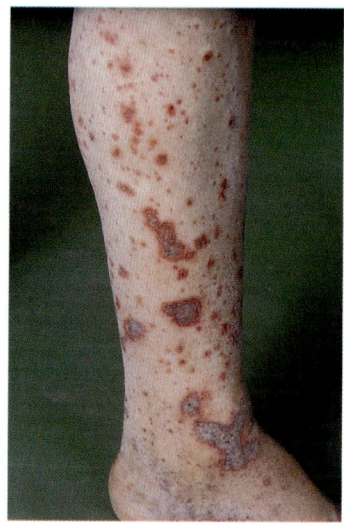

LARGE VESSEL VASCULITIS

High Yield — Large Vessel: Giant Cell Arteritis (GCA)
- Average 70 years of age
- Headaches, scalp tenderness, **jaw claudication**, diplopia, amaurosis fugax (risk of blindness if untreated)
  - Can also present as fever without a source
  - Sometimes presents with other symptoms of large vessel vasculitis (strokes, discrepant blood pressures)
- ESR > 60 mm/hour
- Confirm diagnosis with temporal artery biopsy
  - False negative in up to 44% of biopsies
  - Do not wait for biopsy to start treatment
- Rx: high-dose glucocorticoids, tocilizumab

High Yield — Polymyalgia Rheumatica
- 90% are > 60 years of age
- **Shoulder/Hip girdle pain**
  - **Not** weakness
- High ESR
- Dramatic response to prednisone 12.5–25[6] mg/day
  - High yield: In most patients, an initial dose of prednisone 15 mg/day is suggested
- 20% of patients develop GCA
  - Ask about GCA symptoms in anyone with PMR

AR 10
A 70-year-old female with a PMH of HTN presents with pain in shoulders, hips, and thighs × 8 weeks. She says she takes longer to dress in the mornings because of pain. There are no reports of headaches, visual disturbance, or jaw pain when eating. She denies weakness and swelling of any joints or muscle groups.

Musculoskeletal examination unremarkable for synovitis; range of motion mildly limited at the hips

Labs: WBC 9,500 cells/mm³ (normal differential); Hgb 10.5 g/dL; platelets 450,000 cells/mm³; creatinine 0.6 mg/dL; Glu 92 mg/dL; CPK 70 U/L (50–170); ESR 76 mm/hour

Which of the following is the most appropriate next step in management?

A. Prescribe physical therapy.
B. Prednisone 60 mg daily
C. Prednisone 15 mg daily
D. Temporal artery biopsy
E. Start duloxetine.

Answer:_____

SMALL VESSEL VASCULITIS

Small Vessel Vasculitis — EGPA
- Eosinophilic granulomatosis with polyangiitis (EGPA)
  - Pulmonary-renal syndrome
    - History of asthma
    - Peripheral eosinophilia (> 10%)
    - p-ANCA/MPO antibodies
    - Peripheral neuropathy common
    - Prednisone ± cyclophosphamide
    - Mepolizumab — FDA approved

Small Vessel Vasculitis — GPA
- Granulomatosis with polyangiitis (GPA)
  - Constitutional symptoms (fever, weight loss)
  - ENT: nasal symptoms, sinusitis, tracheomalacia, otitis, hearing loss
  - Pulmonary-renal syndrome
    - Cough, hoarseness, wheezing, hemoptysis, dyspnea
    - CXR: nodules, cavitary lesions, alveolar consolidation, ground-glass opacities
    - Acute kidney injury with red cells, casts, proteinuria
  - Joints, eyes, skin, and nervous system, too!

Granulomatosis with Polyangiitis and Microscopic Polyangiitis
- GPA
  - c-ANCA/antiproteinase-3+ (PR3)
  - Tissue biopsy showing vasculitis
    - **Kidney high yield: pauci-immune crescentic glomerulonephritis**
    - Open lung biopsy: granulomatous inflammation
    - Avoid sinus biopsies or tissue from bronchoscopy: low diagnostic yield
- Treatment
  - Cyclophosphamide + steroids (80–90% remission)
  - Rituximab + steroids
  - Plasmapheresis for pulmonary hemorrhage, acute kidney injury
- MPA can present like GPA
  - MPA is usually p-ANCA/MPO+
  - No granulomas
  - Same treatment as GPA

RHEUMATOLOGY

AR 11

A 37-year-old female with no previous PMH presents with 2 months of nosebleeds and sinus pain, cough with blood-tinged sputum.

No travel history

+ fatigue, + weight loss, joint pain, no rashes, no oral ulcers

Vitals: 100.3°F (37.9°C), BP 110/80 mmHg, HR 110 bpm, RR 22, O_2 sats 88% on 2L O_2

Exam: patient is hoarse; blood in nostrils, sinus tenderness, diffuse rhonchi at the lung bases, no synovitis, no rashes, muscle strength 5/5

Cr 1.8 mg/dL (previous 0.9), Hgb 11.3 g/dL

ESR 88 mm/hour

U/A 1+ protein, > 30 RBC with erythrocyte casts

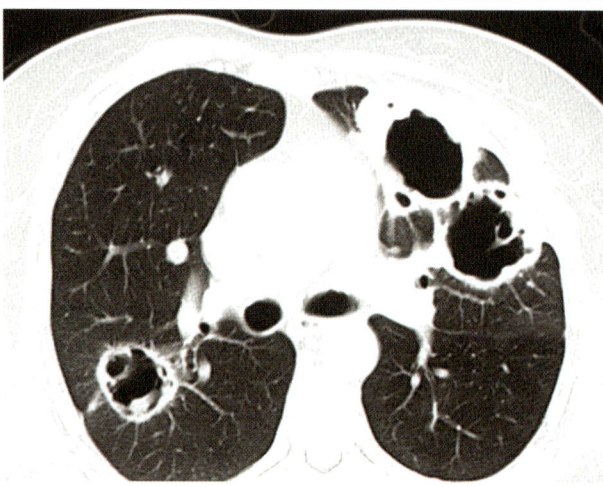

Prominent, bilateral, thick-walled cavitary lesions; multiple scattered lung nodules

Which of the following tests would <u>confirm</u> her diagnosis?

A. Obtain a renal biopsy.
B. Order an ANA test.
C. Obtain a sinus biopsy.
D. Order a TB test.
E. Order ANCA.

Answer:_____

SHOULDER PAIN

Shoulder Pain — Rotator Cuff

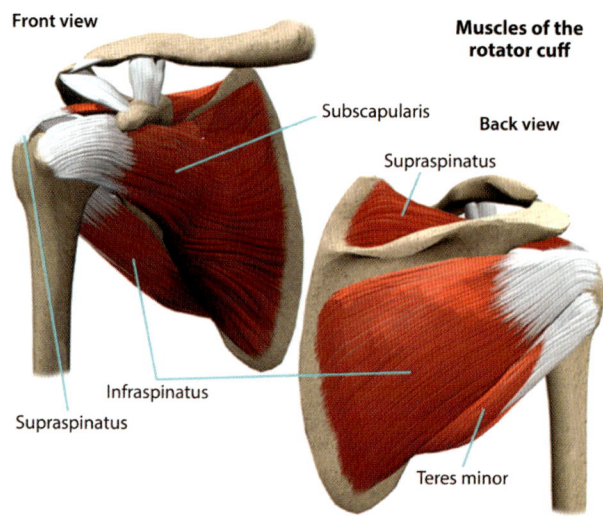

Front view

Muscles of the rotator cuff

Subscapularis

Back view

Supraspinatus

Infraspinatus

Supraspinatus

Teres minor

Shoulder Pain — Exam Pointers
- **If passive range of motion (ROM) is limited**, think about a problem with the glenohumeral joint itself
  - **Glenohumeral OA**
  - **Adhesive capsulitis** ("frozen shoulder")
    - ROM is reduced in all directions
    - Limited active and passive ROM
    - X-ray is normal
- If patient has **objective weakness**, consider a **rotator cuff tear**

Rotator Cuff Impingement Syndrome
- Compression of the subacromial bursa or tendons between the acromion and humeral head (tendinitis, bursitis)
- Pain occurs when patient reaches overhead or pressure on the shoulder
- Diagnosis is clinical
- Exam: Neer test (stabilize scapula, passively forward flex GH joint)
- Hawkins test (elbow flex, arm 90°, internally rotate shoulder)
- Yocum test (patient touches other shoulder, lifts flexed elbow)
- Weakness indicates tear in rotator cuff; Get imaging: MRI or ultrasound

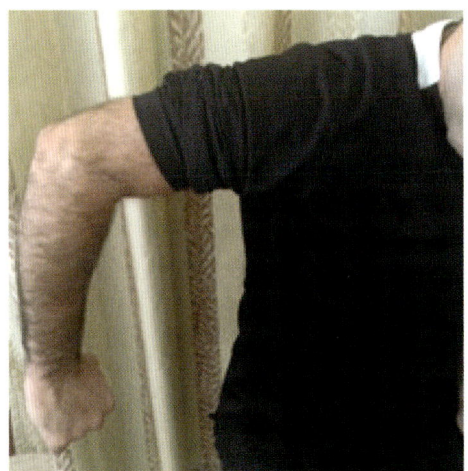

Hawkins test

Rotator Cuff Disorders — Treatment

Disorder	Treatment

Impingement syndrome:
  Rotator cuff tendinitis
  Shoulder bursitis
	Conservative:
	  Oral analgesics
	  Steroid injections
	  Physical therapy

Partial rotator cuff tears	Usually conservative (as above) On occasion, surgery for patients with partial tears who fail conservative Tx
Full thickness rotator cuff tear	**Immediate surgery for tears in younger patients** Conservative Tx in older patients

ELBOW PAIN

I don't play tennis, but my <u>elbow</u> hurts <u>here</u>!

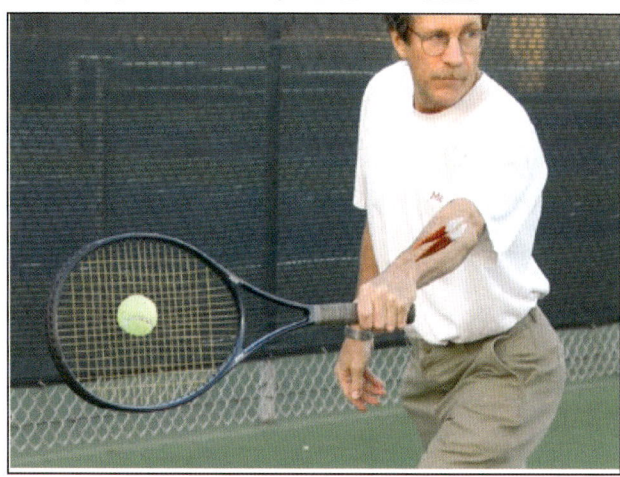

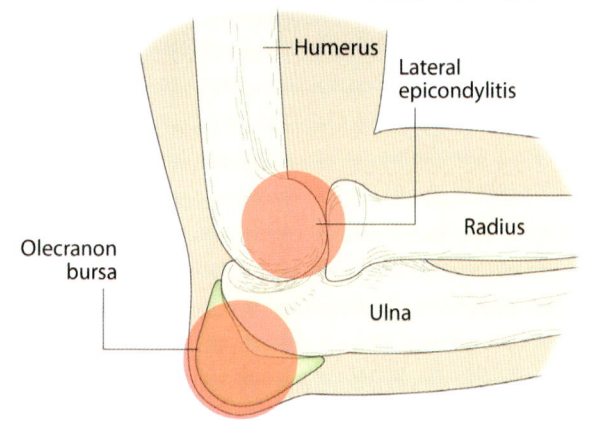

Elbow Pain

Lateral Epicondylitis	Symptoms	Tests	Treatment
Tennis elbow (backhand stroke) Risks: (wrist extension) lifting, turning screwdriver, hitting backhand	***PE: Focal pain distal to the lateral epicondyle, worsened with forced extension of the wrist**	None	**Conservative:** Analgesics Rest/PT Splints Steroid injections controversial: **Not** the answer choice

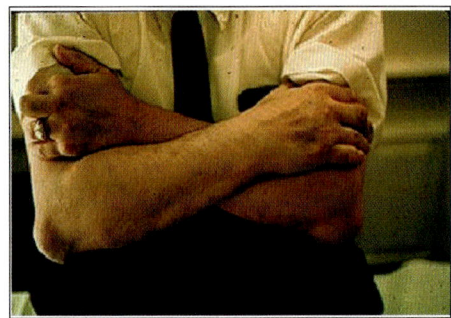

- Olecranon bursitis: diagnostic arthrocentesis to determine underlying cause (infection, gout/RA, traumatic)
- Lateral epicondylitis: pain lateral epicondyle
- Medial epicondylitis: pain on resisted pronation, tenderness medial epicondyle; due to repetitive wrist flexion/pronation

HIP PAIN

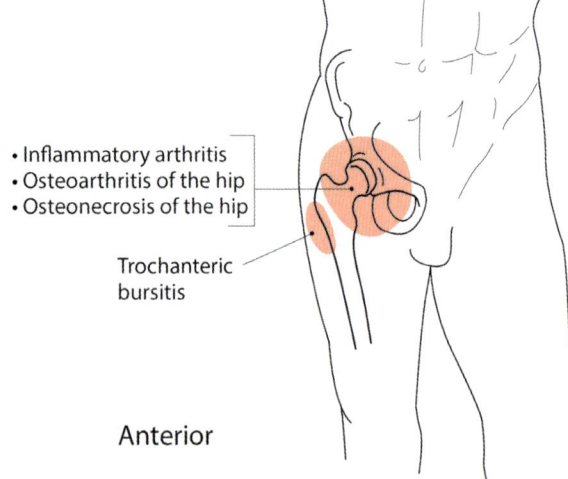

- Inflammatory arthritis
- Osteoarthritis of the hip
- Osteonecrosis of the hip

Trochanteric bursitis

Anterior

- DDx:
  - Hip OA
  - Inflammatory arthritis
  - AVN
  - Femoral impingement syndrome
  - Hip labral tears
  - Greater trochanteric pain syndrome (GTPS; a.k.a. trochanteric bursitis and greater trochanteric bursitis)
  - Iliopsoas syndrome
  - Lumbar radiculopathy

AR 12

A 55-year-old male presents with chronic, severe, achy pain in the left groin with radiation to the inner thigh.

No trauma, numbness, or tingling

History of degenerative disc disease lumbar spine

1 six-pack per day alcohol use

Musculoskeletal exam: normal ROM in the right hip, mild limitation with flexion, abduction and external rotation of the left hip, negative straight-leg raising test

Hip radiographs: normal joint spaces, no osteophytes

Which of the following is the most appropriate next step in patient care?

A. NSAID and rest followed by strength training
B. MRI lumbar spine
C. MRI left hip
D. Inject the trochanteric bursa with glucocorticoids.
E. Referral to interventional radiology for ultrasound-guided glucocorticoid injection left hip

Answer:_____

KNEE PAIN

- Knee OA
- Baker cyst (popliteal cyst)
- Prepatellar bursitis
- Pes anserine bursitis
- Patellofemoral syndrome
- Avascular necrosis
- Pigmented villonodular synovitis (recurrent hemarthrosis)

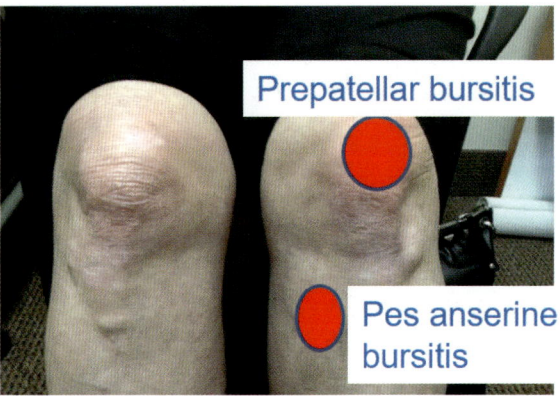

Prepatellar bursitis

Pes anserine bursitis

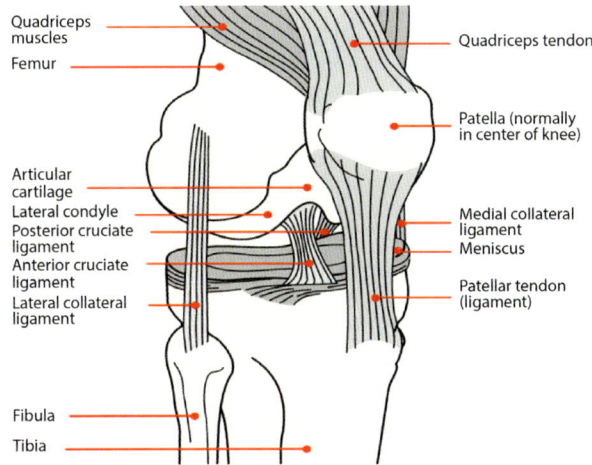

Quadriceps muscles
Femur
Quadriceps tendon
Patella (normally in center of knee)
Articular cartilage
Lateral condyle
Posterior cruciate ligament
Anterior cruciate ligament
Lateral collateral ligament
Medial collateral ligament
Meniscus
Patellar tendon (ligament)
Fibula
Tibia

Iliotibial Band Syndrome

	Symptoms	Tests	Treatment
Buzzword: **Lateral knee pain in a runner** **Due to overuse or malalignment**	**Lateral knee pain, worse with walking down an incline** **PE: Tenderness 2–3 cm proximal to the lateral joint line and along lateral thigh**	X-ray: Not needed for diagnosis	**Conservative:** Analgesics PT Stretch before/after running

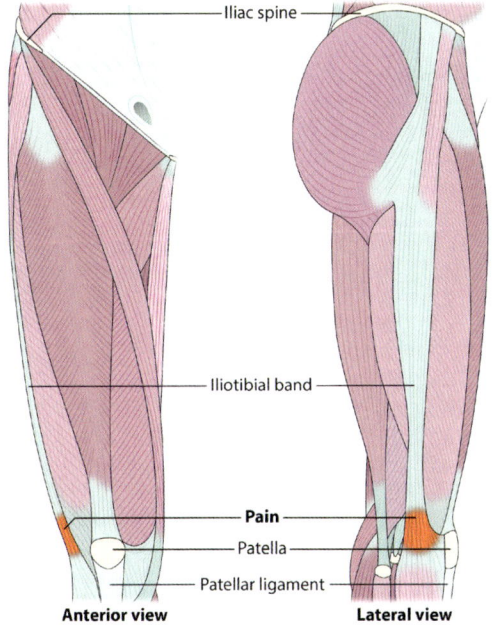

Iliac spine
Iliotibial band
Pain
Patella
Patellar ligament
Anterior view
Lateral view

FOOT PAIN

Foot Pain — Plantar Fasciitis

	Symptoms	Tests	Treatment

Buzzword: Heel pain, worse after first few steps after prolonged rest
 	
Risks: Pes planus, obesity, sedentary lifestyle
	Pain at medial plantar heel, worse in a.m.
	
	PE: Pain worse with dorsiflexion
		X-ray: Not needed for diagnosis	• **Conservative**
			  – Analgesics
			  – PT
			  – Arch support
			  – Heel stretches
			  – Steroid injections controversial

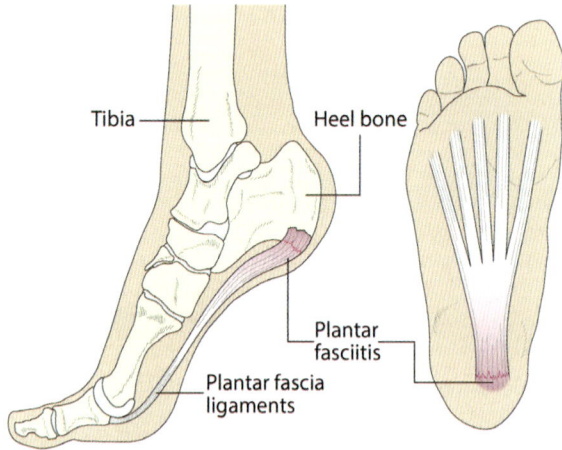

Tibia — Heel bone — Plantar fasciitis — Plantar fascia ligaments

BACK PAIN
- Origin of pain
  1) Vertebra
  2) Disc
  3) Facet joints
  4) Muscle
  5) Nerve root/Spinal cord
- Terms
  1) Spondylosis: OA (DDD/DJD)
  2) Spondylolysis: Defect pars interarticularis/fractures leading to spondylolisthesis
  3) Spondylolisthesis: One vertebra slides over another

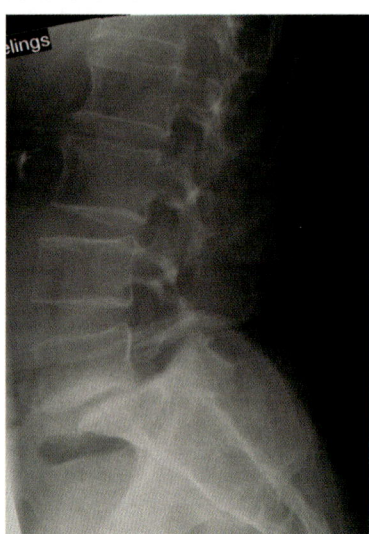

<u>Red flags</u> — <u>Need urgent imaging (MRI)</u>:
- Known cancer diagnosis **or** suspicion for cancer is high
- Recent infection/at risk for infection: injection drug users, +TB exposure
- Urinary retention/fecal incontinence
- Saddle anesthesia
- Progressive motor weakness
- Hemodynamic instability
- <u>DDx back pain</u>
  - Osteoarthritis
  - Muscle strain
  - **Disc herniation***
  - **Spinal stenosis*** (neurogenic claudication)
  - Infection (discitis, osteomyelitis)
  - Malignancy
  - AAA
  - **Compression fracture***
  - Spondyloarthritis
  - DISH

Refractory pain after 1 month conservative Tx → get imaging

*The most common causes of low back pain are spinal stenosis, disc herniation, and compression fractures.

Spinal Stenosis
- Prototypic **spinal stenosis** patient is:
  - A little, old man hunched over a shopping cart to relieve his pseudoclaudication
  - Lower-extremity neuropathy or back pain, which radiates to the legs
  - It is relieved by back flexion (such as ascending stairs or sitting in a chair)

AR 13

A 70-year-old female with RA presents with new-onset severe low back pain.

Meds: methotrexate 20 mg/week and prednisone 10 mg/day for 10 years

She requests permission to increase prednisone to 20 mg/day because she feels her RA is causing the pain. She denies groin pain. Exam reveals RA deformities but without acute synovitis; focal spinal tenderness at L3, L4, L5; no pain with straight-leg raises; no LE motor weakness.

Which of the following is the most appropriate next step in patient care?

A. Increase prednisone to 20 mg daily.
B. Order strict bed rest.
C. Order plain films of the thoracolumbar spine.
D. Prescribe NSAIDs.
E. Prescribe hydrocodone for degenerative disc disease.

Answer:_____

AR 14

A 64-year-old male with ankylosing spondylitis that was previously well controlled on etanercept presents with 4 days of 6/10 back pain that he noticed after he was lifting some boxes.

Exam: Tightness of the paraspinous muscles around L4–5 but no spinal tenderness. There is limited range of motion in the thoracic and lumbar spine with flexion without pain. No buttock tenderness.

Radiographs of the spine 2 years ago revealed bridging syndesmophytes.

Which of the following is the next best step in management?

A. Prescribe high-dose glucocorticoids.
B. Prescribe NSAIDs with physical therapy.
C. Order MRI of the spine.
D. Discontinue etanercept; begin adalimumab.
E. Add methotrexate to his current regimen.

Answer:_____

FIBROMYALGIA

- **Hypersensitivity syndrome**
  - Diffuse pain
  - Fatigue
  - Nonrestorative sleep
  - 2010 ACR diagnostic criteria: widespread pain index (WPI) + symptom severity (SS) Score
- No longer a diagnosis of exclusion!
- Treatment
  - Exercise
  - Sleep restoration (i.e., CPAP if OSA)
  - Stress reduction
  - Nonnarcotic analgesics (NSAIDs, acetaminophen, tramadol)
  - FDA approved: duloxetine, milnacipran, and pregabalin
  - Off-label use: trazodone, TCAs, gabapentin, other antidepressants

AR 15

A 45-year-old female smoker with PMH: irritable bowel syndrome, interstitial cystitis, depression complains of widespread pain in the neck, shoulders, back for the past several months. She reports excessive fatigue and headaches in the morning, sleeps poorly, and has generalized achiness.

Meds: gabapentin, duloxetine

PE: BP 137/87 mmHg, BMI 29 kg/m^2; numerous widespread tender points; tenderness to palpation of the paravertebral muscles of the lumbar spine; strength 5/5 all extremities; reflexes 2+ symmetric; negative straight-leg raise test; sensation to light touch; and normal pinprick throughout

Normal chemistry, CBC, TSH, free T$_4$

Which of the following is the next most appropriate course of action?

A. Start oxycodone/acetaminophen.
B. High-dose ibuprofen
C. Evaluate for psychosocial stressors, including domestic violence.
D. Electromyogram/nerve conduction velocity study
E. Serum ANA and rheumatoid factor

Answer:_____

HIGH-YIELD PEARLS

- Recognize patterns of how diseases present
- Inflammatory arthritis = swelling, heat, pain, redness, morning stiffness > 1 hour, improves with activity
- Osteoarthritis = bony hypertrophy, worse with activity, improves with rest, stiffness < 30 minutes
- Joint fluid WBC > 2000, think inflammatory; > 50,000, think infection
- Remember to add gout flare prophylaxis when starting uric acid lowering therapy
  - Colchicine (preferred), NSAIDs, or low-dose prednisone
- Always perform diagnostic arthrocentesis in a patient who presents with olecranon bursitis
  - Treatment plan depends on the underlying cause (traumatic, gout/RA, infection)
- Methotrexate is the initial drug of choice in patients with new RA
- TNF-inhibitors (biologic DMARDs) for RA are generally well tolerated but have an increased risk for infections
  - Screen for latent TB and HBV/HCV prior to initiating therapy
  - Stop these drugs (and all biologic drugs) in the setting of an active infection
- Be aware of drug-induced lupus secondary to TNF-inhibitors; Stopping the offending drug is the treatment of choice
- In patients with ANCA vasculitis, the diagnostic gold standard is a biopsy (kidney has the highest diagnostic yield) demonstrating nongranulomatous necrotizing pauci-immune vasculitis of small vessels
- In lupus patients who present with kidney disease (new proteinuria/hematuria, acute kidney injury), kidney biopsy is the diagnostic test of choice to assess and categorize kidney disease
  - 6 different classes, significant prognostic and therapeutic implications
- All patients on methotrexate for RA should be on daily folic acid therapy
  - Helps to prevent methotrexate-related oral ulcers and cytopenias
- HLA-B27 should not be used as a screening test for those with back pain given the low sensitivity and specificity for spondyloarthritis; in a patient with a high pretest probability it can help to support the diagnosis
- Start an oral bisphosphonate (alendronate, risedronate, or zoledronic acid) in patients at risk for glucocorticoid-induced osteoporosis
  - At least prednisone 2.5 mg daily for 3 months or more **and**
  - Moderate or high risk Fracture Risk Assessment (FRAX) score

AUDIENCE RESPONSE ANSWERS

Audience Response 1
B. Anti-RNA polymerase III and limited sclerosis

AR 2
B. Seronegative rheumatoid arthritis (RA)

AR 3
A. Erosive osteoarthritis

AR 4
D. Sulfamethoxazole-trimethoprim

AR 5
D. Uveitis

AR 6
C. Start allopurinol and colchicine; target to uric acid goal < 5.0 mg/dL.

AR 7
C. Lupus nephritis

AR 8
B. Malignancy-associated dermatomyositis

AR 9
A. Check creatine kinase (CK) and thyroid function tests.

AR 10
C. Prednisone 15 mg daily

AR 11
A. Obtain a renal biopsy.

AR 12
C. MRI left hip

AR 13
C. Order plain films of the thoracolumbar spine.

AR 14
B. Prescribe NSAIDs with physical therapy.

AR 15
C. Evaluate for psychosocial stressors, including domestic violence.

ENDNOTES

[1]   Used with permission by Dr. Kathryn Dao

[2]   Jonathan Trobe, M.D. [CC BY 3.0 (https://creativecommons.org/licenses/by/3.0)]

[3]   Aringer M, et al. *Arthritis Rheumatol* 2019;71(9):1400-1412.

[4]   Systemic Lupus Erythematosus. Horowitz, Diane; Marder, Galina; Furie, Richard. Published January 1, 2011. Pages 921-942.

[5]   Used with permission by Dr. Kathryn Dao

[6]   https://www.rheumatology.org/Portals/0/Files/2015%20PMR%20guidelines.pdf

MedStudy

INTERNAL MEDICINE REVIEW

Statistics

Presented by

Christopher L. Knight, MD

STATISTICS

TABLE OF CONTENTS

SETTING UP THE 2 × 2 TABLE

Statistics — Diagnostic Test
- Set up table!
- Disease goes on top, + to left of –
- Test goes down the side, + above –
- So, those <u>with disease</u> and have a <u>positive test</u> (true positives) go in upper left corner
- Those <u>without disease</u> and have a <u>negative test</u> (true negatives) go in lower right corner

Interpretation of Test Results

	Disease	No Disease
Test +		
Test –		

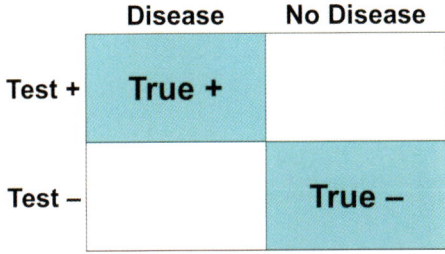

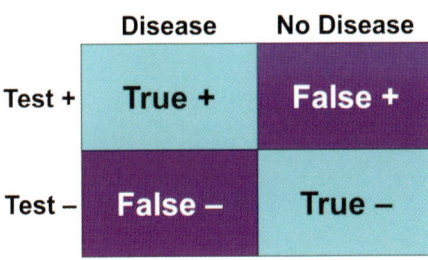

MATH OVERVIEW

- Always true results over total results
- Sensitivity/Specificity: Use **columns**
- PPV/NPV: Use **rows**

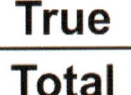

$$\frac{True}{Total}$$

SENSITIVITY

- Proportion of diseased population with positive test results
- TP/(TP + FN)
- Use left column: (Top left) divided by (Total of column)!

$$\frac{True\ +}{Total\ disease}$$

Interpretation of Test Results

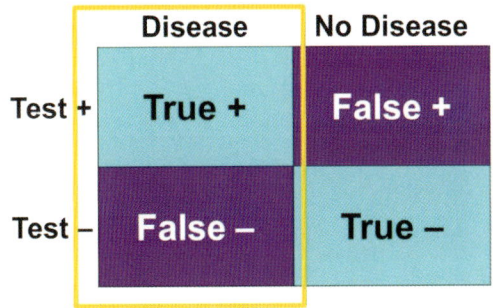

SPECIFICITY

- Proportion of healthy population with negative test results
- TN/(TN + FP)
- Use right column: (Bottom right) divided by (Total of column)!

$$\frac{True\ -}{Total\ healthy}$$

Interpretation of Test Results

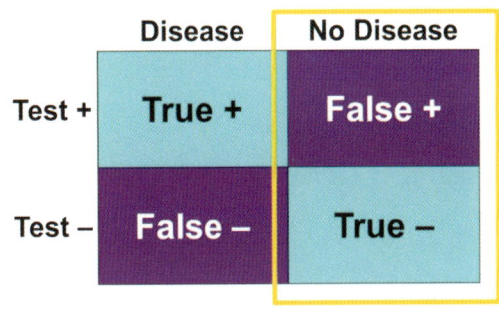

Rules of Thumb
- SpPin: A <u>P</u>ositive result on a <u>Sp</u>ecific test rules disease <u>in</u>
- SnNout: A <u>N</u>egative result on a <u>Sn</u>sitive test rules disease <u>out</u>

Combining Tests
- A good testing strategy is to use a fast/cheap sensitive test followed by a slow/costly specific test
- HIV ELISA followed by WB
- D-dimer followed by CT-PA (CT pulmonary angiography)

STATISTICS

POSITIVE PREDICTIVE VALUE (PPV)

- Positive predictive value is the proportion of patients with positive tests who have the disease

$$\frac{\text{True} +}{\text{Total} +}$$

- PPV = TP/(TP + FP)
- Use top row: (Top left) divided by (total of row)

Interpretation of Test Results

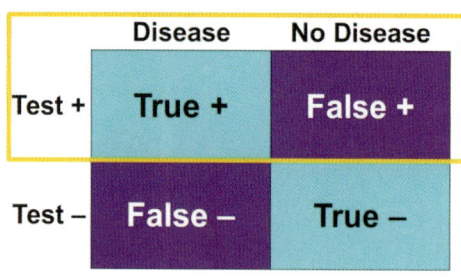

Common — 20% Prevalence

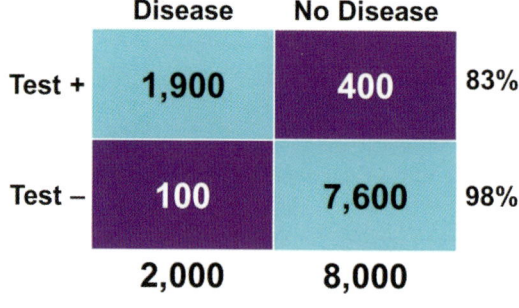

Rare — 0.2% Prevalence

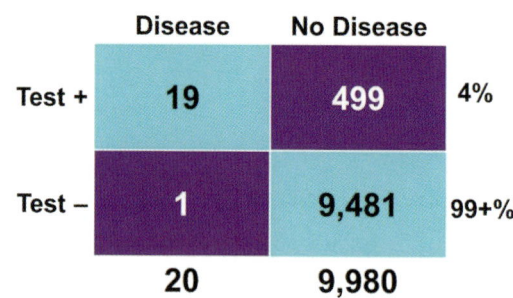

NEGATIVE PREDICTIVE VALUE (NPV)

- Negative predictive value is the proportion of patients with a negative test who are disease free

$$\frac{\text{True} -}{\text{Total} -}$$

- NPV = TN/(FN + TN)
- Use bottom row: (Bottom right) divided by (total of row)

Interpretation of Test Results

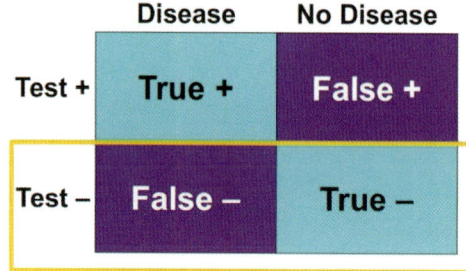

LIKELIHOOD RATIO (LR)

- Different way of looking at tests
- Combines sensitivity & specificity
- **Confusing:** Uses <u>odds</u> instead of <u>probability</u>

Odds — Coin Comes Up Heads

Flips	Probability	Odds
1	1/2	1:1
2	1/4	1:3
3	1/8	1:7
4	1/16	1:15
5	1/32	1:31

Odds — Coin <u>Doesn't</u> Come Up Heads

Flips	Probability	Odds
1	1/2	1:1
2	3/4	3:1
3	7/8	7:1
4	15/16	15:1
5	31/32	31:1

Influence of Disease Prevalence on PPV and NPV
- Prevalence of a disease within a screening population influences the performance of a screening test
- As prevalence of a disease falls, PPV drops and NPV rises
- The less common a disease, the more likely a positive test represents a false positive

Positive Likelihood Ratio (LR+)

- Change in odds of disease being present with **positive** test result
- Posttest odds = pretest odds × LR
- Higher LR+ = more powerful at ruling **in** disease

$$\frac{\text{Sens}}{1 - \text{Spec}}$$

Negative Likelihood Ratio (LR−)

- Change in odds of disease being present with **negative** test result
- Posttest odds = pretest odds × LR
- Lower LR− = more powerful at ruling **out** disease

$$\frac{1 - \text{Sens}}{\text{Spec}}$$

LR for Those with No Calculator

LR	Δ Prob
10	+45%
5	+30%
2	+15%
1	0
0.5 (1/2)	-15%
0.2 (1/5)	-30%
0.1 (1/10)	-45%

Audience Response 1

In a study of 2,271 patients with a history of colon cancer, fecal occult blood testing (FOBT) is done to screen for recurrent colon cancer. 146 patients have positive FOBT, and 2,125 patients have negative FOBT. Colonoscopy is done on all the patients, finding 46 cancers. 12 patients with positive FOBT have colon cancer, and 34 with negative tests have colon cancer.

What is the sensitivity for FOBT?

A. 8.2%
B. 26.1%
C. 94%
D. 98.4%

Answer: _____

Interpretation of Test Results

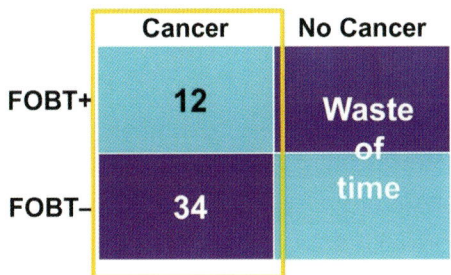

AR 2

A 67-year-old patient comes to the emergency department for cough and shortness of breath for the past 3 days. Past medical history is notable for prior MI and class II HF.

VS: T 99.2° F, 116/78, P 92, R 26, S_pO_2 88% RA

Chest: Crackles and scattered wheezes bilaterally

WBC 12.1, BNP 260

Procalcitonin blood test is positive.

Procalcitonin has a positive LR of 8.2 and a negative LR of 0.7.

Which statement best describes the diagnostic value of procalcitonin?

A. Good for ruling <u>in</u> disease, poor for ruling it out
B. Good for ruling <u>out</u> disease, poor for ruling it in
C. Good for <u>both</u> ruling disease in and out
D. Poor for <u>both</u> ruling disease in and out

Answer: _____

2 × 2 Table for Treatment

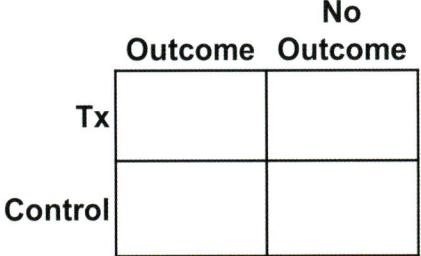

ABSOLUTE / RELATIVE RISK

- Risk in a study arm = number of events/total number of patients in that arm
- Absolute risk **difference** (reduction/increase) = Risk in control arm − risk in treatment arm
- Relative risk is a **ratio** = $\frac{\text{Risk in treatment arm}}{\text{Risk in control arm}}$

STATISTICS

NUMBER NEEDED TO TREAT (NNT)

- Number of people needed to treat to prevent 1 outcome
- NNT = 1/(absolute risk reduction)

Table for Treatment

	Dead	Not Dead	Total	
Tx	150	850	1,000	15%
Cntrl	200	800	1,000	20%
			ARR	5%

RR = 15% / 20% = 0.75
NNT = 1 / 0.05 = 20

AR 3

A study of colchicine for secondary prevention in CAD was recently completed. The treatment group had 250 patients, of whom 50 had an MI. The control group had 300 patients, of whom 90 had an MI.

What is the NNT for colchicine to prevent one MI?

A. 10
B. 25
C. 125
D. 1,000

Answer: _____

Table for Treatment

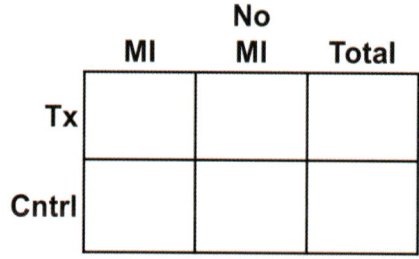

	MI	No MI	Total	
Tx	50	Time	250	20%
Cntrl	90	Sink	300	30%
			ARR	10%

NNT = 1 / 0.10 = 10

p VALUE

- A p value is used to express a study's reliability
- A p value of 0.10 means the likelihood that the results are due to chance is 10%
- p values < 0.05 are generally considered statistically significant; The lower the p value, the better ($p < 0.001$ better than $p < 0.01$)

p Value — Coin Comes Up Heads

Flips	Probability	p
1	1/2	0.5
2	1/4	0.25
3	1/8	0.13
4	1/16	0.06
5	1/32	0.03

95% CONFIDENCE INTERVAL

- Close cousin to p value
- 95% probability that the true result falls within the confidence interval
- Usually applied to the **difference** in outcomes between treatment and intervention group
- More patients in the study usually result in tighter confidence intervals and lower p values

NULL HYPOTHESIS

- The null hypothesis means no difference
- If talking about:
  - Treatment, test result, survival, or morbidity factor — look for "0"; If the confidence interval range includes 0, then it is **not** significant
  - Odds **Ratio**, Hazard <u>Ratio</u>, or <u>Relative</u> Risk — look for "1"; If the confidence interval range includes 1, then it is **not** significant

FOREST PLOTS

Forest Plots Made Simple
- Graphic of results from multiple studies
- Width of the bar represents confidence interval
- **Vertical line is the null hypothesis**
- If the bar touches the line, that study's result was not significant

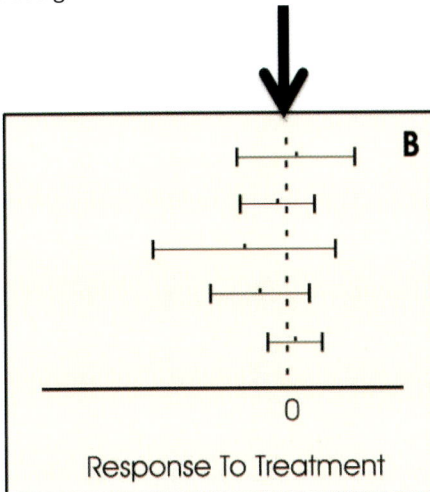

Response To Treatment

Metaanalysis
- Mathematically combines multiple studies into a single result
- Look for a different shape (usually a diamond) at the bottom of the chart: That's the aggregate result
- **If the diamond touches the bar, the result is not significant**

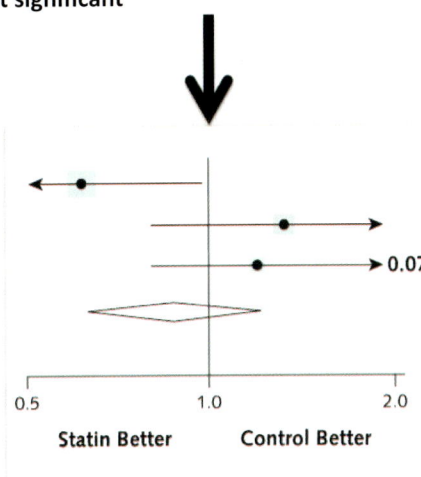

AR 4

A metaanalysis is done to see if ordering diagnostic tests reduces patient anxiety. The forest plot of the odds ratio for reduced anxiety is shown.

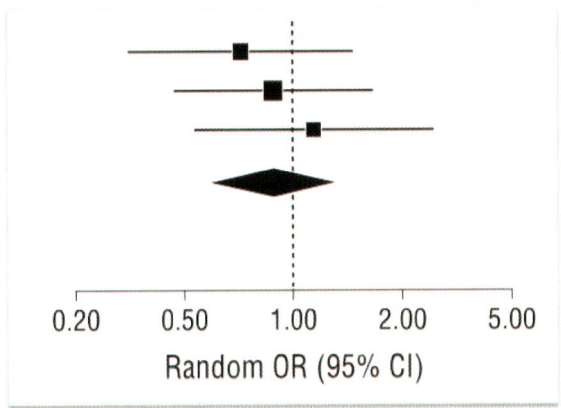

Random OR (95% CI)

What is a correct interpretation?

A. Ordering tests causes a statistically significant reduction in anxiety.
B. There is no significant difference in anxiety from ordering tests.
C. Ordering tests causes a statistically significant increase in anxiety.

Answer: _____

STUDY DESIGNS

- Observational studies
  - Cross-sectional study
  - Cohort study
  - Case-control study
- Intervention studies
  - Randomized controlled trial

Cross-Sectional Study
- Weakest type of study
- Snapshot in time
- Difficult to draw conclusions about causation
- Example: Women have lower rates of MI than men; Maybe it has something to do with estrogen

Cohort Study
- Prospective or retrospective
- Identify **risk factors** first, then see who gets **disease**
- Unmeasured variables can confound results
- Good for potentially harmful exposures
- Example: Women who choose to take hormone replacement therapy have lower risk of MI than women who don't

Case-Control Study
- Always retrospective
- Identify **disease** first, then measure **risk factors**
- Good for initial studies of rare events
- Good for potentially harmful exposures
- Example: Women with endometrial cancer are 2.5× more likely to have taken unopposed estrogen in the past

STATISTICS

Randomized Control Trials
- Always prospective
- Randomize into groups to either receive an intervention or not and blind the patient and the researcher to what was given; this reduces risk of confounding and bias
- Can't use for harmful exposures in humans
- Example: Women randomly assigned to take hormone replacement have **higher** risk of MI than those assigned to take placebo

Breaking It Down
- "Randomized" or "assigned" = intervention trial
- Was study a snapshot in time (cross-sectional), or did it look forward (prospective) or backward (retrospective)?
- What is the outcome/disease being studied?
- Did the authors find patients with risk factors first (cohort) or with outcome/disease first (case-control)?

AR 5
In a group of 99,187 patients with prior MI followed for 5 years, patients who took NSAIDs were found to have an increased risk of death compared to those who didn't; the hazard ratio is 1.59 (95% CI 1.49–1.69).

What type of study was this?

A. Cross-sectional study
B. Cohort study
C. Case-control study
D. Randomized controlled trial

Answer: _____

Audience Response 1
B. 26.1%

AR 2
A. Good for ruling <u>in</u> disease, poor for ruling it out

AR 3
A. 10

AR 4
B. There is no significant difference in anxiety from ordering tests.

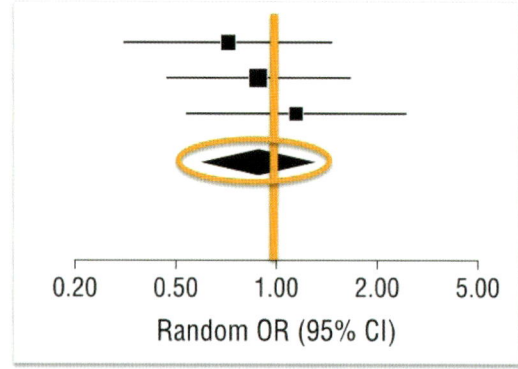

AR 5
B. Cohort study